Dengue: Diagnosis, Treatment and Control

Editor: Bertie Chotae

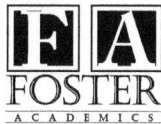

FA FOSTER
ACADEMICS

www.fosteracademics.com

www.fosteracademics.com

FOSTER
ACADEMICS

Cataloging-in-Publication Data

Dengue : diagnosis, treatment and control / edited by Bertie Chotae.
    p. cm.
Includes bibliographical references and index.
ISBN 978-1-63242-484-6
1. Dengue. 2. Dengue--Diagnosis. 3. Dengue--Prevention. 4. Dengue--Treatment. 5. Dengue viruses.
I. Chotae, Bertie.
RC137 .D46 2017
616.918 52--dc23

Foster Academics,
118-35 Queens Blvd., Suite 400,
Forest Hills, NY 11375, USA

ISBN 978-1-63242-484-6 (Hardback)

Printed and bound in the United States of America.

Contents

Permissions

List of Contributors

Index

Preface

The purpose of the book is to provide a glimpse into the dynamics and to present opinions and studies of some of the scientists engaged in the development of new ideas in the field from very different standpoints. This book will prove useful to students and researchers owing to its high content quality.

The virus causing dengue fever is known as the dengue virus. It is a mosquito borne single positive-stranded RNAS virus belonging to the family of Flaviviridae. This book is a compilation of topics that elaborately discuss the different aspects of dengue virus. It aims to provide its reader a broad spectrum of researches that have happened around the world on the nature of the virus and its changing characteristics. The text is an invaluable source of knowledge for those seeking information on the different approaches of immune system interaction and the different vaccines available. Coherent flow of topics, student-friendly language and extensive use of examples make this book a resource guide for students, researchers, experts and professionals associated with this area of study.

At the end, I would like to appreciate all the efforts made by the authors in completing their chapters professionally. I express my deepest gratitude to all of them for contributing to this book by sharing their valuable works. A special thanks to my family and friends for their constant support in this journey.

Editor

Clinical and Virological Descriptive Study in the 2011 Outbreak of Dengue in the Amazonas, Brazil

Valquiria do Carmo Alves Martins[2]*, Michele de Souza Bastos[1,2], Rajendranath Ramasawmy[1,2,3], Regina Pinto de Figueiredo[1], João Bosco Lima Gimaque[1], Wornei Silva Miranda Braga[1,2], Mauricio Lacerda Nogueira[1,4], Sergio Nozawa[3], Felipe Gomes Naveca[5], Luiz Tadeu Moraes Figueiredo[1,6], Maria Paula Gomes Mourão[1,2,3]*

1 Fundação de Medicina Tropical Dr. Heitor Viera Dourado (FMT-HVD), Manaus, Amazonas, Brazil, 2 Universidade do Estado do Amazonas (UEA), Manaus, Amazonas, Brazil, 3 Universidade Nilton Lins, Manaus, Amazonas, Brazil, 4 Faculdade de Medicina de São Jose do Rio Preto (FAMERP), São Jose do Rio Preto, São Paulo, Brazil, 5 Instituto Leônidas & Maria Deane (ILMD), Fundação Oswaldo Cruz (FIOCRUZ), Manaus, Amazonas, Brazil, 6 Centro de Pesquisas em Virologia, Faculdade de Medicina de Ribeirão Preto (FMRP-USP), Ribeirão Preto, São Paulo, Brazil

Abstract

Background: Dengue is a vector-borne disease in the tropical and subtropical region of the world and is transmitted by the mosquito *Aedes aegypti*. In the state of Amazonas, Brazil during the 2011 outbreak of dengue all the four Dengue virus (DENV) serotypes circulating simultaneously were observed. The aim of the study was to describe the clinical epidemiology of dengue in Manaus, the capital city of the state of the Amazonas, where all the four DENV serotypes were co-circulating simultaneously.

Methodology: Patients with acute febrile illness during the 2011 outbreak of dengue, enrolled at the Fundação de Medicina Tropical Dr. Heitor Viera Dourado (FMT-HVD), a referral centre for tropical and infectious diseases in Manaus, were invited to participate in a clinical and virological descriptive study. Sera from 677 patients were analyzed by RT-nested-PCRs for flaviviruses (DENV 1–4, Saint Louis encephalitis virus-SLEV, Bussuquara virus-BSQV and Ilheus virus-ILHV), alphavirus (Mayaro virus-MAYV) and orthobunyavirus (Oropouche virus-OROV).

Principal Findings: Only dengue viruses were detected in 260 patients (38.4%). Thirteen patients were co-infected with more than one DENV serotype and six (46.1%) of them had a more severe clinical presentation of the disease. Nucleotide sequencing showed that DENV-1 belonged to genotype V, DENV-2 to the Asian/American genotype, DENV-3 to genotype III and DENV-4 to genotype II.

Conclusions: Co-infection with more than one DENV serotype was observed. This finding should be warning signs to health authorities in situations of the large dispersal of serotypes that are occurring in the world.

Editor: Dong-Yan Jin, University of Hong Kong, Hong Kong

Funding: This research was financed by Conselho Nacional de Desenvolvimento Científico e Tecnológico (CNPq) and Fundação de Ampara à Pesquisa do Estado do Amazonas (FAPEAM) through grant 887/2010. The funders had no role in study design, data collection and analysis, decision to publish, or preparation of the manuscript.

Competing Interests: The authors have declared that no competing interests exist.

* Email: alvesvalquiria@yahoo.com.br (VdCAM); mariapaula.mourao@gmail.com (MPGM)

Introduction

Dengue virus (DENV) infection may display either benign acute febrile illness or severe disease such as dengue hemorrhagic fever/dengue shock syndrome (DHF/DSS) [1]. Over the last 31 years, Brazil has suffered successive outbreaks of dengue. The incidence of dengue continues to increase, and in the last decade 700,000 cases are reported per year. The mean age of severe dengue patients is decreasing. A high proportion of children are increasingly affected with severe disease [2]. In recent years, dengue outbreaks have displayed many atypical cases such as

myocarditis, hepatitis, meningoencephalitis and acute kidney failure [3]. Fatality rates have also increased.

In Manaus, the capital city of the Amazonas state, circulation of the four DENV serotypes was observed during the 2011 outbreak and is the only city to date to report co-circulation of all four DENV serotypes simultaneously in Brazil, providing a clear evidence of dengue hyperendemicity [4]. The occurrence of severe forms of dengue is commonly related to secondary infections leading to antibody dependent enhancement (ADE) of DENV infection in macrophages [5]. Alternatively, severe forms of

Table 1. Clinical presentation of dengue patients associated to infecting virus serotypes and co-infections.

Clinical presentation	DENV-1		DENV-2		DENV-3		DENV-4		Co-infections (DENV-1/2, DENV-1/4, DENV-2/4 and DENV-3/4)		Total
	N	%	N	%	N	%	N	%	N	%	
Dengue without warning signs	23	89	88	73	18	75	58	75	5	39	192
Dengue with warning signs	2	8	9	8	4	17	6	8	2	15	23
Severe dengue	1	4	23	19	2	8	13	17	6	46*	45
Total	**26**		**120**		**24**		**77**		**13**		**260**

*p = 0.004 Comparison of co-infected patients to mono-infected patients.

Table 2. Clinical aspects of dengue patients associated to the infecting virus serotype and co-infection.

Clinical presentation	DENV-1		DENV-2		DENV-3		DENV-4		Co-infection (DENV-1/2, DENV-1/4, DENV-2/4 and DENV-3/4)		P value
	N	%	N	%	N	%	N	%	N	%	
Headache	6	23	49	41	10	42	30	39	9	69	0.09
Myalgia	5	19	43	36	9	36	30	39	9	69	0.05
Arthralgia	2	8	28	23	5	21	18	23	7	54	0.03*
Rash	6	23	9	8	1	5	4	5	4	31	<0.01*
Ocular pain	4	15	28	23	9	38	15	20	7	54	0.03*
Alarm signs	3	12	32	27	7	29	19	25	8	62	0.02*
Hemorrhagic phenomena	1	4	21	18	5	21	10	13	8	62	<0.01*

*p<0.05 is considered statistically significant. Comparison of co-infected patients to mono-infected patients.

Table 3. Laboratory findings of dengue patients associated with classification of dengue severity.

Variable	Dengue without warning signs		Dengue with warning signs		Severe dengue		P Value
	N	%	N	%	N	%	
Hemoconcentration (45% for males, 42% for females)	46	36	7	35	23	51	0.74
Platelet <100×10³/µL	17	13	16	80	42	93	<0.01*
Leucocytes <3.0×10³/µL	36	29	2	29	2	17	0.66
Albumin <3.5 g/dL	4	4	1	5	6	14	0.03*

*$p < 0.05$ is considered statistically significant. Comparisons between severe dengue patients to Dengue with/without warning signs patients.

dengue could be related to virus mutants that emerge as part of a natural selection process [6]. Molecular epidemiology studies have shown that DENV genome suffers mutations and may lead each virus serotype to differentiate into multiple genotypes [7].

This study describes the clinical epidemiology of dengue in a city where all the four DENV serotypes are co-circulated simultaneously and also provides the opportunity to compare clinical severity to DENV serotypes. The results of the arboviruses surveillance performed by FMT-HVD during a dengue outbreak in 2011 are shown. Simultaneous circulations of the four DENV serotypes and different clades were observed. Dengue co-infection seems to lead to more severe manifestations.

Materials and Methods

Study design

This is a clinical and virological descriptive study to correlate clinical data with DENV serotypes during the 2011 outbreak of dengue in the Amazonas, Brazil. Patients with dengue were recruited from January 2011 through May 2011. A total of 677 patients from Manaus seeking medical assistance at the FMT-HVD agreed to participate in the study.

Setting

All of the patients participating in this study are inhabitants of Manaus and were recruited at the FTM-HVD. The FMT-HVD, located in the Manaus city with almost a population of 2 million inhabitants, is the referral centre for acute febrile illness and tropical infectious diseases.

Study sample

Patients with acute febrile illness but negative for malaria by thick blood smear test and presenting any two of the following symptoms in the first visit: headache, myalgia, arthralgia or malaise, were invited to participate in the present study. All of the patients participating in the study signed a written informed consent form. Parents or responsible party of children less than 18 years were required to sign a written inform consent form. This study was approved by the internal review board of the Ethics Committee of the FMT-HVD under the register number 2015.

Inclusion criteria

Patients with acute febrile illness presenting fever less than 7 days were selected and classified according to the 2012 World Health Organization guidelines for dengue cases (http://www.who.int/denguecontrol/9789241504713/en/).

Group I

Dengue without warning signs. Patients live in/travel to dengue endemic area, with fever and two of the following symptoms: nausea, vomiting, rash, aches and pains; tourniquet test positive; leukopenia.

Group II

Dengue with warning signs. Patients with abdominal pain or tenderness; persistent vomiting; clinical fluid accumulation; mucosal bleed; lethargy, restlessness; liver enlargement >2 cm; increase in haematocrit concurrent with rapid decrease in platelet count.

Group III

Severe dengue. Patients presenting severe plasma leakage leading to shock (DSS); fluid accumulation with respiratory

Table 4. Dengue co-infection prevalence and associated variables.

Variable	N	N+ (%) (95%IC)	OR (95% CI)	P value
Total sample	**260**	**13 (5.0) (2.4–7.6)**	-	-
Severe dengue				
N	247	39 (15.8)	1	
Y	13	6 (46.20)	4.57 (1.43–14.33)	0.004
Arthralgia				
N	247	53 (21.5)	1	
Y	13	7 (53.8)	4.27 (1.38–13.25)	0.013
Rash				
N	247	20 (8.1)	1	
Y	13	4 (30.8)	5.04 (1.43–17.84)	0.023
Ocular pain				
N	247	56 (27.7)	1	
Y	13	7 (53.8)	3.98 (1.28–12.32)	0.018
Hemorrhagic phenomena				
N	247	37 (15.0)	1	
Y	13	8 (61.5)	9.08 (2.82–29.28)	<0.001
Alarm signs				
N	247	61 (24.7)	1	
Y	13	8 (61.5)	4.88 (1.54–15.47)	0.007
Platelet $<100 \times 10^3/\mu L$				
N	182	66 (36.3)	1	
Y	11	9(81.1)	7.91 (1.66–37.71)	0.004
Albumin <3.5 g/dL				
N	144	8 (5.6)	1	
Y	11	3 (27.3)	6.37 (1.41–28.75)	0.032

Odds Ratio (OR) were calculated by Chi-squared test.

distress; severe bleeding, and severe organ involvement including the liver (AST or ALT>1000 U/dL); the central nervous system (impaired consciousness); and the heart [8].

The clinical classification of the patients with dengue was performed by the clinicians according to the 2012 WHO guidelines for dengue on the day of enrollment. All of the severe dengue patients were hospitalized and followed-up until discharge. Furthermore, patients were seen in outpatient clinics 48 hours and 6–7 days after hospital discharge for hospitalized patients. Non-hospitalized patients were seen twice, between 48 hours and 6 days after first clinical assessment.

Biochemical and hematology analysis

Blood sample was collected from all the patients on the day of presentation at the FMT-HVD. The biochemical tests were done with automatic analyzer CT 600i Wiener lab group apparatus while the hematological tests with the ABX pentra DX 120 HORIBA ABX Magnos bc.

PCR screening

Five mL of blood was collected from all the participants on the day of presentation at the FMT-HVD. Serum was separated and RNA was purified from 200 µL using the QIAamp Viral RNA mini kit (Qiagen, Germany) according to the protocol of the kit. The extracted RNAs were stored at −70°C or immediately used for laboratory tests. cDNA was synthesized by reverse transcrip-

tion (RT) with AccessQuick RT-PCR System kit (Promega, USA). The RT mixture consisted of 5 µl of RNA, 1 unit of the enzyme reverse transcriptase, 12.5 µl of AccessQuick Master Mix (2x), 1 µl of Random primer and 20 U of RNase inhibitor (RNaseOUT - Invitrogen, USA) in a final volume of 20 µl completed with RNase free water. The mixture was incubated at 72°C for 5 minutes (min) and at 45°C for 60 min and stored at −20°C until use.

For determining the DENV serotype, the cDNA were tested by a semi-nested multiplex reverse transcription-PCR as described elsewhere [9]. Briefly, each cDNA was subjected to polymerase chain reaction (PCR) amplification with D1 and D2 primers for 35 cycles: 1 min at 94°C, 1 min at 55°C, and 1 min at 72°C, with a final extension for 10 min at 72°C. A second round of amplification was conducted with 10 µl (diluted 1:100) of the first reaction mixture, including DENV serotype-specific reverse primers (TS1–TS4), and the conserved forward primer D1. The same cycling parameters were used as in the first reaction.

All negative samples underwent another screening for DENV and other flaviviruses using the real time RT-PCR with Maxima SYBR GREEN/ROX reagents (Fermentas) [10]. Negative samples by real time RT-PCR were also tested by a conventional RT-PCR with *Flavivirus* genera specific primers followed by multiplex-nested-PCRs with species-specific primers [11]. After the first round of PCR with *Flavivirus* genera specific primers, nested-PCR primers specific for Dengue DENV 1–4, Saint Louis encephalitis virus-SLEV, Bussuquara virus-BSQV and Ilheus

Table 5. Clinical presentation of dengue in co-infected patients.

Patient	Age/Gender	Days of fever	Clinical diagnosis	Hospitalization	Dengue serotype (PCR)	Hemorrhagic events	Cavitary effusion	Abdominal pain	Gallbladder wall thickening
1	25/M	3	I	No	DENV-1/DENV-4	N	N	ND	ND
2	31/M	ND	I	No	DENV-1/DENV-2	N	N	ND	ND
3	17/F	5	II	Yes	DENV-2/DENV-4	Y	N	N	Y
4	64/F	7	III	Yes	DENV-3/DENV-4	Y	N	Y	N
5	38/M	3	I	Yes	DENV-1/DENV-4	Y	N	N	N
6	27/M	4	III	Yes	DENV-2/DENV-4	Y	Y	Y	Y
7	18/F	6	III	Yes	DENV-1/DENV-4	Y	N	Y	N
8	61/F	4	III	Yes	DENV-2/DENV-4	N	N	N	N
9	45/F	ND	I	No	DENV-1/DENV-4	N	N	ND	ND
10	36/F	ND	I	No	DENV-2/DENV-4	N	N	ND	ND
11	28/F	7	III	Yes	DENV-1/DENV-4	Y	N	N	Y
12	17/F	4	II	Yes	DENV-2/DENV-4	Y	N	N	N
13	40/M	6	III	Yes	DENV-2/DENV-4	Y	Y	Y	N

I: dengue without warning signs; II: dengue with warning signs; III: severe dengue; M: male; F: female; Y: yes; N: No; ND: no data.

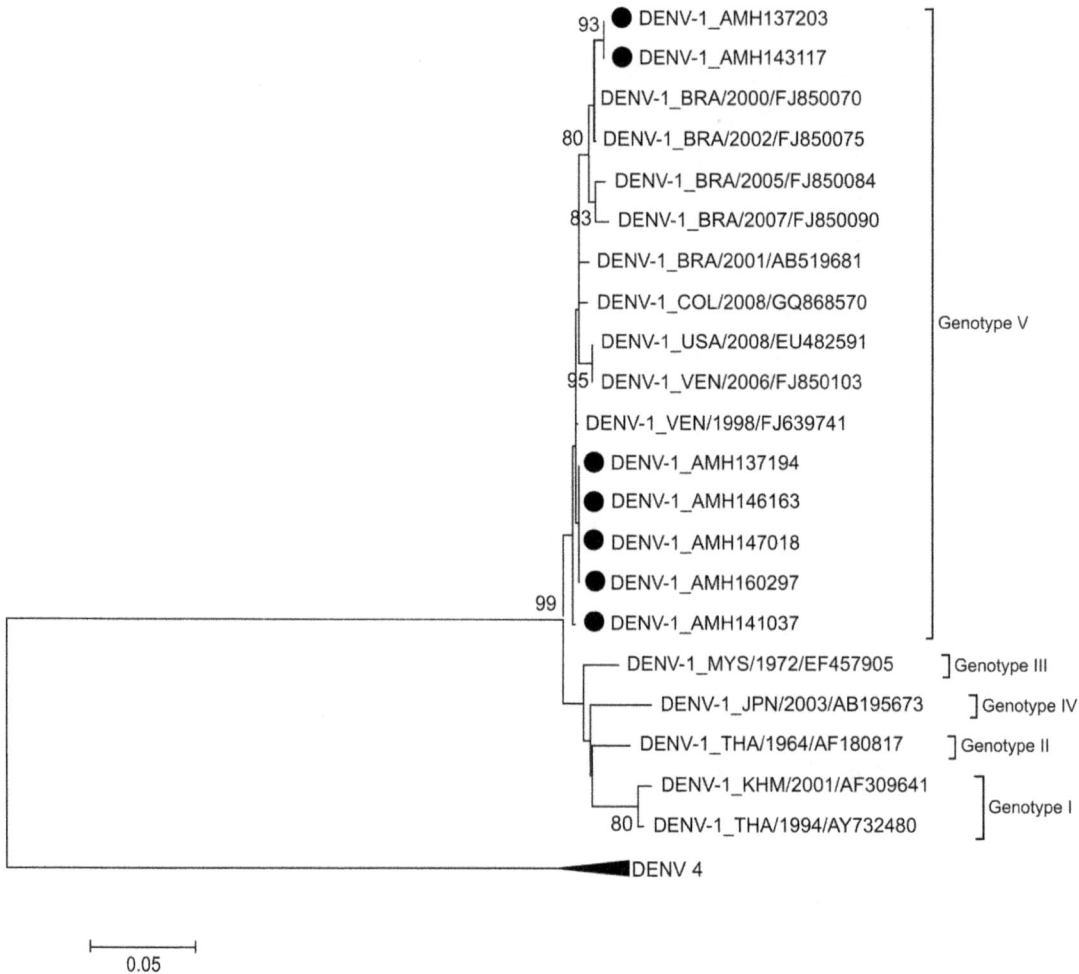

Figure 1. Phylogenetic tree of DENV-1. The neighbor-joining tree was constructed based on the prM-C genome region and sequences were compared to sequences retrieved from Gene-Bank (NCBI, USA). Sequences from this study are marked with dots. Only boot-strap values above 75% are shown in the figure.

virus-ILHV, were used in the Multiplex-PCR. Precautions to avoid contamination were followed. Positive and negative controls were used in all reactions.

Samples previously negative to dengue were also tested for alphaviruses using genera-specific primers followed by a Multiplex-Nested-PCR with species-specific primers, including those for MAYV as previously described elsewhere [12]. For orthobunyaviruses, the samples were tested using genera-specific primers followed by a Nested-PCR with OROV specific primers [13].

All the samples that showed co-infections were reprocessed for RNA purifications from another aliquot of sera and undergone the RT-nested PCR for DENV to confirm co-infections and to avoid any doubt of contaminations.

Nucleotide sequencing and phylogenetics

Nucleotide sequencing of amplicons was performed after treatment with Exonuclease I (20 U/μL) (BioLabs, New England) and Shrimp Alkaline Phosphatase-SAP (1 U/μL) (Fermentas). Briefly, the purification mixture included amplicons, 10 μL of Exo/SAP (0.025 μL SAP, 0.250 μL of Exonuclease I and 9.725 μL of Milli Q water). The mixture was incubated at 37°C for 30 min and 95°C for 5 min. Quantification of amplicons was performed in a NanoDrop 2000/2000c (Termo Scientific).

Purified amplicons were directly sequenced using the Big dye Terminator Cycle Sequencing Kit (Applied Biosystems, EUA), following instructions of the manufacturer in the automatic sequencer ABI 3130L (Applied Biosystems, EUA).

Nucleotide sequences were analyzed by algorithms of the BioEdit Sequence Alignment software [14]. Nucleotide and putative amino acid sequences were compared to other sequences from GenBank for phylogenetic analysis by neighbor-joining method using the Mega 5.05 software with 1000 bootstrap replications [15].

Gene Accession numbers

All the nucleotide sequences were submitted to GenBank and can be accessed with the following numbers: KF417476, KF417479, KF417480, KF417481, KF417478, KF417482, KF417477, KF417485, KF417484, KF417483, KF417488, KF417486, KF417489, KF417487, KF417490, KF417491, KF417496, KF417492, KF417493, KF417495, KF417494.

Correlation of clinical data to DENV serotypes

Laboratory findings and DENV serotypes were crossed blindly to the clinical status of all of the patients.

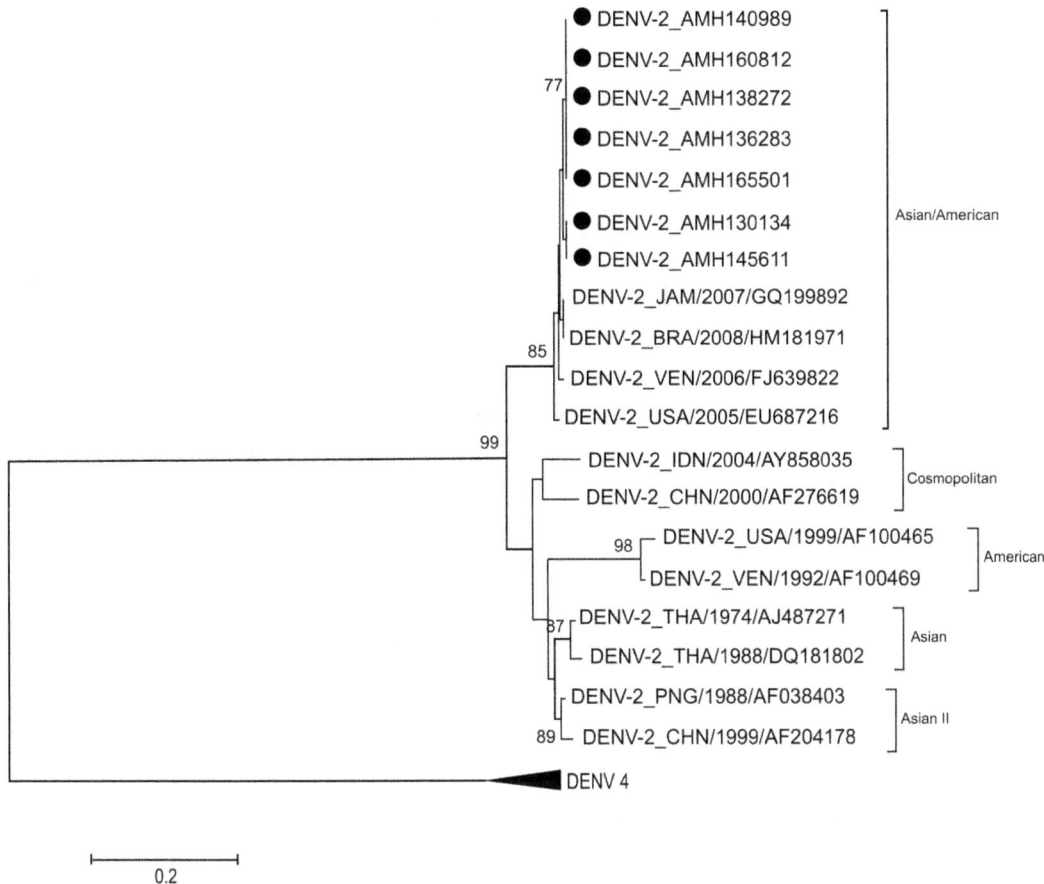

Figure 2. Phylogenetic tree of DENV-2. The neighbor-joining tree was constructed based on the prM-C genome region and sequences were compared to sequences retrieved from Gene-Bank (NCBI, USA). Sequences from this study are marked with dots. Only boot-strap values above 75% are shown in the figure.

Statistical analysis

The Epi Info version 7.3.2 software was used for data handling. Descriptive analyses were performed to calculate means and standard deviation for continuous variable and relative frequency for categorical variable. Statistical analysis was performed using SPSS version 17.0. Chi-Square tests with Yates correction were performed for statistical comparison. Odds Ratio (OR) and 95% confidence interval (CI) were calculated by logistic regression to estimate the effect of co-infection or other clinical variables. Differences were considered significant at $p \leq 0.05$.

Results

General characteristics of the study population

A total of 677 patients with acute febrile illness and negative for malaria were included in the study. The mean age of the infected patients was $35.7 \pm SD$ 15.7 (range 4 to 83 years) and 53.5% (139/260) were females.

Molecular typing

Molecular typing for DENV showed positivity for 260 (38.4%) patients. The DENV serotypes were as follows: 46.2% (120/260) had DENV-2, 29.% (77/260) DENV-4, 10.0% (26/260) DENV-1 and 9.2% (24/260) DENV-3. Thirteen had co-infections: 2.3% (6/260) had DENV-2/4, 1.9% (5/260) DENV-1/4, 0.4% (1/260) DENV-1/2 and 0.4% DENV-3/4. All samples were negative to

other flaviviruses, and also negative to MAYV and OROV. The patients were from different regions of the city and comparison among the regions to DENV serotypes did not show any difference. The co-infected patients were also from different regions.

Based on clinical presentation, dengue patients were classified as 192 dengue without warning signs cases, 45 severe dengue cases (DHF in 37 cases and 8 cases with neurological manifestations as somnolence, irritability and disorientation), and 23 dengue with warning signs cases. Clinical presentations of the dengue patients associated with DENV serotypes are shown in Table 1. Seven of the co-infected patients were classified as dengue with/without warning signs and the other six were hospitalized after initial evaluation. Co-infected patients with more than one DENV serotypes had more severe dengue ($p = 0.004$) compared to mono-infected patients. The serology and the viral load were not performed and it is possible that many of the co-infected patients may be of secondary infections and developed severe disease. Comparison of the different DENV serotypes with severity of the disease showed no statistical difference.

Clinical manifestations associated with dengue serotypes and co-infections are shown in Table 2. Cutaneous rash was more frequent ($p = 0.003$) among patients infected by DENV-1 or patients co-infected compared to patients infected with the other serotypes. Ocular pain ($p = 0.03$) and hemorrhagic phenomena

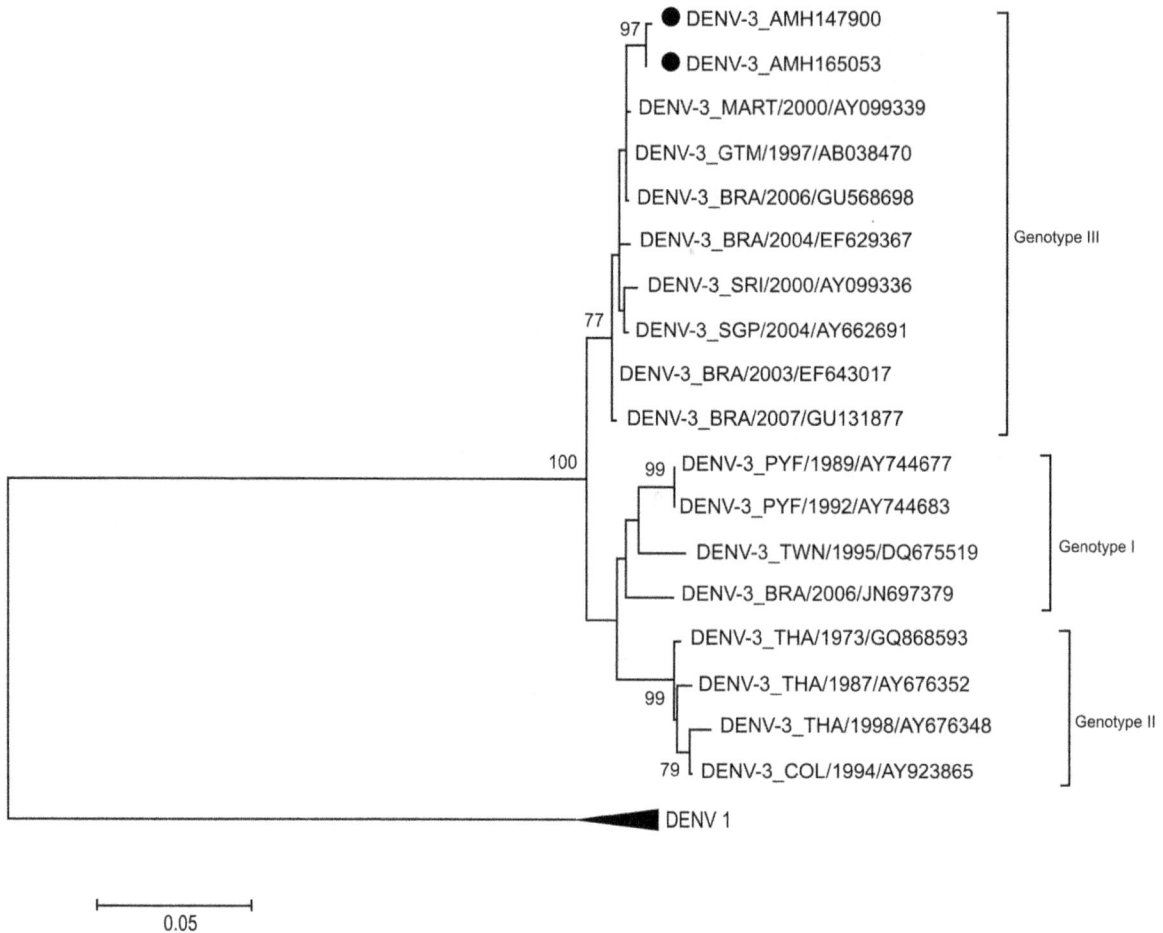

Figure 3. Phylogenetic tree of DENV-3. The neighbor-joining tree was constructed based on the prM-C genome region and sequences were compared to sequences retrieved from Gene-Bank (NCBI, USA). Sequences from this study are marked with dots. Only boot-strap values above 75% are shown in the figure.

($p = 0.01$) were more frequent among patients co-infected with different serotype mixtures.

Laboratory findings associated to clinical severity of dengue are shown in Table 3. Levels of albumin in plasma ($p = 0.03$) and platelet counts $<100.000/mm^3$ ($p<0.01$) were significantly related to severe dengue and dengue with warning signs respectively.

Severe Dengue or minor hemorrhagic phenomena were prevalent among co-infected patients with an OR of 4.57 ($p = 0.004$) and 9.09 ($p<0.001$) respectively as shown in Table 4. Other variables such as arthralgia, rash, ocular pain, alarm signs, platelets counts and serum albumin level were also statistically significant compared to mono-infected patients. In table 5 is described the individual data for each patient co-infected with emphasis in their clinical and epidemiological findings.

Phylogenetics analysis

Nucleotides sequencing of a fragment of 453 base pairs for the region of prM-C of 21 samples (16 cases with dengue without warning signs, 3 with severe dengue and 2 with dengue with warning signs) were performed. Of the 21 samples, 7 were of DENV-1, 7 of DENV-2, 2 of DENV-3 and 5 of DENV-4. Nucleotide sequences were aligned and neighbor joining phylogenetic trees were generated for each DENV serotype, as shown at Figures 1, 2, 3 and 4. DENV-1 (Fig.1), DENV-2 (Fig.2), DENV-3 (Fig.3) and DENV-4 (Fig. 4) belong to the genotype V, Asian/American genotype, genotype III and genotype II respectively. All the nucleotide sequences were submitted to NCBI and the corresponding GenBank accession numbers were generated (Table S1, ALVES VCR 301013 STROBE).

Discussion

In the present study, 677 patients with suspected dengue fever were evaluated and through three different molecular techniques only DENV were detected in 260 patients. All the four DENV serotypes were detected with the predominance of DENV-2 and DENV-4. Thirteen patients were co-infected with more than one DENV serotypes. The co-infected patients manifested severe dengue and dengue with warning signs compare to mono-infected patients. The clinical presentation of dengue without warning signs among co-infected patients was exuberant with cutaneous rash, arthralgia and ocular pain.

No difference was observed between the DENV serotypes and severity of the disease. This is an important finding as DENV-2 in Brazil is related to severe disease [16,17]. Co-infection with more than one DENV serotypes has been gradually reported in the last decade. Rocco and colleagues (1998) were the first to report a case of co-infection by serotypes of DENV-1 and 2 in a 30-year-old resident of Miranda, MS, Brazil in 1996 and Lorono-Pino et al

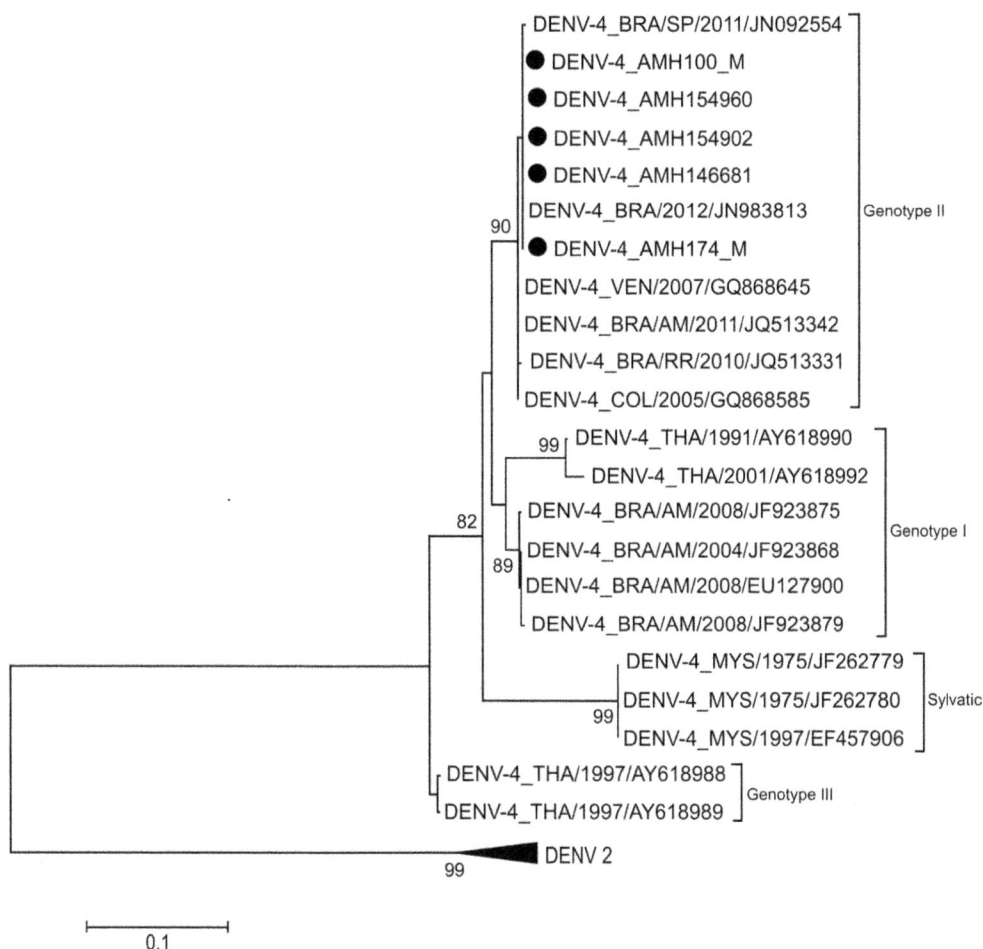

Figure 4. Phylogenetic tree of DENV-4. The neighbor-joining tree was constructed based on the prM-C genome region and sequences were compared to sequences retrieved from Gene-Bank (NCBI, USA). Sequences from this study are marked with dots. Only boot-strap values above 75% are shown in the figure.

(1999) suggested that infections with more than one serotype should be excepted in hyperendemic areas [18,19]. Since then several other authors have been reporting DENV co-infections [20–22].

In this study, co-infections were observed in 13 patients. Different from three previous studies in Brazil where all the six co-infected reported patients were of dengue without warning signs [18,23,24], 61% (8/13) of the co-infected patients in this study had either severe dengue or dengue with warning signs. Some studies have shown that co-infection can cause severe disease. In a study conducted in India, six out of nine co-infected patients had DHF [25].

Altogether it can be suggested that concurrent infections by more than one serotype could influence the clinical expression of dengue. The presence of two DENV serotypes in an individual may possibly increase the DENV viremia levels compare to a mono-infected patient. The number of infected leucocytes in co-infected patients may be higher and can induce a large cytotoxicity phenomena leading to a cytokine storm and progress to severe disease. High viral load and secondary infections may also trigger the development of severe disease. The drawback in our study is that the serology and the viral load were not performed. It cannot be rule out that many of the patients were of secondary infections and developed severe disease.

DENV can cause manifestations of central nervous system and an increasing number of cases have been reported in the last few years [26–29]. In the present study, among 45 patients with severe dengue, eight had neurologic alteration (alteration in consciousness) and were not associated to any DENV serotype or co-infections. All of the patients with neurologic alteration recovered from the disease. These findings underscore the need to investigate dengue in patients with viral meningoencephalitis in Manaus and other endemic areas.

Haematocrit, a parameter associated with capillary leak syndrome, was not significantly increased among patients with severe dengue and dengue with warning signs. It is possible that the oral rehydration therapy offered to all these patients has been started before installation of a marked capillary leak. This intervention certainly has reduced severe cases (only 1% among our patients) and fatalities. However, platelet counts under 100.000/mm^3 were related to severe dengue patients and to dengue with warning signs.

Manaus is relatively isolated from the rest of the country. To identify whether the DENV genotypes that are circulating in the country are similar in Manaus, nucleotide sequencing of the selected samples were performed. All the DENV-1 serotypes were of genotype V, the only genotype detected so far in Brazil [30]. The phylogenetic tree of DENV-1 (Fig. 1) displayed two distinct clades of genotype V from patients in this study, which is supported by a high bootstrap value. In our samples DENV genotypes and clades were not associated with severity of the disease and neither to any region of the city. However, the dataset is small and need to be further characterized to confirm this observation. In fact the co-circulation of different clades and/or clade replacement is related to high genetic diversity of that isolates and can lead to new distinct biological proprieties that may induce more severe disease. Recently, two complete distinct strains (both belonging to genotype V) of DENV-1 were observed in Brazil [30].

DENV-2 serotypes from Manaus were grouped with the Asian/American genotype that is more virulent than the indigenous American genotype and is also the predominant genotype in Brazil [16,31]. DENV-3 belonged to genotype III introduced from the Caribbean Islands and present in Brazil since the last 15 years [32,33]. All DENV-4 analyzed in this study belonged to genotype II. DENV-4 was first described in Manaus in 2008 [34]. It was found that this DENV-4 belonged to the genotype I, which is of Asian origin and was never described in the American Continent [34,35]. Presently, probably, 2 genotypes (I and II) of DENV-4 are circulating in Manaus [36,37].

Conclusions

The co-circulation of multiple serotypes or strains of dengue genotypes are becoming common in endemic region and may increase the risk of major epidemics as observed in Manaus during the 2011 outbreak where more than 50,000 cases of dengue virus infections were reported. Future studies with quantification of viruses and serology test will be needed to understand the mechanism of how co-infection with more than one DENV serotypes may lead to severe dengue disease in the city of Manaus.

Author Contributions

Conceived and designed the experiments: VdCAM MdSB RR FGN LTMF MPGM. Performed the experiments: VdCAM MdSB RPdF JBLG SN FGN. Analyzed the data: VdCAM MdSB RR WSMB LTMF MPGM. Contributed reagents/materials/analysis tools: VdCAM MdSB RR RPdF SN FGN LTMF MPGM. Wrote the paper: VdCAM MdSB RR MLN LTMF MPGM.

References

1. Gubler DJ (2002) The global emergence/resurgence of arboviral diseases as public health problems. Archives of medical research 33: 330–342.
2. Rocha LA, Tauil PL (2009) [Dengue in children: clinical and epidemiological characteristics, Manaus, State of Amazonas, 2006 and 2007]. Rev Soc Bras Med Trop 42: 18–22.
3. Figueiredo LTM (2012) Dengue in Brazil. Revista da Sociedade Brasileira de Medicina Tropical 45: 285–285.
4. Bastos MS, Figueiredo RM, Ramasawmy R, Itapirema E, Gimaque JB, et al. (2012) Simultaneous circulation of all four dengue serotypes in Manaus, State of Amazonas, Brazil in 2011. Rev Soc Bras Med Trop 45: 393–394.
5. Halstead SB (1988) Pathogenesis of dengue: challenges to molecular biology. Science 239: 476–481.
6. Rico-Hesse R, Harrison LM, Salas RA, Tovar D, Nisalak A, et al. (1997) Origins of dengue type 2 viruses associated with increased pathogenicity in the Americas. Virology 230: 244–251.
7. Wu W, Bai Z, Zhou H, Tu Z, Fang M, et al. (2011) Molecular epidemiology of dengue viruses in southern China from 1978 to 2006. Virol J 8: 322.
8. WHO/TDR (2012) Handbook for clinical management of dengue. Geneva, Switzerland World Health Organization. pp. 124.
9. Lanciotti RS, Calisher CH, Gubler DJ, Chang GJ, Vorndam AV (1992) Rapid detection and typing of dengue viruses from clinical samples by using reverse transcriptase-polymerase chain reaction. Journal of clinical microbiology 30: 545–551.
10. Chao DY, Davis BS, Chang GJ (2007) Development of multiplex real-time reverse transcriptase PCR assays for detecting eight medically important flaviviruses in mosquitoes. Journal of clinical microbiology 45: 584–589.
11. de Morais Bronzoni RV, Baleotti FG, Ribeiro Nogueira RM, Nunes M, Moraes Figueiredo LT (2005) Duplex reverse transcription-PCR followed by nested PCR assays for detection and identification of Brazilian alphaviruses and flaviviruses. Journal of clinical microbiology 43: 696–702.
12. Bronzoni RV, Moreli ML, Cruz AC, Figueiredo LT (2004) Multiplex nested PCR for Brazilian Alphavirus diagnosis. Transactions of the Royal Society of Tropical Medicine and Hygiene 98: 456–461.
13. Moreli ML, Aquino VH, Cruz AC, Figueiredo LT (2002) Diagnosis of Oropouche virus infection by RT-nested-PCR. Journal of medical virology 66: 139–142.
14. Hall TA (1999) BioEdit: a user-friendly biological sequence alignment editor and analysis program for Windows 95/98/NT. Nucl Acids Symp Ser 41: 95–98.
15. Tamura K, Peterson D, Peterson N, Stecher G, Nei M, et al. (2011) MEGA5: molecular evolutionary genetics analysis using maximum likelihood, evolutionary distance, and maximum parsimony methods. Mol Biol Evol 28: 2731–2739.
16. Drumond BP, Mondini A, Schmidt DJ, Bronzoni RV, Bosch I, et al. (2013) Circulation of different lineages of dengue virus 2, genotype american/asian in Brazil: dynamics and molecular and phylogenetic characterization. PLoS One 8: e59422.
17. Oliveira MF, Galvao Araujo JM, Ferreira OC Jr., Ferreira DF, Lima DB, et al. (2010) Two lineages of dengue virus type 2, Brazil: Emerg Infect Dis. 2010 Mar;16(3):576–8. doi: 10.3201/eid1603.090996.
18. Rocco IM, Barbosa ML, Kanomata EH (1998) Simultaneous infection with dengue 1 and 2 in a Brazilian patient. Rev Inst Med Trop Sao Paulo 40: 151–154.
19. Lorono-Pino MA, Cropp CB, Farfan JA, Vorndam AV, Rodriguez-Angulo EM, et al. (1999) Common occurrence of concurrent infections by multiple dengue virus serotypes. Am J Trop Med Hyg 61: 725–730.
20. Araújo FMdC, Nogueira RMR, Araújo JMGd, Ramalho ILC, Roriz MLFdS, et al. (2006) Concurrent infection with dengue virus type-2 and DENV-3 in a patient from Ceará, Brazil. Memórias do Instituto Oswaldo Cruz 101: 925–928.
21. Wenming P, Man Y, Baochang F, Yongqiang D, Tao J, et al. (2005) Simultaneous infection with dengue 2 and 3 viruses in a Chinese patient return from Sri Lanka. J Clin Virol 32: 194–198.
22. Yu M, Peng WM, Fan BC, Deng YQ, Qin ED (2004) [Demonstration of simultaneous infection with dengue type 2 and 3 in a Chinese patient]. Wei Sheng Wu Xue Bao 44: 717–719.
23. Figueiredo RM, Naveca FG, Oliveira CM, Bastos Mde S, Mourao MP, et al. (2011) Co-infection of Dengue virus by serotypes 3 and 4 in patients from Amazonas, Brazil. Rev Inst Med Trop Sao Paulo 53: 321–323.
24. dos Santos CL, Bastos MA, Sallum MA, Rocco IM (2003) Molecular characterization of dengue viruses type 1 and 2 isolated from a concurrent human infection. Rev Inst Med Trop Sao Paulo 45: 11–16.
25. Bharaj P, Chahar HS, Pandey A, Diddi K, Dar L, et al. (2008) Concurrent infections by all four dengue virus serotypes during an outbreak of dengue in 2006 in Delhi, India. Virol J 5: 5–1.
26. Soares CN, Cabral-Castro MJ, Peralta JM, Freitas MR, Puccioni-Sohler M (2010) Meningitis determined by oligosymptomatic dengue virus type 3 infection: report of a case. Int J Infect Dis 14: e150–152.
27. Soares CN, Faria LC, Peralta JM, de Freitas MR, Puccioni-Sohler M (2006) Dengue infection: neurological manifestations and cerebrospinal fluid (CSF) analysis. J Neurol Sci 249: 19–24.
28. Domingues RB, Kuster GW, Onuki-Castro FL, Souza VA, Levi JE, et al. (2008) Involvement of the central nervous system in patients with dengue virus infection. J Neurol Sci 267: 36–40.
29. Misra UK, Kalita J, Syam UK, Dhole TN (2006) Neurological manifestations of dengue virus infection. J Neurol Sci 244: 117–122.
30. Drumond BP, Mondini A, Schmidt DJ, Bosch I, Nogueira ML (2012) Population dynamics of DENV-1 genotype V in Brazil is characterized by co-circulation and strain/lineage replacement. Arch Virol 157: 2061–2073.
31. Bona AC, Twerdochlib AL, Navarro-Silva MA (2012) Genetic diversity of dengue virus serotypes 1 and 2 in the State of Parana, Brazil, based on a fragment of the capsid/premembrane junction region. Rev Soc Bras Med Trop 45: 297–300.
32. Alfonso HL, Amarilla AA, Goncalves PF, Barros MT, Almeida FT, et al. (2012) Pylogenetic relationship of dengue virus type 3 isolated in Brazil and Paraguay and global evolutionary divergence dynamics. Virol J 9: 124.
33. Aquino VH, Anatriello E, Goncalves PF, Da Silva EV, Vasconcelos PF, et al. (2006) Molecular epidemiology of dengue type 3 virus in Brazil and Paraguay, 2002–2004. Am J Trop Med Hyg 75: 710–715.

34. Figueiredo RM, Naveca FG, Bastos MS, Melo MN, Viana SS, et al. (2008) Dengue virus type 4, Manaus, Brazil. Emerging infectious diseases 14: 667–669.

35. de Melo FL, Romano CM, de Andrade Zanotto PM (2009) Introduction of dengue virus 4 (DENV-4) genotype I into Brazil from Asia? PLoS neglected tropical diseases 3: 28.

36. de Figueiredo ML, Alfonso HL, Amarilla AA, Figueiredo LT, Aquino VH, et al. (2013) Detection of DENV-4 genotype I from mosquitoes collected in the city of Manaus, Brazil. Virol J 10: 60.

37. Naveca FG, Souza VC, Silva GA, Maito RM, Granja F, et al. (2012) Complete genome sequence of a Dengue virus serotype 4 strain isolated in Roraima, Brazil. J Virol 86: 1897–1898.

2

Comprehensive Multiplex One-Step Real-Time TaqMan qRT-PCR Assays for Detection and Quantification of Hemorrhagic Fever Viruses

Zheng Pang[◑], **Aqian Li**[◑], **Jiandong Li, Jing Qu, Chengcheng He, Shuo Zhang, Chuan Li, Quanfu Zhang, Mifang Liang, Dexin Li***

Key Laboratory of Medical Virology, NHFPC, National Institute for Viral Disease Control and Prevention, China CDC, Beijing, China

Abstract

Background: Viral hemorrhagic fevers (VHFs) are a group of animal and human illnesses that are mostly caused by several distinct families of viruses including *bunyaviruses, flaviviruses, filoviruses* and *arenaviruses*. Although specific signs and symptoms vary by the type of VHF, initial signs and symptoms are very similar. Therefore rapid immunologic and molecular tools for differential diagnosis of hemorrhagic fever viruses (HFVs) are important for effective case management and control of the spread of VHFs. Real-time quantitative reverse transcriptase-polymerase chain reaction (qRT-PCR) assay is one of the reliable and desirable methods for specific detection and quantification of virus load. Multiplex PCR assay has the potential to produce considerable savings in time and resources in the laboratory detection.

Results: Primers/probe sets were designed based on appropriate specific genes for each of 28 HFVs which nearly covered all the HFVs, and identified with good specificity and sensitivity using monoplex assays. Seven groups of multiplex one-step real-time qRT-PCR assays in a universal experimental system were then developed by combining all primers/probe sets into 4-plex reactions and evaluated with serial dilutions of synthesized viral RNAs. For all the multiplex assays, no cross-reactivity with other HFVs was observed, and the limits of detection were mainly between 45 and 150 copies/PCR. The reproducibility was satisfactory, since the coefficient of variation of Ct values were all less than 5% in each dilution of synthesized viral RNAs for both intra-assays and inter-assays. Evaluation of the method with available clinical serum samples collected from HFRS patients, SFTS patients and Dengue fever patients showed high sensitivity and specificity of the related multiplex assays on the clinical specimens.

Conclusions: Overall, the comprehensive multiplex one-step real-time qRT-PCR assays were established in this study, and proved to be specific, sensitive, stable and easy to serve as a useful tool for rapid detection of HFVs.

Editor: Stefan Dübel, Technical University of Braunschweig, Germany

Funding: This work was supported by the National Science and Technology Major Project of China (2011ZX10004-001) and (2013ZX10004-101). The funders had no role in study design, data collection and analysis, decision to publish, or preparation of the manuscript.

Competing Interests: The authors have declared that no competing interests exist.

* E-mail: lidx@chinacdc.cn

◑ These authors contributed equally to this work.

Introduction

Viral hemorrhagic fevers (VHFs) generally describe a severe, variety of viral often fatal diseases characterized by fever and bleeding in humans [1,2], which are caused by several distinct families of enveloped, single-stranded RNA viruses including *Bunyaviridae, Flaviviridae, Filoviridae* and *Arenaviridae*, and a novel rhabdovirus associated with acute hemorrhagic fever found in Central Africa in 2012 [3–9]. After transmission from their reservoir hosts or vectors to humans, or even spread from person to person, many of hemorrhagic fevers viruses (HFVs) cause severe, life-threatening diseases [10,11]. The clinical symptoms in the early phase of VHFs are very similar irrespective of the causative viruses and resemble a flu-like illness or common enteritis, often including marked fever, fatigue, dizziness, muscle aches, loss of strength, and exhaustion [12,13]. Therefore, it is too difficult to distinguish the various etiologic agents based on clinical signs and symptoms, which makes the accurate and timely laboratory detection of viruses important in early diagnosis of VHFs.

In view of its identifying the selected target gene of RNA viruses rapidly and specifically, probe-based real-time quantitative reverse transcription-polymerase chain reaction (qRT-PCR) assay is widely used for virus detection [14,15]. Quite a lot of such methods for detection of hemorrhagic fever viruses have been published, which provides useful references for people working on VHFs [16–20]. However, most of these qRT-PCR assays may cover limited virus strains or apply under different cycling conditions. Therefore, a panel of reliable comprehensive one-step real-time qRT-PCR assays covering all important pathogens, suitable for multiplex screening or specific quantitative identification with fast turn-around time and identical cycling parameters is still urgently needed, so that the unknown samples can be tested simultaneously and effectively.

Here, we established a series of one-step real-time qRT-PCR assays for multiplex detection of 28 viruses, which covered nearly all the important viral pathogens that cause VHFs, including Hantaan virus (HTNV), Seoul virus (SEOV), Puumala virus (PUUV), Dobrava virus (DOBV), Tula virus (TULV), Black creek canal virus (BCCV), Andes virus (ANDV), Sin nombre virus (SINV), Crimean-congo hemorrhagic fever virus (CCHFV), Rift valley fever virus (RVFV), Severe fever with thrombocytopenia syndrome virus (SFTSV), Heartland virus (HLV), Omsk hemorrhagic fever virus (OHFV), Kyasanur forest disease virus (KFDV), Dengue virus (DENV), Yellow fever virus (YFV), Marburg virus (MARV), Ebola Zaire virus (ZEBOV), Ebola Sudan virus (SEBOV), Ebola Cote d'Ivoire virus (CEBOV), Junin virus (JUNV), Machupo virus (MACV), Guanarito virus (GTOV), Sabia virus (SABV), Chapare virus (CHAV), Lassa virus (LASV), Lujo virus (LUJV) and Bas-Congo virus (BASV). All assays were optimized at a universal thermal cycling condition, and evaluated under monoplex or multiplex condition for detection and absolute quantification of viral RNAs, which were proved to be reliable molecular tools of early diagnosis and consequently addressing the threat of viral hemorrhagic fevers.

Results

Selection of Primers and Probes

Genomic sequences of all representative strains of each viral species were downloaded from the GenBank database (Supplementary Table S1). Alignments were performed with Clustal W using complete sequences of listed HFVs. After visual inspection of the sequence alignments, targeted genomic regions with high conservation were chosen, which located at encoding gene of nucleocapsid protein (NP) of viruses from *Bunyaviridae*, *Filoviridae* and BASV, non-structural protein 5 (NS5) of viruses from *Flaviviridae*, and glycoprotein (GP) of viruses from *Arenaviridae*. In total, 27 primer-probe pairs were designed and appraised, and all primers/probes were grouped into seven groups based on the related diseases or virus families. Of them, ANDV and SINV were designed to share the same primers/probe set in Group B (Table 1). BLAST analysis was also performed among chose viral target sequences in NCBI database to confirm the specificities of the primer-probe sets.

Preparation of Viral RNA Standards

To evaluate the designed primers/probe and optimize the real-time PCR assay, viral RNA standards were needed. Firstly double-stranded DNA fragments of the complete open reading fragments (ORFs) of NP coding gene of the viruses from *Bunyaviridae* and *Filoviridae*, partial ORF of NP coding gene of BASV, complete ORFs of GP coding gene of the viruses from *Arenaviridae*, and partial ORFs of NS5 coding gene of the viruses from *Flaviviridae* were obtained through chemical synthesis or RT-PCR amplification from viral isolates (HTNV, SEOV, SFTSV, DENV and YFV). After the introduction of T7 promoter sequence to the 5′ or 3′ terminus of these DNA fragments using PCR amplification, the PCR products were used as DNA templates for *in vitro* transcription of positive- or negative-sense viral RNA standards corresponding to related viruses. The resulted 28 RNA transcripts were purified and measured by NanoDrop Spectrophotometer. The 260 nm/280 nm ratios were all between 2.0 and 2.1, indicating that the RNA products were highly pure. The concentration of RNA transcripts were quantified with ranging from 200 to 1185 ng/μL, and the copy numbers were calculated respectively according to the concentration and size of each single-stranded RNA fragment (Supplementary Table S2). Then, a serial dilution (10^1 to 10^8 copies/μL) of purified viral RNA transcripts was used to create RNA standard templates for development of one-step real-time qRT-PCR.

Development of One-step Real-time qRT-PCR Assays

The goal was to obtain one universal system able to detect effectively all 28 common hemorrhagic fever viruses listed above. Thus we performed numerous assays to optimize the concentrations of primers/probe and experimental condition, which consequently resulted a developed one-step real-time RT-PCR assay.

The optimized reaction system of 25 μL total volume consisted of 12.5 μL of 2× RT-PCR buffer, 400 nM of each primer, 120 nM of each probe, 1 μL of Enzyme Mix and 5 μL of viral RNA transcripts or RNA extracts. The optimal reaction conditions of a one-step assay were used as follows: 50°C for 30 min, 95°C for 10 min, then 40 cycles of 15 s at 95°C and 45 s at 60°C. The CT value for a positive sample was set at 35 cycles according to a liner range of a typical standard curve for each virus detection assay, which was also a strict standard for positive determination.

Using the developed reaction system, we tested each primers-probe set in the monoplex assays, and then combined them into 4-plex reactions for multiplex one-step real-time qRT-PCR assays according to Table 1.

Specificities and Qualitative Ability of Assays

To assess the specificity of the multiplex one-step real-time qRT-PCR, the cross-reactivity of the monoplex primers/probe was examined first using all the *in vitro* transcribed viral RNA standards with the concentration of 10^6 copies/μL, RNA extracts from viral isolates and human serum (140 μL of each sample producing 40 μL RNA extract) as templates. According to the criteria of qualitative determination in this study, the detection results of all the samples were determined. For testing of synthetic RNA standards, no cross-amplification reaction for any other virus was observed. All of the specific reactions had high positive fluorescence signals, and mean CTs were in the range of 15.22–20.13 (Table 2). In addition, there was also no significant non-specific amplification plots obtained in the testing of viral RNA extracts and healthy human sera (Table 3). The specificities of these 28 qRT-PCR assays were suggested to be 100% at a cut-off C_t value ≤ 35. It was indicated that the specificity of the developed one-step real-time qRT-PCR assay is considered satisfactory, and the primers/probe sets will be applicable for the multiplex assays.

Sensitivities and Detection Limits of Assays

To evaluate sensitivity, 10-fold serial dilutions of RNA standards (from 10^1 to 10^8 copies/μL) were used to estimate the detection limits of viral RNA copy load for the developed one-step real-time qRT-PCR assay. The amplification efficiencies of the monoplex assays for the 28 HFVs were all above 90%. The standard curves showed a high correlation coefficient, $R^2 > 0.99$, for all the viruses detections (Supplementary Figure S1). The potential limits of detection (LODs) of these assays were determined to be at a range from 30 to 160 RNA copies/PCR (Table 4).

The synthesized RNA standards were then used for the multiplex assay testing, and standard curves of detections for each virus RNA transcripts were also constructed and showed high correlation coefficient, $R^2 > 0.99$ (Figure 1). The results showed that the multiplex one-step real-time qRT-PCR assays could detect all the listed HFVs confirmed positive samples and no cross-reaction with the other examined RNA viruses was observed. In

Table 1. Primers, probes, and amplicon sizes of the one-step real-time qRT-PCR assays.

Group	Viruses	GenBank Accession No.	Forward Primers	Reverse Primers	Probes	Amplicon size (bp)
A	HTNV	NC_005218	F(771–793): GCTTCTTCCAGATACAGCAGCAG	R(862–884): GCCTTTGACTCCTTTGTCTCAT	P(811–839): FAM-CCTGCAACAAACAGGGAYTACTTACGGCA-BHQ1	114
	SEOV	NC_005236	F(217–237): GATGAACTGAAGCGCCAACTT	R(272–291): CCCTGTAGGATCCCGGTCTT	P(239–263): HEX-CCGACAGGATTGCAGCA GGGAAGAA-BHQ1	76
	PUUV	NC_005224	F(181–201): AGGCAACAAACAGTGTCAGCA	R(334–359): GCATTTACATCAAGGACATTTCCATA	P(278–304): Texas Red-CTGACCCGACTGG GATTGAACCTGATG-BHQ2	179
	DOBV	NC_005233	F(755–772): TGACCTCCCRTGCAARCT	R(801–818): GGTGGATGGGCCTTTGGT	P(777–803): Cy5-TCTGAGCCATCWCCAA CRTCTTTGACC-BHQ2	65
B	TULV	NC_005227	F(181–199): AGACGGGCAGCTGTGTCAG	R(286–303): ATCCGGCTCAAGCCCAGT	P(215–239): Texas Red -GGCAGACTTCAA GAGGCAGCTTGC-BHQ2	126
	BCCV	L39949	F(818–842): CGACAAATGGTGCTTACTTTATGAA	R(884–909): TGATTCAGCAGTGTCAATTAGGTCTA	P(847–875): Cy5-CAGACACAGGTTGAAG AGTCAAAGGTGCA-BHQ2	92
	ANDV/SINV	NC_003466	F(81–102): ACACGAACAACAGCTCGTGACT	R(278–299): GGTTCAATCCCTGTTGGATCAA	P(197–224): FAM-CTRCATTGGAGACCAA ACTCGGRGAACT-BHQ1	219
C	CCHFV	NC_005302	F(726–747): GCCGTTCAGGAATAGCACTTGT	R(869–889): TGTTATCATGCTGTCGGCRCT	P(750–777): HEX-CAACAGGCCTTGCYAAG CTYGCAGAGAC-BHQ1	164
	RVFV	NC_014395	F(1254–1275): CATGGTWGTCCCAGTGACAGGA	R(1330–1355): GATGAGTGACTCTATCACGAGTGC	P(1276–1303): Cy5-AGCCACTCACTCAAG ACGACCARAGCCT-BHQ2	102
	SFTSV	HM745932	F(1104–1125): GGGTCCCTGAAGGAGTTGTAAA	R(1155–1178): TGCCTTCACCAAGACTATCAATGT	P(1127–1146): Texas Red -TTCTGTCTTGCTG GCTCCGCGC-BHQ2	75
D	HLV	JX005842	F(1457–1484): GCATTCTTCTTCAGCTCATAGACTCTAG	R(1525–1549): GAACAAGATAGTGAAAGCATGTGGC	P(1495–1525): FAM-CATCCTCTCAGCGCCTT TCTTAGACATCTTG-BHQ1	93
	OHFV	NC_005062	F(9557–9579): TCGAGGCTACAGACTCACACAAC	R(9614–9633): AAGGCGTTCTTCTCCGTGGT	P(9588–9611): FAM-CGCAGCCACCTCTCC ACTCGTAGC-BHQ1	77
	KFDV	NC_004355	F(9416–9434): GAGGCTGCGTCATGGACAT	R(9487–9508): CCTTGATGTTCGTGAGGGTGTT	P(9451–9473): HEX-CAACGTGGTTCAGGC CAGGTGGT-BHQ1	93
	DENV	NC_001474	F(8977–9002): GGAAGTAGAGCAATATGGTACACATGTG	R(9157–9179): CCGGCTGTGTCATCAGCATAYAT	P(9082–9109): Texas Red -TGTGCAGTCC TTCTCCTTCCACTCCACT-BHQ2	203
E	YFV	NC_002031	F(9858–9878): GAGGAAGGGTGTCCAGGAA	R(9911–9932): ACATGTTGGCATAGGCTTTGCT	P(9883–9910): CY5-CTGGATGATCAAG GAAACAGCTTGCCTC-BHQ2	75
	MARV	NC_001608	F(1179–1203): AACAATTCCACCTTCAGAAAACTGA	R(1310–1331): GTGACACCGATTCTGTGATTG	P(1209–1236): Cy5-CACACAGTCAGACAY TNGCCGTCCTCAG-BHQ2	153
	ZEBOV	NC_002549	F(501–521): CGCCGAGTCTCACTGAATCTG	R(609–633): AGTTGGCAAATTTCTTCAAGATTGT	P(578–608): FAM-CGGCAAAGAGTCATC CCAGTGTATCAAGTAA-BHQ1	133
	SEBOV	NC_006432	F(1832–1855): GTTGACCCGTATGATGATGAGAGT	R(1915–1934): CATCGTCGTCGTCCAAATTG	P(1870–1894): HEX-CTACGAGGATTCG GCTGAAGGCACC-BHQ1	103
	CEBOV	NC_014372	F(2030–2051): CGAAACCCGACTAATATGCCAA	R(2095–2117): TGTTATCCCTGGCGTATTCTTGA	P(2055–2085):Texas Red -AAGACTCCA CACAAACAATGACAATCCTGC-BHQ2	88
F	JUNV	NC_005081	F(1135–1158): TGATGAGTGTCCCYTACTGCAATT	R(1251–1276):AATATCCAGTCATTACGGAAGTCAGA	P(1192–1220): FAM-CAGGACAACACTC ATTRCCAAGGTGCTGG-BHQ1	142
	MACV	NC_005078	F(1388–1411): GTTGAYATTTGTTTCTGGAGCACA	R(1478–1497): TGAGGCAAAGGACCAGGCTTC	P(1456–1479): HEX-CACCCATCGACAC CTCAAAGGCGA-BHQ1	110

Table 1. Cont.

Group	Viruses	GenBank Accession No.	Forward Primers	Reverse Primers	Probes	Amplicon size (bp)
	GTOV	NC_005077	F(847–867): TGACATGCCAGGTGGTTACTG	R(919–941): TCAAATTACACTTGGCRACAGCT	P(865–893): Texas Red -CAGCAACCAA CATCCACCTYTCAAGACAG-BHQ2	95
	SABV	NC_006317	F(882–905): TTGAAAGATGGATGCTAGTGACGT	R(961–983): TCAACATGTCACAGAATTCCGAA	P(928–959): Cy5-CACAGACTAGCAAAA TGTAACCTTGACCACG-BHQ2	102
G	CHAV	NC_010562	F(1109–1133): GACACTCCCTACTGCAACTACACAA	R(1176–1196): TAACCATCCAACAGCGTGGAA	P(1144–1171): HEX-TGTCAACCACAC CATCACAGGAGAGCAT-BHQ1	88
	LASV	NC_004296	F(2380–2402): ATGGCTTGTTTGTTGAAGTCRAA	R(2488–2509): TGACCAGGTGGATGCTAATTGA	P(2412–2442): Texas Red -CATGTCA CAAAATTCTTCATCGTGCTTCTCA-BHQ2	130
	LUJV	NC_012776	F(571–591): GGCCCATGATGACAAGAACTG	R(637–661): CCTCACTTTGTAGTGGGTTTCTGAA	P(599–628): Cy5-CTACACCCATTGAAC TACCTGAGGCTCCTG-BHQ2	91
	BASV	JX297815	F(763–785): GGACTGGGATTGGTCACTAGGTC	R(842–865): TGGATCTGTCTGAATGAAGGACTG	P(794–819): FAM-CTGCATCGGCCTGT TCCAACCTGTAC-BHQ1	103

most multiplex assays (26 out of 28 virus detections), the LODs were at a range from 45 to 150 RNA copies/PCR, which was similar to that in the monoplex assays (Table 4). Besides, HTNV and RVFV detection assays showed a little lower sensitivity with the LODs of 174.3 and 215.6 copies/PCR, respectively. The analysis of the LOD indicated that the strategy of multiplex detection ensures the sensitivity of the assay system.

Reproducibility of Multiplex One-step Real-time qRT-PCR Assay

To assess the reproducibility of the multiplex one-step real-time qRT-PCR assay, mean C_T values were calculated at a serial dilution of viral RNA transcript standards (from 10^1 to 10^8 copies/ μL), and the variations within and between runs in the linear range of the assays were statistically analyzed (Supplementary Table S3). The coefficients of variation (CVs) of C_T values were all less than 5% with 0.03–4.84% for intra-assays and 0.07–4.98% for inter-assays (Figure 2), suggesting that the developed multiplex one-step real-time qRT-PCR assay is reproducible.

Evaluation using Clinical Specimens

To evaluate sensitivity and specificity of the multiplex one-step real-time qRT-PCR assays on clinical specimens, healthy human sera and sera from the respective patients infected with individual viruses were collected, in which HFRS patients, SFTS patients and Dengue fever patients were included. Three related groups of multiplex qRT-PCR assays, including Group A, Group C and Group D. were performed for test the diagnostic specificity and sensitivity in comparison with monoplex qRT-PCR assays. For the tested sera from 11 HFRS patients infected with HTNV and 48 SFTS patients infected with SFTSV, the assay sensitivity was 100% with all tested samples detected HTNV positive (11/11) in Group A or SFTSV positive (48/48) in Group C respectively, and the rest viruses in Group A (0/11) or C (0/48) were detected negative for above collected clinical samples (Table 5). The test of 53 sera collected from Dengue fever patients showed 96.2% sensitivity (51 out of 53 detected DENV positive) with only two negative samples (Table 5). There were no false positive results observed in the unrelated patients sera and healthy human sera, suggesting 100% specificity in all the three tested groups of multiplex assays (Table 5).

Discussion

VHFs are often fatal in spite of modern intensive care, especially some HFVs can be transmitted from human to human and consequently threat to cause epidemics with high mortality rates [21,22]. Due to the unspecific clinical characters at the early phase of VHFs, a rapid and reliable laboratory testing appeared to be of utmost importance in diagnosis. Molecular assays based on RT-PCR have been successfully applied in the diagnosis of many types of VHFs [16–20]. However, most of these published methods only covered part of vial pathogens that caused VHFs. In this study, a multiplex quantitative real-time RT-PCR assay for detection of 28 HFVs which could be carried out in the same 96 wells plate was developed and evaluated. The assay sensitivity and specificity for diagnosis of HTNV, SFTSV and Dengue fever virus infection in patient sera were reliable and desirable. The assay system permits to use a universal reactive condition simultaneously to detect nearly all the hemorrhagic fever viral pathogens. Primers and probes were designed based on alignments of all possible representative viral genomic sequences in recent updated GenBank database, and optimized to react effectively under the same thermal cycling condition, which makes it possible to group

Table 2. Specificity analysis using in vitro transcribed viral RNAs.

Assay	In vitro transcribed target viral RNA (5×10⁶ copies/PCR)																											
	HTNV	SEOV	PUUV	DOBV	TULV	BCCV	ANDV	SINV	CCHFV	RVFV	SFTSV	HLV	OHFV	KFDV	DENV-2	YFV	MARV	ZEBOV	SEBOV	CEBOV	JUNV	MACV	GTOV	SABV	CHAV	LASV	LUJV	BASV
HTNV	20.13	–	–	–	–	–	–	–	–	–	–	–	–	–	–	–	–	–	–	–	–	–	–	–	–	–	–	–
SEOV	–	17.69	–	–	–	–	–	–	–	–	–	–	–	–	–	–	–	–	–	–	–	–	–	–	–	–	–	–
PUUV	–	–	18.25	–	–	–	–	–	–	–	–	–	–	–	–	–	–	–	–	–	–	–	–	–	–	–	–	–
DOBV	–	–	–	17.53	–	–	–	–	–	–	–	–	–	–	–	–	–	–	–	–	–	–	–	–	–	–	–	–
TULV	–	–	–	–	19.51	–	–	–	–	–	–	–	–	–	–	–	–	–	–	–	–	–	–	–	–	–	–	–
BCCV	–	–	–	–	–	17.67	–	–	–	–	–	–	–	–	–	–	–	–	–	–	–	–	–	–	–	–	–	–
ANDV/SINV	–	–	–	–	–	–	18.87	18.92	–	–	–	–	–	–	–	–	–	–	–	–	–	–	–	–	–	–	–	–
CCHFV	–	–	–	–	–	–	–	–	18.31	–	–	–	–	–	–	–	–	–	–	–	–	–	–	–	–	–	–	–
RVFV	–	–	–	–	–	–	–	–	–	19.01	–	–	–	–	–	–	–	–	–	–	–	–	–	–	–	–	–	–
SFTSV	–	–	–	–	–	–	–	–	–	–	18.46	–	–	–	–	–	–	–	–	–	–	–	–	–	–	–	–	–
HLV	–	–	–	–	–	–	–	–	–	–	–	17.58	–	–	–	–	–	–	–	–	–	–	–	–	–	–	–	–
OHFV	–	–	–	–	–	–	–	–	–	–	–	–	18.11	–	–	–	–	–	–	–	–	–	–	–	–	–	–	–
KFDV	–	–	–	–	–	–	–	–	–	–	–	–	–	18.62	–	–	–	–	–	–	–	–	–	–	–	–	–	–
DENV	–	–	–	–	–	–	–	–	–	–	–	–	–	–	18.55	–	–	–	–	–	–	–	–	–	–	–	–	–
YFV	–	–	–	–	–	–	–	–	–	–	–	–	–	–	–	17.65	–	–	–	–	–	–	–	–	–	–	–	–
MARV	–	–	–	–	–	–	–	–	–	–	–	–	–	–	–	–	17.39	–	–	–	–	–	–	–	–	–	–	–
ZEBOV	–	–	–	–	–	–	–	–	–	–	–	–	–	–	–	–	–	18.93	–	–	–	–	–	–	–	–	–	–
SEBOV	–	–	–	–	–	–	–	–	–	–	–	–	–	–	–	–	–	–	17.52	–	–	–	–	–	–	–	–	–
CEBOV	–	–	–	–	–	–	–	–	–	–	–	–	–	–	–	–	–	–	–	17.69	–	–	–	–	–	–	–	–
JUNV	–	–	–	–	–	–	–	–	–	–	–	–	–	–	–	–	–	–	–	–	18.82	–	–	–	–	–	–	–
MACV	–	–	–	–	–	–	–	–	–	–	–	–	–	–	–	–	–	–	–	–	–	17.25	–	–	–	–	–	–
GTOV	–	–	–	–	–	–	–	–	–	–	–	–	–	–	–	–	–	–	–	–	–	–	17.92	–	–	–	–	–
SABV	–	–	–	–	–	–	–	–	–	–	–	–	–	–	–	–	–	–	–	–	–	–	–	17.83	–	–	–	–
CHAV	–	–	–	–	–	–	–	–	–	–	–	–	–	–	–	–	–	–	–	–	–	–	–	–	18.32	–	–	–
LASV	–	–	–	–	–	–	–	–	–	–	–	–	–	–	–	–	–	–	–	–	–	–	–	–	–	18.13	–	–
LUJV	–	–	–	–	–	–	–	–	–	–	–	–	–	–	–	–	–	–	–	–	–	–	–	–	–	–	17.92	–
BASV	–	–	–	–	–	–	–	–	–	–	–	–	–	–	–	–	–	–	–	–	–	–	–	–	–	–	–	18.9

The number indicates Ct value determined from three replicates;

The minus represents a negative detection;

Table 3. Specificity analysis using viral isolates and healthy human sera.

Assay	Viral isolates						Healthy human serum (positive/tested)
	HTNV	SEOV	SFTSV	DENV1–4*	YFV	CHIKV	
HTNV	19.07	–	–	–	–	–	0/200
SEOV	–	17.33	–	–	–	–	0/200
PUUV	–	–	–	–	–	–	0/200
DOBV	–	–	–	–	–	–	0/200
TULV	–	–	–	–	–	–	0/200
BCCV	–	–	–	–	–	–	0/200
ANDV/SINV	–	–	–	–	–	–	0/200
CCHFV	–	–	–	–	–	–	0/200
RVFV	–	–	–	–	–	–	0/200
SFTSV	–	–	16.28	–	–	–	0/200
HLV	–	–	–	–	–	–	0/200
OHFV	–	–	–	–	–	–	0/200
KFDV	–	–	–	–	–	–	0/200
DENV	–	–	–	16.47, 18.12, 19.07, 15.13	–	–	0/200
YFV	–	–	–	–	15.22	–	0/200
MARV	–	–	–	–	–	–	0/200
ZEBOV	–	–	–	–	–	–	0/200
SEBOV	–	–	–	–	–	–	0/200
CEBOV	–	–	–	–	–	–	0/200
JUNV	–	–	–	–	–	–	0/200
MACV	–	–	–	–	–	–	0/200
GTOV	–	–	–	–	–	–	0/200
SABV	–	–	–	–	–	–	0/200
CHAV	–	–	–	–	–	–	0/200
LASV	–	–	–	–	–	–	0/200
LUJV	–	–	–	–	–	–	0/200
BASV	–	–	–	–	–	–	0/200

The number indicates Ct value determined from three replicates;
The minus represents a negative detection;
*DENV1-4, 4 types of dengue virus, viral strains of Hawaii, New Guinea, H87 and H241 were used.

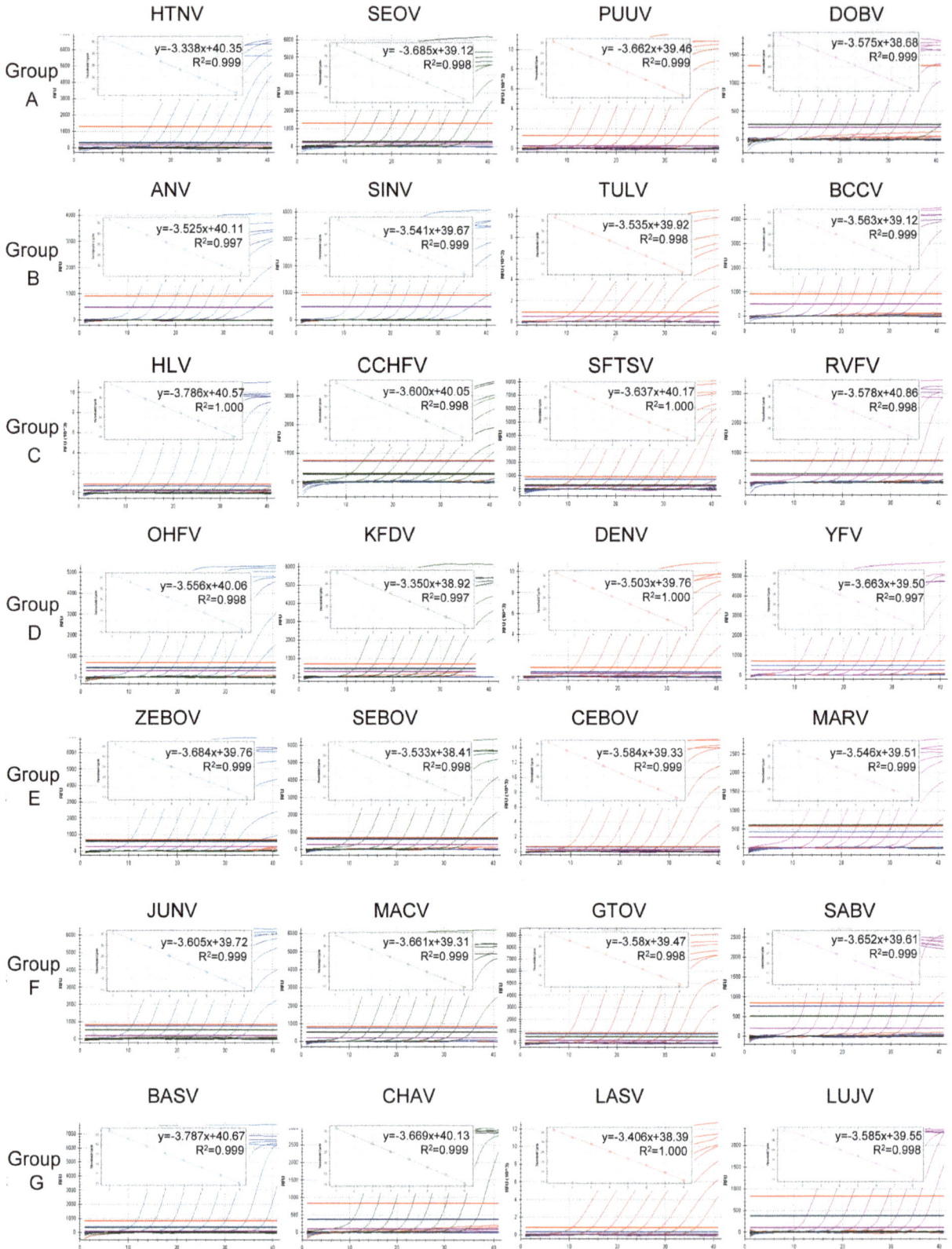

Figure 1. Amplification plots and standard curves of multiplex one-step real-time TaqMan RT-PCR assays. The multiplex one-step real-time TaqMan RT-PCR assays were tested using synthesized in vitro target viral RNA transcripts ranging from 10^1 to 10^8 copies/μL. A PCR baseline subtractive curve fit view of the data is shown with relative fluorescence units (RFUs) plotted against cycle numbers. Standard curves generated from the Ct values obtained against known concentrations, the coefficient of determination (R^2) and slope of the regression curve for each assay are indicated.

Table 4. Detection limits of multiplex one-step real time qRT-PCR assays.

Group	Detected Viruses	Limits of detection (SEM) (Copies/PCR)			
		Monoplex assays		Multiplex assays	
A	HTNV	100.1	(19.1)	174.3	(22.3)
	SEOV	48.2	(8.1)	56.7	(11.5)
	PUUV	85.7	(14.9)	94.1	(10.6)
	DOBV	52.9	(6.1)	55.7	(4.7)
B	TULV	143.9	(14.3)	143.5	(17.6)
	BCCV	64.9	(12.7)	65.5	(10.5)
	ANDV	103.7	(18.3)	148.5	(14.6)
	SINV	86.3	(22.8)	124.3	(14.9)
C	CCHFV	133.5	(10.2)	114.4	(12.5)
	RVFV	155.7	(24.9)	215.6	(3.8)
	SFTSV	94.3	(18.5)	134.8	(2.5)
	HLV	103.5	(9.3)	146.0	(23.3)
D	OHFV	78.1	(14.8)	107.1	(23.2)
	KFDV	53.0	(16.8)	73.6	(1.2)
	DENV	114.2	(15.4)	124.8	(13.6)
	YFV	31.2	(24.9)	66.4	(25.2)
E	MARV	56.5	(3.1)	70.8	(19.6)
	ZEBOV	116.9	(9.4)	110.4	(14.5)
	SEBOV	46.1	(5.2)	46.5	(2.6)
	CEBOV	58.4	(7.4)	64.8	(14.1)
F	JUNV	105.6	(13.5)	116.5	(18.4)
	MACV	45.9	(9.6)	63.5	(14.0)
	GTOV	69.1	(16.4)	86.3	(11.8)
	SABV	68.0	(10.9)	82.3	(15.9)
G	CHAV	84.2	(5.8)	115.6	(18.9)
	LASV	53.2	(6.3)	50.0	(5.0)
	LUJV	62.2	(20.9)	75.8	(15.0)
	BASV	137.8	(23.2)	149.7	(7.4)

these assays as required for broad-range multiplex screening of viral pathogens. It was difficult to obtain specific primers and probes to distinguish ANDV and SINV, thus these two viruses had to share the same primers/probes set to ensure that ANDV and SINV could be detected successfully and rapidly in the established universal system, and other detection methods could be used for further identification. For this point, the system we established in this study still remains to get improvement.

All the assays showed standard curves with high amplification efficiencies and strong linear correlations. The specificity and the reproducibility of the assays were demonstrated and the sensitivity of the systems was acceptable. No significant non-specific amplification was observed among the testing of 28 *in vitro* transcribed viral RNAs (Table 2), RNA extracts of Viruses isolates and 200 healthy human sera (Table 3), which suggested the high specificity of the primers/probe sets. In the multiplex assays testing, there was also no cross-amplification found in RNA transcripts of other viruses, indicating that the developed multiplex one-step real-time qRT-PCR assays were reliable in specificity. The CV of Ct values were all less than 5% in each dilution of synthesized viral RNAs for both intra-assays and inter-assays, suggesting that the multiplex assays were of good reproducibility

(Figure 2). The LODs of these assays were determined in terms of viral RNA copy numbers, ranged from 30 to 160 RNA copies/PCR in the monoplex assays. In the followed multiplex assays, the main range of LODs was from 45 to 150 RNA copies/PCR, which covered more than 90% detected HFVs (Table 4). For HTNV detection assay, the LOD were influenced slightly by viral family based grouping of primers and probes into 4-plex reactions. It resulted in a lower sensitivity of HTNV detection in the multiplex testing with the LOD of 174.3 copies/PCR (Table 4). Another LOD beyond the main range was observed in the RVFV detection (215.6 copies/PCR). It may be, to some extent, due to the relative higher LOD of RVFV detection (155.7 copies/PCR) in the corresponding monoplex assay (Table 4). However, the overall of the sensitivities of multiplex assays was satisfactory, which made it possible to screen VHFs pathogens in one or two steps without requiring of large amount of clinical samples.

So far, most HFVs occurred in limited areas in the world, thus it is difficult to collect clinical samples of all of these 28 viral infections for assays evaluation and validation. The assays developed here were evaluated mostly based on chemically synthesized viral RNA standards, isolated viral RNAs from HFV strains (HTNV, SEOV, SFTSV, DENV 1–4 types, YFV and

A

B

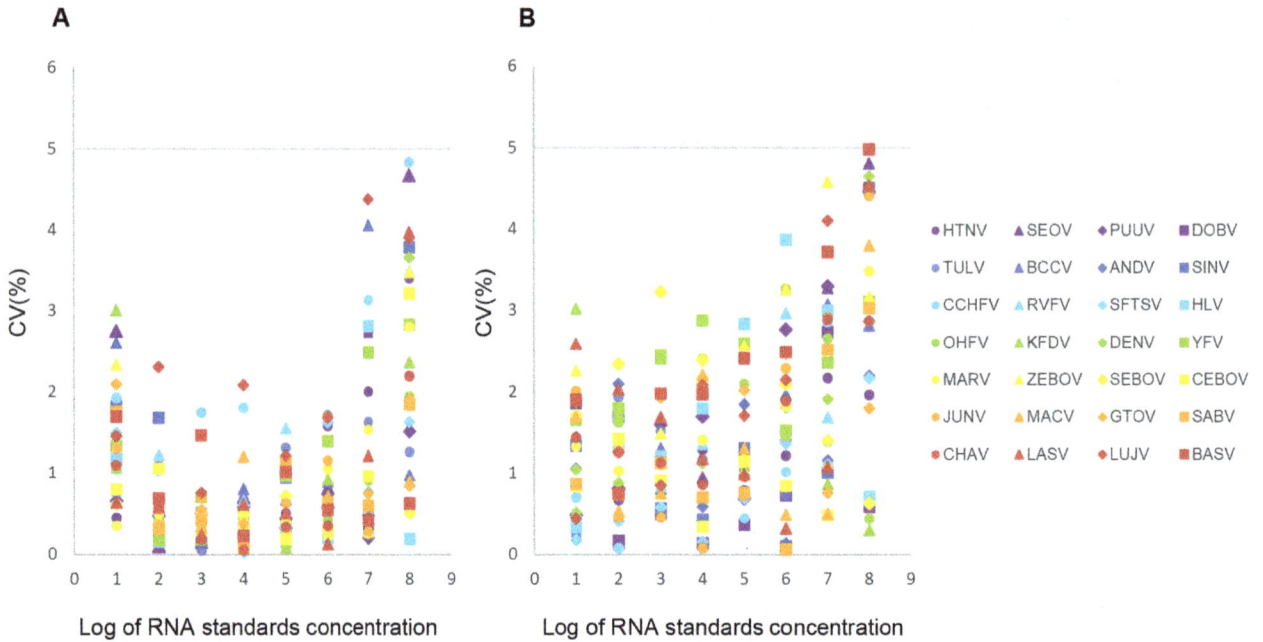

Figure 2. Coefficients of variation of Ct values in the multiplex one-step real-time RT-PCR assays. The multiplex one-step real-time RT-PCR assays were performed in three independent experiments of replicates. The Coefficients of variation (CV) of Ct values were calculated in both intra-assays (A) and inter-assays (B), and showed all less than 5%.

CHIKV) and healthy donor sera as negative control. It still remains the limitations of the assays to evaluate the specificities and sensitivities of the clinical diagnostic for those viruses included in this study because of the lack of clinical specimens. However, It is noteworthy that the LOD was determined by the linearity with statistically proved, resulting in representing the minimal number of copies that will be detected in 100% of the assays. The LODs and standard curves may be extended for quantitative analysis of clinical samples that are from infections caused by hemorrhagic fever viruses. Furthermore, evaluation with clinical samples of patients from three of hemorrhagic fever diseases, including HFRS

caused by HTNV, SFTS caused by SFTSV and Dengue fever caused by DENV (Table 5) showed the reliable specificities and sensitivities for laboratory detection of the infections with these viruses and provided potential use for clinical diagnosis.

In conclusion, the comprehensive multiplex one-step real-time TaqMan qRT-PCR assays for rapid detection of 28 HFVs was established and evaluated in this study, which nearly covered all the hemorrhagic fever viruses. The developed multiplex one-step real-time qRT-PCR assay was tested using different simulate samples and showed excellent parameters in the followed statistical analysis. Therefore, this assay proved to be specific, sensitive and,

Table 5. Evaluation of the multiplex real-time qRT-PCR assays using clinical specimens.

Group	Detected Viruses	Patients sera* (positive/tested)			Healthy human sera (positive/tested)
		HFRS	SFTS	Dengue fever	
A	HTNV	11/11	0/48	0/53	0/100
	SEOV	0/11	0/48	0/53	0/100
	PUUV	0/11	0/48	0/53	0/100
	DOBV	0/11	0/48	0/53	0/100
C	CCHFV	0/11	0/48	0/53	0/100
	RVFV	0/11	0/48	0/53	0/100
	SFTSV	0/11	48/48	0/53	0/100
	HLV	0/11	0/48	0/53	0/100
D	OHFV	0/11	0/48	0/53	0/100
	KFDV	0/11	0/48	0/53	0/100
	DENV	0/11	0/48	51/53	0/100
	YFV	0/11	0/48	0/53	0/100

*Patient types were confirmed by sera detection using the corresponding monoplex assays.

apparently, convenient for rapid and simultaneous identification in laboratory, and could be certainly extended to routine diagnosis and epidemiological detection of VHF infections.

Materials and Methods

Primers and Probes Design

Genomic sequences used in the study were all retrieved from the GenBank database of NCBI (http://www.ncbi.nlm.nih.gov/nuccore/), including the nucleotide sequences of the full genome of the HFVs in the families of *Flaviviridae* and *Filoviridae*, the S segments of the viruses in the families of *Bunyaviridae* and *Arenaviridae*, and the only one genomic sequence of BASV. The multiple alignments of genomic sequences were carried out respectively using Clustal W within the sequence editor package BioEdit (version 7.0.9) to identify conserved regions by visual inspection of the sequence alignments [23]. Primers and probe for each virus were designed using a Primer Express software (version 3.0, Applied Biosystems), and optimized using DNASTAR software by analysis of potentials for dimerization, cross-linking and secondary structures. The specificity of primer and probe sequences was further confirmed using primer–BLAST (NCBI). The probes were differently labeled with the fluorescent dyes, FAM, HEX, TEXAS RED or CY5. All oligonucleotides were synthesized by Shanghai Sangon Biotech Co., Ltd.

Viruses and Samples

Viral isolates propagated in C6/36 or Vero cells, including HTNV (84Fli strain), SEOV (L99 strain), SFTSV (HB29 strain), DENV 1–4 types (Hawaii, New Guinea, H87 and H241 strains), YFV (17D strain) and Chikungunya fever virus (CHIKV, SD08Pan strain), were prepared. Human serum samples from healthy adult donors (n = 200) were assembled from samples library of Chinese National Institute for Viral Diseases Control and Prevention. Among them, CHIKV isolates and healthy human sera were used as negative control in all the tests, whereas the other viral isolates were implied as positive or negative control in the detection assays for different viruses. The human sera from HFRS patients (N = 11), SFTS patients (N = 48) and Dengue fever patients (N = 53) in the acute phase were from our laboratory collections, which were all confirmed by monoplex real-time qRT-PCR assays, and other specific detection methods (virus isolation or IgG detection).

RNA Extraction

RNAs from sera and the culture supernatant of virus-infected cells were extracted from 140 µL of each sample using QIAamp Viral RNA Mini Kit (Qiagen) according to the manufacturer's instructions, then eluted in 40 µL sterilized RNase free water and stored at −80°C before use.

Preparation of Viral RNA Standards

Preparation of viral RNA standards was initiated with viral genomic DNA fragments obtained through chemical synthesis or RT-PCR amplification from viral isolates (HTNV, SEOV, SFTSV, DENV and YFV). The T7 promoter sequence was then introduced into the 5′ terminus (for positive-strand viruses) or 3′ terminus (for negative-strand viruses) of these DNA fragments via PCR amplification. The PCR products were purified using the Gel Extraction Kit (Qiagen) and used for *in vitro* transcription with a RiboMAX™ Large Scale RNA Production Systems-T7 (Promega). The synthetic RNA transcripts were purified by RNeasy Mini Kit (Qiagen), followed by concentration calculation using a NanoDrop ND-1000 spectrophotometer (NanoDrop Technolo-

gies) and analysis by 2% agarose gel electrophoresis, and then stored at −80°C. Dilutions of viral RNA standards ranging from 10^1 to 10^8 copies/µL were prepared by 10-fold serial dilution of RNA transcripts in sterilized RNase free water according to the concentration and length of each transcript.

One-step Real-time qRT-PCR Assays

One-step real-time qRT-PCR reactions were performed using AgPath-ID™ one-step RT-PCR Kit (Applied Biosystems), and contained 12.5 µL of 2× RT-PCR buffer, 400 nM of each primer, 120 nM of each probe, 1 µL of Enzyme Mix and 5 µL of viral RNA transcripts or RNA extracts in a final volume of 25 µL. Total RNA extracted from Hela cells was used as negative control. Real-time qRT-PCR cycling was performed on Bio-Rad CFX96 system as follows: 50°C for 30 min, 95°C for 10 min, then 40 cycles of 15 s at 95°C and 45 s at 60°C. The fluorogenic signal emitted was collected at the end of annealing-extension step. A threshold was automatically set and the threshold cycle value (C_t) was consequently determined. Three replicates of the assay within or between runs were performed. Multiplex assays were assembled by grouping the primers and probes according to the hosts/vectors or viral families (Supplementary Table S3), reaction conditions were as same as described above.

Specificity, Sensitivity and Reproducibility

To assess the specificities of the developed one-step real-time qRT-PCR assays, each pair of primers and probe was tested in triplicate against all the other *in vitro* synthetic viral RNA transcripts with the concentration of 10^6 copies/µL, RNA extracts of HTNV, SEOV, SFTSV, DENV, YFV and CHIKV, as well as serum RNA from a panel of 200 sera from human without VHFs.

To evaluate sensitivity of monoplex and multiplex one-step real-time qRT-PCR assays, each group of 10-fold serial dilutions of 28 *in vitro* synthetic target viral RNA transcripts, ranging from 10^1 to 10^8 copies/µL, were used as standard preparations to assess the detection limits of viral RNA copy load. Three replicates of the assay within or between runs were performed to assess the reproducibility, and the intra-assay and inter-assay variations over the linear range of the assays were statistically calculated.

Statistical Analysis

Regression, reproducibility and the coefficient of variation (CV) of the mean C_t value for each standard concentration within and between individual PCR runs were statically calculated by using GraphPad Prism version 5.01 (GraphPad Software, San Diego, CA; http://www.graphpad.com/prism/Prism.htm) to evaluate linearity and determine the quantitative performance of each assay.

Ethical Consideration

According to the medical research regulation of National Health and Family Planning Commission, China, all studies involved in human samples were reviewed and approved by the ethics committee of China Center for Disease Control and Prevention, which uses international guidelines to ensure confidentiality, anonymity, and informed consent. The written informed consent was agreed by the donors.

Supporting Information

Figure S1 Amplification plots and standard curves of monoplex one-step real-time TaqMan qRT-PCR assays. The monoplex one-step real-time TaqMan RT-PCR assays were performed with synthesized in vitro target viral RNA transcripts ranging from 10^1 to 10^8 copies/μL to evaluate the specificity and the sensitivity of each primers/probe set. A PCR baseline subtractive curve fit view of the data is shown with relative fluorescence units (RFUs) plotted against cycle numbers. Standard curves generated from the Ct values obtained against known concentrations, the coefficient of determination (R^2) and slope of the regression curve for each assay are indicated.

Author Contributions

Conceived and designed the experiments: DXL MFL JDL. Performed the experiments: ZP AQL JQ CCH. Analyzed the data: ZP AQL. Contributed reagents/materials/analysis tools: ZP AQL JQ CCH SZ CL QFZ. Wrote the paper: ZP AQL MFL DXL.

References

1. Bray M, Johnson KM (2009) Viral Hemorrhagic Fevers: a Comparative Appraisal. Clinical Virology, Third Edition.
2. Geisbert TW, Jahrling PB (2004) Exotic emerging viral diseases: progress and challenges. Nat Med 10: S110–121.
3. Le Guenno B (1995) Emerging viruses. Sci Am 273: 56–64.
4. Charrel RN, de Lamballerie X (2003) [The Alkhurma virus (family Flaviviridae, genus Flavivirus): an emerging pathogen responsible for hemorrhage fever in the Middle East]. Med Trop (Mars) 63: 296–299.
5. Bray M (2005) Pathogenesis of viral hemorrhagic fever. Curr Opin Immunol 17: 399–403.
6. Delgado S, Erickson BR, Agudo R, Blair PJ, Vallejo E, et al. (2008) Chapare virus, a newly discovered arenavirus isolated from a fatal hemorrhagic fever case in Bolivia. PLoS Pathog 4: e1000047.
7. Briese T, Paweska JT, McMullan LK, Hutchison SK, Street C, et al. (2009) Genetic detection and characterization of Lujo virus, a new hemorrhagic fever-associated arenavirus from southern Africa. PLoS Pathog 5: e1000455.
8. McMullan LK, Folk SM, Kelly AJ, MacNeil A, Goldsmith CS, et al. (2012) A new phlebovirus associated with severe febrile illness in Missouri. N Engl J Med 367: 834–841.
9. Grard G, Fair JN, Lee D, Slikas E, Steffen I, et al. (2012) A novel rhabdovirus associated with acute hemorrhagic fever in central Africa. PLoS Pathog 8: e1002924.
10. Khan AS, Maupin GO, Rollin PE, Noor AM, Shurie HH, et al. (1997) An outbreak of Crimean-Congo hemorrhagic fever in the United Arab Emirates, 1994–1995. Am J Trop Med Hyg 57: 519–525.
11. Centers for Disease C, Prevention (2001) Outbreak of Ebola hemorrhagic fever Uganda, August 2000-January 2001. MMWR Morb Mortal Wkly Rep 50: 73–77.
12. Drosten C, Kummerer BM, Schmitz H, Gunther S (2003) Molecular diagnostics of viral hemorrhagic fevers. Antiviral Res 57: 61–87.
13. Anderson PD, Bokor G (2012) Bioterrorism: pathogens as weapons. Journal of Pharmacy Practice 25: 521–529.
14. Mackay IM, Arden KE, Nitsche A (2002) Real-time PCR in virology. Nucleic Acids Res 30: 1292–1305.
15. Espy MJ, Uhl JR, Sloan LM, Buckwalter SP, Jones MF, et al. (2006) Real-time PCR in clinical microbiology: applications for routine laboratory testing. Clin Microbiol Rev 19: 165–256.
16. Drosten C, Gottig S, Schilling S, Asper M, Panning M, et al. (2002) Rapid detection and quantification of RNA of Ebola and Marburg viruses, Lassa virus, Crimean-Congo hemorrhagic fever virus, Rift Valley fever virus, dengue virus, and yellow fever virus by real-time reverse transcription-PCR. J Clin Microbiol 40: 2323–2330.
17. Weidmann M, Muhlberger E, Hufert FT (2004) Rapid detection protocol for filoviruses. J Clin Virol 30: 94–99.
18. Aitichou M, Saleh SS, McElroy AK, Schmaljohn C, Ibrahim MS (2005) Identification of Dobrava, Hantaan, Seoul, and Puumala viruses by one-step real-time RT-PCR. J Virol Methods 124: 21–26.
19. Moureau G, Temmam S, Gonzalez JP, Charrel RN, Grard G, et al. (2007) A real-time RT-PCR method for the universal detection and identification of flaviviruses. Vector Borne Zoonotic Dis 7: 467–477.
20. Trombley AR, Wachter L, Garrison J, Buckley-Beason VA, Jahrling J, et al. (2010) Comprehensive panel of real-time TaqMan polymerase chain reaction assays for detection and absolute quantification of filoviruses, arenaviruses, and New World hantaviruses. Am J Trop Med Hyg 82: 954–960.
21. Bossi P, Tegnell A, Baka A, Van Loock F, Hendriks J, et al. (2004) Bichat guidelines for the clinical management of haemorrhagic fever viruses and bioterrorism-related haemorrhagic fever viruses. Euro Surveill 9: E11–12.
22. Whitehouse CA (2004) Crimean-Congo hemorrhagic fever. Antiviral Res 64: 145–160.
23. Hall TA. BioEdit: a user-friendly biological sequence alignment editor and analysis program for Windows 95/98/NT; 1999. 95–98.

3

Demographic and Clinico-Epidemiological Features of Dengue Fever in Faisalabad, Pakistan

Faiz Ahmed Raza[1,2]*, **Shafiq ur Rehman**[2], **Ruqyya Khalid**[3], **Jameel Ahmad**[4], **Sajjad Ashraf**[5], **Mazhar Iqbal**[1], **Shahida Hasnain**[2]

1 Pakistan Medical Research Council, Research Centre, Punjab Medical College, Faisalabad, Pakistan, 2 Department of Microbiology and Molecular Genetics, University of the Punjab, Quaid-e-Azam Campus, Lahore, Pakistan, 3 School of Biological Sciences, University of the Punjab, Quaid-e-Azam Campus, Lahore, Pakistan, 4 Department of Pathology, Allied Hospital, Faisalabad, Pakistan, 5 Nano Bio Energy Engineering School of Integrative Engineering, Chung-Ang University, Seoul, Korea

Abstract

This cross-sectional study was carried out to explore the epidemiological and clinical features of dengue fever in Faisalabad, Pakistan during 2011 and 2012. During the study period, anti-dengue IgM positive cases were reported in the post-monsoon period during the months of August–December. Certain hotspots for the dengue infection were identified in the city that coincide with the clusters of densely populated urban regions of the city. Out of total 299 IgM positive patients (male 218 and female 81); there were 239 dengue fever (DF) and 60 dengue hemorrhagic fever (DHF) patients. There was decrease in the median age of dengue patients from 31 years in 2011 to 21.5 years in 2012 (p<0.001). Abdominal pain was seen in 35% DHF patients followed by nausea in 28.3%, epistaxis in 25% and rash in 20% patients (p<0.05). Patients reported to be suffering from high-grade fever for an average of 8.83 days in DHF as compared to 5.82 days in DF before being hospitalized. Co-morbidities were found to be risk factor for the development of DHF in dengue patients. Clinical and laboratory features of dengue cases studied could be used for the early identification of patients at risk of severe dengue fever.

Editor: Douglas M. Watts, University of Texas at El Paso, United States of America

Funding: This work was supported by Pakistan Medical Research Council (www.pmrc.org.pk) via Grant No. 4-23-4/11/Dengue/RDC/PMC/3495. The funders had no role in study design, data collection and analysis, decision to publish, or preparation of the manuscript.

Competing Interests: The authors have declared that no competing interests exist.

* E-mail: faiz.raza@gmail.com

Introduction

Dengue is an arthropod-borne arboviral disease becoming major public health concern, both in the tropical and subtropical regions of the world. It is estimated that 50 to 100 million cases of dengue virus (DENV) infection reported annually; which leads to 250,000 to 500,000 cases of dengue hemorrhagic fever (DHF) or dengue shock syndrome (DSS) and 20,000–25,000 deaths. The causative agent belongs to family Flaviviridae; currently there are 4 distinct serotypes: DENV-1, DENV-2, DENV-3 and DENV-4; being transmitted to humans principally by *Aedes aegypti* and *Aedes albopictus* mosquitoes. Dengue infection results in a wide spectrum of clinical symptoms ranging from mild dengue fever (DF) to the very severe form of the disease, DHF and DSS [1,2].

Pakistan, the sixth most populated country (185 million people) of the world located in south Asia between latitudes 23.45° and 36.75° north and longitudes 61° and 75.5° east. Due to its subtropical location and suitable climatic conditions for vectors, it has been source of many vector born diseases including malaria, leishmaniasis, Crimean Congo hemorrhagic fever, dengue hemorrhagic fever, West Nile virus infection, Japanese encephalitis and scrub typhus [3,4]. Although dengue virus exists in this region even before creation of Pakistan [5], the first outbreak of DF due to DENV-1 and DENV-2 was reported in 1994 leading to morbidity in thousands [6]. Decade after first outbreak, a second outbreak involving DENV-3 occurred in 2005 in Karachi with a

sudden increase in number of DHF patients. The increase in disease severity might be contributed by infection with DENV-3, in a population sensitized previously with DENV-1 and DENV-2, through antibody dependent enhancement (ADE) [7]. Afterwards, another outbreak occurred in 2006 affecting the population in the north to south of Pakistan leading to 3500 confirmed cases and 52 deaths. Analysis of the selected samples revealed co-circulation of DENV-2 and DENV-3 in the population [8]. During 2010 and 2011, Pakistan was hit by devastating floods that had not only destroyed property and lives but also provided breeding sites for dengue virus vectors, resulting in worst outbreaks during these years [6].

Various small scale and large scale studies had been carried out previously in various cities of Pakistan [7–9]. However, there is severe deficiency of thorough studies related to dengue outbreaks in Faisalabad. In this direction, we present comprehensive dengue infection epidemiology in the Faisalabad city during 2011–2012. The patient's data was used to identify possible hotspots for the dengue infection in the city during the two years of study. The possible effect of prevailing weather conditions, at the time of epidemic, on the frequency of dengue cases was investigated. In addition, patient's demographic and clinical features were studied that can facilitate in the early identification of patients suffering from severe form of dengue fever.

Materials and Methods

Ethical Clearance

Ethical clearance was taken from institutional ethical review committee of Punjab Medical College, Faisalabad before starting the study. Written informed consent was taken from all patients or legal guardians.

Study Setting and Patient Data

Faisalabad, the second largest city in the province of Punjab and third largest city of Pakistan, located between latitudes 31.41°N and longitude 73.11°E, having a population of more than 2.6 million [10], is considered as an industrial hub of Pakistan. Two major public sector hospitals in the city are Allied Hospital (1150 beds) and DHQ Hospital (600 beds). This cross-sectional study was carried out in 2011 and 2012. All clinically confirmed cases of dengue fever who were admitted to the high dependency unit of Allied Hospital and DHQ Hospital Faisalabad for its management were included in the study. Diagnosis of dengue was confirmed if apart from high grade fever these patients also had positive anti-dengue IgM antibodies. All patients were interviewed for signs and symptoms related to dengue fever and they were followed daily till their discharge from the hospital for any change in their clinical signs and laboratory parameters. The data for confirmed cases of dengue included their demographics, co-morbidity, previous exposure, length of hospital stay, hemorrhagic manifestations and clinical signs and symptoms.

Dengue cases were classified into Dengue Fever (DF) and Dengue Hemorrhagic Fever (DHF) according to World Health Organization (WHO) classification and case definition [11]. A patient was considered as a confirmed case of DF if presented with fever of 2–7 days duration and having two or more of the following symptoms: headache, retro-orbital pain, myalgia/arthralgia, rash, hemorrhagic manifestations (petechiae and positive tourniquet test) and, leukopenia. The patients of DHF were distinguished from DF if they had (1) fever for 2–7 days; (2) one or more hemorrhagic manifestations (positive tourniquet test, petechiae, ecchymosis or purpura, bleeding from mucosa, injection sites or other sites); (3) Thrombocytopenia (platelet count $<100,000/mm^3$); and (4) evidence of plasma leakage. A patient was confirmed to have dengue virus infection if IgM anti-dengue antibodies were detected in the patient's serum after 5 days of fever. Dengue IgM antibodies were measured by indirect IgM enzyme linked immunosorbant assay (ELISA), using commercially available kit (Human GmbH, Wiesbaden, Germany). Antibody index of >0.496 was considered as positive for dengue virus infection. Patients having an index value less than the cutoff and reported with other febrile illness were excluded from the study. Furthermore, data for the patients having co-morbidities is discussed separately to the data for the patients with dengue infection alone.

Diagnostic Laboratory Values

Platelet count less than 150,000 cells/mm^3 blood was defined as thrombocytopenia. Leukocyte count of less than 4.5 cells/mm^3 was defined as leucopenia. Hematocrit (HCT) of $>48\%$ was considered as elevated. Hemoglobin (Hb) concentration less than 13 and 12 g/L was considered as decreased in males and females respectively while in children values less than 11.2 g/L was considered as low. The values of alanine aminotransferase (ALT) and aspartate aminotransferase (AST) above 45 U/ml and 36 U/ml respectively were considered as elevated.

Cluster Map for Dengue Infection

Google Earth^{TM} was used to build map of the Faisalabad city in which polygons represent residential units (towns, colonies etc.) whereas placemarks indicate areas from which dengue cases were reported. Number on the placemarks represent frequency of dengue cases from the specified area. Boundaries of individual residential units were determined in Google Maps^{TM}.

Statistical Analysis

Statistical Package for Social Sciences (SPSS) (Chicago, IL), version 19 was used for data entry, processing and statistical analysis. p value was calculated by Wilcoxon test for age, temperature, hematocrit and fluid therapy, while χ^2 test was used for all other categorical variables. A 2-tailed p value≤0.05 was considered to be statistically significant.

Results

This two years cross-sectional study was carried out in 2011 and 2012. A total of 393 confirmed dengue patients, including 353 in 2011 and 40 in 2012, were enrolled in the study. Amongst them 94 (23.9%) cases of dengue fever were reported with single/multiple co-morbidities, which are discussed separately.

Patient Characteristics

Out of 299 patients, 218 (72.9%) were males and 81 (27.1%) were females. The median age of the patients was 30 years and age ranged from 6 to 90 years, including 27 (9%) children (till 16 years) and 272 (91%) adults. However, no child was reported under the age of 6, during both years. There were 132 (48.5%) young adults (17 to 30 years old) among adult patients. There was decrease in the median age of patients from 31 years in 2011 to 21.5 years in 2012 (p<0.001). The highest prevalence of dengue patients was observed between 16 to 30 years (Figure 1). Table 1 gives yearly distribution of dengue cases according to different age groups and disease severity. Within age group of 6–15 years there was 20% increase in the prevalence of dengue patients, while there was 23.9% increase in DHF within age group of 6 to 30 years, in 2012 than the previous year. Table 2 presents demographic features, clinical characteristics and laboratory findings of dengue patients according to severity of the disease. DF was diagnosed in 239 patients (184 males, 55 females) and DHF in 60 patients (34 males, 26 females), with highest incidence (p = 0.03) of infection in male population. The median age of DF patients was 30 years and 24.5 years in DHF patients. DHF was reported more commonly in younger population (p = 0.05).

Clinical Signs and Symptoms

Myalgia was present in 87.3% patients, followed by headache (76.9%), vomiting (52.2%), abdominal pain (18.4%), nausea (17.7%), cough (9.7%), rash (9.4%), retro-orbital pain (8.7%), sore throat (7.4%), anorexia (7.4%), restlessness (6%), diarrhea (5.4%), periorbital puffiness (3.3%) and cold/clammy skin (3%) patients. Out of 299 patients, 143 (47.8%) patients presented with various types of hemorrhage, which included epistaxis in 9.7% patients, followed by gingivitis (9.4%), melena (7%), hematemesis (7%), petechiae (6.4%) and hematuria (3.3%) patients. Spleen and liver were enlarged in 29 (9.7%) and 30 (10%) patients, respectively.

Although, headache, myalgia/arthalgia and vomiting were the most common symptoms observed but they were not significantly different amongst DF and DHF patients. Conversely, abdominal pain, nausea, rash, cold/clammy skin and periorbital puffiness were significantly (p<0.05) different in DHF. Retro-orbital pain and restlessness were mostly, but not significantly, associated with

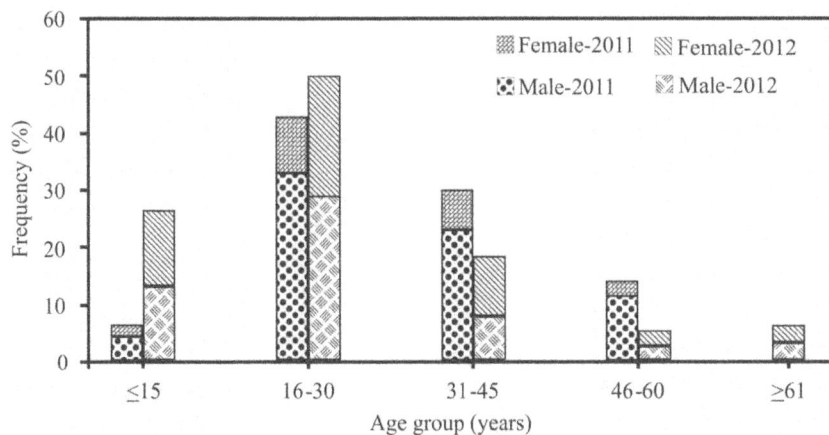

Figure 1. Gender wise distribution of dengue patients according to different age groups.

DHF. Furthermore, spontaneous hemorrhages, abdominal tenderness, splenomegaly and hepatomegaly were most frequently ($p \leq 0.05$) observed in DHF (Table 2).

Laboratory Findings

Liver involvement, as indicated by abnormal levels of liver enzymes, was observed in various dengue patients. Alanine aminotransferase (ALT) was raised 55.3%, whereas aspartate aminotransferase (AST) was raised in 68.4% patients. Increase in the levels of liver enzymes (AST and ALT) was most frequently associated with DHF. ALT levels were raised in 74.2% ($p = 0.032$), while AST levels were raised in all DHF patients ($p = 0.077$). ALT was 2.7 times higher, while AST was 10 times higher than the normal values in DHF patients. Majority of the patients (96%) presented with thrombocytopenia at time of admission. Low hemoglobin and leucopenia were observed in 49.6% and 71.8% of all patients, respectively. Median hematocrit level for all dengue patients was 41.3. Amazingly the hematocrit, an indicator of capillary leakage, was higher in DF patients (42%) in contrast to DHF patients (36%; $p < 0.001$), at the time of hospitalization.

Dengue Case Management

Table 3 presents data related to impact of severity of the disease on length of hospitalization, course of illness and management of dengue patients. Proper diagnosis and treatment of dengue patients is a primary clinical goal that could contribute significantly in the reduction of length of hospitalization and treatment

Table 1. Year Wise Distribution of Patients Suffering From Dengue Fever (DF) and Dengue Hemorrhagic Fever (DHF) According to Different Age Groups.

Age group (years)	Year-2011		Year-2012	
	DF (%)	DHF (%)	DF (%)	DHF (%)
≤15	9 (3.3)	5 (1.8)	3 (10.7)	6 (21.4)
16 to 30	98 (36.2)	23 (8.5)	10 (35.7)	5 (17.9)
31 to 45	67 (24.7)	13(4.8)	3 (10.7)	1 (3.6)
46 to 60	34 (12.5)	5 (1.8)	0.0	0.0
>60	15 (5.5)	2 (0.7)	0.0	0.0

costs but could also affect the outcome of the disease. DF patients were reported with high grade fever from average 6.7 days before being hospitalized. Mean length of hospital stay for DF was 3.8 days. However, severe form of the disease (DHF) has contributed substantially towards longer course of illness (8.83 fever days) and length of stay (4.9 days). Fluid replacement therapy was administered in case of hypotension, while whole blood and/or platelet concentrates were infused in those having severe thrombocytopenia, low hematocrit and capillary leakage. Furthermore, total 12 deaths were recorded (case fatality rate 2.5%) due to severe form of dengue fever (DHF/DSS), in 2011 only. The victims were suffering from multiple co-morbidities and were mostly died due to multiple organ failure.

Co-morbidities and Outcome of Dengue Infection

Table 4 shows the frequency of various co-morbidities in dengue infection. Total 94 (23.9%) cases of dengue fever were reported with single or multiple co-morbidities, including 70 (74.5%) males and 22 (25.5%) females. Their median age was 33.4 years, including 16 (17%) children (till 16 years) and 78 (83%) adults. Attack rates with multiple co-morbidities increased constantly with the age and was highest among the age group of 46 to 50 years. Low hemoglobin and thrombocytopenia at time of admission were observed in 41 (87%) and 94 (100%) dengue patients, respectively. Splenomegaly, hepatomegaly and severe thrombocytopenia (platelet count $\leq 15,000$ cells/mm^3) were most frequently observed ($p < 0.05$) in patients with co-morbidities as compared to DF patients. Low hemoglobin was observed most commonly, although not significantly ($p = 0.089$), in patients with co-morbidities than with DF. Hypotension, severe thrombocytopenia, low hematocrit and capillary leakage in patients with co-morbidities were managed with average 4.39 liters of intravenous fluids, 1.4 ± 0.5 whole blood transfusions and 2 ± 1.2 platelets transfusions. Fluid replacement therapy, number of whole blood and platelets transfusions were significantly higher ($p < 0.05$) in patients with co-morbidities than in DF patients. DF was diagnosed in 62 (49 males, 13 females) and DHF in 32 (21 males, 11 females) patients.

Among the co-morbidities 53 (56.4%) of the dengue patients were co-infected with hepatitis C virus (HCV), including one with diabetes mellitus, hypertension, typhoid, ischemic heart disease and abdominal tuberculosis; one with hepatitis B virus co-infection; one with typhoid and another one with malarial parasite. Data for the 49 dengue patients with HCV co-infection

Table 2. Characteristics Presented by Patients Suffering from Dengue Fever (DF) and Dengue Hemorrhagic Fever (DHF) Patients.

Characteristics	DF (%)	DHF (%)	N	p value[1]
Demographics				
Age [median (interquartile range)]	30 (22)	24.5 (17)	299	0.05
Gender				
Male	184 (77)	34 (56.7)	299	0.03
Female	55 (23)	26 (43.3)		
Clinical Presentation				
Headache	184 (77)	46 (76.7)	299	>0.05
Myalgia/arthralgia	212 (88.7)	49 (81.6)	299	0.191
Vomiting	121 (50.6)	35 (58.3)	299	0.314
Abdominal pain	34 (14.2)	21 (35)	299	0.001
Nausea	36 (15.1)	17 (28.3)	299	0.023
Rash	16 (6.7)	12 (20)	299	0.005
Diarrhea	11 (4.6)	5 (8.3)	299	0.331
Anorexia	13 (5.4)	9 (15)	299	0.22
Sore throat	16 (6.7)	6 (10)	299	0.407
Retro-orbital pain	17 (7.1)	9 (15)	299	0.07
Cough	22 (9.2)	7 (11.6)	299	0.625
Cold skin/clammy skin	4 (1.7)	5 (8.3)	299	0.018
Restlessness	11 (4.6)	7 (11.6)	299	0.062
Periorbital puffiness	5 (2.1)	5 (8.3)	299	0.031
Hemorrhages				
Epistaxis (Nose bleed)	14 (5.9)	15 (25)	299	<0.001
Gingivitis (Gum Bleed)	17 (7.1)	11 (18.3)	299	0.012
Melena (blood in stool)	9 (3.8)	12 (20)	299	<0.001
Hematemesis (vomiting blood)	13 (5.4)	8 (13.3)	299	0.045
Hematuria (blood in urine)	5 (2.1)	5 (8.3)	299	0.031
Petechiae (small spots)	12 (5)	7 (11.7)	299	0.074
Other*	8 (3)	7 (11.7)	299	0.016
Clinical Signs				
Temperature [median (SD)]	37 (0.2)	37.22 (1.1)		0.108
Abdominal tenderness	7 (2.9)	8 (13.3)	299	0.003
Splenomegaly (Spleen enlargement)	15 (6.3)	14 (23.3)	299	<0.001
Hepatomegaly (Liver enlargement)	12 (5)	18 (30)	299	<0.001
Laboratory Findings				
Thrombocytopenia at presentation	226 (96.2)	57(95)	295	0.715
Low hemoglobin	104 (44.1)	43 (71.7)	296	<0.001
Hematocrit level on admission [median (SD)]	42.05 (8.3)	36 (17.9)	296	<0.001
Leukopenia	172 (72.3)	42 (70)	298	0.749
Increased ALT	112/213 (52.6)	23/31 (74.2)	244	0.032
Increased AST	08/14 (57.1)	05/05 (100)	19	0.077

[1]p-value was calculated by non-parametric (Mann-Whitney U) test for age, temperature, and hematocrit. The χ^2-test was used for all other categorical variables; p value less than 0.05 was considered as significant.
*Menstrual bleed, Sub-conjunctival bleed, Ear Bleed, Hemoptysis, Purpura, Ecchymosis.

was compared exclusively with the patients with dengue infection alone. No significant (p>0.05) difference was observed in the clinical signs and symptoms in the dengue patients and those with the HCV co-infection. However, hemorrhagic tendencies were significantly higher (p = 0.02) in patients with HCV co-infection. DF was diagnosed in 36 (73.5%) and DHF in 17 (26.5%) HCV co-infected dengue patients.

Total 12 (9 males, 3 females) patients were reported with *Plasmodium vivex* co-infection, among them one was also co-infected with HCV and HBV; one with HBV alone and one with *Salmonella typhae* alone. 50% of the dengue patients with malarial parasite (MP) co-infection developed DHF. Among the three female patients having malarial co-infection two were pregnant (38 weeks pregnancy). Both of them were diagnosed as cases of DHF with

Table 3. Impact of Disease Severity on Length of Hospitalization, Course of Illness and Management of Dengue Patients [mean (SD)].

Characteristics	DF	DHF	N	p value[1]
Days of fever (at presentation)	5.82 (2.7)	8.83 (6.2)	299	<0.001
Length of stay (days)	3.56 (1.4)	4.90 (2.5)	299	<0.001
Fluid administered (liters)	3.36 (2.1)	5.45 (5)	253	0.001
Number of blood transfusions	1.3 (1)	2.2 (2.1)	78	0.073
Number of platelet transfusions	1.23 (0.4)	1.5 (1)	54	0.494

[1]p value was calculated by non-parametric (Mann-Whitney U) test; p value less than 0.05 was considered as significant.

severe internal bleeding (HCT<29%), various hemorrhages, ulcers on the lips and anemia, resulting in intrauterine death of the fetuses.

Clusters of Dengue Infection in the City

Figure 2 shows possible hot spots in Faisalabad city from which dengue infections were reported more frequently. The patients were reported from 14 adjoining and 3 distant districts of province Punjab, including the major share from Faisalabad city alone, followed by other neighboring districts. The cases reported from Faisalabad city were from both of its less populated peripheral regions, as well as, from its densely populated central regions. Comparing the data for both years indicate high incidence of infection from various overlapping regions in the Faisalabad city. Furthermore, these hot spots coincide with the clusters of densely populated central regions. More recently, infections from new areas adjacent to these hot spots reported around the city.

Environmental Factors and Frequency of Dengue Cases

Figure 3 gives monthly average humidity, temperture and frequency of dengue patients reported during the study period. The onset of dengue virus epidemics during the study period coincide with the post-monsoon era, starting from August, reaching its peak in September/October and declining in November/December, both years. The highest and the lowest monthly temperature was recorded during June (35°C), and December (14°C) respectively in both years. Similarly, the highest and the lowest monthly relative humidity (RH) was recorded during September (71%) and June (31%) respectively. In contrast to subsequent year, second peak of dengue virus infection was observed in November-2011 with highest prevalence (36.7%) in that year. Mid of 2012 was warmer (average temperature during June–Sep was 33°C) and dryer (average RH during June–September was 53%) than the previous year (average temperature 31.5°C; RH 63.3%), accompanied by rapid decline in temperature by the end of year.

Discussion

The dengue virus has threatened half of the world's population, hence becoming a major public health problem especially in tropical countries [12]. The central place of Faisalabad city amongst surrounding districts having underdeveloped health settings makes it a hotspot for health care seekers. Dengue patients were reported from the densely populated central regions of the Faisalabad city. Certain hotspots were also detected from which dengue cases were reported more frequently both years. In

Table 4. Frequency of Different Co-morbidities in Dengue Patients.

	A	B	C	D	E	F	G	H	I	J	K
A	48										
B	1	1									
C	0	0	1								
D	1	0	0	7							
E	1	1	0	1	9						
F	0	0	0	0	0	2					
G	0	0	0	0	0	4	3				
H	0	0	0	0	0	2	1	0			
I	0	0	0	0	0	0	1	0	0		
J	0	0	0	0	0	0	0	0	0	1	
K	0	0	0	0	0	0	0	0	0	0	1
L	1	0	0	0	0	0	0	0	0	0	0
M	1	0	0	0	0	0	0	1	0	0	0

A, Hepatitis C; **B**, Hepatitis B; **C**, Hepatitis A; **D**, Typhoid; **E**, Malaria; **F**, Diabetes; **G**, Hypertension; **H**, Ischemic heart disease; **I**, Urinary tract infection; **J**, Cancer; **K**, Hepatitis C, Malaria, Typhoid, Abdominal tuberculosis, Diabetes, Hypertension and Ischemic heart disease; **L**, Hepatitis B and Malaria; **M**, Diabetes and Hypertension.

addition, new cases of dengue fever from adjacent regions of these hot spots show the spread of dengue infection to adjacent areas. Both year data also indicate outwards progression of dengue infection from the populated central areas to adjoining less-populated regions of the city.

The dynamics of the dengue fever epidemic are influenced by the complex interactions among virus, vector, host and directly dependent on climatic and environmental conditions [13]. The peak incidence of dengue virus infection was observed from September to November during both years of study. Seasonal humidity and temperature variations have role in vector survival that ultimately linked with emergence of dengue epidemics. This study has also provided the evidence for influence of environmental conditions on dengue virus infection. The observed average humidity and temperature during the study period indicates that less hot and humid conditions favor dengue virus infections, which might have linked with better vector growth.

The higher proportion of male victims as compared to females among the effected patients is evident in this study. Similar observations were also reported by a recent study, conducted for the analysis of dengue incidence in six Asian countries [14]. Different other studies conducted in different regions of Asia also reported the similar observations [15–17]. These observations indicate the gender specific difference among the dengue incidence, which might be related to exposure of dengue vector or by some unknown factor. Interestingly, the incidence of dengue infection in North America is reported either equal proportions of both females and males or females in higher proportions [18–20]. The phenomenon of gender specificity in relation to dengue infection might have been contributed by social, cultural (women being covered) and exposure reasons.

There is conflicting data regarding the age of affected people from dengue. Studies conducted previously in Asia, using surveillance data, correlated the age of affected patients with the severity of disease. Recent studies conducted in Pakistan suggested decrease in the median age of dengue patients during 2003–2007 and the reported age of affected individuals was 11 to 25 years

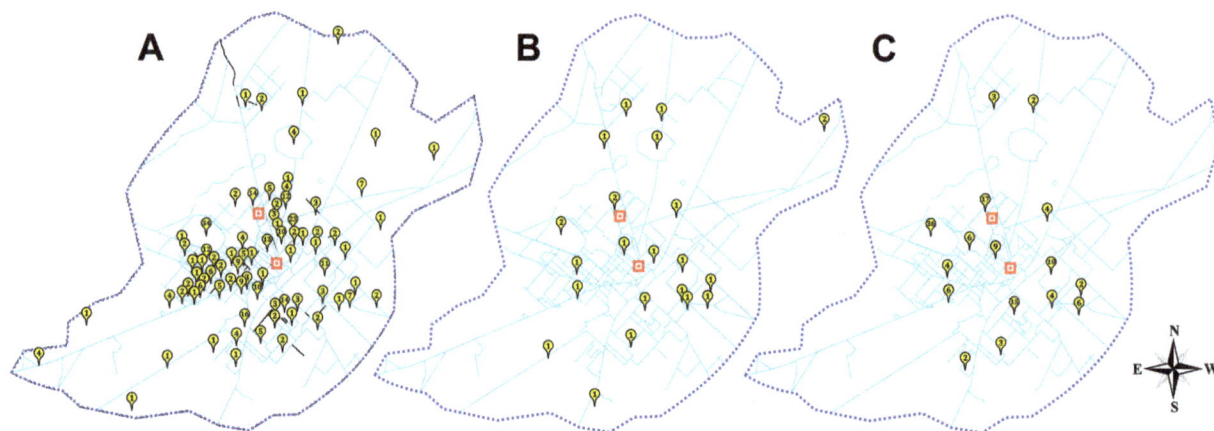

Figure 2. Hot spots for dengue infection in Faisalabad city. The distribution of dengue cases reported from Faisalabad city. A) Map of Faisalabad city showing areas from which dengue cases were reported in 2011, B) in 2012 and during both years. Squared place marks represents location of medical centers in the city.

[21]. Similarly, a study conducted previously in Indonesia during 1975 to 1984 reported increase in incidence of dengue infections in younger population [22]. In compliance to previous studies the median age of affected individuals was decreased from 31 years in 2011 to 21.5 years in 2012 (p<0.001), respectively. Decrease in the median age of infection suggests the development of immunity against majority of population, due to the circulation of multiple serotypes over a period of time. Additionally, severe form of disease (DHF) was reported more commonly in the younger population (Figure 2). There was increase in the frequency of DHF patients in 2012 compared with 2011; which might be contributed by infections with more virulent virus. Attack rates were highest among the age group of 31 to 45 years, while the attack rates were lowest in the younger population (till 15 years). In contrast, the children are reportedly the highly effected group by dengue virus infection [23,24]. The high frequency of cases in the age group of 16 to 30 years in this study was due to larger population size in that age category.

Identification of diagnostic markers to predict the DHF during dengue infection is important for disease management. The clinical symptoms are helpful in diagnosing the DHF according to the WHO criteria [25]. In the current study, different clinical features and hematological abnormalities which were significantly different (p<0.05) in both DF and DHF include abdominal pain, nausea, rash, cold/clammy skin, periorbital puffiness, epistaxis, gingivitis, melena, hematemesis, hematuria, splenomegaly and hepatomegaly. While all of these features were also presented by DF patients, the clinical significance of these abnormalities in predicting the disease severity is restricted. However combination of these rare symptoms could be used as predictors of DHF [21,25]. Periorbital puffiness, referred to swelling of the orbits due to fluid buildup around the eyes is a new observation in this study, associated significantly with DHF. However further research is required to determine the clinical significance of this sign in determining disease severity.

Most patients in this study had thrombocytopenia, leucopenia, elevated liver enzymes and hematological abnormalities. The ALT levels were up to 2.7 times higher than normal in DHF patients 74.2% (p = 0.032) while AST levels were raised up to 10 times than normal in all DHF patients; which indicates their significance in predicting the disease severity. The liver injury is very common in Dengue virus infection, which is being mediated by the infection

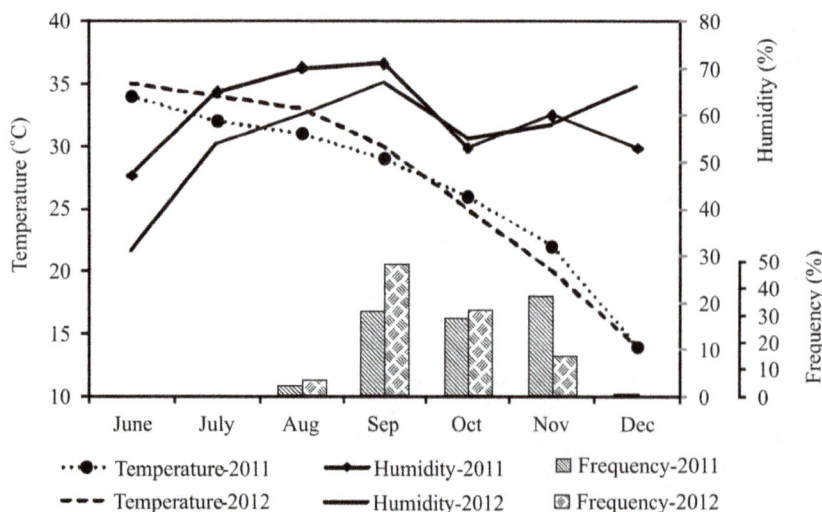

Figure 3. Effect of humidity and temperature on the frequency of dengue cases. Solid and dotted lines represents humidity and temperature respectively, whereas vertical bars represents frequency of dengue cases during the months of July to December.

of hepatocytes and Kupffer cells by the virus [26,27]. Likewise the use of ALT and AST levels are suggested recently for evaluating the severity of dengue virus infection. Different studies have reported the prediction of disease severity using the AST and ALT levels [21,28] other than that, Splenomegaly was significantly ($p<0.05$) higher in DHF patients. Dengue virus replicates predominantly in spleen, thymus and lymph nodes, resulting in lymphadenopathy and splenomegaly in DHF. Splenic rupture may occur as a more sever complication of splenomegaly [28]. Amazingly hematocrit, an indicator of capillary leakage was higher in DF (42.05 ± 8.25) than DHF (36 ± 17.8) patients, the phenomenon might be contributed by overt/occult bleed [11].

Preexisting co-morbidities in dengue infection are considered to be risk factor for the development of severe dengue fever (DHF) [29]. Moreover, higher case fatalities were significantly associated with co-morbidities [30]. The odds to develop severe dengue fever (DHF/DSS), in the present study, were significantly higher (OR 2.05, 95% CI 1.2 to 3.4, $p = 0.005$) in patients with co-morbidities as compared to dengue infection alone. Previously diabetes, hypertension and allergies were shown to be associated with sever manifestations of dengue fever [29,30,31], however there is scarcity of the data available on this topic, especially with hepatitis C virus or malarial parasite co-infection. HCV co-infection significantly contributed in the severity of the dengue infection.

Odds to develop severe dengue fever was significantly higher (OR 2.1, 95% CI 1.1 to 4.1, p 0.02) in patients with HCV co-infection than in dengue infection alone. However, these results cannot be generalized due to limited sample size and further studies are warranted to confirm the outcome of dengue infection in multiple co-morbidities.

Conclusions

Demographic, clinical and laboratory features of dengue cases studied could be used for the early diagnosis and treatment of the patients at risk of severe dengue fever. Abdominal pain, nausea, rash, cold/clammy skin, periorbital puffiness, elevated liver enzymes and visceromegaly could be used as predictors of DHF. The areas spotted in this study from which dengue cases reported more frequently, could be focused by policy makers, educationists and health professionals for the control of dengue fever in the city. Co-morbidities in dengue infection are considered to be risk factors for DHF.

Author Contributions

Conceived and designed the experiments: FAR SR. Performed the experiments: FAR JA SA MI. Analyzed the data: FAR RK SH. Wrote the paper: FAR SR RK JA SA MI SH.

References

1. Gubler DJ (2002) Epidemic dengue/dengue hemorrhagic fever as a public health, social and economic problem in the 21st century. Trends in microbiology 10: 100–103.
2. Laughlin CA, Morens DM, Cassetti MC, Costero-Saint Denis A, San Martin JL, et al. (2012) Dengue research opportunities in the Americas. J Infect Dis 206: 1121–1127.
3. Anonymous (2003) Country Report Pakistan. Vector-borne diseases in Pakistan. In: Inter-country workshop on developing a regional strategy for integrated vector management for malaria and other vector-borne diseases. Islamabad: Directorate of Malaria Control, Government of Pakistan; 21e23 January 2003. Khartoum, Sudan.
4. Nishtar S, Boerma T, Amjad S, Alam AY, Khalid F, et al. (2013) Pakistan's health system: performance and prospects after the 18th Constitutional Amendment. Lancet 381: 2193–2206.
5. Barraud PJ (1934) The fauna of British India, including Ceylon and Burma. Diptera. Family Culicidae. Tribe Megarhinini and Culicinae. London: Taylor and Francis.
6. Rasheed SB, Butlin RK, Boots M (2013) A review of dengue as an emerging disease in Pakistan. Public Health 127: 11–17.
7. Jamil B, Hasan R, Zafar A, Bewley K, Chamberlain J, et al. (2007) Dengue virus serotype 3, Karachi, Pakistan. Emerg Infect Dis 13: 182–183.
8. Khan E, Hasan R, Mehraj V, Nasir A, Siddiqui J, et al. (2008) Co-circulations of two genotypes of dengue virus in 2006 out-break of dengue hemorrhagic fever in Karachi, Pakistan. J Clin Virol 43: 176–179.
9. Akram DS, Igarashi A, Takasu T (1998) Dengue virus infection among children with undifferentiated fever in Karachi. Indian J Pediatr 65: 735–740.
10. World-Gazetteer. Faisalabad population data. Available: http://world-gazetteer.com. Accessed 2013 May 28.
11. World Health Organization. Dengue: guidelines for diagnosis, treatment, prevention and control-New edition. 2009: 1–147. Available: http://www.who.int/rpc/guidelines/9789241547871/en/. Accessed 2013 May 28.
12. Bhatty S, Shaikh NA, Fatima M, Sumbhuani AK (2009) Acute acalculous cholecystitis in dengue fever. J Pak Med Assoc 59: 519–521.
13. Descloux E, Mangeas M, Menkes CE, Lengaigne M, Leroy A, et al. (2012) Climate-based models for understanding and forecasting dengue epidemics. PLoS Negl Trop Dis 6: e1470.
14. Anker M, Arima Y (2011) Male-female differences in the number of reported incident dengue fever cases in six Asian countries. Western Pacific Surveillance and Response Journal 2: 17–23.
15. Shekhar KC, Huat OL (1992) Epidemiology of dengue/dengue hemorrhagic fever in Malaysia–a retrospective epidemiological study. 1973–1987. Part II: Dengue fever (DF). Asia Pac J Public Health 6: 126–133.
16. Ooi EE, Goh KT, Gubler DJ (2006) Dengue prevention and 35 years of vector control in Singapore. Emerg Infect Dis 12: 887–893.
17. Yew YW, Ye T, Ang LW, Ng LC, Yap G, et al. (2009) Seroepidemiology of dengue virus infection among adults in Singapore. Ann Acad Med Singapore 38: 667–675.
18. Trravassos da Rosa AP, Vasconcelos PF, Travassos Da Rosa ES, Rodrigues SG, Mondet B, et al. (2000) Dengue epidemic in Belem, Para, Brazil, 1996–97. Emerg Infect Dis 6: 298–301.
19. Garcia-Rivera EJ, Rigau-Perez JG (2003) Dengue severity in the elderly in Puerto Rico. Rev Panam Salud Publica 13: 362–368.
20. Gunther J, Ramirez-Palacio LR, Perez-Ishiwara DG, Salas-Benito JS (2009) Distribution of dengue cases in the state of Oaxaca, Mexico, during the period 2004–2006. J Clin Virol 45: 218–222.
21. Khan E, Kisat M, Khan N, Nasir A, Ayub S, et al. (2010) Demographic and clinical features of dengue fever in Pakistan from 2003–2007: a retrospective cross-sectional study. PLoS One 5: e12505.
22. Seneviratne SL, Malavige GN, de Silva HJ (2006) Pathogenesis of liver involvement during dengue viral infections. Trans R Soc Trop Med Hyg 100: 608–614.
23. Hammond SN, Balmaseda A, Perez L, Tellez Y, Saborio SI, et al. (2005) Differences in dengue severity in infants, children, and adults in a 3-year hospital-based study in Nicaragua. Am J Trop Med Hyg 73: 1063–1070;
24. Guzman MG, Kouri G, Bravo J, Valdes L, Vazquez S, et al. (2002) Effect of age on outcome of secondary dengue 2 infections. Int J Infect Dis 6: 118–124.).
25. Carlos CC, Oishi K, Cinco MT, Mapua CA, Inoue S, et al. (2005) Comparison of clinical features and hematologic abnormalities between dengue fever and dengue hemorrhagic fever among children in the Philippines. Am J Trop Med Hyg 73: 435–440.
26. Murgue B, Deparis X, Chungue E, Cassar O, Roche C (1999) Dengue: an evaluation of dengue severity in French Polynesia based on an analysis of 403 laboratory-confirmed cases. Trop Med Int Health 4: 765–773.
27. de Souza LJ, Nogueira RM, Soares LC, Soares CE, Ribas BF, et al. (2007) The impact of dengue on liver function as evaluated by aminotransferase levels. Braz J Infect Dis 11: 407–410.
28. Gulati S, Maheshwari A (2007) Atypical manifestations of dengue. Trop Med Int Health 12: 1087–1095.
29. Pang J, Salim A, Lee VJ, Hibberd ML, Chia KS, et al. (2012) Diabetes with hypertension as risk factors for adult dengue hemorrhagic fever in a predominantly dengue serotype 2 epidemic: a case control study. PLoS Negl Trop Dis 6(5): e1641.
30. Thein T-L, Leo Y-S, Fisher DA, Low JG, Oh HML, et al. (2013) Risk Factors for Fatality among Confirmed Adult Dengue Inpatients in Singapore:A Matched Case-Control Study. PLoS ONE 8(11): e81060.
31. Figueiredo MAA, Rodrigues LC, Barreto ML, Lima JWO, Costa MCN, et al. (2010) Allergies and Diabetes as Risk Factors for Dengue Hemorrhagic Fever: Results of a Case Control Study. PLoS Negl Trop Dis 4(6): e699.

4

Spatial and Temporal Patterns of Locally-Acquired Dengue Transmission in Northern Queensland, Australia, 1993–2012

Suchithra Naish[1]*, Pat Dale[2], John S. Mackenzie[3], John McBride[4], Kerrie Mengersen[5], Shilu Tong[1]

1 School of Public Health and Social Work & Institute of Health and Biomedical Innovation, Queensland University of Technology, Kelvin Grove campus, Brisbane, Queensland, Australia, **2** Environmental Futures Centre, Australian Rivers Institute, Griffith School of Environment Griffith University, Brisbane, Queensland, Australia, **3** Australian Biosecurity CRC and Faculty of Health Sciences, Curtin University, Perth, Western Australia, Australia, **4** School of Medicine and Dentistry, James Cook University, Cairns, Queensland, Australia, **5** Mathematical Sciences, Queensland University of Technology, Gardens Point campus, Brisbane, Queensland, Australia

Abstract

Background: Dengue has been a major public health concern in Australia since it re-emerged in Queensland in 1992–1993. We explored spatio-temporal characteristics of locally-acquired dengue cases in northern tropical Queensland, Australia during the period 1993–2012.

Methods: Locally-acquired notified cases of dengue were collected for northern tropical Queensland from 1993 to 2012. Descriptive spatial and temporal analyses were conducted using geographic information system tools and geostatistical techniques.

Results: 2,398 locally-acquired dengue cases were recorded in northern tropical Queensland during the study period. The areas affected by the dengue cases exhibited spatial and temporal variation over the study period. Notified cases of dengue occurred more frequently in autumn. Mapping of dengue by statistical local areas (census units) reveals the presence of substantial spatio-temporal variation over time and place. Statistically significant differences in dengue incidence rates among males and females (with more cases in females) ($\chi^2 = 15.17$, d.f. = 1, p<0.01). Differences were observed among age groups, but these were not statistically significant. There was a significant positive spatial autocorrelation of dengue incidence for the four sub-periods, with the Moran's *I* statistic ranging from 0.011 to 0.463 (p<0.01). Semi-variogram analysis and smoothed maps created from interpolation techniques indicate that the pattern of spatial autocorrelation was not homogeneous across the northern Queensland.

Conclusions: Tropical areas are potential high-risk areas for mosquito-borne diseases such as dengue. This study demonstrated that the locally-acquired dengue cases have exhibited a spatial and temporal variation over the past twenty years in northern tropical Queensland, Australia. Therefore, this study provides an impetus for further investigation of clusters and risk factors in these high-risk areas.

Editor: Yury E. Khudyakov, Centers for Disease Control and Prevention, United States of America

Funding: Authors would like to acknowledge ARC grant (#DP 110 100 651). The funders had no role in study design, data collection and analysis, decision to publish, or preparation of the manuscript.

Competing Interests: The authors have declared that no competing interests exist.

* E-mail: s.naish@qut.edu.au

Introduction

Dengue is emerging and resurging as a worldwide public health problem since the 1950s, affecting more than 110 countries today, and is a leading cause of hospitalisation and morbidity among children in the tropics and subtropics [1]. It is a mosquito-borne viral disease caused by one of four dengue viruses transmitted by *Aedes* mosquitoes. Currently mosquito control is the only available mitigation strategy but *Wolbachia* and the genetic manipulation of mosquitoes to lead to male sterility, may change this in the intermediate future. *Aedes aegypti* is the most common dengue-transmitting mosquito in the state of Queensland in Australia. *Aedes albopictus* (Asian tiger mosquito) another mosquito able to transmit dengue is currently threatening the Australian mainland

having been detected on a number of Torres Strait islands [2]. *Ae. aegypti* typically breeds in human-made container habitats such as water storage jars in and around human settlements including those in dense urban areas [3]. *Ae. albopictus* breeds in the same containers as *Ae. aegypti* but also breeds in natural containers in the bush such as tree holes, cut bamboo, banana trees and coconut shells. However, both these mosquitoes breed in fresh waters, but not in swamps or creeks. The recent arrival of the exotic species *Ae. albopictus* is of great concern because, if *Ae. albopictus* colonises the mainland, it could extend to the southern states due to its tolerance of more temperate conditions [2].

In Australia, dengue re-emerged in north Queensland during 1992–1993, after disappearing for about 10 years, i.e., 1981–1991 [4]. Since then, outbreaks and epidemics of dengue, with locally-acquired cases, were reported in Cairns and Port Douglas [4]. These are located in the north-east (urban tropical) coastal regions in Queensland. From January 1993 to June 2012, a total of 2,398 locally-acquired cases were documented in Queensland by Queensland Health. Outbreaks of dengue occur primarily in areas where *Ae. aegypti* mosquitoes are found. Dengue viruses may be introduced into areas by travellers who become infected while visiting other areas of the tropics where dengue commonly exists [5].

Most mosquito-borne diseases exhibit spatial and temporal variations in their distribution [6]. Spatial analyses using geostatistics such as spatial autocorrelations, variograms, interpolations, and temporal analyses using chi-squared statistics and time series models are commonly applied to highlight patterns of disease incidence [7,8].

Geographic information systems (GIS) play an important role in disease surveillance and control of the mosquito-borne diseases as they assist in the analysis of potential risk factors associated with the disease through the geo-coding processes [8] and facilitate maps that are useful for the identification of spatially and temporally localised areas of potential high-risk populations [7–11]. The visualised information represented in different types of maps based on GIS enables simultaneous observation of both the attribute and geographical relationships [12–14]. Maps also help policy decision-makers and public health officials to communicate with the public and policy decision-makers about complex information in an easily interpretable format [15,16].

GIS can provide not only an opportunity to improve our understanding of the distribution patterns of dengue, but can also provide an environmentally and socially informed platform to develop the elements of an early warning system towards control and prevention of dengue [8]. The advancement of geographical information systems (GIS) and spatial statistics has greatly improved the understanding of dengue dynamics, including its dependence on ecological factors. Hence, in this study, we examined the spatial and temporal patterns of locally-acquired dengue transmission in northern Queensland, Australia using GIS tools and geostatistical techniques.

Methods

Study area

Queensland is the third largest state by population size in Australia (after New South Wales and Victoria), occupying a total area of 1,723,936 km^2 with a total population of 4.56 million people (20% of Australia's total population) and is the fastest growing state with 23.9% of population growth in Australia to June 2012 [17]. Northern Queensland, a tropical region which is 100 km north of the Tropic of Capricorn (Figure 1) is selected as the study area as it had the largest total number of recorded notifications (n = 2,273) in Queensland, and the largest compared any other Australian state and territory, during the period 2005–2012 [18]. Northern Queensland has a tropical climate, with average temperatures in summer ranging from 24–33 degrees Celsius, and in winter 14–26.

Data collection

Dengue data. Dengue is a notifiable disease and all positive cases are required to be reported by laboratories to the state government (Queensland Health), by the Public Health Act 2005. These records are archived by the Data Custodians, Communicable Disease Branch (CDB) unit in Queensland Health under the National Notifiable Disease Surveillance System (NNDSS). The NNDSS was established in 1990 under the auspices of the Communicable Diseases Network Australia. Vector-borne diseases notified to the NNDSS include mosquito-borne diseases caused by alphaviruses, such as Ross River virus (RRV), Barmah Forest virus (BFV) and the flavivirus, Dengue.

In Australia, dengue outbreaks are a combination of locally-acquired and overseas- or imported-cases. According to government of Queensland Health, a dengue outbreak is declared when there is one or more locally-acquired dengue cases are confirmed. An overseas- or imported-case is defined as someone who is infected with dengue overseas (i.e., viraemic traveller) and arrives Australia with the virus in their blood [19]. A locally-acquired case is defined as when a local dengue mosquito bites this overseas dengue infected person and it passes the virus on to other people by biting them [19].

We obtained computerised and anonymous notification data (data that does not contain any identifiers such as name, street and house number or Medicare number or other medical insurance number) on locally-acquired dengue cases from January 1993 to June 2012 (approximately 20 years) for the study area from the CDB, Queensland Health. Dengue data included date of notification, age group (e.g., <1, 1–4, 5–9, 10–14 etc.), gender, post code of residence and statistical local area (SLA) (census unit) name. SLA is an Australian Standard Geographical Classification (ASGC) defined area which consists of one or more collection districts (the smallest geographical unit) in Australian census. Therefore, we have analysed the data based on age group.

Population data. Population data for the SLAs for the national census years 2001, 2006 and 2011 were obtained from the Australian Bureau of Statistics. For the remaining years during 1993 to 2012, the annual population data were estimated based on linear interpolation. We have adjusted SLA boundaries to match earlier censuses.

The study was approved by the Data Custodians, Human Research Ethics Committee under Chapter 6, Part 4, Section 280 of the Public Health Act 2005, CDB of Queensland Health and following the ethical considerations of the Research Ethics Unit, Queensland University of Technology (Number: 1100001110).

Statistical analyses

The study period was divided into four time periods, with five years in each time period for the ease of the analysis and to visualise the spatial and temporal patterns more clearly and precisely: Period 1: 1993–1997, Period 2: 1998–2002, Period 3: 2003–2007 and Period 4: 2008–2012. Population data for each period were attached to each SLA in the maps and these were used as the denominator in the computation of incidence rates. Period-wise distribution maps were produced on dengue cases and incidence rates by SLA. MapInfo Professional (version 11) incorporated with Vertical Mapper (version 3.7) was used to produce the final outputs as tables and maps.

Spatial and temporal analyses

To investigate the spatial and temporal patterns of dengue disease and to determine the risk of dengue disease, monthly incidence rates were calculated at both SLA and state levels. Incidence rates for each age group and gender were also calculated from the total number of dengue cases notified in each age group for each SLA in different time periods, divided by the respective total person-years and then multiplied by 100,000. These incidence rates were expressed as: total number of dengue cases/total population*100,000. Differences between age- and gender-specific incidence rates were tested using chi-square analyses (SPSS version 21).

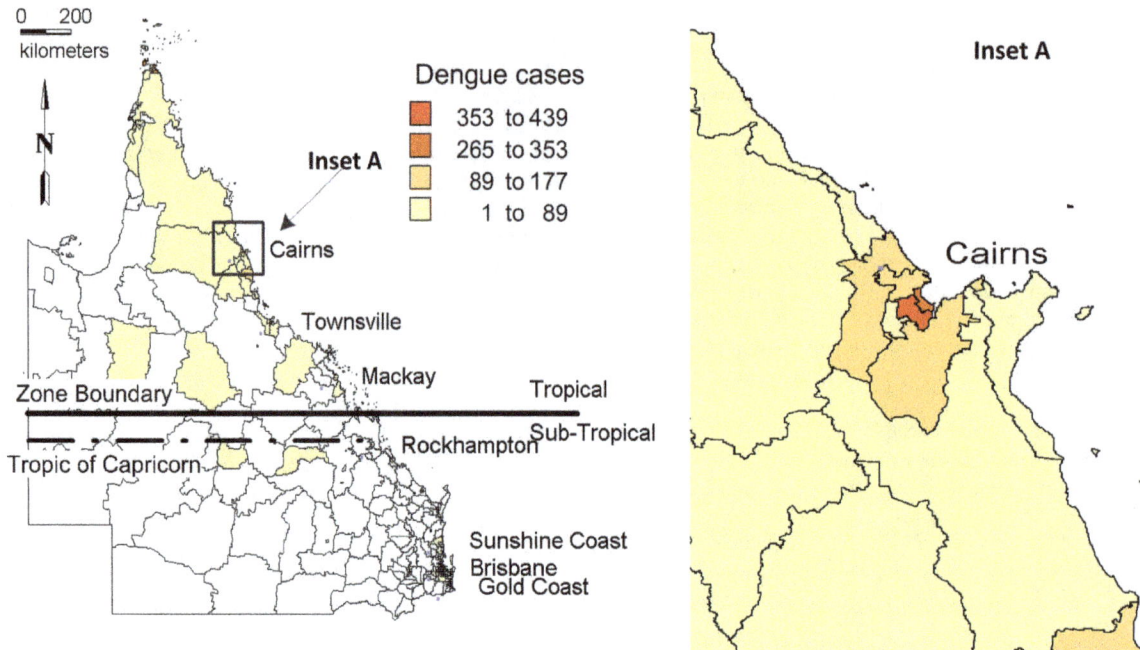

Figure 1. Study area showing the spatial distribution of dengue cases in northern Queensland, Australia, 1993–2012.

Age- and gender-standardised incidence rates (SIRs) were calculated for each SLA, using the direct method (based on Queensland population as a "reference"), adjusted for differences in the age and gender distribution. For example, dengue was high among the 25–29 year old age group so a SLA with a higher proportion of this age group would have a higher overall incidence rate of dengue. The equation for calculating SIR is:

$$SIR = \frac{\sum e_i}{\sum d_i^{(comparison)}} \text{ (expressed per 100,000 people)}$$

Where $\sum e_i$ is the total number of expected cases generated using the reference population rates for each SLA; $\sum d_i^{(comparison)}$ is the total population in the comparison group.

Further, the SIR estimates were mapped to identify the spatial differences. A significant difference between the observed and expected number of cases is indicated if the confidence interval (CI) does not contain zero. Differences between observed and expected number of cases for age and gender were tested using chi-square analyses.

Spatial analysis. We conducted spatial analysis comprising three components: 1) spatial autocorrelations, 2) semi-variogram models and 3) interpolations of SIR values (kriging).

Spatial autocorrelations. The global Moran's I test statistic was used to assess the presence of significant spatial autocorrelation of dengue overall incidence rates in each of the four time periods of 1993–1997, 1998–2002, 2003–2007 and 2008–2012. Moran's I ranges from -1 to 1: a value close to 0 indicates spatial randomness while a positive value indicates positive spatial autocorrelation, and a negative one indicates a negative autocorrelation, that is clustering of observations, and similarly a negative value indicates negative spatial autocorrelation, that is, repulsive behaviour between observations. Statistical significance was tested using randomisation based on 999 permutations [20]. The neighbourhood matrix used for the computation of spatial

autocorrelation statistics, was based on Queen contiguity and Euclidean distance [20].

Semi-variogram analysis. We used semi-variogram modelling analysis to explore the spatial structure and spatial autocorrelation of SIRs of dengue and age. The semi-variogram is a graphical representation of the variation among observations as the distance between the observations increases. If the variation, measured in terms of semi-variance, is distinctly small for low values of lag distance, it is considered as an indication of positive spatial autocorrelation, i.e., values at short distance from each other are more alike than those at larger distances. The best-fit semi-variogram model was identified by using Vertical Mapper within MapInfo Professional to identify the smallest differences in the model [21].

Kriging interpolation. Since the semi-variogram illustrates the spatial dependency between the observed measurements as a function of the distance between them, it allows us to estimate the SIR value of dengue at any point from the observed data. This interpolation was based on the best-fit semi-variogram using a kriging method [22–24] with inverse distance weighting [25]. Inverse distance weighting interpolation has been employed in other analyses of mosquito-borne diseases [26–28]. The kriged SIR values were obtained using the interpolation method in Vertical Mapper within MapInfo Professional and mapped to better visualise the distribution of spatially related patches of dengue.

Temporal analysis. To examine temporal patterns, epidemic curves were produced by calculating the annual incidence rate of dengue (annual dengue cases for each year divided by total population for each year * 100,000 people) and monthly cases of dengue during the period 1993–2012. Monthly differences between incidence rates for the study period were tested using Chi-square test. The statistical significance was set at <0.05.

Results

Descriptive statistics

Table 1 shows summary descriptive statistics for the dengue cases for the four time periods across SLAs in northern Queensland, Australia. Overall, the average number of dengue cases was 6.82 cases per year in northern Queensland. The SLAs notified with dengue cases varied over the four time periods. There were 13 SLAs with dengue cases (n = 34) in 1993–1997, 11 SLAs in 1998–2002 (n = 130 cases), 58 SLAs in 2003–2007 (n = 1042 cases) and 58 SLAs in 2008–2012 (n = 1192 cases). In all these periods, seasonal differences were observed between the dengue cases (Table 1). During 1998–2002 and 2008 to 2012, higher number of dengue cases (n = 86 and 773, respectively) were documented in summer whereas during 1993–1997 and 2003 to 2007, higher number of dengue cases (n = 29 and 625, respectively) were recorded in autumn.

Figure 2 shows the age- and gender-specific distribution of dengue incidence rates (per 100,000 people) during 1993–2012 for northern Queensland. The age and gender distributions are comparable with the last national population census data in 2011 [29]. The median age of the dengue cases was 44 years (range <1–80 above years). The incidence rate increased steadily with increasing age (children aged 5–9 years to those aged 50–54 years). Females in the younger (20–25 year) age groups had slightly higher incidence rates than males in the same age groups whereas in all other age groups males had slightly higher incidence rates compared with females. This difference was statistically significant (χ^2 = 15.17, d.f. = 1, p<0.01). Differences were observed among age groups, but these were not statistically significant.

Temporal analysis

Figure 3 displays the temporal epidemic patterns of dengue cases and incidence rates for four time periods in northern Queensland, including four major outbreaks in 2003, 2004, 2005 and 2009. The annual incidence rates fluctuated from 5.65 per 100,000 people (in 2000) to 82.84 per 100,000 people (in 2005).

The distribution of dengue cases and incidence rates was highly seasonally sensitive over the whole study period and in each of the four time periods. The incidence rates of dengue for the years 1993 to 2012 in northern Queensland indicates a strong seasonal pattern (χ^2 = 8.357, d.f. = 1, p<0.01), with a peak in Autumn (i.e., March) and reduction in Winter (i.e., August), with striking differences (Fig 4) among the four time periods. This supports the observed differences in cases in Table 1.

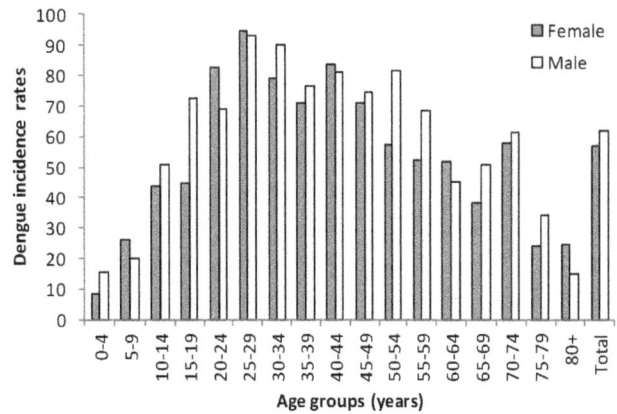

Figure 2. Dengue incidence rates by age and gender in northern Queensland, Australia, 1993–2012.

Spatial analysis

Figure 5 depicts the spatial patterns of dengue incidence rates in the four time periods during 1993–2012. Overall and in each period, the far north Queensland regions had the highest incidence rates: SLAs with highest incidence rates were Torres followed by Cairns City (central suburbs) for the years 2008 to 2012. Other relatively large incidence rates were reported in south Townsville and Cairns central suburbs. In all the time periods, incidence rates were high in Torres, Cairns City (central suburbs), Cairns - Mt Whitfield, South Townsville, Currajong, North Ward - Castle Hill, South Flinders and Rowes Bay - Belgian Gardens. Overall, dengue appears to have spread dramatically from Cairns regions to north Queensland regions during 1993–2012. In general, dengue occurred for 15 consecutive years from 1998 primarily in the same SLAs along the coastal northern Queensland regions and gradually expanded into newer SLAs, with the highest number of cases (n = 956) reported in 2009 during January to April.

Spatial autocorrelation. Table 2 shows the results of the calculation of global autocorrelation statistics for dengue cases for the four time periods in northern Queensland. The results of the global Moran's I tests for dengue incidence rates for all four periods are statistically significant and indicate spatial heterogeneity. There was an increase in spatial autocorrelation over the period 2003–2007, reaching the highest value during 2008–2012.

Standardised incidence rates. Standardised incidence rates (SIRs) of dengue for each SLA in northern Queensland over the the study period were calculated and mapped (Fig 6). Geograph-

Table 1. Descriptive statistics of dengue cases among SLAs in northern Queensland, Australia, 1993–2012.

Indicators	1993–1997	1998–2002	2003–2007	2008–2012	Total
No. of SLAs positive	13	11	58	58	140
Total cases in all SLAs	34	130	1042	1192	2398
In summer	3	86	233	773	1095
In autumn	29	43	625	350	1047
In winter	1	0	50	17	68
In spring	1	1	134	52	188

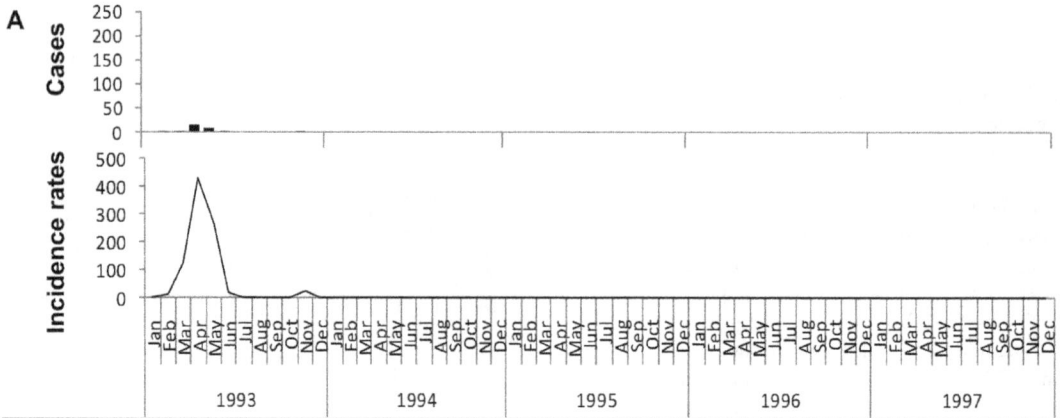

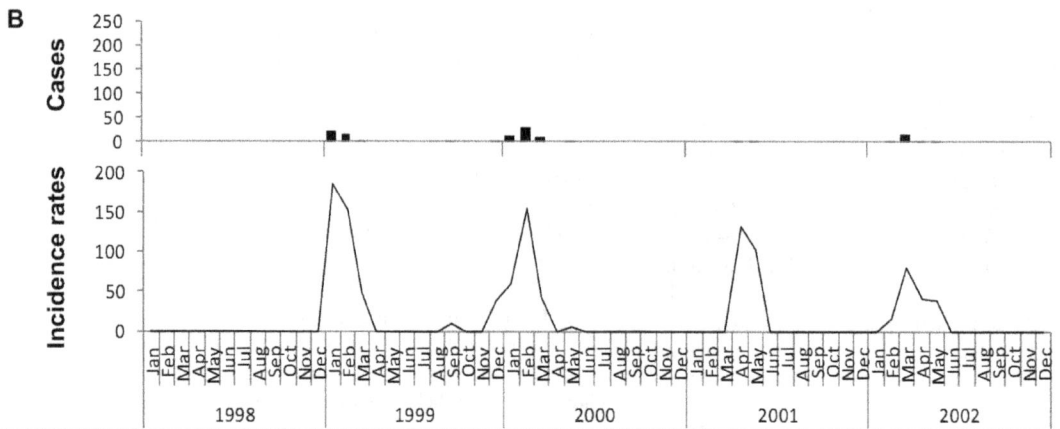

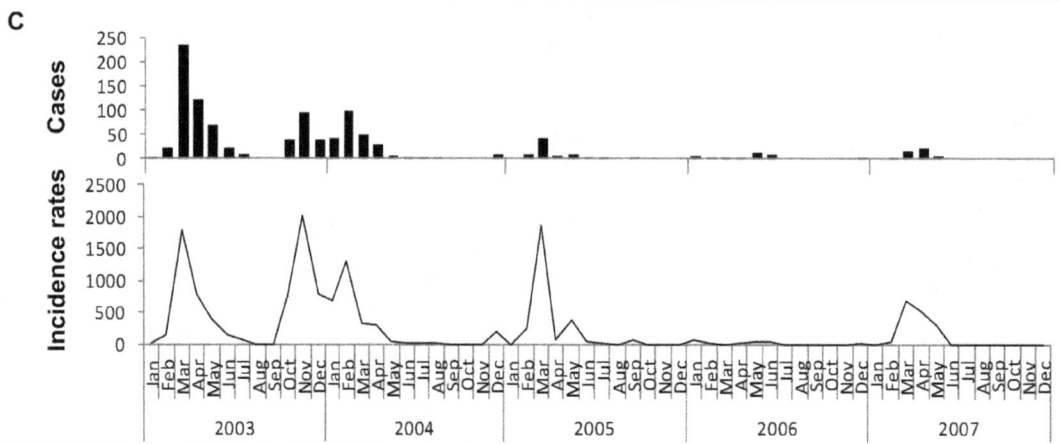

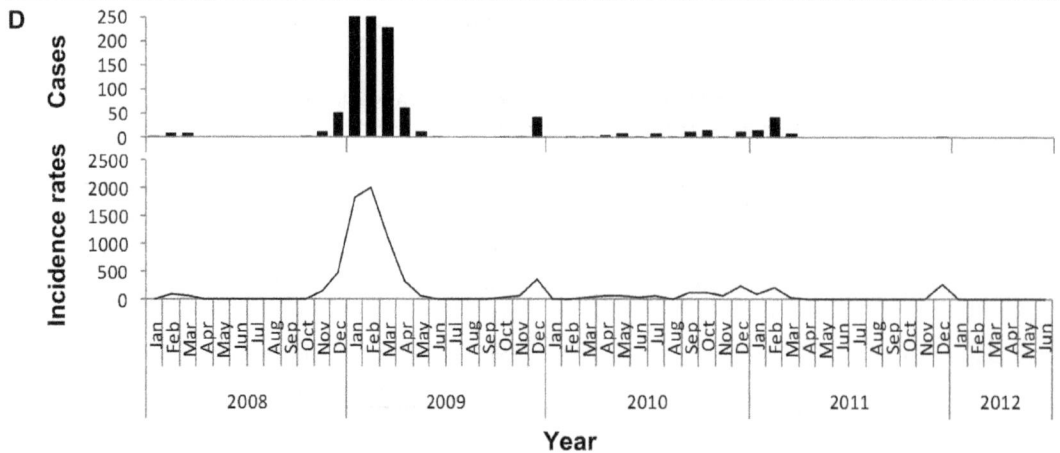

Year

Figure 3. Temporal distribution of dengue cases (depicting bar) and incidence rates (depicting line) for different time periods (A: 1993–1997, B: 1998–2002, C: 2003–2007 and D: 2008–2012).

ically, the largest SIRs were observed in the coastal areas; with the peak SIR of 180/100,000 for Cairns City (central suburbs) while the average SIR in northern Queensland was 2.06/100,000.

Semi-variogram analysis and kriging. Spatial dependence of dengue SIRs was evaluated using semi-variograms. A quadratic model was fitted to the semi-variogram using a sill and nugget of 400 and 0, respectively and a range of 5 degrees (Fig 7). This best-fit semi-variogram model was then used in the kriging procedure to map the SIRs. The map of the kriged SIR is shown in Figure 7. This provides visual confirmation that the pattern of SIRs of dengue disease is not homogeneous across the northern Queensland.

Discussion

This study reveals the spatial and temporal characteristics of dengue in northern Queensland using GIS tools and geostatistical analytical techniques. These methods have been applied to other vector-borne infectious diseases to study the distribution patterns of the disease, to identify the high-risk areas or hot spots, and to determine the risk factors for the transmission of the disease [26,30–35]. Locally-acquired dengue cases only occurred in northern Queensland where the vector was common and where the virus was commonly introduced by viraemic travellers [36]. Our results indicate that dengue incidence rates had an uneven spatial distribution in northern Queensland and thus the disease was spatially heterogeneous. In addition, the GIS maps clearly revealed spatial expansion of dengue transmission in northern Queensland over recent years (i.e., 2008–2012). For example,

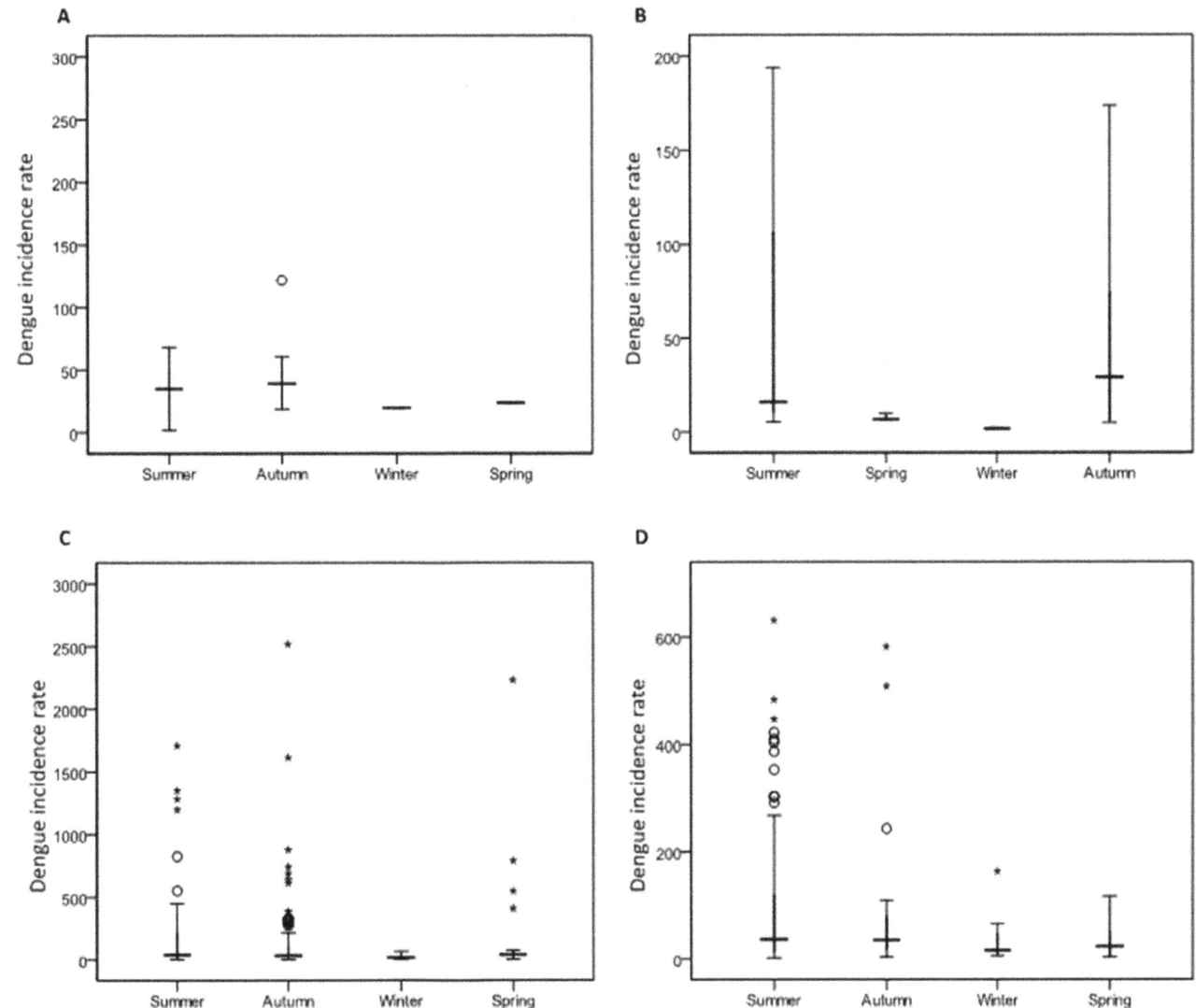

Figure 4. Box-plots showing the seasonal distribution of dengue cases for the different periods: A: 1993–1997, B: 1998–2002, C: 2003–2007 and D: 2008–2012.

A 1993-1997 Inset A

B 1998-2002 Inset A

C 2003-2007 Inset A

D 2008-2012 Inset A

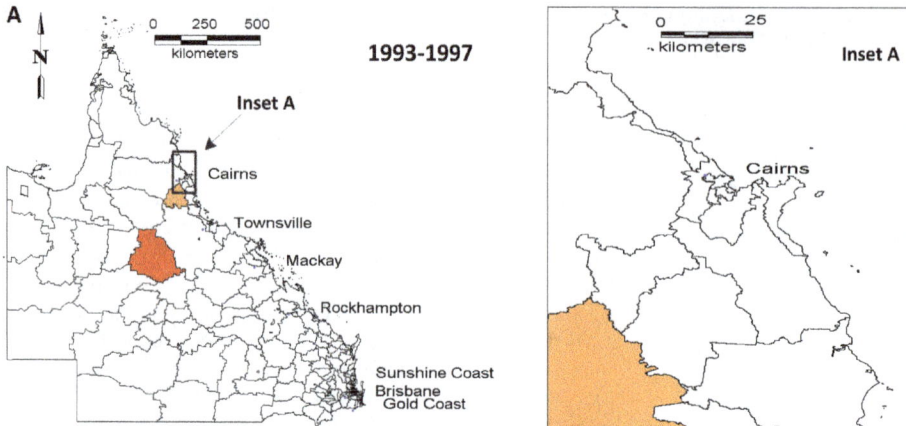

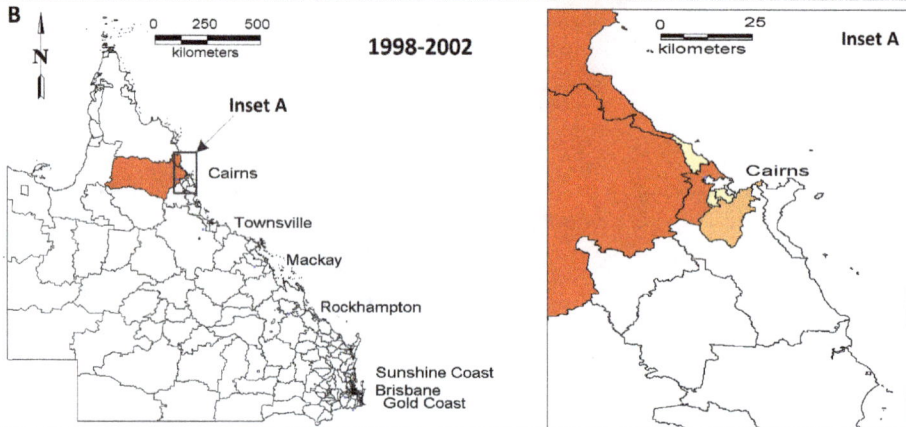

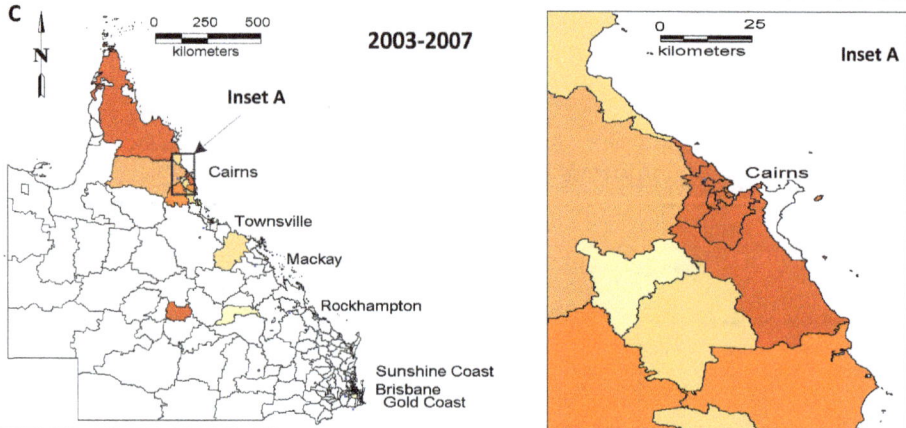

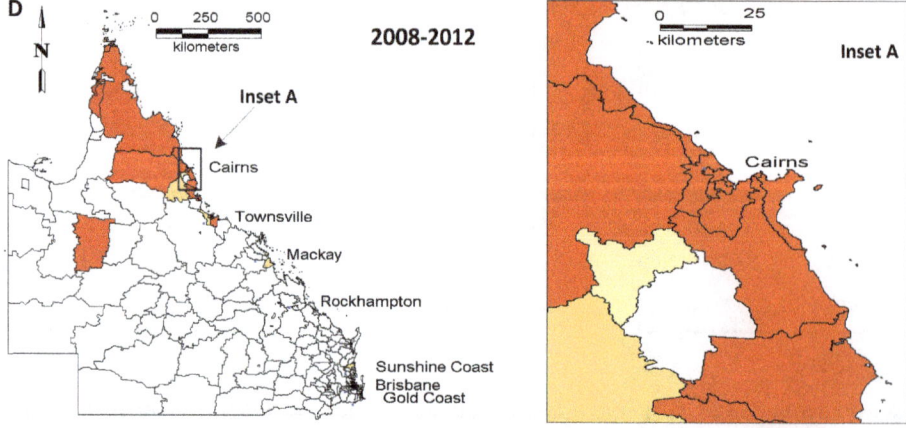

0.1 - 10   >10 - 20   >20 - 30   >30 - 40   >40 – 10,000

Figure 5. Maps showing the dengue incidence rates by SLA over different periods (A: 1993–1997, B: 1998–2002, C: 2003–2007 and D: 2008–2012).

dengue transmission has increasingly spread from Cairns regions to a wider area.

Temporally, significant differences were noticeable across different time periods in the study area. Our findings demonstrate that the annual incidence rates fluctuated considerably, with the two largest peaks in 2003 and 2009 (see Fig 2). It is important to understand the influence of annual seasons on transmission cycles. Our results also show that there has been an increasing trend in the incidence rates of dengue during the study period. The overall temporal pattern of dengue incidence in northern Queensland indicates two general peaks per annum: the first short peak in summer (i.e. extending for two months in November and December), and a second long peak in autumn (i.e. four months from January to April). These two peaks may be preceded by peaks of mosquito densities in December and May, following the normal typical wet season. Our findings strongly support previous studies that have suggested an increase in mosquito population in summer, with a lagged impact on the seasonal variation of dengue [37,38]. However, whether this corresponds to the peaks of tourists who might introduce the virus is still unknown.

The study results indicate that dengue outbreaks usually occur during the rainy season (i.e., November to April) in northern tropical Queensland, which generally has a lower temperature by a few degrees and higher humidity than during the hot dry season. These small environmental fluctuations may possibly increase the female mosquito longevity and survival, thus increase the likelihood of dengue transmission. Our findings strongly support previous studies that have reported a strong seasonal pattern of dengue [2,37,39].

The spatial and temporal differences may due partly to occurrence of epidemics due to introduced cases, mosquito distribution, local changes in climate and people's culture and behaviour towards personal protection, human adaptation to forecasted drought (e.g., water storage facilities) and housing conditions and life-style activities [2,40] and partly to local vector control programs such as dengue mosquito management plan and dengue alert response team activities [4]. Thus, further research is needed to investigate the social mobilisation, entomological surveillance, vector biology, dengue viruses, local people's behaviour and the local climatic factors on the transmission of dengue in the northern Queensland region.

In this study, locally-transmitted dengue was reported in a small number of SLAs across the study area. The study results reveal that quite a few numbers of SLAs had the highest incidence rates and SIRs (see Figs 4 & 7). This may be due to the several conditions that favour vector, density, distribution, survival and longevity [2,39,41]. A combination of flooding and heavy rainfall

Table 2. Moran's *I* values for the dengue incidence rates in northern Queensland, Australia, 1993–2012.

Period	Moran's *I* value	p-value
1993–1997	0.0116	0.03
1998–2002	0.0019	0.001
2003–2007	0.1362	0.001
2008–2012	0.4639	0.001

has resulted in dengue epidemics across Australia [2,4,40]. In addition, local factors such as the climate and socio-ecological conditions may be more suitable for the local mosquitoes and thus the transmission of dengue. Therefore, it is evident that further studies on the environmental and socio-ecological factors on dengue mosquitoes and dengue virus would assist in identifying the reasons behind this phenomenal variation.

In this study, dengue incidence occurred in all age groups, but was highest among males and females of age group 25–29 (see Fig 3). The reasons for the differences in incidence rates among age and gender groups are unknown, but may include different exposure rates or other behavioural risk factors such as increased internal (domestic) travel, immigration, work and leisure related activities [29], however, this kind of information is unavailable in this study. The possible reasons could be increased levels of time spent outdoors for recreation (e.g., fishing and walking) and leisure (e.g., sport and exercise) activities and internal (within the state) travel due to work and family commitments. Clearly, the relationships between the incidence rate of dengue, age and gender needs to be understood in order to better manage and reduce incidence spikes in certain age groups.

Epidemiologists normally use the ratio of case numbers at a particular time to past case occurrences using the mean or median [42]. However, since dengue cases vary from one place to another, the spatial and temporal component must also be taken into consideration. In disease surveillance and public health surveys, spatial and temporal patterns are one of the most important components influencing the distribution of diseases. Although spatial analytical techniques rarely provide reasons for the occurrences of spatial patterns, they do identify the geographical locations of the occurrence of spatial pattern. Within this realm, it provides a useful means to hypothesise about factors that may influence health outcomes or to identify spatial issues that need to be further investigated [43]. The evaluation of spatial distributions as a measure of disease risk may provide etiological insights [44]. Regular time series models are difficult to fit to our data, given the epidemic and irregular seasonal patterns of dengue incidence. Thus, we haven't pursued these models in this study.

In this study, the global Moran's *I* statistic is used to measure the degree of spatial autocorrelation and map the geographic patterns of the areal units. To appropriately use dengue notification data aggregated according to SLAs, it is important to choose the spatial autocorrelation technique for the specification of local neighbourhoods. This is defined by the spatial weights matrix. In general, the spatial autocorrelation may be the strongest between the nearest neighbours. As the neighbourhoods increase in number, this autocorrelation weakens. However, a recognised guide for choosing a proper spatial weight matrix has not yet been developed. In this study, an appropriate spatial weight matrix was chosen after a comparison of the connectivity distributions of neighbours obtained with the distance-based contiguity and the first order Queen's contiguity methods [20].

Spatial autocorrelation and semi-variogram analysis are valuable tools to study spatial patterns over time. The semi-variogram estimators used in this paper directly account for population size, attenuating the influence of less reliable rates recorded in sparsely populated areas. Maps created from kriging interpolation revealed that dengue was spatially and temporally distributed. Further studies of local environmental and socio-environmental factors that operate at fine spatial scales are crucial for improving the

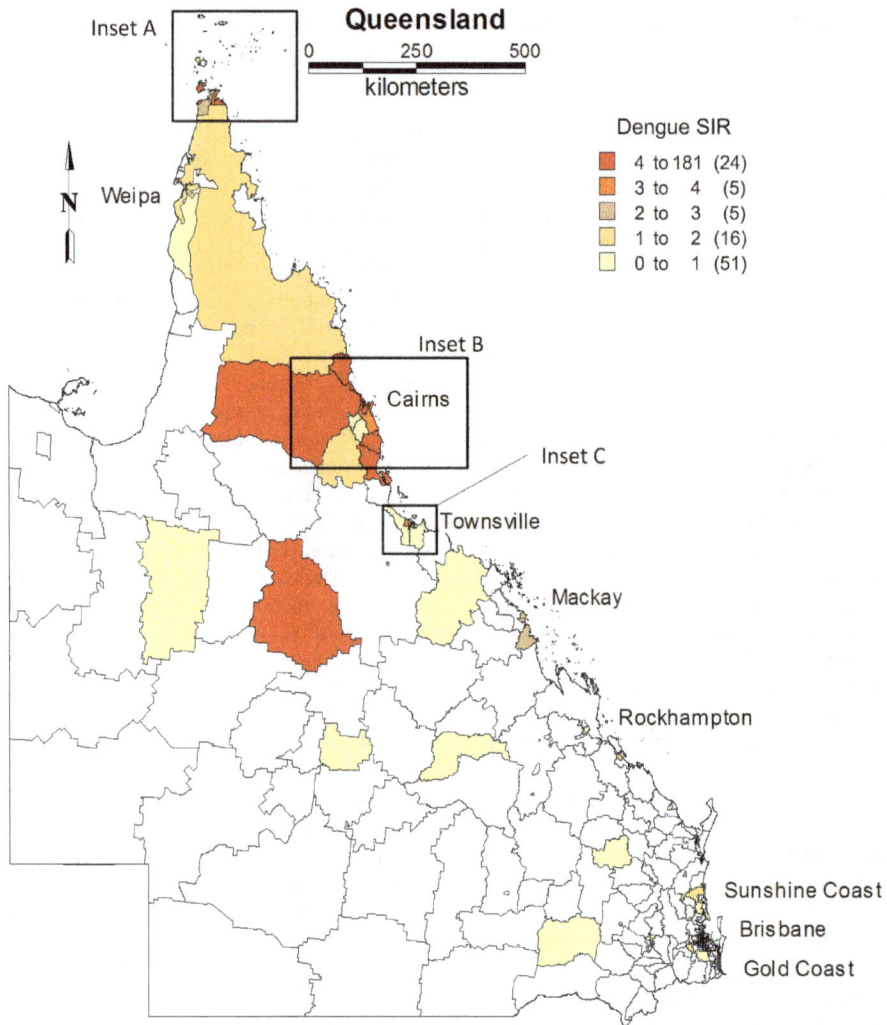

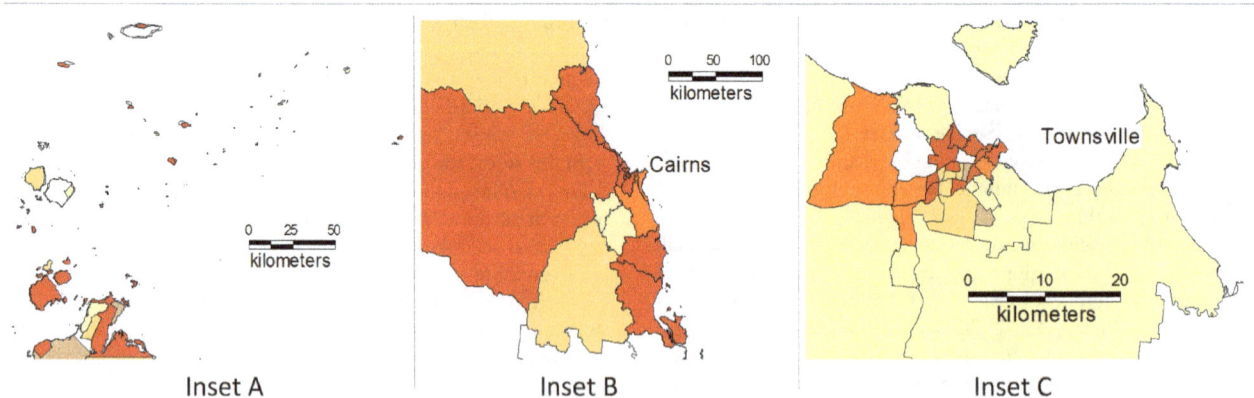

Figure 6. Map showing the standardised incidence rates of dengue by SLA in northern Queensland, Australia, 1993–2012.

understanding of the spatial and temporal patterns of dengue. Moreover, further investigation is warranted to understand the effect of climatic and topographic factors on dengue local transmission in the study area.

Vector-borne infectious diseases such as dengue present complex and dynamic transmission patterns, which include vector related factors such as type, density, distribution, breeding places and human related factors such as population density, behaviour and immunity, and virus related factors such as circulating multiple virus serotypes DENV 1 to DENV 4, and environmental factors such as temperature and rainfall [1,11,45]. Several dengue outbreaks by different serotypes may occur in the same population, and there is a large range of factors in intra-urban areas which may favour the maintenance of potential breeding sites of mosquitoes.

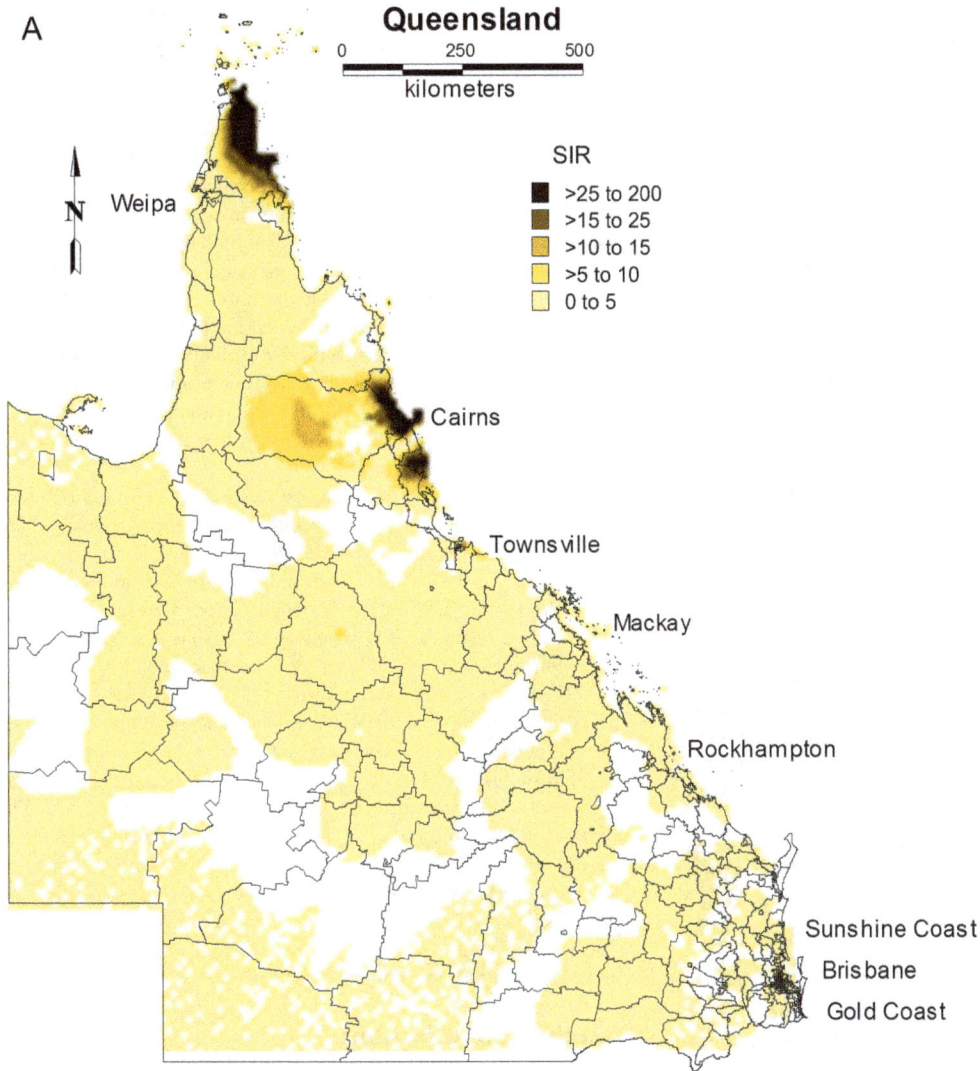

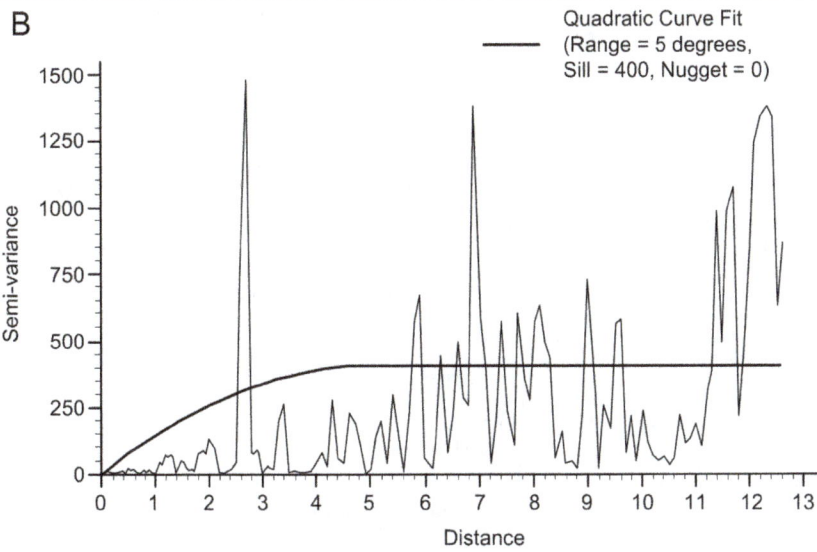

Figure 7. The smoothed map of standardised incidence rates of dengue using kriging (Panel A) and a semi-variogram model (Panel B).

We acknowledge that there could be issues in monitoring and reporting dengue locally-acquired notification data. For this study, the clinically proven cases on dengue were provided by Queensland Department of Health. Dengue is one of the notifiable diseases in Australia, and is required to be reported to the local health, by law. Data reliability issues for mosquito-borne diseases have previously been discussed by Russell [46]. Underreporting is also likely to occur when people infected with dengue do not seek medical attention. For example, it is likely that there was considerable underreporting in 1992 and 1993 but we have evidence to suggest that in more recent epidemics the publicly notified cases are not a gross underestimate of the total number of cases. Nevertheless, these issues cannot entirely account for the geographic distribution of dengue across northern Queensland.

This study has three major strengths. Firstly, this is the first study to examine the geographic variation of dengue across geo-political borders (i.e., SLAs) in northern Queensland using GIS tools and geostatistical techniques. This study is an impetus for future investigations on the spatial and temporal risk factor analysis of dengue including multiple factors on environmental, entomological, ecological and socio-demographic variables. Secondly, the results of this study demonstrate that GIS mapping techniques may be used as a tool to quickly display information and generate maps to highlight dengue risk-prone areas for developing strategies towards dengue management. The maps could be used by policy-decision makers to suggest particular geographical localities or communities where further investigation should be focused, to identify whether increased disease surveillance measures or possible control activities are warranted. Moreover, the corresponding statistical analyses can limit over-reaction or unwarranted action based on purely visual assessment, for example unsubstantiated identification of so-called 'clusters' of cases and putative source identification. Finally, dengue data used in this study are quite comprehensive, covering northern Queensland for approximately 20 years.

The study has also two key limitations. First, the quality of the dengue surveillance system may vary with place and time as the awareness of dengue among medical professionals and public may have increased over recent years. However, spatiotemporal variation of dengue infers that the dengue distribution is unlikely to be entirely accounted for by a detection/surveillance. Second, the exact place/location (i.e., residential address) where dengue cases were notified may vary from those where they were infected/

acquired (i.e., exact place/location), particularly during holiday periods. However, all the cases involved in this study were locally-acquired and were not imported.

The maps produced in this study would provide useful information to health authorities and could assist in focusing and implementing control and preventive activities to monitor and control the incidence of dengue precisely and effectively, especially in the event when there is no report on dengue cases. The study suggests that local surveillance teams should be vigilant at all times, particularly after the wet season, not only in the epidemic period, as dengue mosquitoes live with the human population. Furthermore, this study provides a new dimension to the health authorities in northern Queensland, specifically in the potential of using GIS applications to develop locally appropriate and eco-environmentally friendly strategies for the implementation of preventive and control activities, not only for dengue, but also for other vector-borne diseases in Queensland.

In conclusion, this study has revealed that the spatio-temporal patterns of dengue differ significantly in northern Queensland and the study has highlighted that there are different transmission patterns in SLAs between regions. This study has also concluded that the spatial distribution of dengue appears to have expanded over recent years. This is based on the results (see Tables 1 & 2) and on the observation that dengue has spread from Cairns regions to a wider area during 1993–2012. Autocorrelation function can be beneficial for public health officials or policy-developers to visualise and understand the distribution and trends of diffusion patterns of dengue and to prepare warnings over high-risk areas only rather than for a whole state or a whole region. This may save time and cost and make public health authorities efforts more efficient.

Future research should focus on the spectrum of dengue risk factors and the prediction of future dengue transmission which are necessary to improve the effectiveness and efficiency of dengue local prevention and control programs.

Author Contributions

Conceived and designed the experiments: SN. Performed the experiments: SN. Analyzed the data: SN. Contributed reagents/materials/analysis tools: SN. Wrote the paper: SN PD JM JMB KM ST. Wrote the manuscript, reviewed critically and accepted for publication: SN PD JM JMB KM ST.

References

1. WHO (2013) Dengue - Neglected tropical diseases research Available: http://www.who.int/tdr/research/ntd/dengue/en/index.html. Accessed 6 February, 2013.
2. Russell RCCB, Lindsay MD, Mackenzie JS, Ritchie SA, Whelan PI (2009) Dengue and climate change in Australia: predictions for the future should incorporate knowledge from the past. Med J Aust 190: 265–268.
3. Tsuzuki AVT, Higa Y, Nguyen TY, Takagi M (2009) Effect of peridomestic environments on repeated infestation by preadult Aedes aegypti in urban premises in Nha Trang City, Vietnam. Am J Trop Med Hyg 81: 645–650.
4. Queensland Health. (2013) Dengue fever. Available: http://www.health.qld.gov.au/dengue/outbreaks/current.asp. Accessed 20 January, 2013.
5. Schwartz E, Weld LH, Wilder-Smith A, von Sonnenburg F, Keystone JS, et al. (2008) Seasonality, annual trends, and characteristics of dengue among ill returned travelers, 1997–2006. Emerg Infect Dis 14: 1081–1088.
6. Lloyd CD, Atkinson PM (2009) Cartographic veracity in medieal mapping:analyzing geographic variation in the Gough map of Great Britain. Ann Asso Am Geo 99: 27–48.
7. Fotheringham AS, Rogerson PA, editors (2009) The Sage Handbook of Spatial Analysis. London: Sage Publications. 183–206 p.
8. Lloyd C (2010) Spatial data analysis - An introduction for GIS users. Oxford: Oxford University Press.
9. Collinge SK (2010) Spatial Ecology and Conservation. Nature 1: 69.
10. Haining R (2003) Spatial Data Analysis: Theory and Practice. Cambridge: Cambridge University Press.

11. Githeko AK (2012) Advances in developing a climate based dengue outbreak models in Dhaka, Bangladesh: Challenges & opportunities. Indian J Med Res 136: 7–9.
12. Cleveland WS (1993) Visualising data: Summit, N.J. Hobart Press.
13. Indaratna K, Hutubessy R, Chupraphawan S, Sukapurana C, Tao J, et al. (1998) Application of geographical information systems to co-analysis of disease and economic resources: dengue and malaria in Thailand. Southeast Asian J Trop Med Public Health 29: 669–684.
14. Keim DA (2002) Information visualization and visual data mining. IEEE Transaction on Visualization and Computer Graphics 7: 100–107.
15. Kitron U (2000) Risk maps: Transmission and burden of vector-borne diseases. Parasitoly Today 16: 324–325.
16. Rezaeian M (2008) How to Visualize Public Health Data? Part Two: Direct and Indirect Standardization Methods. Middle East Journal of Family Medicine 7: 42–44.
17. Queensland Treasury and Trade (2013) Population growth highlights and trends, Queensland. Available: http://www.oesr.qld.gov.au/products/publications/pop-growth-highlights-trends-qld/pop-growth-highlights-trends-qld-2013.pdf. Accessed 2013, 10 August.
18. National Notifiable Disease surveillance system N (2013) Number of notifications of dengue virus infection received from State and Territory health authorities in the period of 1991 to 2012 and year-to-date notifications for 2013. Department of Health and Ageing.

19. Queensland Health (2013) Mosquito-borne diseases. Available: www.health.qld. gov.au. Accessed 2013, 20 November.

20. Anselin L, Syabri I, Kho Y (2006) GeoDa: An introduction to spatial data analysis. Geographical Analysis 38: 5–22.

21. MapInfo Professional Software version 10.5.2. (2011) MapInfo Vertical Mapper, version 3.7, MapInfo Corporation

22. Fotheringham AS, Rogerson PA, editors (2009) The Sage Handbook of Spatial Analysis. London: Sage Publications. 183–206 p.

23. Lloyd CD, Shuttleworth IG (2005) Analysing commuting using local regression techniques: scale, sensitivity and geographical pattterning. Environment and Planning A: 81–103.

24. Longley PA, Goodchild MF, Maguire D, Rhind DW (1999) Geographical Information Systems New York: John Wiley & Sons.

25. Isaaks EH, Srivastava RM, editors (1989) An introduction to applied geostatistics. Oxford, United Kingdom: Oxford University Press. 249–277 p.

26. Naish S, Hu W, Mengersen K, Tong S (2011) Spatio-temporal patterns of Barmah Forest virus disease in Queensland, Australia. PLoS ONE 6: e25688.

27. Quinn HE, Gatton ML, Hall G, Young M, Ryan PA (2005) Analysis of Barmah forest virus disease activity in Queensland, Australia, 1993–2003: Identification of a large, isolated outbreak of disease. J Med Entomol 42: 882–890.

28. Woodruff RE, Guest CS, Garner MG, Becker N (2006) Early warning of Ross River virus epidemics: combining surveillance data on climate and mosquitoes. Epidemiology 17: 569–575.

29. ABS (2012) Census of Population and Housing - Basic community profiles, Commonwealth of Australia, Canberra, Australian Bureau of Statistics, ABS. Available: www.abs.com.au. Accessed 10 December, 2012.

30. Naish S, Hu W, Mengersen K, Tong S (2011) Spatial and temporal clusters of Barmah Forest virus disease in Queensland, Australia. Trop Med Int Health 16: 884–893.

31. Russell RC (1998) Vectors vs. humans in Australia-who is on top down under? An update on vector-borne disease and research on vectors in Australia. J Vector Ecol 23: 1–46.

32. Earnest A, Tan SB, Wilder-Smith A (2012) Meteorological factors and El Niño Southern Oscillation are independently associated with dengue infections. Epidemiology and Infection 140: 1244–1251.

33. Huang FZS, Zhang S, Zhang H, Li W (2011) Meteorological Factors-Based Spatio-Temporal Mapping and Predicting Malaria in Central China. Am J Trop Med Hyg 85: 560–567.

34. Impoinvil DE, Solomon T, Schluter WW, Rayamajhi A, Bichha RP, et al. (2011) The Spatial Heterogeneity between Japanese Encephalitis Incidence Distribution and Environmental Variables in Nepal. PLoS ONE 6: e22192.

35. Rochlin ITD, Gomez F, Ninivaggi DV, Campbell SR (2011) Predicitve mapping of human risk for West Nile Virus (WNV) based on environmentala dn socioeconomic factros. PLoS ONE 6: e23280.

36. Knope KGC (2013) Increasing notifications of dengue in Australia related to overseas travel, 1991 to 2012. Commun Dis Intell 37: E5–E7.

37. Hu W, Clements A, Williams G, Tong S (2010) Dengue fever and El Nino/ Southern Oscillation in Queensland, Australia: a time series predictive model. Occup Environ Med 67: 307–311.

38. Hu W, Clements A, Williams G, Tong S, Mengersen K (2012) Spatial patterns and socioecological drivers of dengue fever transmission in Queensland, Australia. Environ Health Perspect 120: 260–266.

39. Beebe NW, Cooper RD, Mottram P, Sweeney AW (2009) Australia's dengue risk driven by human adaptation to climate change. PLoS Negl Trop Dis 3: e429.

40. Williams CR, Bader CA, Kearney MR, Ritchie SA, Russell RC (2010) The Extinction of Dengue through Natural Vulnerability of Its Vector. PLoS Negl Trop Dis 4: e922.

41. Jansen CC, Beebe NW (2010) The dengue vector Aedes aegypti: what comes next. Microbes Infect 12: 272–279.

42. Nakhapakorn KJS (2006) Temporal and spatial autocorrelation statistics of dengue fever. Dengue Bull 30: 177–183.

43. Er ACRM, Asmahani A, Mohamad Naim MR, Harsuzilawati M (2010) Spatial mapping of dengue incidence: A case study in Hulu Langat District, Selangor, Malaysia. International Journal of Human and Social Sciences 5: 410–414.

44. Moore DA, Carpenter TE (1999) Spatial analytical methods and geographic information systems: use in health research and epidemiology. Epidemiologic Reviews 21 143–161.

45. WHO (2012) Global strategy for dengue prevention and control, 2012–2020. Available: Accessed 5 February, 2013.

46. Russell RC (1994) Ross River Virus: disease trends and vector ecology in Australia. Bulletin of Social and Vector Ecology 19: 73–81.

5

Fusion of Protegrin-1 and Plectasin to MAP30 Shows Significant Inhibition Activity against Dengue Virus Replication

Hussin A. Rothan[1]*, **Hirbod Bahrani**[1], **Zulqarnain Mohamed**[2], **Noorsaadah Abd Rahman**[3], **Rohana Yusof**[1]

1 Department of Molecular Medicine, Faculty of Medicine, University of Malaya, Kuala Lumpur, Malaysia, **2** Genetics and Molecular Biology Unit, Institute of Biological Science, Faculty of Science, University of Malaya, Kuala Lumpur, Malaysia, **3** Department of Chemistry, Faculty of Science, University of Malaya, Kuala Lumpur, Malaysia

Abstract

Dengue virus (DENV) broadly disseminates in tropical and sub-tropical countries and there are no vaccine or anti-dengue drugs available. DENV outbreaks cause serious economic burden due to infection complications that requires special medical care and hospitalization. This study presents a new strategy for inexpensive production of anti-DENV peptide-fusion protein to prevent and/or treat DENV infection. Antiviral cationic peptides protegrin-1 (PG1) and plectasin (PLSN) were fused with MAP30 protein to produce recombinant antiviral peptide-fusion protein (PG1-MAP30-PLSN) as inclusion bodies in *E. coli*. High yield production of PG1-MAP30-PLSN protein was achieved by solubilization of inclusion bodies in alkaline buffer followed by the application of appropriate refolding techniques. Antiviral PG1-MAP30-PLSN protein considerably inhibited DENV protease (NS2B-NS3pro) with half-maximal inhibitory concentration (IC_{50}) 0.5 ± 0.1 μM. The real-time proliferation assay (RTCA) and the end-point proliferation assay (MTT assay) showed that the maximal-nontoxic dose of the peptide-fusion protein against Vero cells is approximately 0.67 ± 0.2 μM. The cell-based assays showed considerable inhibition of the peptide-fusion protein against binding and proliferating stages of DENV2 into the target cells. The peptide-fusion protein protected DENV2-challeged mice with 100% of survival at the dose of 50 mg/kg. In conclusion, producing recombinant antiviral peptide-fusion protein by combining short antiviral peptide with a central protein owning similar activity could be useful to minimize the overall cost of short peptide production and take advantage of its synergistic antiviral activities.

Editor: Wenzhe Ho, Temple University School of Medicine, United States of America

Funding: This project was funded by the University of Malaya and Ministry of Science, Technology and Innovation (ERGS Grant ER016-2013A). The funders had no role in study design, data collection and analysis, decision to publish, or preparation of the manuscript.

Competing Interests: The authors have declared that no competing interests exist.

* E-mail: rothan@um.edu.my

Introduction

Dengue virus is a member of the *Flaviviridae* family, transmitted by the mosquito vector *Aedes aegypti* [1]. Dengue virus infects 50–100 million people worldwide each year and causes various clinical symptoms such as dengue fever (DF) that may later develop to severe dengue haemorrhagic fever (DHF), and dengue shock syndrome (DSS) [2–4]. Annually, there are approximately 0.5 million cases of DHF and DSS that lead to more than 20,000 deaths worldwide [5].The severe syndromes caused by dengue infection translate to serious economic burden in more than 100 tropical and sub-tropical countries [5]. Moreover, countries plagued with the dengue virus epidemic are mostly classified by World Bank as low income countries [6]. In view of that, there is an increased interest globally in developing new inexpensive vaccines and drugs as well as diagnostic tests that can be used for clinical management, and this would also be seen as a significant increase on the current support for new neglected tropical diseases technologies [7,8].

Short cationic peptides have been considered as best drug leads for designing and developing new antiviral therapies [9–10]. The main reason for the interest in these peptides is that they possess high specificity and selectivity in their interactions and this ultimately reduce the possible side effects and maximize the potencies of action [11]. Previous studies reported significant inhibition of viral entry by synthetic peptides designed to target the last stage of virus fusion [12]. In addition, antimicrobial cationic peptides like Protegrin-1 (PG1) have been shown to inhibit the dengue NS2B-NS3pro that in turn impairs viral replication in the host cells [13]. One of the main hindrances for successful production of these peptides using chemical synthesis are the high costs involved, and is currently deemed uneconomic especially to achieve the required volumes for epidemic response. As an alternative, production of these peptides in recombinant form would be cost-effective if a suitable expression system is establish to be scalable and well suited for mass production of bioactive peptides.

Escherichia coli and its various strains have been widely used as economic expression systems to produce numerous foreign proteins. Unfortunately, there are considerable limitations in using this system to produce bioactive antiviral peptides. One of these limitations is the low efficiency in the formation of disulphide bonds for cysteine-rich peptides that is important for antimicrobial bioactivity [14]. In addition, short peptides are almost always produced in soluble form and are often misfolded. This necessitates additional steps like in-column refolding and purification, and thus represents a considerable problem to large-scale production efforts [15]. Producing antiviral peptides in *E. coli* as inclusion bodies could represent an attractive solution to the problem above, and to facilitate high yield production. This approach requires only a few washing steps to isolate the inclusion bodies, and this is then followed by the appropriate refolding technique [16,17]. Our previous work reported production of the plectasin peptide in inclusion bodies by tandem fusion of two peptide units separated by a protease recognition site [16]. This strategy required extra steps of enzyme digestion and elimination of enzyme residues from the final products. The current study presents a new approach in which functional recombinant cationic peptides are produced as parts of a peptide-fusion protein. This protein was designed to harbour antiviral peptides fused to a central antiviral protein. The central protein MAP30, an antiviral protein isolated and purified from the fruit and seeds of the Momordica charantia (or commonly known as bitter gourd, has been previously shown to be successfully produced in *E. coli* as inclusion bodies [18].

In this study, the short cationic peptides protegrin-1 (PG1) and plectasin (PLSN) were doubly fused with a central protein, MAP30, to produce a recombinant antiviral peptide-fusion protein (PG1-MAP30-PLSN). PG1 is originally isolated from porcine white blood cells and has been considered as a potent antibiotic agent against a broad range of microorganisms [19,20]. PLSN, on the other hand is the first antimicrobial fungus-derived defensin, produced by the fungus *Pseudoplectania nigrella* with secondary structures similar to those of defensins found in other organisms [10,21]. These two peptides PG1 and PLSN are fused to MAP30 as an anchoring central antiviral protein. MAP30 is a 30 kDa type-I ribosome inactivating protein (RIP) possessing anti-HIV activities [22,23]. In terms of their antiviral activity, both PG1 and PLSN have been previously shown to possess considerable inhibition potential against dengue NS2B-NS3 serine protease and virus replication *in vitro* [13,16]. There are currently no reports on whether or not MAP30 possesses an inhibition potential towards dengue virus. As such, this study was also designed to address this question.

Methods

Design of antiviral peptide-fusion protein

The peptide-fusion protein consisted of PG1 and PLSN as flanking peptides fused to MAP30 as a central protein. The peptide-fusion protein PG1-MAP30-PLSN protein was constructed by joining the C-terminal of PG1 with the N-terminal of MAP30 by using a ten amino-acid linker, and the C-terminal of MAP30 was joined to the N-terminal of PLSN by using another ten amino-acid linker.

Production of recombinant proteins in *E. coli*

The recombinant peptide-fusion protein (PG1-MAP30-PLSN) was produced in *E. coli*. For comparison purposes, the PLSN peptide and MAP30 were produce in recombinant form as previously described [16,18] while PG1 was chemically manufactured by standard solid-phase peptide synthesis [13]. The DNA sequence of the peptide-fusion protein (*PG1-MAP30-PLSN*) (Fig.1A) was obtained by reverse translating the amino acid sequence and optimized to *E. coli* preferred codons as previously describe [24,25] using software available online. Alternating sense and antisense oligos of 60-mers in length (with 15 bp overlap region) were designed to span the entire PG1-MAP30-PLSN expression cassette and synthesized commercially (1stbase, Kuala Lumpur–Malaysia) (Data S1). Splicing and synthesis of the entire PG1-MAP30-PLSN expression cassette was achieved using

Klenow-*Pfu* DNA polymerase method [26]. The PG1-MAP30-PLSN expression cassette (and the individual MAP30 gene) was amplified using forward and reverse primer that were designed to include *Bam*HI and *Hind*III restriction sites respectively. Then, the PG1-MAP30-PLSN expression cassette or MAP30 was digested with *Bam*HI and *Hind*III enzymes to facilitate cloning into an appropriate *E. coli* expression vector (pTrc-His-A, Invitrogen, Cat. no. V360-20). To isolate inclusion bodies, bacterial cells were harvested and lysed by sonication in lysis buffer. Following a centrifugation step, the isolated inclusion bodies were subjected to excessive washing steps and solubilized by NaOH. This was then followed by protein refolding steps as described previously [27]. Further purification was carried out using column chromatography to eliminate host cell contamination from the final product.

Dengue NS2B-NS3 protease (NS2B-NS3pro) assay

The assay was carried out to examine the ability of antiviral peptides to inhibit DENV2 dengue serine protease (NS2B-NS3pro) [13, 15 and 16]. In brief, a single chain NS2B (G_4-T-G_4) NS3pro was produce as a recombinant protein in *E. coli* [28,29]. The end point reaction mixture was performed in black 96-well plates which contained 2 μM recombinant NS2B-NS3pro, 100 μM fluorogenic peptide substrate (Boc-Gly-Arg-Arg-AMC) and antiviral peptides of varying concentrations, buffered at pH 8.5 with 200 mM Tris-HCl with total volume of 200 μl. The reaction mixture without antiviral peptides, substrate with antiviral peptides, enzyme and different concentrations of antiviral peptides were used as controls. Thereafter, all reaction mixtures were incubated at 37°C for 30 minutes and the substrate was added to the specific reaction mixtures and incubated at the same temperatures for another 30 minutes. Measurements were performed in triplicates using Tecan Infinite M200 Pro fluorescence spectrophotometer (Tecan Group Ltd., Switzerland). Substrate cleavage was normalized against buffer only (control) at the emission of 440 nm upon excitation at 350 nm. The IC_{50} was calculated from nonlinear regression fitting of signal *vs.* concentration data points to the standard dose–response equation $Y = Bottom + ((Top - Bottom) \div 1 + 10(X - \log IC50))$. In this equation, X was the log of compound concentration, Y was the response signal, and bottom and top refer to plateaus of the sigmoid response curve. All assays were performed in triplicate and repeated twice. The inhibition percentage was calculated using the following formula: $\% \, DENV2 \, protease \, activity = 100 - \dfrac{(\text{intensity of enzyme activity} - \text{intensity left after inhibition})}{\text{intensity of enzyme activity}} \times 100$

Maximum non-toxic dose test (MNTD)

The MNTD assay was carried out to determine the maximal concentration with lessen cytotoxic effects of the antiviral peptides. The MNTD test was initiated by seeding Vero cells at 1×10^4 cells/well in triplicates, at optimal conditions (37°C, 5% CO_2 in humidified incubator) in 96 well plates with blank control (media only) and cells control (cells only). After overnight incubation, the cells were treated with increased concentrations of each antiviral peptide with DMEM media supplemented with 2% FBS. The cell culture was analyzed after 72 h using Non-Radioactive Cell Proliferation assay (Promega, USA) according to the manufacturer's protocol. The MNTD was calculated from dose-response curves and the percentage of cell viability was calculated as follows:

(A)

| T7 promoter | His Tag | Protegrin-1 | Linker | Map 30 | Linker | Plectasin |

PG1-MAP30-PLSN Chimeric protein MW 37.7kDa

RGGRLCYCRRRFCVCVGR<u>VPGVGVPGVG</u>DVNFDLSTATAKTYTKFIEDFRATLPFSHKVY
DIPLLYSTISDSRRFILLNLTSYAYETISVAIDVTNVYVVAYRTRDVSYFFKESPPEAYN
ILFKGTRKITLPYTGNYENLQTAAHKIRENIDLGLPALSSAITTLFYYNAQSAPSALLVL
IQTTAEAARFKYIERHVAKYVATNFKPNLAIISLENQWSALSKQIFLAQNQGGKFRNPVD
LIKPTGERFQVTNVDSDVVKGNIKLLLNSRASTADENFITTMTLLGESVVN<u>VPGVGVPGV</u>
<u>G</u>GFGCNGPWDEDDMQCHNHCKSIKGYKGGYCAKGGFVCKCY

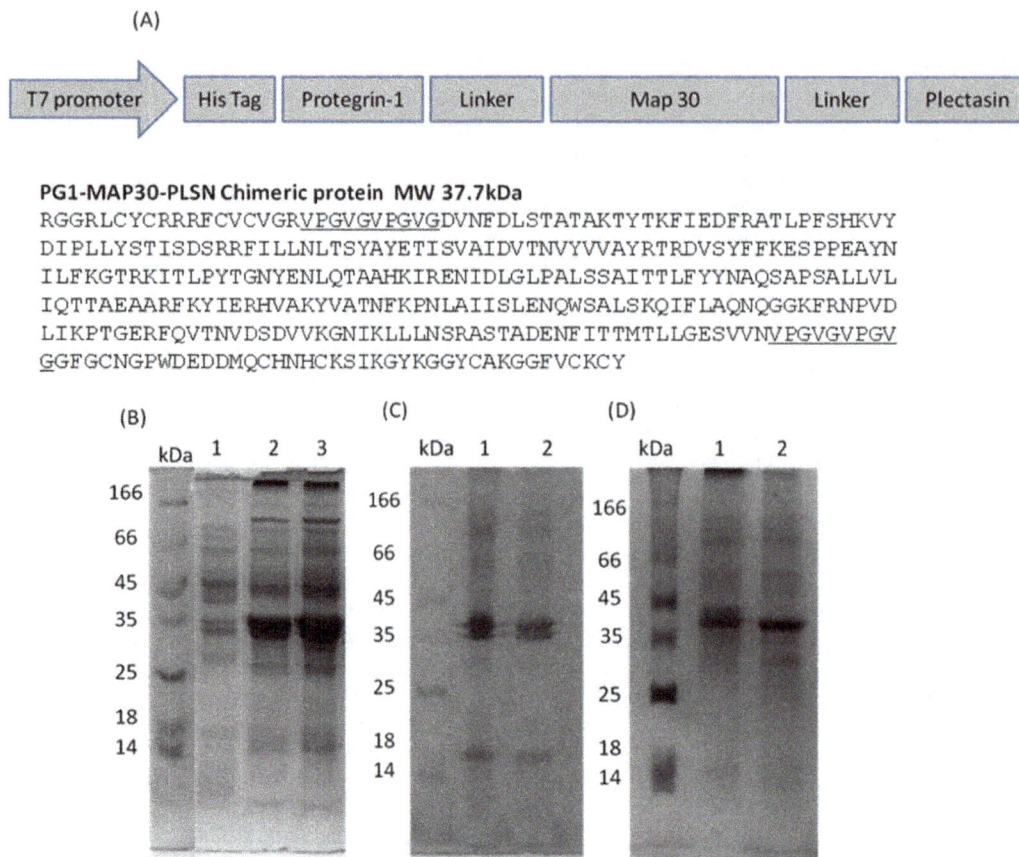

Figure 1. Production of recombinant peptide-fusion protein (PG1-MAP30-PLSN) in *E. coli* as inclusion bodies. (A) Design of peptide-fusion protein: PG1 peptide was joined with N-terminal of MAP30 by 10-amino-acid linkers (underlined) and PLSN peptide was joined to the C-terminal of MAP30 by similar linkers. (B) The peptide-fusion protein was produced insolubly as inclusion bodies: Lane 1, before induction with IPTG; Lane 2, expression of peptide-fusion protein after induction; Lane 3, expression of MAP30 after induction. (C) Isolation of inclusion bodies by multiple washing steps: Lane 1, peptide-fusion protein; Lane 2, MAP30. (D) Inclusion bodies were solubilized and refolded in an alkaline buffer containing redox agents: Lane 1, peptide-fusion protein; Lane 2, MAP30.

100-(Absorbance of treated cells ÷

Absorbance of untreated cells) × 100

Real-Time Cell Proliferation Assay (RTCA assay)

This assay was carried out to test the real time effects of the peptide-fusion protein on cell viability. Cell proliferation was measured using xCELLigence Real-Time Cellular Analysis (RTCA) system (Roche, Germany) as described previously [30]. Cell viability and growth was monitored continuously after applying increased concentrations of PG1-MAP30-PLSN protein. Briefly, background measurements were taken after adding 100 µl of the culture medium to the wells. Next, cells were seeded at a density of 1×10^4 cell/well on a 16-well plate with electrodes for 18 h to allow cells to grow to the log phase. Cells were treated with different concentrations of the compounds dissolved in cell culture media and continuously monitored for up to 100 h. Cell sensor impedance was expressed as an arbitrary unit called the Cell Index. Cell index were recorded every 5 min by RTCA analyzer. To eliminate variation between wells, cell index values were normalized to the value at the beginning of treatment time-point.

Treatment of DENV2-infected cells with antiviral peptides

To infect Vero cell lines with dengue virus (DENV2-isolate Malaysia M2, GenBank Toxonomy No.: 11062), the cells were cultured in 24-well plates (1.5×10^5 cells/well) for 24 h at 37°C and 5% CO_2. Virus supernatant was added to the cells at multiplicity of infection (MOI) of 0.2 followed by incubation for 1 h with gentle shaking every 15 min for optimal virus to cell contact. The cells were washed twice with fresh serum-free DMEM media after removing the virus supernatant. Then, new complete DMEM media mixed with each peptide were separately added and the cultures were incubated for 24, 48 and 72 h. Afterwards, cellular supernatants were collected and stored at −80°C for viral load quantification.

Virus binding assay

This test was carried out to examine the ability of the peptides in inhibiting virus binding to the host cells. Vero cells were grown in six-well microplates (1.5×10^6 cells/well) for 24 h. Cell culture media were removed and the cells were washed three times with PBS. Then, new media containing virus supernatant mixed with each peptide were separately added and the cells were incubated for 1 h at 4°C. The media were removed and the cells were washed extensively with cold PBS to remove the unadsorbed virus.

Cells were harvested at 24, 48 and 72 h and the viral RNA was quantified by qReal time-PCR.

Virus quantification by plaque formation assay

To determine the virus yield after treatment with different concentrations of the peptides, culture supernatants were collected and serially diluted to reduce the effects of drug residues. A 10-fold serial dilution of medium supernatant was added to new Vero cells grown in 24-well plate (1.5×10^5 cells) and incubated for 1 h at 37°C. The cells were then overlaid with DMEM medium containing 1.1% methylcellulose. Viral plaques were stained with crystal violet dye after five-day incubation. Virus titers were calculated according to the following formula: Titer (p.f.u./ml) = number of plaques/volume of diluted virus added to the well × dilution factor of the virus used to infect the well in which plaques were enumerated.

Quantitative real-time PCR

After treatment with antiviral peptides, the RNA copies of DENV2 were quantified using One-step Real-time PCR as previously described [13]. In brief, a standard curve was generated by 10-fold serial dilution of known copies of DENV2 RNA. Then, viral RNA was extracted from culture supernatant using QIAmp viral RNA extraction kit (QIAGEN, Germany). The qRT-PCR was carried out using SyBr Green Master Kit (Qiagen, Germany) in quadruple experiments and absolute quantification was performed using ABI7500 machine (Applied Biosystems, Foster City, CA). Results were analyzed using Sequence Detection Software Version 1.3 (Applied Biosystems, Foster City, CA).

Indirect immunostaining

In order to examine the uptake of the peptide-fusion protein by Vero cells, the cells were grew on the cover slide in 6 well plates and treated with the peptide-fusion protein for 24 h. Then, the cells were washed three times with PBS to remove the residues of the peptide and fixed with ice-cold methanol for 15 min at −20°C. After washing steps, the cells were incubated with coating buffer for 1 h at room temperature. Mouse anti-His tag antibody was added and the cells were incubated overnight at 4°C. The cells were washed three times with PBS and incubated for 30 min with anti-mouse IGg labelled with FITC fluorescence dye and the Hoechst dye was added at the last 15 min of the incubation period.

Animal experiments

ICR mice were handled in accordance with University of Malaya guidelines on the care and use of laboratory animals. The Animal Ethics Committee of the University of Malaya approved all experimental procedures that were used in the present study. Mice were used at 3 to 5 weeks of age and average body weight of approximately 30 g. The animals were firstly used to evaluate the lethal dose of the peptide- fusion protein that kills 50 percent of the animals (LD_{50}). Two groups of animals (n = 12 each, 6 females and 6 males) were intraperitoneally administrated with 5 mg/kg as a low dose (0.25 ml of 0.6 mg/ml of the peptide-fusion protein) and 50 mg/kg as a high dose (0.25 ml of 6 mg/ml of the peptide-fusion protein). The animals were observed for 24 h without any signs of toxicity, after 14 days post- treatment, the animals were healthy and no signs of toxicity or death cases were recorded. Then, four groups of animals (n = 6 each) were intraperitoneally inoculated with 4×10^3 plaque-forming units (PFU) of the purified DENV2 (DENV2-isolate Malaysia M2, GenBank Taxonomy No.: 11062). Simultaneously, three groups were individually

administrated with 12.5, 25 and 50 mg/kg of the peptide-fusion protein by intraperitoneal administration; while the forth group was administrated with PBS as a mock-administrated group. Mice were observed for 7 days post-infection and the death cases were recorded and Kaplan-Meier analysis was used to generate survival curves with Prism software 5.01 (GraphPad Software, San Diego, CA).

Statistical analysis

All the assays were done in triplicates and the statistical analyses were performed using GraphPad Prism version 5.01 (GraphPad Software, San Diego, CA). P values of <0.05 were considered significant. Error bars are expressed as ± SD.

Results

Production of recombinant peptide-fusion protein (PG1-MAP30-PLSN)

PG1 peptide was joined to the N-terminal portion of MAP30 by using a 10-amino-acid linker and PLSN peptide was joined to the C-terminal of MAP30 using a similar linker. The DNA sequence coding the peptide-fusion protein expression cassette (PG1-MAP30-PLSN) was optimized for *E. coli* preferred codon and constructed *in vitro* using Klenow-*Pfu* DNA polymerase procedure. The molecular weight of the resulting peptide-fusion protein was approximately 37.7 kDa (Fig. 1A). The peptide-fusion protein was produced insolubly as inclusion bodies at high levels reaching approximately 80% of the total bacteria protein (Fig. 1B). Inclusion bodies were isolated by washing steps to eliminate host cell proteins (Fig. 1C). In order to retrieve the bioactivity of recombinant peptide-fusion protein, isolated inclusion bodies was solubilized and refolded in alkaline-based buffer containing redox agents (Fig. 1D). The recombinant peptide-fusion protein was designed to include 6X His-tag to facilitate purification by Ni-affinity chromatography. The antimicrobial activity of the recombinant protein was confirmed as it showed high inhibition potential against gram-positive and gram-negative bacteria (data not shown).The total amount of recombinant peptide-fusion protein was approximately 30 mg per litre of *E. coli* cell culture.

Inhibition of dengue protease by antiviral peptide-fusion protein

Dengue NS2B-NS3 protease (NS2B-NS3pro) assay was carried out to evaluate the inhibition potential of the peptides individually or as peptide-fusion protein. The results showed that all peptides exhibited significant dose-dependent inhibition against dengue NS2B-NS3pro (Fig. 2). The peptide-fusion protein showed significantly higher inhibition potential against dengue NS2B-NS3pro (IC_{50}, 0.50 ± 0.1 μM) compared to individual MAP30 (IC_{50}, 2.3 ± 0.5 μM), PG1 (IC_{50}, 11.6 ± 2.1 μM) and PLSN (IC_{50}, 10.0 ± 1.8 μM) (Fig. 2).

Evaluation of peptide cytotoxicity

Toxicity was measured to determine the maximum non-toxic dose (MNTD) of the inhibitory peptides. Besides the undesired effect, toxicity could induce cellular alterations that decrease the formation of plaques leading to false interpretation of antiviral activity. Toxic effects ranged from no evidence to minimal toxicity for different peptides when compared to untreated control cells. In order to evaluate the anti-dengue properties of the peptide-fusion protein in comparison to the peptides acting individually, all peptides were first subjected to a toxicity test. In this study, the MNTD values were determined using serially diluted peptides

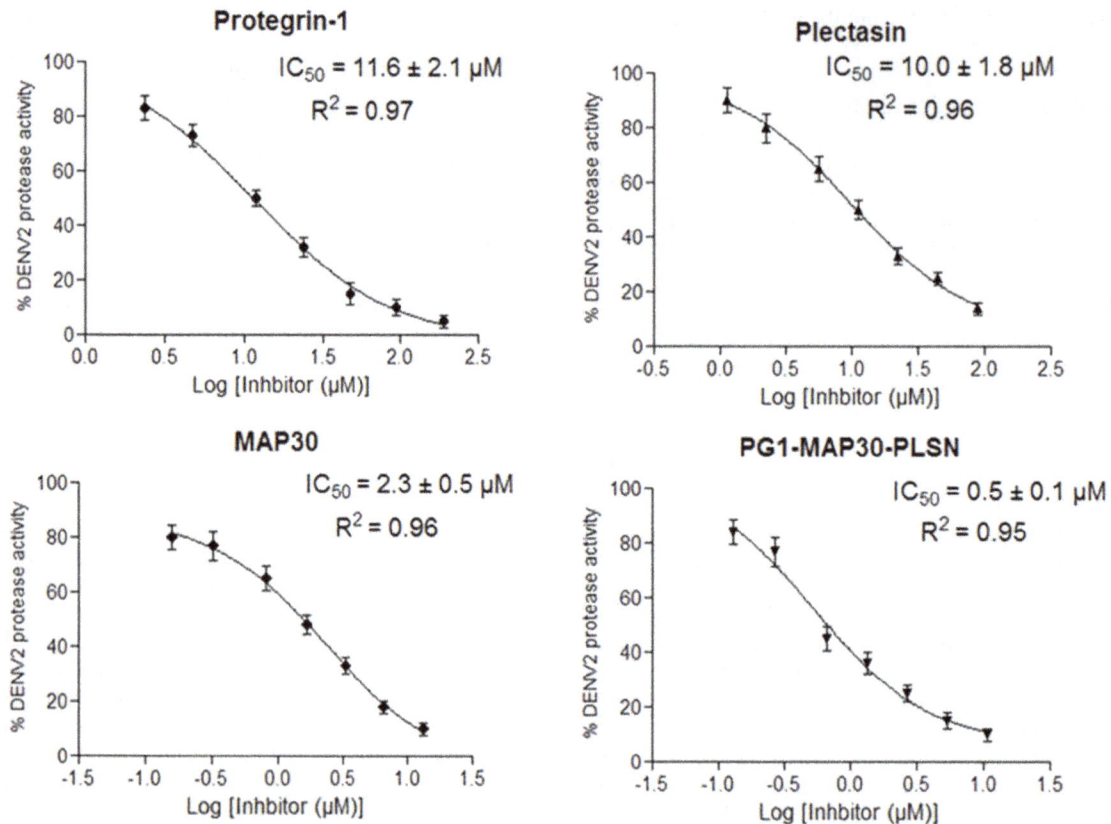

Figure 2. Evaluation of the inhibitory effects of the peptide-fusion protein and the individual antiviral peptides against dengue NS2B-NS3 protease. Recombinant dengue NS2B-NS3pro was produce in *E. coli* and used in an end point reaction mixture with fluorogenic peptide substrate, antiviral peptides of varying concentrations and buffer. The antiviral peptides showed significant dose-dependent inhibition towards dengue NS2B-NS3pro. The peptide-fusion protein inhibited dengue protease at IC_{50} value lower than MAP30, PG1 and PLSN.

followed by further optimization in order to achieve a specific cytotoxic concentration. The MNTD value of each peptide obtained through the optimization steps are presented in Figure 3. The MNTD value of PG1 (25.0 ± 4.1 μM), PLSN (20.0 ± 3.2 μM), MAP30 (0.80 ± 0.2 μM) and PG1-MAP30-PLSN (0.67 ± 0.2 μM) were used in the following experiments.

Cellular uptake of the peptide-fusion protein and real-time cell proliferation assay

To evaluate the internalization of the peptide-fusion protein into Vero cells, the intracellular PG1-MAP30-PLSN protein was targeted by anti-His tag antibody and secondary antibody conjugated with FITC. The result showed that the targeted protein was distributed around the cells nuclei (Fig. 4A). As mentioned earlier, our antiviral peptide-fusion protein (PG1-MAP30-PLSN) contains MAP30 as a central protein, which possesses ribosome-inactivation activities [23]. This activity of MAP30 could induce cellular alterations that decrease the formation of plaques leading to false interpretation of antiviral activity. To clarify this issue, we examined the effects of increased concentrations of the peptide-fusion protein on real time cell proliferation using the Real-Time Cellular Analysis (RTCA) system. The cells were incubated for 20 h without treatment and then treated with increased concentration of the peptide-fusion protein. The results showed that the effects of peptide-fusion protein on cell proliferation were insignificant at the dose of 25 μg/ml (0.67 μM) for 82 h as the cell index was similar with

untreated control cells. Cell proliferation was considerably decreased at the dose of more than 50 μg/ml (1.35 μM) (Fig. 4).

Assessment of antiviral activity

The effectiveness of the peptides was verified by testing the antiviral activity of the peptides against DENV2 using plaque formation assay and qRT-PCR analysis. The results showed significant ($p<0.001$) reduction in the DENV2 load that was expressed as plaque forming units per ml (p.f.u./ml) after treatment with all the peptides compared to untreated cells (Fig. 5A and 5B). The peptide-fusion protein showed the highest reduction in the viral load ($1.21\pm0.3 \times10^7$, $0.93\pm0.2\times10^7$ and $0.82\pm0.2\times10^7$ p.f.u./ml at 24, 48 and 72 h respectively) compared with untreated control ($7.40\pm0.8\times10^7$, $8.10\pm0.6\times10^7$ and $8.41\pm0.7\times10^7$ at 24, 48 and 72 h respectively). While, MAP30 showed the lowest antiviral activity amongst the other peptides ($5.41\pm0.6\times10^7$, $4.23\pm0.9\times10^7$, $4.11\pm0.7\times10^7$ p.f.u./ml at 24, 48 and 72 h respectively). Interestingly, both of PG1-MAP30-PLSN and MAP30 showed significant ($p<0.05$) time-dependent antiviral activity. The inhibition potential of PG1 and PLSN was approximately similar, which was significantly ($p<0.001$) higher than MAP30 and lower than PG1-MAP30-PLSN with insignificant time-dependent effects.

These results were further verified by quantification of viral copy number by evaluating viral RNA levels using qRT-PCR analysis. The results showed that the peptide-fusion protein was significantly ($p<0.001$) able to inhibit virus replication in Vero

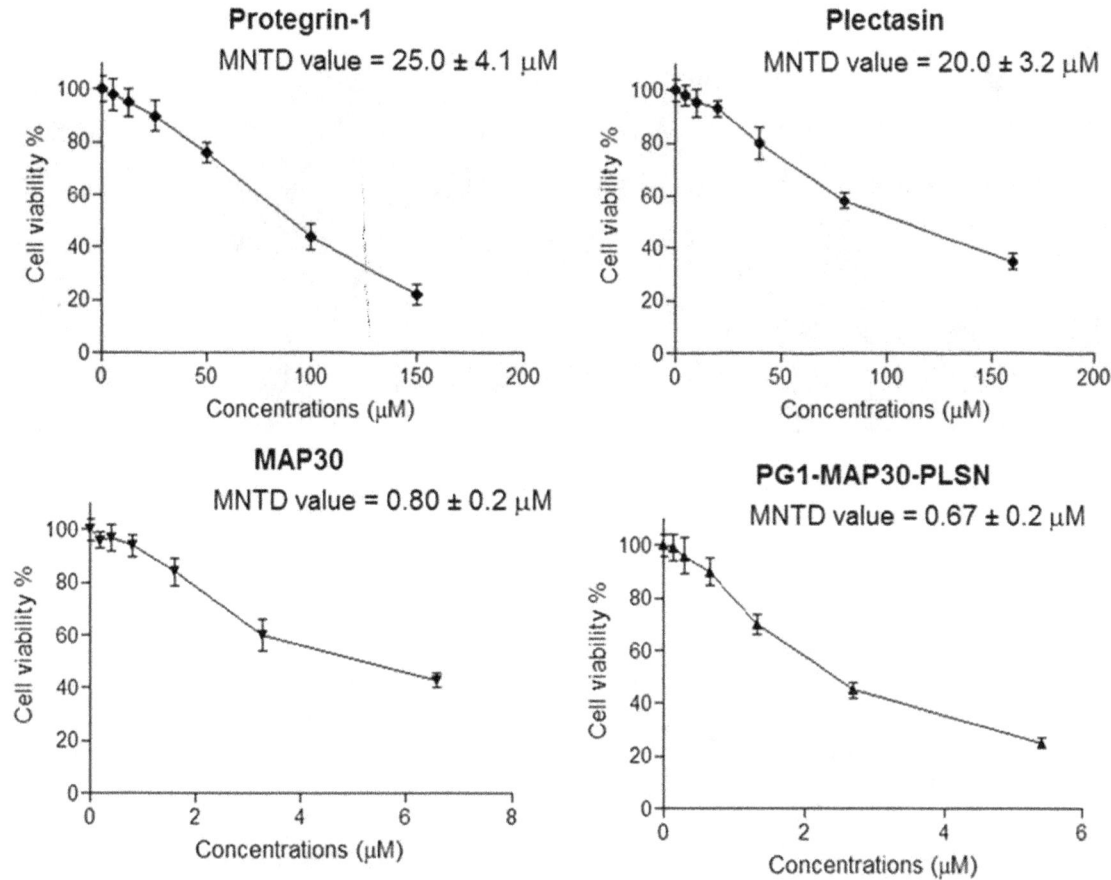

Figure 3. Evaluation of peptide cytotoxicity. Toxicity was measured to determine the maximal non-toxic dose test (MNTD) value of the inhibitory peptides, which is the highest concentration of the peptide that causes minimal toxic effects on the cells. This assay was carried out by seeding Vero cells at 1×10^4 cells/well in triplicates and treated with increased concentrations of antiviral peptides. The cell culture was analyzed after 72 h using Non-Radioactive Cell Proliferation assay. In this study, the peptide concentration that showed 90% and above of the cell viability was considered as the MNTD value, assuming that approximately 90% of the cells were healthy.

cells by reducing viral copy number ($1.20\pm0.3\times10^6$, $0.78\pm0.2\times10^6$ and $0.67\pm0.2\times10^6$ at 24, 48 and 72 h respectively) compared with untreated control ($7.30\pm0.9\times10^6$, $7.91\pm0.7\times10^6$ and $8.22\pm0.6\times10^6$ at 24, 48 and72 h). In addition, MAP30 showed the lowest inhibitory effect ($p<0.001$) amongst the other peptides ($5.41\pm0.6\times10^6$, $4.23\pm0.9\times10^6$ and $4.11\pm0.7\times10^6$ at 24, 48 and 72 h respectively). In parallel with the results of plaque formation assay, both PG1-MAP30-PLSN and MAP30 showed time- dependent inhibitory effects. However, PG1 and PLSN showed insignificant time-dependent effects. Both of PG1 and PLSN showed similar inhibition activities that were lower than PG1-MAP30-PLSN and higher than MAP30 (Fig. 6A).

The results also showed significant ($p<0.001$) reduction in viral copy number when DENV2 was individually incubated with each peptide to examine the effect of the peptides on virus binding to the target cell. The peptide-fusion protein (PG1-MAP30-PLSN) potentially inhibited virus binding to the target cell as evidenced by a considerable reduction in the viral copy numbers ($0.74\pm0.2\times10^5$, $0.65\pm0.1\times10^5$ and $049\pm0.1\times10^5$ compared with untreated control $6.70\pm0.9\times10^5$, $6.98\pm0.8\times10^5$ and $7.10\pm0.9\times10^5$ at 24, 48 and 72 h respectively). However, there was insignificant ($p>0.05$) effect of MAP30 on virus binding to the target cell while PG1 and PLSN significantly ($p<0.001$) inhibited virus binding to the target cell as presented in Figure 6A and 6B.

Determination of the antiviral peptide-fusion protein effective dose

Dose response curves were generated for the recombinant peptide-fusion protein in comparison with MAP30 against DENV2 to determine the effective dose that inhibits 50% of the viral activity (EC_{50}). The inhibitory activity increased with increasing concentrations of both recombinant proteins. Interestingly, the peptide-fusion protein showed a maximum inhibition activity against DENV2 of $18.6\%\pm7.2$ at 0.75 μM with EC_{50} about 0.43 μM, while MAP30 showed a maximum inhibition activity against DENV2 of $68.9\%\pm6.7$ at 0.75 μM with EC_{50} more than 0.75 μM as shown in Figure 7.

Protection against DENV2 infection

The ICR mice were intraperitoneally administrated with low dose (5 mg/kg) and high dose (50 mg/kg) of the peptide-fusion protein. The animals were kept for 14 days post-administration with no signs of toxicity or death cases were observed. Therefore, we assumed that the LD_{50} value of the peptide- fusion protein could be more than 50 mg/kg. Based on that, the doses that were used in the following experiment were equal or less than 50 mg/kg to eliminate the possible cytotoxic effect of the peptide-fusion protein that may cause animal death. DENV2-chalenged animals were simultaneously treated with 12.5, 25 and 50 mg/kg of the

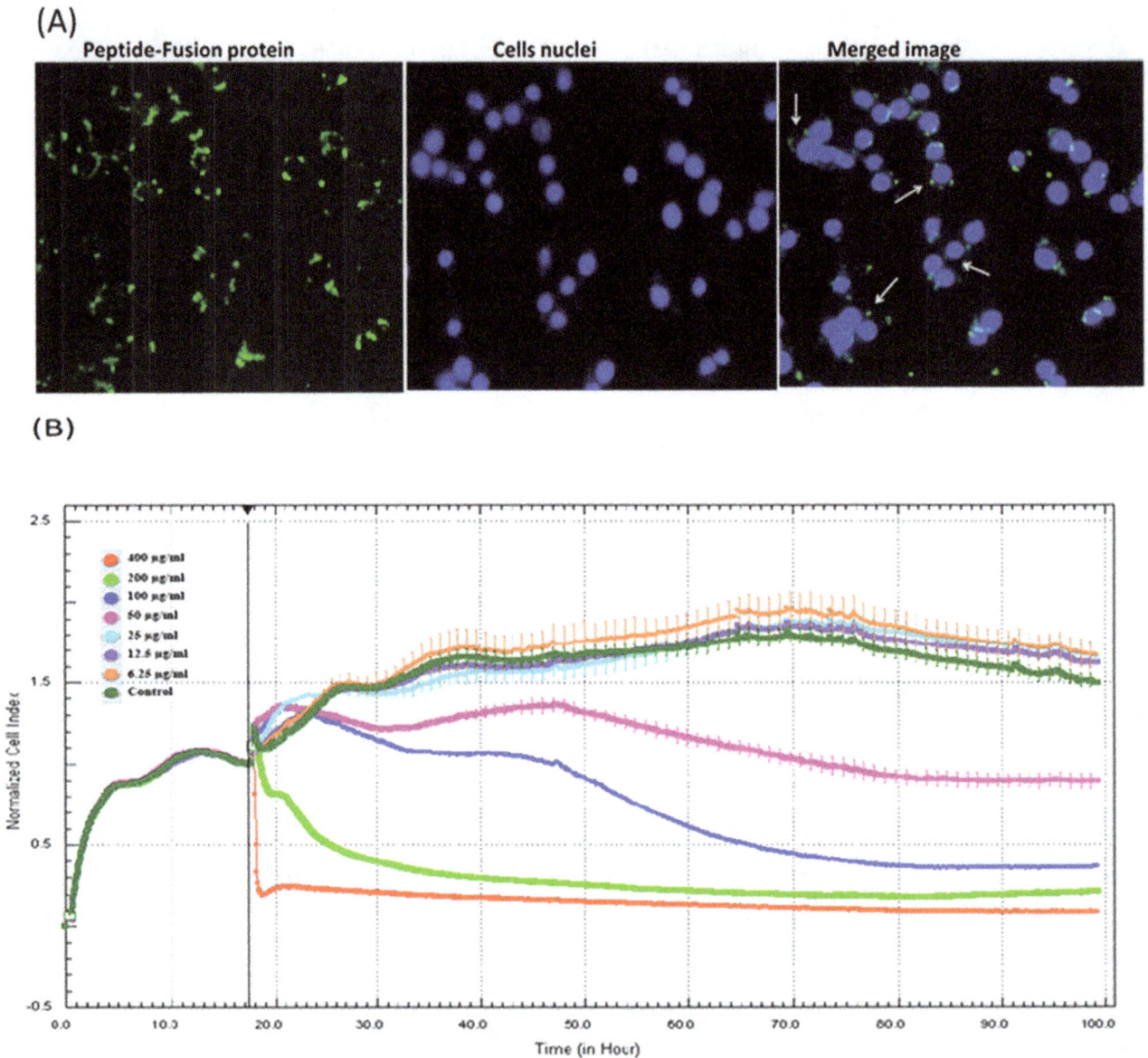

Figure 4. Peptide-fusion protein uptake and real time cell proliferation assay. (A) Cellular uptake of the peptide-fusion protein was analyzed by immunostaining images that show localization of peptide-fusion protein around cells nuclei. (B) Cell proliferation was measured using xCELLigence Real-Time Cellular Analysis (RTCA) system. Cell viability and growth was monitored continuously after incubating the cells for 18 h at standard condition and applying increased concentrations of the PG1-MAP30-PLSN protein (6.25, 12.5, 25, 50, 100, 200 and 400 μg/ml or 0.17, 0.34, 0.67, 1.35, 2.70, 5.40 and 10.81 μM).The effects of the peptide-fusion protein on cell proliferation were insignificant at the doses less than 25 μg/ml (0.67 μM) for 82 h as the cell index was similar with untreated control cells. Cell proliferation was considerably decreased at the dose more than 50 μg/ml (1.35 μM).

peptide fusion protein and kept for 7 days post-infection. The results showed that the peptide-fusion protein protected DENV2-challenged animals in a dose-dependent manner. All the animals of the mock-administrated group were died at the period of 4 days post-infection and 5 of 6 animals that administrated with 12.5 mg/kg of the peptide- fusion protein were died at the period of 5 days post-infection (Fig. 8A). However, only one animal of the group that was administrated with 25 mg/kg was died at the seventh day of the experiment (Fig. 8B). Interestingly, the peptide-fusion protein showed 100% of survival at the dose of 50 mg/kg as presented in Figure 8C.

Discussion

Our previous studies have shown that PG1 and PLSN exhibited significant inhibition against dengue serine protease (NS2B-NS3pro) and dengue replication in infected cells. We then hypothesized that the design and construction of a recombinant antiviral peptide-fusion protein by fusing these peptides to a central antiviral protein will provide two significant advantages over conventional approaches. Firstly, the recombinant peptide-fusion protein can synergistically result in amplified antiviral activity. Secondly, the use of MAP30, a protein already known to be successfully expressed through inclusion bodies, as the

(A)

(B)

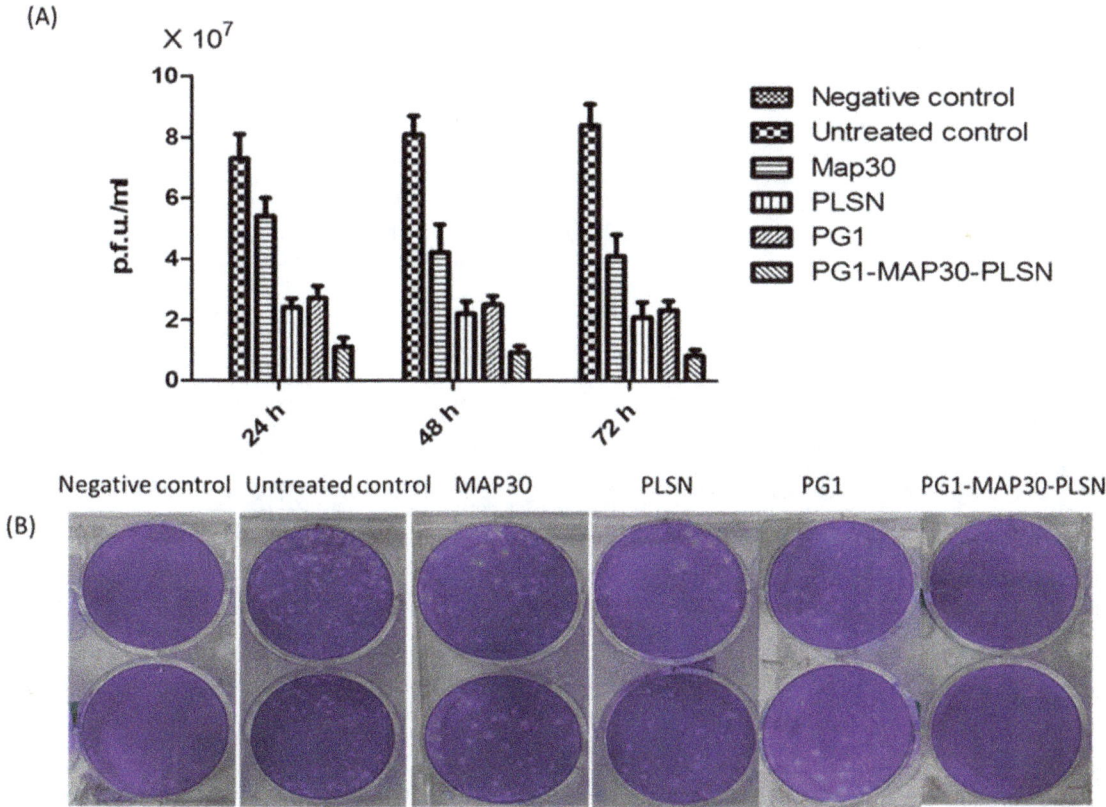

Figure 5. Evaluation of the peptides antiviral activities using plaque formation assay. (A) Virus load expressed as plaque forming units per ml (p.f.u/ml) was significantly reduced after treatment with all the peptides compared to untreated cells. The peptide-fusion protein (PG1-MAP30-PLSN) showed the highest inhibition potential compared with the other peptides. (B) Plaque formation assay shows the reduction of plaque generation after the treatment of the infected cells with the peptides. (Two-way ANOVA with Bonferroni post-test, $p < 0.001$).

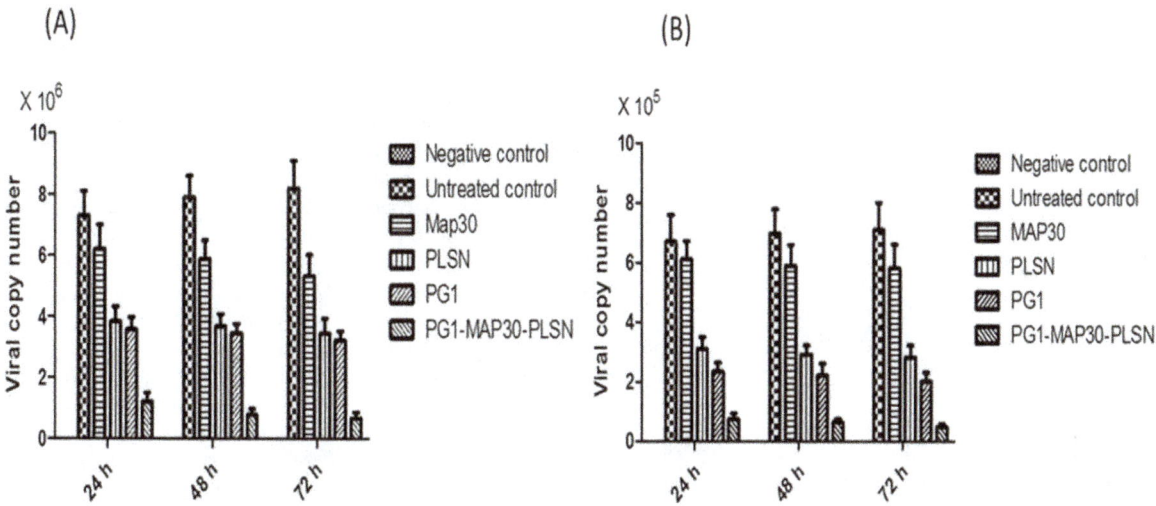

(A)   (B)

Figure 6. Evaluation of the peptides antiviral activities using qRT-PCR. Viral RNA levels were quantified by qRT-PCR to determine the level of viral copy number after the treatment of DENV2-infected cells with the antiviral peptides. (A) Viral copy number was reduced after the treatment with the peptides compared with untreated control. The peptide-fusion protein (PG1-MAP30-PLSN) showed the highest reduction in the viral copy number amongst the other peptides in a time-dependent manner. (B) Inhibition of virus binding to the target cells that led to reduce dengue virus copy number after the treatment with the peptides. The peptide-fusion protein potentially inhibited virus binding to the target cell by considerable reduction in the viral copy number compared with untreated control. However, there was insignificant ($p > 0.05$) effect of MAP30 on virus binding to the target cell. PG1 and PLSN similarly inhibited virus binding at significant levels. Results are expressed as mean ± SD from a representative experiment performed in quadruple experiments. (Two-way ANOVA with Bonferroni post-test, $p < 0.001$).

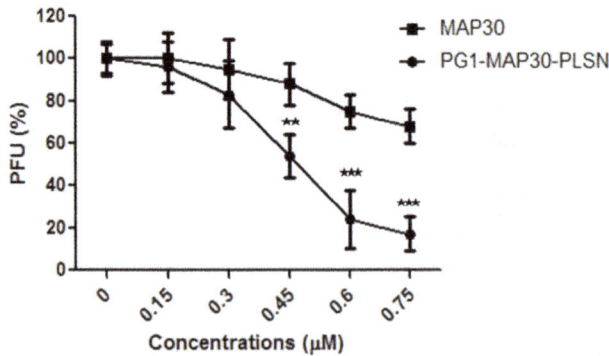

Figure 7. Dose-response curves for peptide-fusion protein and MAP30. The figure shows the effect of increasing concentrations of the peptide-fusion protein and MAP30 peptides against DENV2. The peptide-fusion protein showed a maximum inhibitory activity against DENV2 of 18.6%±7.2 at 0.75 µM with EC$_{50}$ about 0.43 µM. MAP30 showed a maximum inhibition activity against DENV2 of 68.9%±6.7 at 0.75 µM with EC$_{50}$ more than 0.75 µM. Results are expressed as mean ± SD from a representative experiment performed in triplicate. Asterisk denotes statistically significant differences between peptide-fusion protein and MAP30. (Two-way ANOVA with Bonferroni post-test, p<0.001).

anchoring central protein would facilitate high yield production in *E. coli*.

Producing antiviral peptides in inactive and insoluble (inclusion bodies) form by *E. coli* has considerable advantages over active and soluble form. Producing recombinant protein in inclusion bodies is considered a scalable strategy for recombinant protein production which has been applied for the production of high quantities of recombinant globular adiponectin [17]. Furthermore, formation of inclusion bodies is also important to protect the host cells from the toxic effects of the expressed product. This strategy was useful in producing recombinant phage T4 restriction endoribonuclease which is highly toxic to the host cells [31]. As such, antiviral activity of the peptide-fusion protein was retrieved after solubilization of inclusion bodies in alkaline buffer followed by refolding of the soluble protein in buffer containing redox agents. It is important to note that the activity of antiviral peptides almost always depends on its secondary structure which is maintained by the formation of intra-molecule disulphide bonds [32]. Therefore, reformation of disulphide bones was achieved in this study by reducing the existence bonds and reforming it in the presence of reduced and oxidized glutathione as previously reported [27].

The results of this study showed that the peptide-fusion protein (PG1-MAP30-PLSN) as well as, to a lesser extent, its individual components significantly inhibited dengue NS2B-NS3pro. Inhibition of dengue NS2B-NS3pro has been considered as a target to develop anti-dengue drugs [4]. It is now known that the post-translational proteolytic cleavage of viral precursor protein is largely dependent on dengue NS2B-NS3pro and host cell proteases. This process results in the formation of three structural proteins and seven non-structural viral proteins that is later required for dengue virus propagation [33–34]. Therefore, inhibition of dengue NS2B-NS3pro leads to impaired production of viral proteins which eventually leads to reduced virus replication capabilities. Importantly, the binding between dengue protease subunits depends on the interaction between negatively charged amino acids of NS2B and positively charged amino acids of NS3 [35]. The possible action of cationic peptides like PG1 and PLSN is to interrupt the binding of NS3 with its co-factor that leads to

reduce enzyme activity. Other peptides that contain α-helical structure similar to the PLSN peptide have shown considerable inhibitory effects against HIV-1 due to an actual interference with the virus assembly stage in the viral life cycle [36]. Similarly, the PG1 peptide that possess a strong positive charge, have shown considerable antiviral activity against the dengue virus protease that is important for post-translational processes [13]. Therefore, the antiviral activity of the PLSN and PG1 peptides against dengue is proposed to be due to their interference with the viral replication stages into the host cells. Consequently, the inhibition potential of peptide-fusion protein (PG1-MAP30-PLSN) against dengue NS2B-NS3pro might be one of the main causes of viral reduction in cell culture after treatment with peptide-fusion protein.

The current study showed considerable inhibition of MAP30 and higher inhibition potential of peptide-fusion protein (PG1-MAP30-PLSN) against viral replication. Besides, the data of this study also confirmed our previous findings of the inhibition potential of PG1, PLSN against dengue virus replication [13,16]. It has been shown that these peptides exhibited similar antiviral activities against different viruses. For example, PG1 showed antiviral activities against human immunodeficiency virus (HIV) [37], while MAP30 showed antiviral activity against herpes simplex virus (HSV) [38], HIV [39] and Kaposi's sarcoma-associated virus [40]. Based on our knowledge, there are no available studies illustrating the antiviral potential of PLSN except against dengue virus [16]. PG1 and PLSN were selected in this study based on their known inhibition potential against dengue NS2B-NS3pro. However, the results of viral binding assay showed that these peptides as well as the peptide-fusion protein also exhibited considerable inhibition against virus binding to the host cells. It could be possible that PG1 and PLSN individually or in fusion form may also act like some other cationic peptides such as retrocyclin which is effective in blocking viral attachment to host cell through its binding ability to heparan sulfate on the cell membrane [41,42]. In parallel, the antiviral activity of MAP30 may depend on its ability in inhibiting host cells protein machinery (such as that shown by RIP) [23] and modulating some cellular genes necessary for viral and cell proliferation and apoptosis [40]. It is important to examine whether or not the antiviral activity of the peptide-fusion protein depends on the effects of MAP30 on cell growth and apoptosis. The results of real time proliferation assay showed that the peptide-fusion protein inhibited virus replication in infected cells with minimal effects on cell proliferation. These data are helpful to conclude that the antiviral activity of the peptide-fusion protein was independent from the possible effects of MAP30 on cell proliferation and apoptosis that have been reported by other studies [43,44].

Based on the findings of this study, we assume that the peptide-fusion protein could potentially interrupt dengue life cycle. The considerable inhibition was observed at the binding stage and post-translational processes of the viral ploygenome, as evidenced by the inhibition of dengue NS2B-NS3pro. Such inhibition of viral protease could hinder flaviviruses replication and virion assembly, as evidenced by the lack of production of infectious virions in mutants carrying inactivating viral proteases [45]. However, other potentials such as the interruption of virus assembly and release from the infected cells need further investigations. Because the peptide-fusion protein consists of three different peptides, its mechanism of antiviral activity still requires additional examinations. Intriguingly, our study showed an evidence of potential efficacy of the peptide-fusion protein against viral propagation in mice challenged with lethal dose of DENV2. The results of the animal experiments demonstrate that the peptide-fusion protein

(A)

(B)

(C)

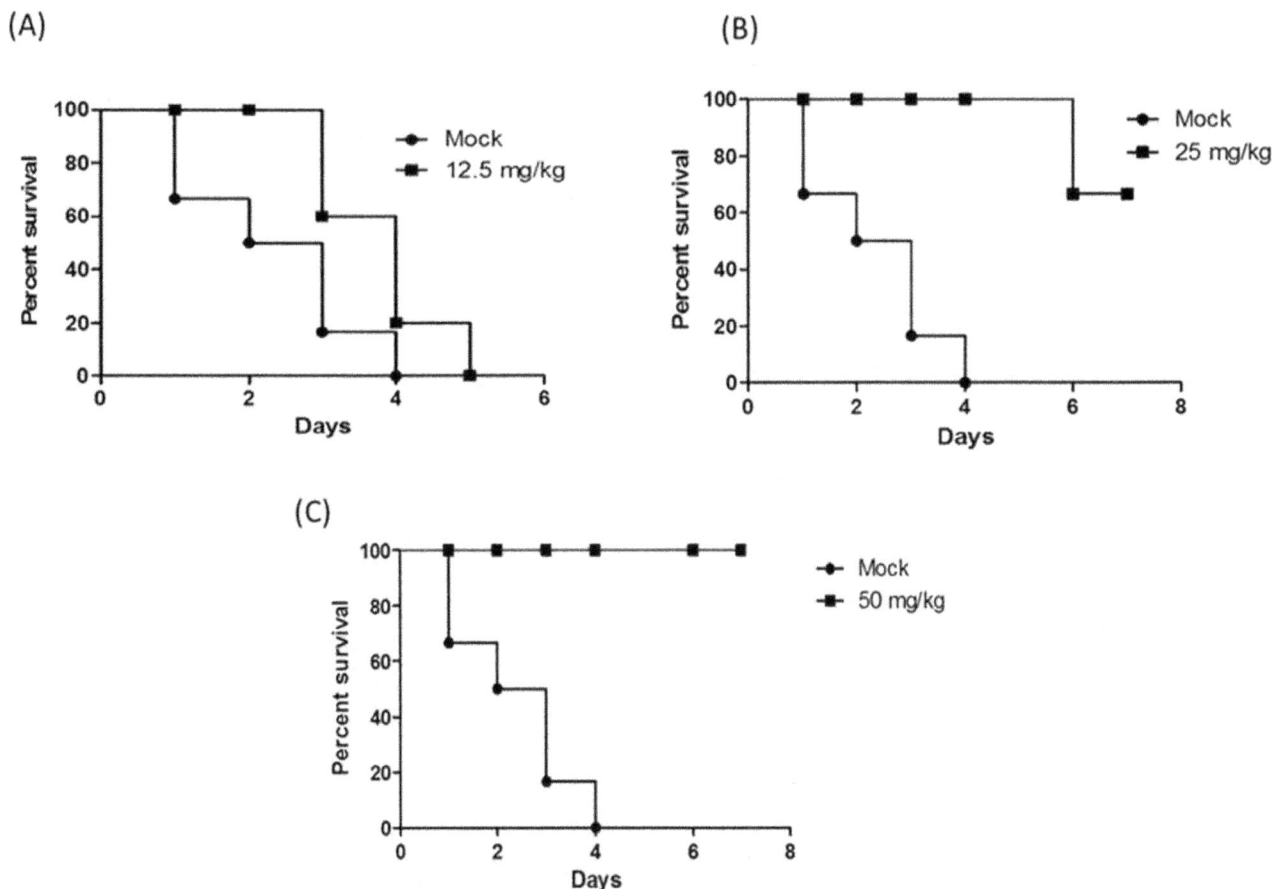

Figure 8. The percentage of survival of DENV2-challenged mice administered with peptide-fusion protein. The lethal dose of the peptide- fusion protein that kills 50 percent of the animals (LD_{50}) was evaluated to be more than 50 mg/kg. Then, four groups of the animals (n = 6) were inoculated with 4×10^3 plaque-forming units (PFU) of the purified DENV2 (DENV2-isolate Malaysia M2, GenBank Toxonomy No.: 11062) and treated with 12.5, 25 and 50 mg/kg of the peptide-fusion protein by intraperitoneal administration; while the forth group was treated with PBS as a mock-administrated group. (A), (B) and (C) The survival percentage of the animals that were administrated with 12.5, 25 and 50 mg/kg of the peptide-fusion protein respectively, compared with the mock-administrated group. Kaplan- Meier analysis was performed to generate survival curves with Prism software 5.01 (GraphPad Software, San Diego, CA).

exhibited significant antiviral efficacy against DENV2 propagation in the mice when the drug was intraperitoneally administered. These encouraging results warrant a need to further examine the efficacy of the peptide-fusion protein against dengue serotypes in sub-human primates, in which antiviral efficacy might be expected owing to the outstanding similarities with human in sites of virus replication.

In conclusion, individually MAP30, PG1 and PLSN showed considerable inhibition potential against dengue NS2B-NS3pro and dengue replication in cell culture. This activity was synergistically amplified in the recombinant peptide-fusion PG1-MAP30-PLSN protein. Our works suggests that identifying novel peptide-fusion protein with anti-dengue activity could lead to improved prevention and/or treatment strategies towards dengue infection. This finding could pave the way to the successful development of therapeutic anti-dengue agents.

Supporting Information

Data S1 Peptide fusion protein and DNA sequences and oligos design and characteristics that were used for DNA construction.

Table S1 Design and characteristics of the oligos that were used to construct the peptide-fusion protein (PG1-MAP30-PLSN).

Author Contributions

Conceived and designed the experiments: HAR. Performed the experiments: HAR HB. Analyzed the data: HAR RY. Contributed reagents/materials/analysis tools: HAR HB. Wrote the paper: HAR ZM NAR RY.

References

1. Rigau-Pérez JG, Clark GG, Gubler DJ, Reiter P, Sanders EJ, et al. (1998) Dengue and dengue haemorrhagic fever. The Lancet 352 (9132): 971–977.
2. Monath TP (1994) Dengue: the risk to developed and developing countries. Proc Natl Acad Sci U S A 91: 2395–2400.
3. Gubler DJ (2002) Epidemic dengue/dengue hemorrhagic fever as a public health, social and economic problem in the 21st century. Trends Microbiol10: 100–103.
4. Botting C, Kuhn RJ (2012) Novel approaches to flavivirus drug discovery. Expert Opin Drug Discov 7: 417–428.

5. Gubler DJ (2002) Epidemic dengue/dengue hemorrhagic fever as a public health, social and economic problem in the 21st century. Trends Microbiol10: 100–103.
6. The World Bank data, country and landing groups, country classification table. Available: http://data.worldbank.org/about/country-classifications/country-and-lending-groups. Accessed 2013 July 15.
7. Hotez PJ (2011) New antipoverty drugs, vaccines, and diagnostics: a research agenda for the US President's Global Health Initiative (GHI). PLoS Negl Trop Dis 5(5): 1133. doi:10.1371/journal.pntd.0001133
8. Peeling RW, Artsob H, Pelegrino JL, Buchy P, Cardosa MJ, et al. (2010) Evaluation of diagnostic tests: dengue. Nature Rev Microbiol S30–S37. doi:10.1038/nrmicro2459
9. Zasloff M (2002) Antimicrobial peptides of multicellular organisms. Nature 415: 389–395.
10. Mygind PH, Fischer RL, Schnorr KM, Hansen MT, Sonksen CP, et al. (2005) Plectasin is a peptide antibiotic with therapeutic potential from a saprophytic fungus. Nature 437, 975–980.
11. David JC, David PF, Spiros L, David P (2013) The Future of Peptide-based Drugs Chem Biol Drug Des 81: 136–147.
12. Schmidt AG, Yang PL, Harrison SC (2010) Peptide inhibitors of dengue-virus entry target a late-stage fusion intermediate. PLoS Pathog. doi: 10.1371/journal.ppat.1000851
13. Rothan HA, Abdulrahman AY, Sasikumer PG, Othman S, Rahman NA, et al. (2012) Protegrin-1 inhibits dengue NS2B-NS3 serine protease and viral replication in MK2 cells. J Biomed Biotechnol 25: 1482.
14. Lai JR, Huck BR, Weisblum B, Gellman SH (2002) Design of non-cysteine-containing antimicrobial β-hairpins: structure-activity relationship studies with linear protegrin- 1 analogues. Biochem 41: 12835–12842.
15. Rothan HA, Han HC, Ramasamy TS, Othman S, Rahman NA, et al. (2012) Inhibition of dengue NS2B-NS3 protease and viral replication in Vero cells by recombinant retrocyclin-1. BMC Infect Dis 12: 314.
16. Rothan HA, Mohamed Z, Rahman NA, Yusof R (2013) Anti-viral cationic peptides as a strategy for innovation in global health therapeutics for dengue virus: high yield production of the biologically active recombinant plectasin peptide. OMICS J Integr Biol 17. doi: 10.1089/omi.2013.0056
17. Heiker JT, Klöting N, Bluher M, Beck-Sickinger AG (2010) Access to gram scale amounts of functional globular adiponectin from E. coli inclusion bodies by alkaline-shock solubilization. Biochem Biophys Res Commun. 16, 398(1): 32–37. doi:10.1016/j.bbrc.2010.06.020
18. Lee-Huang S, Huang PL, Chen HC, Bourinbaiar A, Huang HI, et al. (1995) Anti-HIV and anti-tumor activities of recombinant MAP30 from bitter melon. Gene 161: 151–156.
19. Kokryakov VN, Harwig SSL, Panyutich EA, Shevchenko AA, Aleshina GM, et al. (1993) Protegrins: leukocyte antimicrobial peptides that combine features of corticostatic defensins and tachyplesins. FEBS Letters 327 (2): 231–236.
20. Miyasaki KT, Lehrer RI (1998) β-sheet antibiotic peptides as potential dental therapeutics. Int J Antimicrob Agents 9 (4): 269–280.
21. Schmitz J, Holzgrabe U (2010) Plectasin: a new peptide antibiotic with high therapeutic potential. Pharm Unserer Zeit 39: 336–338.
22. Lee-Huang S, Huang PL, Nara PL, Chen HC, Kung HF, et al. (1990) MAP 30: a new inhibitor of HIV-1 infection and replication. FEBS Lett. 272: 12–18.
23. Wang YX, Neamati N, Jacob J, Palmer I, Stahl SJ, et al. (1999) Solution structure of anti-HIV-1 and anti-tumor protein MAP30: structural insights into its multiple functions. Cell 99: 433–442.
24. Puigb P, Guzmn E, Romeu A, Garcia-Vallv S (2007) OPTIMIZER: A web server for optimizing the codon usage of DNA sequences. Nucleic Acids Research 35: 126–131.
25. Puigb P, Romeu A, Garcia-Vallv S (2008) HEG-DB: a data base of predict highly expressed genes in prokaryotic complete genomes under translational selection. Nucleic Acids Research 36: 524–527.
26. Holowachuk EW, Ruhoff MS (1995) Efficient gene synthesis by Klenow assembly/extension-Pfu polymerase amplification (KAPPA) of overlapping oligonucleotides. Genome Res 4: 299–302.
27. Sijwali PS, Brinen L, Rosenthal PJ (2001) Systematic optimization of expression and refolding of the Plasmodium falciparum cysteine protease falcipain-2. Protein Expr Purif 22: 128–134.
28. Yusof R, Clum S, Wetzel M, Murthy HM, Padmanabhan R (2000) Purified NS2B/NS3 serine protease of dengue virus type 2 exhibits cofactor NS2B dependence for cleavage of substrates with dibasic amino acids in vitro. J Biol Chem 275: 9963–9969.
29. Yon C, Teramoto T, Mueller N, Phelan J, Ganesh VK, et al. (2005) Modulation of the nucleoside triphosphatase/RNA helicase and 5'-RNA triphosphatase activities of Dengue virus type 2 nonstructural protein 3 (NS3) by interaction with NS5, the RNA-dependent RNA polymerase. J Biol Chem 280: 27412–27419.
30. Atienzar FA, Tilmant K, Gerets HH, Toussaint G, Speeckaert S, et al. (2011) The use of real-time cell analyzer technology in drug discovery: defining optimal cell culture conditions and assay reproducibility with different adherent cellular models. J Biomol Screen 16(6): 2011. doi: 10.1177/1087057111402825
31. Saida F, Uzan M, Odaert B, Bontems F (2006) Expression of highly toxic genes in E. coli: special strategies and genetic tools. Curr Protein Pept Sci 7(1): 47–56.
32. Tang YQ, Yuan J, Osapay G, Ösapay K, Tran D, et al. (1999) A cyclic antimicrobial peptide produced in primate leukocytes by the ligation of two truncated α-Defensins. Science 286: 498–502.
33. Chanprapaph S, Saparpakorn P, Sangma C, Niyomrattanakit P, Hannongbua S, et al. (2005) Competitive inhibition of the dengue virus NS3 serine protease by synthetic peptides representing polyprotein cleavage site. Biochem Biophys Res Commun 33: 1237–1246.
34. Stocks CE, Lobigs M (1998) Signal peptidase cleavage at the flavivirus C-prM junction: dependence on the viral NS2B-3 protease for efficient processing requires determinants in C, the signal peptide, and prM. J Virol 72: 2141–2149.
35. Erbel P, Schiering N, D'Arcy A, Renatus M, Kroemer M, et al. (2006) Structural basis for the activation of flaviviralNS3 proteases from dengue and West Nile virus. Nat Struct Mol Biol 13: 372–373.
36. Zhang H, Curreli F, Zhang X, Bhattacharya S, Waheed AA, et al. (2011) Antiviral activity of a-helical stapled peptides designed from the HIV-1 capsid dimerization domain. Retrovirol 8, 28. doi: 10.1186/1742-4690-8-28
37. Tamamura H, Murakami T, Horiuchi S, Sugihara K, Otaka A, et al. (1995) Synthesis of protegrin-related peptides and their antibacterial and anti-human immunodeficiency virus activity. Chemical and Pharmaceutical Bulletin 43: 853–858.
38. Bourinbaiar AS, Lee-Huang S (1996) The activity of plant-derived antiretroviral proteins MAP30 and GAP31 against herpes simplex virus in vitro. Biochem Biophys Res Commun. 219: 923–929.
39. Lee-Huang S, Huang PL, Bourinbaiar AS, Chen HC, Kung HF (1995) Inhibition of the integrase of human immunodeficiency virus (HIV) type 1 by anti-HIV plant proteins MAP30 and GAP31. Proc Natl Acad Sci USA 92: 8818–8822.
40. Sun Y, Huang PL, Li JJ, Huang YQ, Zhang L, et al. (2001) Anti-HIV agent MAP30 modulates the expression profile of viral and cellular genes for proliferation and apoptosis in AIDS-related lymphoma cells infected with Kaposi's sarcoma-associated virus. Biochem Biophys Res Commun 287: 983–994.
41. Munk C, Wei G, Yang OO, Waring AJ, Wang W, et al. (2003) The theta-defensin, retrocyclin, inhibits HIV-1 entry. AIDS Res Hum Retroviruses 19: 875–881.
42. Hazrati E, Galen B, Lu W, Wang W, Ouyang Y, et al. (2006) Human alpha- and beta-defensins block multiple steps in herpes simplex virus infection. J Immunol 177: 8658–8666.
43. Fang EF, Zhang CZ, Wong JH, Shen JY, Li CH (2012) The MAP30 protein from bitter gourd (Momordica charantia) seeds promotes apoptosis in liver cancer cells in vitro and in vivo. Cancer Lett. 1, 66–74. doi: 10.1016/j.canlet.2012.05.005
44. Lee-Huang S, Huang PL, Chen HC, Bourinbaiar A, Huang HI, et al. (1995) Anti-HIV and anti-tumor activities of recombinant MAP30 from bitter melon. Gene 161: 151–156.
45. Chambers TJ, Nestorowicz A, Amberg SM, Rice CM (1993) Mutagenesis of the yellow fever virus NS2B protein: effects on proteolytic processing, NS2B-NS3 complex formation, and viral replication. J Virol 67: 6797–6807.

6

The Prevalence and Endemic Nature of Dengue Infections in Guangdong, South China: An Epidemiological, Serological, and Etiological Study from 2005–2011

Ru-ning Guo[1], Jin-yan Lin[2], Lin-hui Li[1], Chang-wen Ke[3], Jian-feng He[4]*, Hao-jie Zhong[4], Hui-qiong Zhou[3], Zhi-qiang Peng[4], Fen Yang[4], Wen-jia Liang[4]

1 Public Health Emergency management office, Center for Disease Control and Prevention of Guangdong Province, Guangzhou, China, 2 Center for Disease Control and Prevention of Guangdong Province, Guangzhou, China, 3 Institute of Pathogenic Microorganisms, Center for Disease Control and Prevention of Guangdong Province, Guangzhou, China, 4 Institute of Infectious Disease Prevention and Control, Center for Disease Control and Prevention of Guangdong Province, Guangzhou, China

Abstract

Objectives: Frequent outbreaks of dengue are considered to be associated with an increased risk for endemicity of the disease. The occurrence of a large number of indigenous dengue cases in consecutive years indicates the possibility of a changing dengue epidemic pattern in Guangdong, China.

Methods: To have a clear understanding of the current dengue epidemic, a retrospective study of epidemiological profile, serological response, and virological features of dengue infections from 2005–2011 was conducted. Case data were collected from the National Notifiable Infectious Diseases Reporting Network. Serum samples were collected and prepared for serological verification and etiological confirmation. Incidence, temporal and spatial distribution, and the clinical manifestation of dengue infections were analyzed. Pearson's Chi-Square test was used to compare incidences between different age groups. A seroprevalence survey was implemented in local healthy inhabitants to obtain the overall positive rate for the specific immunoglobulin (Ig) G antibody against dengue virus (DENV).

Results: The overall annual incidence rate was 1.87/100000. A significant difference was found in age-specific incidence (Pearson's Chi-Square value 498.008, P<0.001). Children under 5 years of age had the lowest incidence of 0.28/100000. The vast majority of cases presented with a mild manifestation typical to dengue fever. The overall seroprevalence of dengue IgG antibody in local populations was 2.43% (range 0.28%–5.42%). DENV-1 was the predominant serotype in circulation through the years, while all 4 serotypes were identified in indigenous patients from different outbreak localities since 2009.

Conclusions: A gradual change in the epidemic pattern of dengue infection has been observed in recent years in Guangdong. With the endemic nature of dengue infections, the transition from a monotypic to a multitypic circulation of dengue virus in the last several years will have an important bearing on the prevention and control of dengue in the province and in the neighboring districts.

Editor: Jose Antonio Stoute, Pennsylvania State University College of Medicine, United States of America

Funding: The study was supported by Research Base of Key Laboratory of Surveillance and Early-warning on Infectious Disease in China CDC, Health department of Guangdong province (project number: C2012017), and also supported by Public Health Emergency Management and Filed Epidemiology Training Program of key medical subjects of 'Twelfth Five Year Plan' in Guangdong, China. The funders had no role in study design, data collection and analysis, decision to publish, or preparation of the manuscript.

Competing Interests: The authors have declared that no competing interests exist.

* E-mail: hjf_2003@163.com

Introduction

Dengue is a mosquito-borne infectious disease caused by 4 distinct, but closely related serotypes of the dengue virus (DENV-1, 2, 3, 4). Coinciding with the distribution pattern of its mosquito vectors, dengue has been reported as endemic in over 100 tropical and subtropical countries of the world [1,2]. The World Health Organization currently estimates about 2.5 billion people at risk of dengue infection globally.

For an area that experiences dengue epidemics, there are often 2 patterns of infection and transmission: endemicity (one or multiple serotypes present) and non-endemicity (no virus sustained). An endemic area often has the following common features: young age groups at a greater risk of infection [3–5], co-existence of multiple serotypes of dengue virus in local areas [2,3,5,6], a higher seroprevalence of DENV antibodies (as high as 80%) in local inhabitants [3,7] compared to that in non-endemic regions [8,9], and a continuous spectrum of dengue severity identified, with children often at a higher risk of developing a severe form [3–5], whereas travelers often experience typical or mild dengue fever [10,11].

Guangdong province is located in South China, with a hot and humid sub-tropical weather. It has the highest incidence of dengue in mainland China [12]. Since the first laboratory-confirmed DENV-4 epidemic in Fo-shan of Guangdong in 1978 [12,13], periodical infections and transmission of all 4 serotypes of dengue have been recorded in the past 30 years [12]. However, DENV-1 has become the most prevalent serotype in circulation since 1990 [12], causing epidemics and outbreaks in 1991 and from 1995–2010.

Although affected localities seemingly varied alternatively by year [14,15], frequent outbreaks may influence the transmission dynamics and facilitate the endemic process [12,16]. Epidemiological and limited phylogenetic analysis of virus isolates from 1979–2005 showed that dengue epidemics in Guangdong were closely associated with those in Southeast Asian countries, especially Philippines, Indonesia, and Thailand, indicating that dengue infections in Guangdong were still largely triggered by cases imported from overseas [14,17,18].

However, the circulation of DENV-1 over consecutive years in Guangdong reminds us of the possibility of a changing profile of dengue epidemic and endemicity in Guangdong as a large number of locally acquired dengue cases were consistently reported among the inhabitants [19–21]. The transition of a dengue epidemic pattern from non-endemic to hypo-endemic (one serotype present), or even hyper-endemic (multiple serotype present), might have been underway in Guangdong [21]. Evidenced-based epidemiological, serological, and virological studies are needed to illustrate this issue.

As a notifiable infectious disease in China, the prevention and control of dengue has been given high priority in Guangdong since 1978. Nevertheless, routine active surveillance was not conducted until 2003, and prior to 2003, dengue control relied almost solely on subsequent vector control and passive reporting and management of the patients. In 2005, virus monitoring in patients and serology surveillance targeted at healthy populations were initiated. On the basis of the surveillance results from the last 8 years in combination with earlier findings, our study aims to improve our understanding of the current epidemiological characteristics of dengue infections in Guangdong, South China, to evaluate the endemicity issue of dengue that has been posed by researchers since 2005.

Materials and Methods

Study area

Guangdong province is located in South China with typical hot and humid sub-tropical weather. It has an area of 179.8 thousand square kilometers and is divided into 4 regions: Pearl-River-Delta Area (PRDA, containing 10 prefectures), East Area (EA, containing 4 prefectures), West Area (WA, containing 3 prefectures), and Mountain Area (MA, containing 5 prefectures). Comprising a population of 104.3 million people, including millions of foreigners (2010 census data), and being located adjacent to Hong Kong and Macao Special Administrative Region, Guangdong has frequent economic and cultural communication with Southeast Asia and countries bordering the Western Pacific Ocean. Being a coastally developed district, Guangdong is also the transportation hub between mainland China and abroad. Therefore, Guangdong, with the most densely populated urban environment and a largely mobile population, has the natural and social conditions for mosquito vector breeding and reproduction. *Aedes albopictus*, as the primary vector, occupies the majority of the prefectures and counties in Guangdong, while the secondary vector—*Aedes aegypti*—only occupies one prefecture of Guangdong [12].

Case data collection and specimen detection

Data from dengue cases from 2005–2011 were collected from the National Notifiable Infectious Diseases Reporting Network that was established in 2003. A suspected case was identified either by clinical doctors in medical institutions or by field epidemiologists during active case searching when outbreaks or epidemics occurred. Serum samples were collected and sent to the local prefectural Center for Disease Control and prevention for further serology verification and/or etiology confirmation. For acute-phase sera collected within 5 days of onset, TaKaRa One Step Prime Script TM reverse-transcriptase polymerase chain reaction (RT-PCR) kit (Perfect Real Time) was used for nucleic acid detection, and C6/36 or Baby Hamster Kidney (BHK21) cells (Shanghai Bioleaf Biotech Co., Ltd, China) were used for virus culture and isolation. RT-PCR was used for further subtype identification. The detection step was performed according to the manufacturer instructions. For sera collected beyond 5 days of onset, a dengue immunoglobulin (Ig) M/IgG enzyme-linked immunoassay kit (Zhong-shan Biological Engineering Co., Ltd., China) was used for antibody IgM/IgG testing. Convalescent sera (10–14 days) were also required for IgM/IgG verification.

A face-to-face case survey with a detailed structured questionnaire was administered to each suspected patient by well-trained field investigators to obtain the following information: age, sex, occupation, address, exact dates of onset and sampling, clinical presentation and duration, travel history, and mosquito bite exposure 2 weeks prior to symptom onset. When clusters of cases outnumbered 50, for practical purposes, the index case (clinically or epidemiologically), severe cases, and the first 50 patients of a cluster were administered the detailed questionnaire survey, and additional patients received a simpler form of the questionnaire that only obtained the primary demographic, clinical, and epidemiologic exposure information, according to the Provincial Dengue Surveillance and Prevention and Control Guideline.

A suspected, probable, or confirmed case of dengue was determined according to Dengue Diagnostic Criteria enacted by the China Health Criteria Committee in 2005, as outlined below. I. A suspected case is defined by the presence of clinical manifestations and epidemiologic exposure history (stay and mosquito bite history in the dengue-affected area within 2 weeks before the onset of illness). II. A probable case of dengue is defined as a suspected case meeting with the following 2 conditions: low white blood cell and platelet counts, and single serum positive for specific IgM or IgG antibodies. III. A confirmed case of dengue is defined as a probable case presenting with any of the following lab test results: a 4-fold increase in specific IgG antibody titer, positive result on a PCR test or a virus isolation and identification test. In addition, an outbreak is confirmed as the occurrence of 3 epidemiologically linked cases within 2 weeks in a limited area, according to the National Dengue Surveillance and Prevention and Control Guideline. To distinguish cases with different origins of infection, an imported case was defined as a patient who recently travelled to dengue epidemic/endemic countries 2 weeks prior to symptom onset. An indigenous case was defined as a patient whose source of infection was clearly in local areas within China, as opposed to imported cases.

Seroprevalence study in healthy population

To assess the extent of dengue virus exposure in the population, a seroprevalence survey was conducted in healthy inhabitants from

2003 to 2011. Taking into consideration the infection history, and simultaneously accounting for other factors, such as geographical location, economic development, degree of urbanization and adherence to a surveillance program, 4 sentinel cities in Guangdong province were selected, including Guangzhou and Zhong-shan city in PRDA, Zhanjiang city in WA, and Shantou city in EA, which are all high-risk areas for dengue epidemic. With an expected seroprevalence of 5% (range, 1.1%–7.7%) in a non-endemic or hypo-endemic dengue area [9,22,23], an allowable error of 25%, and a significance level of 0.1, a sample size of 800 sera was predicted to be necessary by the simple random sampling method.

The seroprevalence survey was conducted twice a year, in April–May (pre-epidemic) and in December–January (after-epidemic). The epidemic season for dengue was considered to be July–October, during which time a strong association was observed between vector mosquito density and dengue incidence [14].

Two hundred sera samples from healthy local inhabitants (with no specific age requirements) were randomly collected during physical examination of the population in community clinics each sentinel year. A total of over 800 specimens were prepared and analyzed for specific IgG antibodies against DENV throughout recent years (except in 2003 and 2004, as a standardized surveillance was not performed until 2005). An IgG ELISA Kit (Zhong-shan Biological Engineering Co., Ltd., China) was used to test for the IgG antibody targeting serotypes 1, 2, 3, and 4. The sensitivity and specificity of the IgG ELISA Kit was determined to be over 95% [24]. The detection step was performed according to the manufacturer instructions.

Statistical analysis

The database of dengue cases in 2005–2011 was set up using Epi data software and was used for descriptive epidemiological analysis. The annual incidence of dengue infections was obtained by using new cases of dengue identified that year as the numerator and mid-year population in the corresponding year as the denominator. Age-specific cumulative incidences were calculated by using the total new cases identified during 2005–2011 as the numerator, and the mean population during the period as the denominator. Pearson's Chi-Square test was used to compare incidences between different age groups. The positive rate for specific IgG antibodies against DENV was calculated.

Ethical statements

The ethical review committees of the Center for Disease Control and Prevention of Guangdong province granted the ethical approval for this study. Under the premise of ensuring no violation of the Declaration of Helsinki for the protection of human subjects, oral informed consent was obtained from each suspected dengue patient whose serum sample was collected. For the suspected patients who were minors/children, informed consent was obtained from their guardians (parents, next of kin, or caretakers). An oral consent form was adopted, as the collection of sera samples is the routine and necessary clinical diagnostic test for dengue infections, as well as a normal public health response. Participants fully understood the significance of the blood collection procedure and its implied risks, as directly reflected and documented in the corresponding case investigation form. Written informed consent was obtained from each subject who participated in the seroprevalence study for the dengue IgG antibody. The whole process, along with the case investigation, did not reveal the participants' personal information; patients' privacy, confidentiality, rights, and interests were not violated.

Results

Age-specific incidences: no higher incidence found in younger individuals

A total of 1779 dengue cases were reported between 2005 and 2011. Teenagers and adults aged 10–59 years accounted for 86.73% of the total patients (1543/1779). The overall incidence rate was 1.87/100,000. A significant difference was found between age-specific incidences (Pearson's Chi-Square value, 498.008; P<0.001). Adults 30–39 years of age had the highest incidence of 3.55/100,000, followed by those 20–29 years old (2.87/ 100,000), 40–49 years old (2.63/100,000), and 60–69 years old (2.28/100,000). Young children under 5 years of age had the lowest incidence of 0.28/100,000 (Figure 1).

Temporal and spatial patterns: co-existence of imported cases and indigenous cases

In total, 176 cases (9.89%) were imported and 1603 cases (90.11%) were indigenous. Imported cases were detected throughout the year with a sporadic distribution pattern, whereas indigenous cases were concentrated in July–November during which period 99.06% (1588/1603) of the indigenous cases occurred. A spatial distribution analysis of indigenous cases found that 71.9% (1153/1603) of these cases were identified in PDRA, with the metropolis capital city Guangzhou as a high-risk center (comprising 55.1%, 884/1603). Zhan-jiang prefecture in WA and Shan-tou prefecture in EA were the other 2 clustered areas, respectively accounting for 12.8% (205/1603) and 11.2% (179/ 1603; Figures 2 and 3).

Clinical features: the vast majority of cases presented with symptoms of mild and typical dengue fever

A total of 686 dengue patients who were administered the detailed questionnaires underwent clinical spectrum analysis. The majority of these patients presented with typical or mild manifestations, with a sudden fever (98.4%), headache (72.2%), myalgia (51.0%), and rash (39.6%) being the primary clinical symptoms. The mean axillary temperature was 38.9°C. In total, 81.4% (322/394) of the patients had leukopenia and 71.4% (275/ 385) had thrombocytopenia (Figure 4).

There were a small number of severe cases that presented with epistaxis (2.3%), hematemesis (1.8%), blood in the stool (1.8%), hematuria (1.4%), dental bleeding (1.4%), coma (0.3%), and shock (0.2%); however, no cases of dengue hemorrhagic fever, dengue shock syndrome [22,23], or death were reported between 2005–2011.

Seroprevalence of DENV specific IgG in healthy population

A total of 5,586 sera samples from local healthy inhabitants were collected during 2003–2011 in Guangdong. The overall positive rate of IgG antibody was 2.43% (136/5586). The year 2007 had the highest rate of 5.42% (45/830), followed by 2003 with 4.81% (9/187), 2008 with 2.91% (29/995), and 2004 with 2.65% (18/680). For all other years, the IgG antibody positivity rate remained below 2%. Two small conspicuous peaks were observed, in 2003 and 2007, followed by a diminishing trend in the other years (Figure 5).

Etiological surveillance results

A total of 1603 indigenous cases were detected from 2006 to 2011. Only imported cases were identified in 2005. Of the 337 acute-phase sera analyzed, 188 were positive for virus isolation or

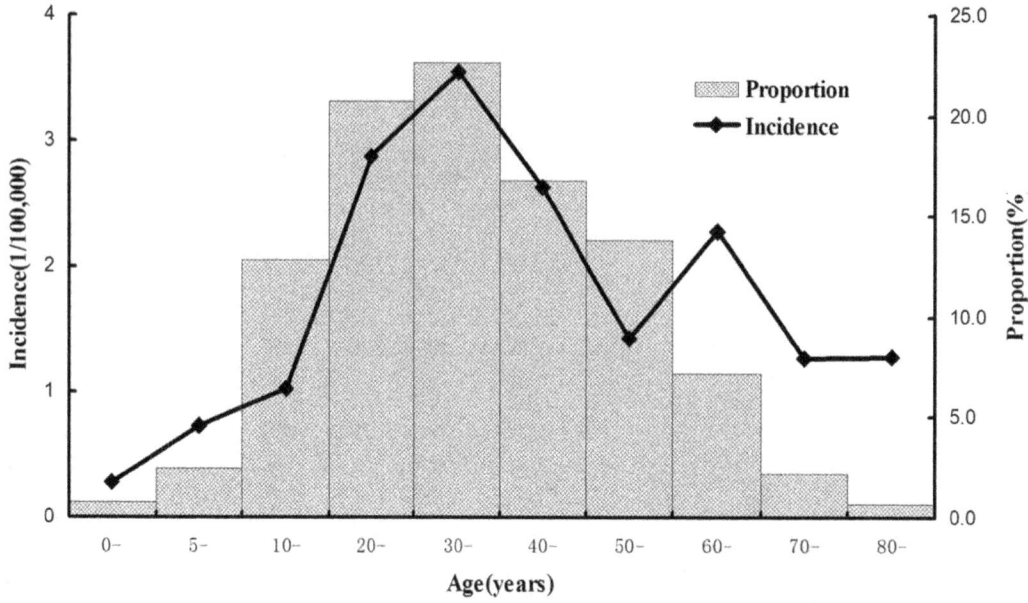

Figure 1. Age-specific incidence of dengue infections in Guangdong, China, 2005–2011. Incidences were indicated with the line chart. The proportion of age-specific cases to the total number was shown with the bar chart.

PCR nucleic acid detection. DENV-1 was the predominant serotype in 78.2% of positive specimens (147/188). Before 2009, DENV-1 was the only serotype detected in indigenous dengue cases, except in 2001 when DENV-1 and DENV-2 were both isolated in different prefectures of Guangdong. From 2009 to 2012, all 4 serotypes (DENV-1, DENV-2, DENV-3, and DENV-4) were derived from autonomous patients from different outbreak localities (as of September 15, 2012; Figure 6).

Discussion

Our epidemiological, serological, and etiological study during 2005–2011 provided a good understanding of the current epidemiological situation of dengue infections in Guangdong. In spite of the exposure to a weak force of infection, as reflected in the low seroprevalence of the IgG antibody, the predominant circulation of DENV-1 for consecutive years and the co-existence of multiple serotypes since 2009 indicates the endemicity of dengue infections in Guangdong.

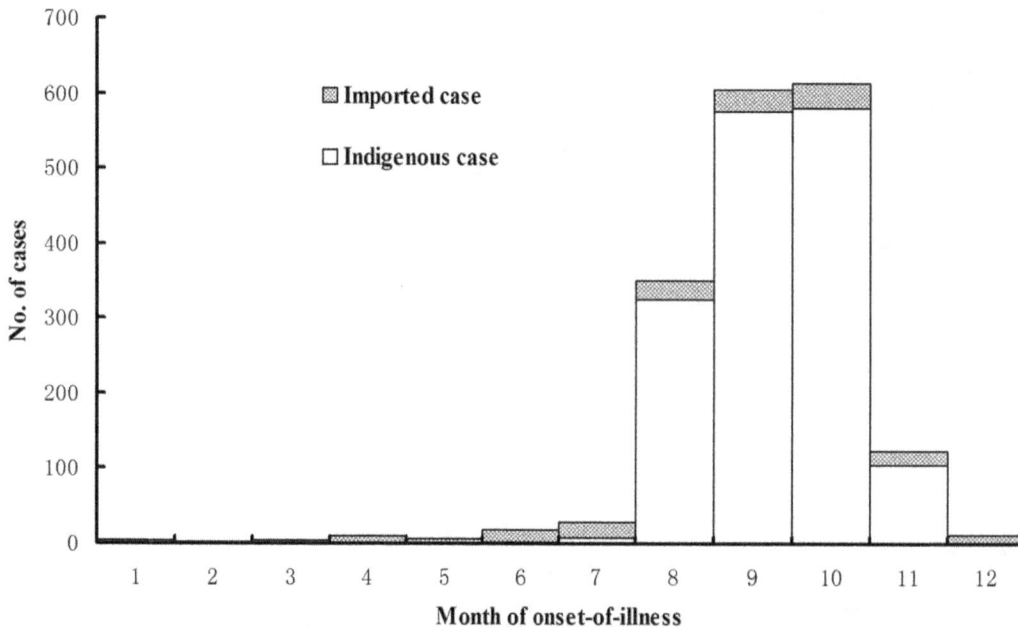

Figure 2. Onset month of dengue cases by infection origin in Guangdong, China, 2005–2011. Imported and indigenous dengue cases were shown with the stacked bar chart using different filling patterns.

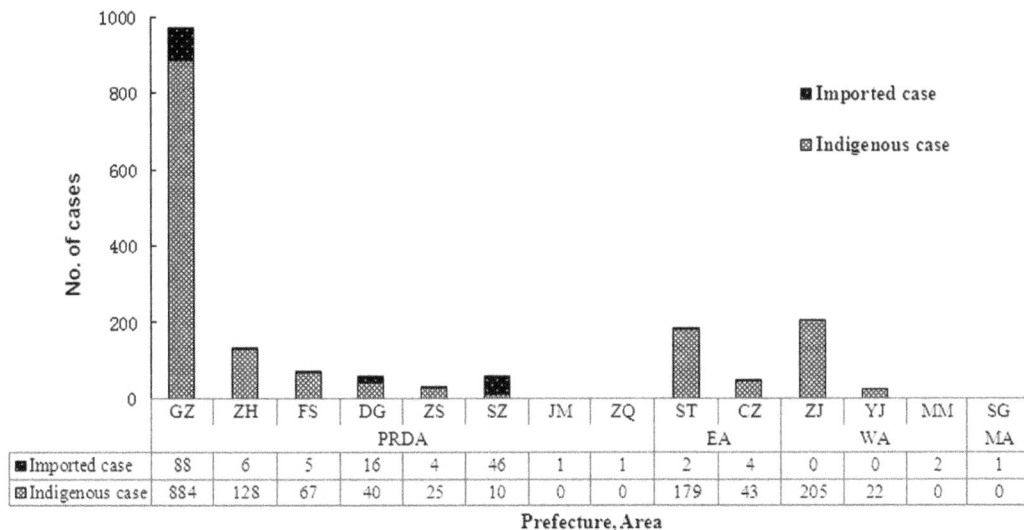

Prefecture, Area	PRDA								EA		WA		MA	
	GZ	ZH	FS	DG	ZS	SZ	JM	ZQ	ST	CZ	ZJ	YJ	MM	SG
■ Imported case	88	6	5	16	4	46	1	1	2	4	0	0	2	1
▨ Indigenous case	884	128	67	40	25	10	0	0	179	43	205	22	0	0

Figure 3. Spatial distribution of dengue cases by infection origin in Guangdong, China, 2005–2011. X-axis represents different prefectures (e.g. GZ,ZH,FS) and areas (PRDA, EA, WA, MA) of Guangdong province: Data tables were shown under the chart to display the case number of imported and indigenous cases. GZ (the metropolis capital city of Guangdong) in PRDA, ST in EA, and ZJ in WA were the top 3 clustered areas.

This study showed that there was no increased risk of acquiring dengue infections among younger individuals, and adults aged 20–59 years had a comparatively higher incidence of infection; this finding is different from the age distribution pattern observed in many dengue-endemic areas, where the shift towards a higher incidence in younger patients was reported [3,25]. However, this may still be a cause for concern, as dengue can be endemic in areas where a great number of adults are affected. It is also noteworthy that the periodic outbreaks and epidemics in Guangdong in recent years were largely led by the predominant DENV-1 serotype, which is considered to have a much lower risk of causing severe dengue compared to DENV-2, DENV-3, and DENV-4 [26,27]. This finding might explain why the vast majority of dengue infections in Guangdong presented as mild or typical dengue fever instead of severe forms of the disease.

It is notable that the years 2003 and 2007 had a relatively higher seroprevalence of IgG antibody against DENV than the other years included in this study, indicating an unusual circulation state of DENV during those years. This can be explained by the large-scale outbreaks and epidemics in preceding years (in 2002 and 2006, respectively) in PDRA, WA, and EA of Guangdong province [28,29]. Fortunately, the overall low seroprevalence of IgG antibody ($<5\%$) in healthy populations suggested the presence of an average weak force of infections in Guangdong.

The epidemic pattern of dengue in Guangdong to date is seemingly different from that in hyper-endemic areas, given the

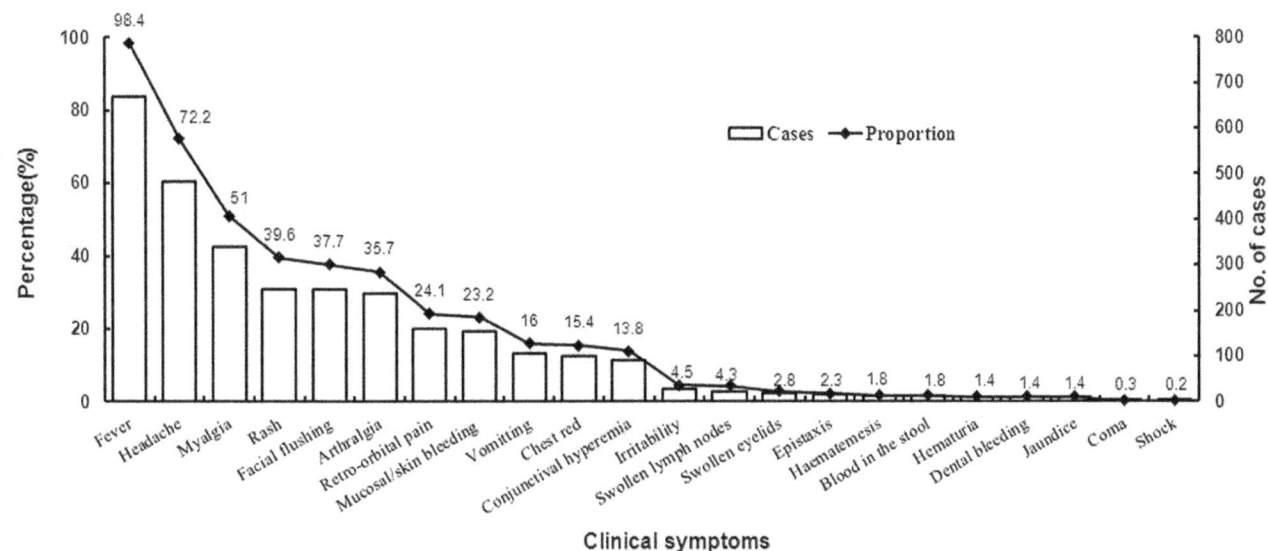

Figure 4. Clinical presentations of dengue infections in Guangdong, China, 2005–2011. Percentage of certain clinical symptom was shown with the line chart. Case number was shown with the bar chart. Data labels of percentage were appended to the line chart.

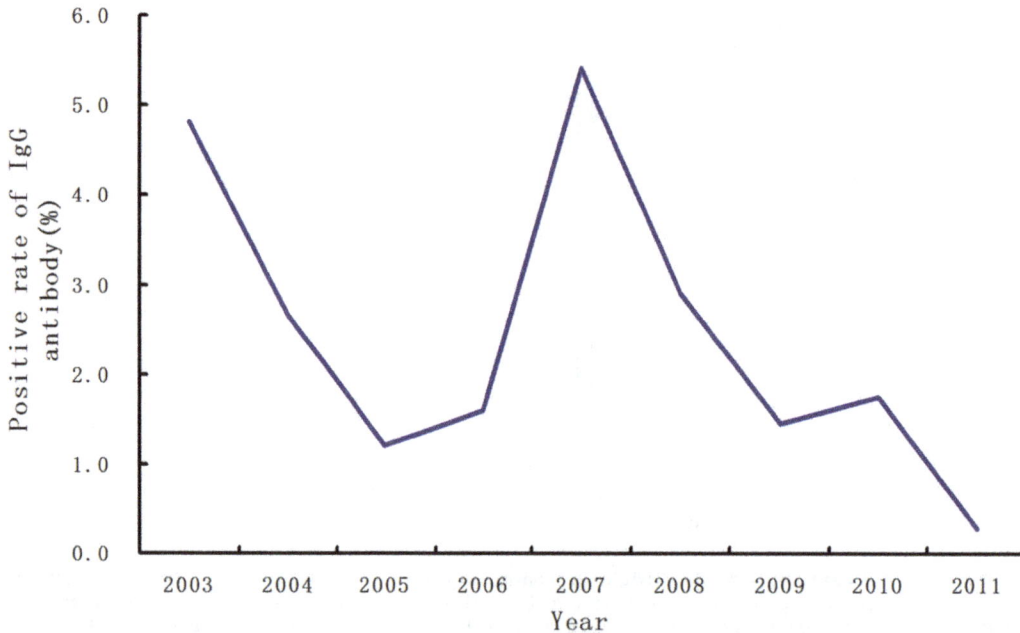

Figure 5. Seroprevalence of specific immunoglobulin (Ig) G antibody against dengue virus among healthy inhabitants. Data were collected through 2003–2011 in 4 sentinel cities of Guangdong, south China. Seroprevalence rate of IgG antibody by year was shown with the line chart. The average positive rate of IgG antibody was 2.43%.

age profile, clinical spectrum of patients, and the low seroprevalence of the dengue IgG antibody. However, the monotypic circulation state for continuous years may presage the hypo-endemicity of dengue infections. In addition, more evidence in favor of endemicity has been observed since 2009. Multiple serotypes of viruses were identified in outbreak localities [15,30–33], changing the monotypic situation led by the predominant DENV-1 serotype for 7 years (from 2002–2008). In 2010 and 2012, all 4 serotypes were detected one after another in indigenous outbreak locations.

These results remind us of the possibility of a changing circulation pattern in Guangdong, from non-endemicity (no virus sustained), to hypo-endemicity (one serotype present), and even hyper-endemicity (multiple serotype present) of dengue infections [21,34]. It is important to have a clear understanding of the current dengue epidemic in Guangdong, which is the most densely populated province in southern China, surrounded by large number of dengue-endemic countries, and which has a subtropical climate, providing the optimal environmental, social, and biological circumstances for vector mosquito breeding and reproduction

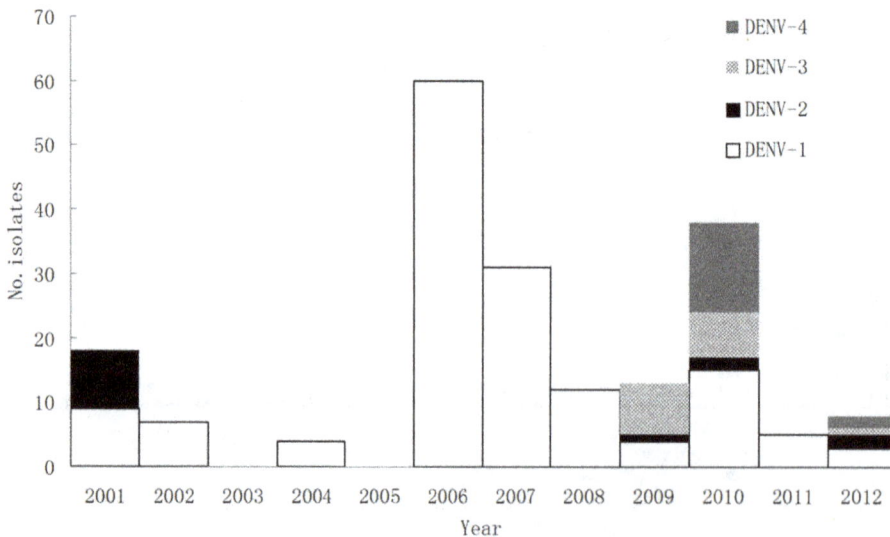

Figure 6. Serotypes of dengue virus identified in autonomous dengue patients from outbreak localities of Guangdong. Etiology data were collected from 2001 to 2012 (as of September 15, 2012). No viruses were isolated from indigenous cases in 2003 and 2005. Stacked bar chart was used to show the different serotypes of dengue viruses with different filling patterns.

[1]. The change from monotypic to multitypic circulation of DENV in previous years might have an important bearing on the epidemiology of dengue in Guangdong, especially for the capital city of Guangzhou. As the hardest hit location in terms of reported cases and clustered areas, Guangzhou is confronted with a particular challenge for the prevention and control of dengue transmission, particularly taking into account the favorable factors of a dense population and a high degree of urbanization.

Through the analysis of the characteristics of dengue infections in Guangdong, our findings affirm the endemic nature of this disease on the basis of the patients, virus, and serology surveillance in recent years. However, we have to address several limitations of our study. Firstly, patients were identified through the National Notifiable Disease Reporting Network, which mainly relies on the reporting of diseases by medical practitioners. Although this passive surveillance network covers over 99.5% of the hospitals and clinics in the province, the possible omission of cases associated with healthcare providers (due to awareness of diagnosis and reporting and a sense of responsibility) could not be completely excluded. However, the impact on the reliability of our data owing to self-reporting should be very small. Secondly, we cannot obtain age-specific seroprevalence rates for dengue, owing to the lack of age stratification during sampling. A more stringently designed serology survey (with age-stratified sampling and a bigger sample size) is needed to have a better assessment of infection status. Thirdly, the majority of sera samples were collected beyond the acute phase of dengue infection, resulting in a lack of acute-phase samples for etiology diagnostic testing; an even smaller percentage of samples were obtained for further molecular evolution analysis. Fourthly, the lack of phylogenetic analysis for viral isolates from local places and surrounding dengue-endemic countries made it difficult to understand their phylogenetic relationships and to determine the source of infections.

Although it has its limitations, our study helps to illustrate the epidemiological situation of dengue infection in Guangdong, China. Our findings describing the endemic nature in the last several years will have important implications for the prevention and control of dengue in the province. A well-designed serological and etiological surveillance program targeting patients, the healthy population, and vector mosquitos should be considered. Furthermore, phylogeographic analysis of viral isolates derived from outbreak localities in Guangdong and the surrounding Southeast Asian countries is needed to clearly determine the evolutionary relationship of dengue viruses.

Acknowledgments

The authors wish to thank all participants in local prefectural Center for Disease Control and Prevention, for their great support in data and specimens collection. Thanks also go to Dr. Benjamin M. Althouse and other anonymous reviewers for their thoughtful suggestions and insights, which have enriched the manuscript and produced a more balanced and better account of the research.

Author Contributions

Conceived and designed the experiments: RNG JYL JFH. Performed the experiments: CWK HQZ. Analyzed the data: RNG WJL FY. Contributed reagents/materials/analysis tools: LHL HJZ ZQP. Wrote the paper: RNG LHL JFH.

References

1. Kyle JL, Harris E (2008) Global spread and persistence of dengue. Annu Rev Microbiol 62: 71–92.
2. Ong SH, Yip JT, Chen YL, Liu W, Harun S, et al. (2008) Periodic re-emergence of endemic strains with strong epidemic potential - a proposed explanation for the 2004 Indonesian dengue epidemic. Infect Genet Evol 8: 191–204.
3. Rodriguez-Barraquer I, Cordeiro MT, Braga C, de Souza WV, Marques ET, et al. (2011) From re-emergence to hyperendemicity: the natural history of the dengue epidemic in Brazil. PLoS Negl Trop Dis 5: e935.
4. Siddiqui FJ, Haider SR, Bhutta ZA (2009) Endemic dengue fever: a seldom recognized hazard for Pakistani children. J Infect Dev Ctries 3: 306–312.
5. Halstead SB (2007) Dengue. Lancet 370: 1644–1652.
6. Raghwani J, Rambaut A, Holmes EC, Hang VT, Hien TT, et al. (2011) Endemic dengue associated with the co-circulation of multiple viral lineages and localized density-dependent transmission. PLoS Pathog 7: e1002064.
7. Yamashiro T, Disla M, Petit A, Taveras D, Castro-Bello M, et al. (2004) Seroprevalence of IgG specific for dengue virus among adults and children in Santo Domingo, Dominican Republic. Am J Trop Med Hyg 71: 138–143.
8. Iturrino-Monge R, Avila-Aguero ML, Avila-Aguero CR, Moya-Moya T, Canas-Coto A, et al. (2006) Seroprevalence of dengue virus antibodies in asymptomatic Costa Rican children, 2002–2003: a pilot study. Rev Panam Salud Publica 20: 39–43.
9. Vairo F, Nicastri E, Meschi S, Schepisi MS, Paglia MG, et al. (2012) Seroprevalence of dengue infection: a cross-sectional survey in mainland Tanzania and on Pemba Island, Zanzibar. Int J Infect Dis 16: e44–46.
10. Wilder-Smith A (2012) Dengue infections in travellers. Paediatr Int Child Health 32 Suppl 1: 28–32.
11. Freedman DO, Weld LH, Kozarsky PE, Fisk T, Robins R, et al. (2006) Spectrum of disease and relation to place of exposure among ill returned travelers. N Engl J Med 354: 119–130.
12. Wu JY, Lun ZR, James AA, Chen XG (2010) Dengue Fever in mainland China. Am J Trop Med Hyg 83: 664–671.
13. Huang MT, Li XD, Du F (1981) Etiological and serological study of a dengue outbreak in Foshan of Guangdong province Acta Microbiologica Sinica 21: 239–246.
14. Jian-feng H, Hui-ming L, Wenj-jia L, Kui Z, Min K, et al. (2007) Epidemic situation of dengue fever in Guangdong province, China, 1990–2005. Dengue Bulletin 31.
15. Luo L, Liang HY, Hu YS, Liu WJ, Wang YL, et al. (2012) Epidemiological, virological, and entomological characteristics of dengue from 1978 to 2009 in Guangzhou, China. J Vector Ecol 37: 230–240.
16. McBride WJ (2010) Dengue fever: is it endemic in Australia? Intern Med J 40: 247–249.
17. Luo H, He J, Zheng K, Li L, Jiang L (2002) [Analysis on the epidemiologic features of Dengue fever in Guangdong province, 1990–2000]. Zhonghua Liu Xing Bing Xue Za Zhi 23: 427–430.
18. Zheng K, Jiang L, Luo H, He J, Dong X (2002) [Nucleotide sequencing of E/NS1 gene segment of dengue type 1 viruses isolated in Guangdong Province]. Zhonghua Shi Yan He Lin Chuang Bing Du Xue Za Zhi 16: 382–384.
19. Zheng K, Zhou HQ, Yan J, Ke CW, Maeda A, et al. (2009) Molecular characterization of the E gene of dengue virus type 1 isolated in Guangdong province, China, in 2006. Epidemiol Infect 137: 73–78.
20. Jin Y, Hui-qiong Z, De W, Chan-wen K (2009) Phylogenetic analysis of the E gene of dengue virus isolated in Guangdong province from 2006–2007. CHin J Microbiol Immunol 29: 121–125.
21. Fu-chun Z, Yan-qing C, Ye-chen L, Jian W, Wan-shan C, et al. (2005) Analysis on clinical and epidemiological characteristics of 1032 patients with dengue fever in Guangzhou. CHINESE JOURNAL OF EPIDEMIOLOGY 26: 421–423.
22. Lo CL, Yip SP, Leung PH (2013) Seroprevalence of dengue in the general population of Hong Kong. Trop Med Int Health.
23. Ratnam I, Black J, Leder K, Biggs BA, Matchett E, et al. (2012) Incidence and seroprevalence of dengue virus infections in Australian travellers to Asia. Eur J Clin Microbiol Infect Dis 31: 1203–1210.
24. Hui-qiong Z, Li-min J, Kui Z, Yao-liang G, Wen-yan L, et al. (2006) Analysis on the sensitivity and specificity of the recombinant dengue antigens reacting with anti-dengue IgG-antibody. Chinese Journal of Zoonoses 22: 665–667.
25. Gupta E, Dar L, Kapoor G, Broor S (2006) The changing epidemiology of dengue in Delhi, India. Virol J 3: 92.
26. Ocazionez RE, Cortes FM, Villar LA, Gomez SY (2006) Temporal distribution of dengue virus serotypes in Colombian endemic area and dengue incidence. Re-introduction of dengue-3 associated to mild febrile illness and primary infection. Mem Inst Oswaldo Cruz 101: 725–731.
27. Ocazionez RE, Gomez SY, Cortes FM (2007) [Dengue hemorrhagic fever serotype and infection pattern in a Colombian endemic area]. Rev Salud Publica (Bogota) 9: 262–274.
28. Luo L, Yang ZC, Wang YL (2008) [Comparison on epidemic characters of dengue fever between 2002 and 2006, Guangzhou City, China]. Zhonghua Liu Xing Bing Xue Za Zhi 29: 203.
29. Yang F, Luo HM, He JF, Liang WJ (2007) dengue Epidemiological analysis of dengue in Guangdong Province, 2006 South China Journal of Preventive Medicine 33: 8–10.

30. Zhao H, Yu XD, Zhang XY, Jiang T, Hong WX, et al. (2012) Complete genome sequence of a dengue virus serotype 4 strain isolated in guangdong, china. J Virol 86: 7021–7022.

31. Jing QL, Yang ZC, Luo L, Xiao XC, Di B, et al. (2012) Emergence of dengue virus 4 genotype II in Guangzhou, China, 2010: Survey and molecular epidemiology of one community outbreak. BMC Infect Dis 12: 87.

32. Jiang T, Yu XD, Hong WX, Zhou WZ, Yu M, et al. (2012) Co-circulation of two genotypes of dengue virus serotype 3 in Guangzhou, China, 2009. Virol J 9: 125.

33. Xiao X-l, Zhan L-h, Luo X-f, Luo L, Zeng W-b, et al. (2011) Investigation of a family cluster of dengue infections caused by DENV-III in Guangzhou China tropical medicine 11: 969–970.

34. Gibbons RV, Vaughn DW (2002) Dengue: an escalating problem. BMJ 324: 1563–1566.

7

Acute Undifferentiated Febrile Illness in Rural Cambodia: A 3-Year Prospective Observational Study

Tara C. Mueller[1], Sovannaroth Siv[2], Nimol Khim[3], Saorin Kim[3], Erna Fleischmann[1], Frédéric Ariey[4], Philippe Buchy[5], Bertrand Guillard[6], Iveth J. González[7], Eva-Maria Christophel[8], Rashid Abdur[9], Frank von Sonnenburg[1], David Bell[10], Didier Menard[3]*

1 Department of Tropical Medicine and Infectious Diseases, University of Munich, Munich, Germany, 2 National Center for Parasitology, Entomology, and Malaria Control, Phnom Penh, Cambodia, 3 Malaria Molecular Epidemiology Unit, Institut Pasteur in Cambodia, Phnom Penh, Cambodia, 4 Parasitology and Mycology Department, Institut Pasteur, Paris, France, 5 Virology Unit, Institut Pasteur in Cambodia, Phnom Penh, Cambodia, 6 Medical Laboratory, Institut Pasteur in Cambodia, Phnom Penh, Cambodia, 7 Foundation for Innovative New Diagnostics (FIND), Geneva, Switzerland, 8 WHO Regional Office for the Western Pacific (WPRO), Manila, Philippines, 9 WHO Country Office, Phnom Penh, Cambodia, 10 Intellectual Ventures Laboratory, Seattle, Washington, United States of America

Abstract

In the past decade, malaria control has been successfully implemented in Cambodia, leading to a substantial decrease in reported cases. Wide-spread use of malaria rapid diagnostic tests (RDTs) has revealed a large burden of malaria-negative fever cases, for which no clinical management guidelines exist at peripheral level health facilities. As a first step towards developing such guidelines, a 3-year cross-sectional prospective observational study was designed to investigate the causes of acute malaria-negative febrile illness in Cambodia. From January 2008 to December 2010, 1193 febrile patients and 282 non-febrile individuals were recruited from three health centers in eastern and western Cambodia. Malaria RDTs and routine clinical examination were performed on site by health center staff. Venous samples and nasopharyngeal throat swabs were collected and analysed by molecular diagnostic tests. Blood cultures and blood smears were also taken from all febrile individuals. Molecular testing was applied for malaria parasites, *Leptospira*, *Rickettsia*, *O. tsutsugamushi*, Dengue- and *Influenza* virus. At least one pathogen was identified in 73.3% (874/1193) of febrile patient samples. Most frequent pathogens detected were *P. vivax* (33.4%), *P. falciparum* (26.5%), pathogenic *Leptospira* (9.4%), *Influenza* viruses (8.9%), *Dengue* viruses (6.3%), *O. tsutsugamushi* (3.9%), *Rickettsia* (0.2%), and *P. knowlesi* (0.1%). In the control group, a potential pathogen was identified in 40.4%, most commonly malaria parasites and *Leptospira*. Clinic-based diagnosis of malaria RDT-negative cases was poorly predictive for pathogen and appropriate treatment. Additional investigations are needed to understand their impact on clinical disease and epidemiology, and the possible role of therapies such as doxycycline, since many of these pathogens were seen in non-febrile subjects.

Editor: Luzia H. Carvalho, Centro de Pesquisa Rene Rachou/Fundação Oswaldo Cruz (Fiocruz-Minas), Brazil

Funding: The authors thank USAID, World Health Organization/Western Pacific Regional Office and the Foundation for Innovative New Diagnostics (FIND) for funding this study. The funders had no role in study design, data collection and analysis, decision to publish, or preparation of the manuscript.

Competing Interests: The authors have declared that no competing interests exist.

* E-mail: dmenard@pasteur-kh.org

Introduction

Fever is the main clinical symptom of various tropical infectious diseases. In rural areas of developing countries, where diagnostic facilities are limited, etiologies of acute febrile illness remain largely unknown. Malaria has long been considered the most important infectious disease in the Mekong Region in terms of public health impact and it's elimination has become an international priority with the emergence of artemisinin-resistant parasites along the Thai-Cambodian border [1]. In the past decade, the Cambodian government, with the support of the World Health Organization (WHO) Mekong Malaria Program, successfully implemented diverse strategies to control *falciparum* malaria. Over the last 13 years there was a steady reduction of around 10% per year for diagnosed cases and 8.5% for case fatality rates [2]. By 2010 the overall malaria incidence was 4.07 cases/1,000 population and the mortality rate was 0.98/100,000 population. The relative proportion of *P. vivax* cases rose among reported cases over this time, from 8% in 2000 to 37% in 2011 [3,4]. The introduction and wide use of malaria rapid diagnostic tests (RDTs), together with the declining overall malaria incidence, has raised the relative importance of non-malarial febrile illness (NMFI) in routine case management. However, the absence of clear guidelines on management of acute undifferentiated fever, and a lack of tools to diagnose non-malarial pathogens to provide information on their prevalence, has resulted in a management dilemma and the suspicion of inappropriate prescription of antimalarial and antimicrobial drugs. A number of infectious diseases such as leptospirosis, scrub typhus, rickettsial diseases, typhoid fever, dengue fever and influenza have been recognized previously among causes of NMFI in the region [5–21]. As a first step towards the development of algorithms that could guide clinical management of malaria-negative fever at the peripheral health care level, it is crucial to determine the prevalence and epidemiology of the causative pathogens.

In this context, we designed a cross-sectional prospective observational study to investigate the causes of NMFI in three rural areas of Cambodia. Our primary objective was to detect pathogens in samples taken from febrile outpatients in the remote areas where malaria persists, and where malaria RDTs are the only available diagnostic tool for health workers. We also aimed to determine priorities for diagnostic tools applicable in field conditions and guide the improvement of case management algorithms. Additionally, this study aimed to build capacity for operational research and pathology testing within Cambodia and develop a prototype study design useable in similar settings in other tropical countries.

Materials and Methods

Ethics Statement

The study protocol was reviewed and approved by the Cambodian National Ethics Committee on Health Research. An informed written consent was provided by the parents/guardians of all participants before testing. All samples were anonymized prior to laboratory testing.

Study Sites and Participants

Three outpatient health centers (HCs) in remote areas in western (Soun Kouma and Ou Chra, Pailin Province) and eastern Cambodia (Snoul, Kratie Province) were selected as study sites (Figure 1). These sites were chosen to demonstrate potential geographical differences in pathogen distribution (east and west). Pailin Province is known to be an area of low malaria transmission, whereas Kratie province is an area of intermediate transmission. Further considerations for choice of sites were availability of staff and sample transportation service which were coordinated by the National Malaria Control Program (CNM).

From January 2008 to December 2010, all male and female patients, aged from 7 to 49 years, who had an acute febrile illness (tympanic membrane temperature on admission >38.0°C, and a history of fever not longer than 8 days), and who were eligible to be tested for malaria by RDT according to the national guidelines (CareStart Malaria HRP2/pLDH (Pf/PAN) Combo G0131, Access Bio Inc. USA) were invited to participate in the study. Patients with severe illness warranting immediate transfer to a hospital were excluded.

In parallel, a group of non-febrile accompanying persons, aged 7–49 years, with a tympanic membrane temperature <38.0°C, no recent history of febrile illness, and providing written informed consent, were recruited as controls.

Field Procedures

In both groups (cases and controls groups) a physical examination and malaria RDT (CareStart Malaria HRP2/pLDH (Pf/PAN) COMBO G0131, Access Bio Inc. USA) were performed as per routine practice by the clinical staff. History of illness and results of the physical examination (for case group) were recorded on standardized and simplified forms in Cambodian language, provided by the National Malaria Control Programme (Figure S1). Whole blood (10–15 ml), a blood smear and a nasopharyngeal throat swab were collected from each study participant. Blood samples were separated immediately, with 5 ml of whole blood collected in an EDTA tube, stored at 4°C, and transported to the Institut Pasteur in Cambodia (IPC) in Phnom Penh within 24 hours. Another 5 ml of blood was centrifuged on site and the plasma stored in liquid nitrogen, as were the throat swab samples before shipment to IPC. An additional 5 ml of whole blood from febrile patients was immediately incubated in an aerobic blood culture bottle (Pharmaceutical Factory No. 2, Vientiane, Lao PDR), sent to Phnom Penh in an insulated box (with an electronic temperature monitor), and incubated and monitored at 37°C, for 5 days. The patient's data and the specimens were anonymized on site. Clinical data forms were sent to CNM where translation and data entry were performed.

Laboratory Procedures

At the IPC in Phnom Penh, EDTA blood samples were centrifuged at 2000 rpm for 10 minutes and DNA extraction was performed on 200 μl of packed blood cells, using the QIamp DNA Mini Kit (Qiagen, Hilden, Germany), according to the manufacturer's instructions. Nested-PCRs and nucleotide sequencing were applied to detect DNA sequences of *Plasmodium* (*cytb* gene [22]), *Leptospira* (*16srRNA* gene [23]), *O. tsutsugamushi* (*47 kDa* gene [24]) and *Rickettsia* (*gltA* and *ompB* genes [24]). After purification by filtration with a NucleoFast 96 PCR plate (Macherey-Nagel, Düren, Germany), sequencing reactions were performed for both strands by using the ABI Prism BigDye terminator cycle sequencing ready reaction kit run on a 3730 xl genetic analyzer (Applied Biosystems, Courtaboeuf, France). Electrophoregrams were visualized and analyzed with CEQ2000 genetic analysis system software (Beckman Coulter, Villepinte, France). Nucleotide sequences were compared to the *P. falciparum* 3D7 sequence (GenBank accession number AY282930), *Leptospira interrogans* 16sRNA sequence (GenBank accession number EU581713), *Orientia tsutsugamushi* 47 kDa sequence (GenBank accession number L11697) and *Rickettsia* sp. OmpB and GltA sequences (GenBank accession numbers EF219461 and AB444098). Plasma and throat swab samples were processed for RNA extraction using the QIamp Viral RNA Mini Kit (Qiagen, Hilden, Germany) on 200 μl of plasma and from 140 μl of throat swab-sample, according to the manufacturer's instructions. In-house multiplex Reverse-Transcriptase (RT) PCR assays were performed on plasma and throat swab RNA extracts, for detection of Dengue (*PrM/E* gene [25]) and Influenza-Virus (*M* gene [26]), respectively [27]. In case of detection of Influenza A virus, sub-typing was performed by real-time-PCR [27]. Positive and negative samples were used as controls in each run.

The thresholds of detection for each PCR/RT-PCR were assessed by using dilutions of positive controls (Table S1). External quality control assurance system was also set up between Phnom Penh and Vientiane (Lao-Oxford-Mahosot Hospital-Wellcome Trust Research Unit - LOMWRU, Microbiology Laboratory, Mahosot Hospital, Vientiane, Lao PDR). C-reactive-protein (CRP) was also quantified on plasma using latex bead immuno-turbidimetric method adapted on Integra 400 (Ref 0764930, Roche Diagnostics, Indianapolis, Ind., USA) and calibrated controls, according to the manufacturer instructions. Finally, blood smears were analyzed by a single WHO Level 1 qualified microscopist for comparative malaria diagnostics.

Patient Management

Available laboratory results which may have had a direct bearing on patient management were immediately sent back to the HCs. Immediate decisions on the use of antimalarial or antimicrobial drugs were taken by qualified personnel at the HCs as per usual practice.

Statistical Analysis

Data were entered and verified using Microsoft Excel software and analyzed using XLSTAT (Addinsoft, France) and MedCalc (MedCalc 9.1.0.1, Belgium). The Mann-Whitney U test or Kruskal-Wallis method were used for non-parametric compari-

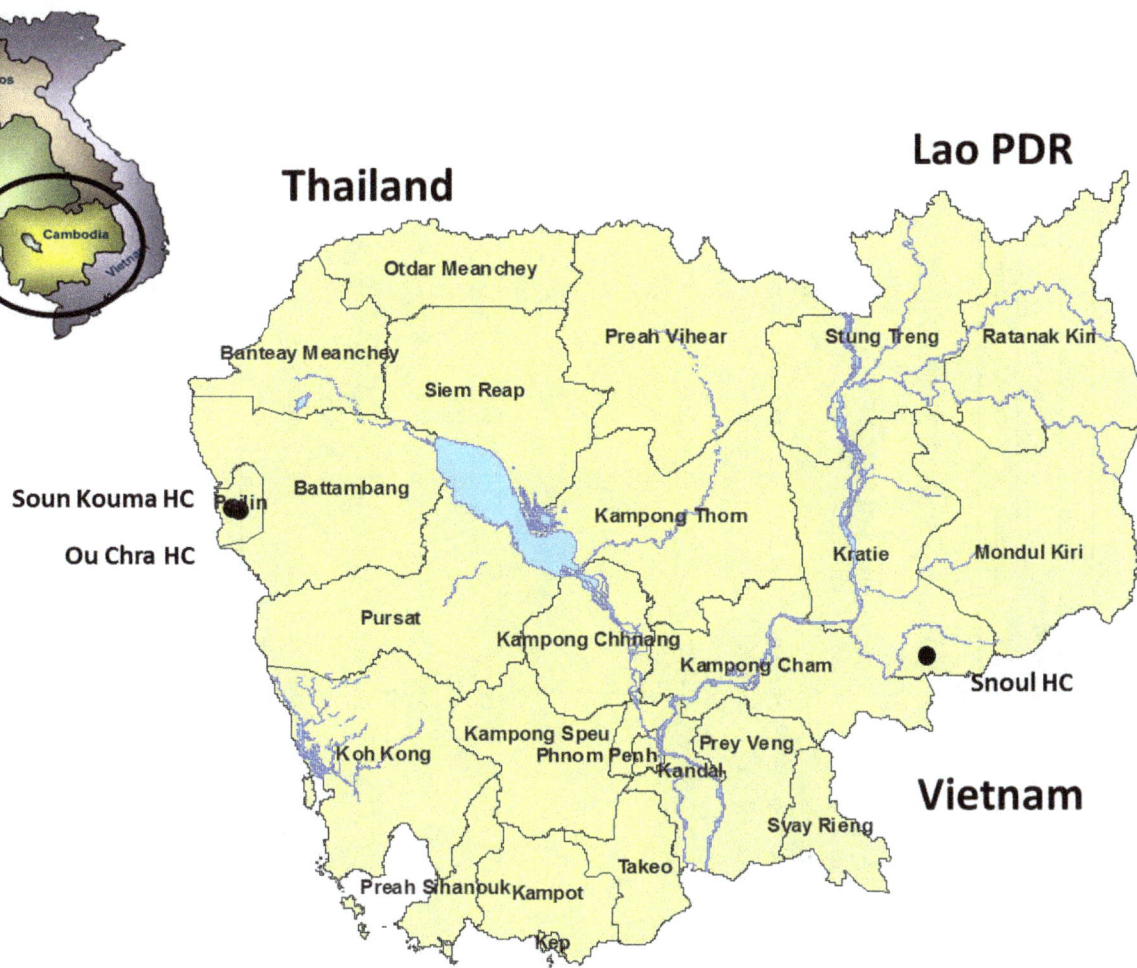

Figure 1. Map of Cambodia displaying the location of the study sites in remote areas in western (Soun Kouma and Ou Chra) and eastern Cambodia (Snoul).

sons, and Student's t test or one-way analysis of variance for parametric comparisons. For categorical variables, Chi-squared or Fisher's exact tests were used to assess significant differences in proportions. Odd ratios (OR) and their 95% confidence intervals (CI) were measured to compare prevalence of pathogens between case and control groups. The Attributable Fraction among case (AFe) was assessed for each pathogen using the following formula: [(OR-1)/OR] ×100. Hypothesis testing was made using risk differences, exact 95% confidence intervals, and p-values. A p-value (two-tailed) of less than 0.05 was considered statistically significant.

Results

Study Population

From January 2008 to December 2010, 1475 individuals were recruited. Among them, 1193 (80.8%) were febrile patients (case group): 621 in Soun Kouma HC and 650 in Ou Chra HC in Pailin Province and 204 in Snoul HC in Kratie Province, and 282 (19.1%) non-febrile individuals (control group) (Figure S2). As presented in Table 1, significant differences in patient characteristics were found between sites: (i) mean temperature on admission was higher in Soun Kouma HC (p<0.0001), (ii) time delay in days between the onset of the fever and the consultation was higher in

Snoul HC (p<0.0001), (iii) sex ratio (M/F) was higher in Snoul HC (p<0.0001) and (iv) mean age of febrile patients was lower in Soun Kouma HC (p<0.0001). The frequency of clinical symptoms of febrile patients on admission also differed between sites (p< 0.0001). The most common symptoms observed were sore throat (612/1193, 51.3%), cough (585/1193, 49.0%), and running nose (259/1193, 21.7%).

Clinical Diagnosis and Management of Febrile Diseases

Of febrile cases, 383/1193 (32.1%) had a positive malaria-RDT on admission (Figure 2) and were treated according to national guidelines [28]. Febrile individuals that had a negative malaria-RDT were clinically diagnosed by health centre staff using normal procedure as: (i) acute upper respiratory infections (AURI) (619/810, 76.4%), (ii) enteric fever (137/810, 16.9%), (iii) malaria (49/810, 6.0%) and (iv) acute lower respiratory infections (ALRI) (5/810, 0.6%). Patients in the AURI group were usually treated with the following antimicrobial drugs: amoxicillin (AMX) (478/619, 77.2%), sulfamethoxazol/trimethoprim (SMX) (89/619, 14.4%), penicillin (30/619, 4.8%), erythromycin (8/619, 1.3%) and cloxacillin (6/619, 1.0%). Metronidazol was used in 3 cases and chloroquine (CQ) in 2 cases. The remaining 3 patients received paracetamol only. Patients clinically diagnosed with enteric fever were treated with metronidazol (60/137, 43.8%), SMX (48/137,

Table 1. Characteristics of patients and controls in each study sites.

Characteristic and on-site management		Soun Kouma HC		Ou Chra HC		Snoul HC		Total		p-value*
		Cases	Controls	Cases	Controls	Cases	Controls	Cases	Controls	
Number		450	171	576	74	167	37	1193	282	n/a
Temperature	Mean (SD), °C	39.0 (0.5)	-	38.8 (0.5)	-	38.8 (0.5)	-	38.9 (05)	-	<0.0001
Duration of fever	Mean (SD), days	2.4 (1.0)	-	2.7 (1.0)	-	3.0 (1.6)	-	2.6 (1.1)	-	<0.0001
Sex	M	254	63	404	8	143	34	801	105	<0.001
	F	196	108	172	66	24	3	392	177	
	Ratio (M/F)	1.3	0.6	2.3	0.1	6.0	11.0	2.0	0.6	<0.001
Age	Mean (SD) years	21.1 (10.7)	34.5 (11.6)	24.6 (10.6)	25.7 (7.5)	25.3 (9.5)	28.1 (10.0)	23.4 (10.6)	31.4 (11.2)	<0.0001
Clinical symptoms	Fever (>37,5°C)	100	-	100	-	100	-	100	-	<0.0001
	Sore throat (%)	67.8	-	46.4	-	24.0	-	51.3	-	
	Cough (%)	59.1	-	46.4	-	31.1	-	49.0	-	
	Running nose (%)	42.0	-	7.3	-	16.8	-	21.7	-	
	Diarrhoea (%)	17.6	-	22.2	-	10.8	-	18.9	-	
	Vomiting (%)	25.3	-	16.1	-	3.6	-	17.9	-	
	Ear ache	13.6	-	0.2	-	2.4	-	5.5	-	
	Headache (%)	6.4	-	0.5	-	1.8	-	2.9	-	
Clinical diagnosis on-site	Malaria (%)	23.6	-	37.5	-	65.9	-	36.2	-	<0.0001
	Enteric fever (%)	1.4	-	18.9	-	13.2	-	11.5	-	
	UARI (%)	74.4	-	43.6	-	19.7	-	51.9	-	
	LARI (%)	0.6	-	0.0	-	1.2	-	0.4	-	
Treatment on-site	Antifebrile drugs (%)	100	-	100	-	98.8	-	99.8	-	<0.0001
	Antimalarial drugs (%)	23.2	-	37.7	-	66.5	-	36.1	-	
	Antimicrobial drugs (%)	75.9	-	62.7	-	34.1	-	63.7	-	
	No drug (%)	0.9	-	0	-	0	-	0.34	-	

n/a: Not calculated;
*among cases between sites.

35.0%), fluoroquinolones (21/137, 15.3%), AMX (4/137, 3.0%), nalidixic acid (1/137, 0.7%), erythromycin (1/137, 0.7%), CQ (1/137, 0.7%) or mebendazol (1/137, 0.7%). Patients clinically diagnosed as malaria, despite negative RDT (49/810) were treated with antimalarials according to the national guidelines. All patients with lower acute respiratory infections (5/810) were treated with AMX.

Detection of Potential Pathogens

In total, 754/1475 (51.1%) enrolled individuals were malaria positive by PCR. The observed prevalence was almost 2-fold higher in the case group (676/1193, 56.7%) compared to the control group (78/282, 27.7%, p<0.01). The attributable fraction among cases (AFe) was estimated to 70% (Table 2). Nucleotide sequencing revealed that the predominant species was *P. vivax* (389/754, 51.6%) followed by *P. falciparum* (306/754, 40.6%). Both *Plasmodium spp.* were more frequently detected in the case than in the control group (p<0.01), with AFe values of 72% and 61%, respectively. In 7.4% of all malaria positive samples (56/754), *P. falciparum/P. vivax* mixed infections were detected without difference in term of frequency between the groups (p = 0.07). Two human cases of the emerging simian malaria parasite *P. knowlesi* were also detected, one in the case and one in the control group. *P. ovale* was found only once, in the control group (Table 2).

All positive malaria RDT individuals (383/1475, 25.9%) belonged to the case group (383/1193, 32.1%) and 376/383 (98.2%) of them were confirmed positive by malaria-PCR. In addition, 300 patients from the case group with negative malaria RDT results were also positive by malaria PCR.

Leptospira spp. were identified as the second most frequent pathogens. Globally, 167/1475 samples were positive by PCR (11.3%). The ratio between pathogenic and non-pathogenic *Leptospira* was 140/27. The distribution of the main pathogenic species determined by sequencing was as following: *L. interrogans* (85, 60.8%), *L. weilii* (47, 33.6%), *L. kmetyi* (3, 2.1%), *L. kirschneri* (1, 0.7%), *L. santarosai* (1, 0.7%), *L. wolffii* (1, 0.7%), *L. genomospecies1* (1, 0.7%) and *L. noguchii* (1, 0.7%) (Table 2). The overall prevalence of pathogenic leptospirosis was not significantly different between the three sites, but there was an uneven distribution between species (p<0.01): *L. interrogans* was the most prevalent species in Snoul (22/23) compared to Pailin (29/74). Interestingly, the prevalence of *L. interrogans* was higher in the control group (24/282, 8.5%) than in the case group (61/1193, 5.1%) (OR = 0.60, 95% CI: 0.37–0.98, p = 0.04), while the prevalence of other pathogenic *Leptospira* spp.

was higher in cases than controls (4.3% *vs.* 1.4%, OR = 2.5, 95% CI: 1.1–5.6, p = 0.02). The AFe were not evaluated.

O. tsutsugamushi was detected in 54/1475 samples (3.7%). Its prevalence was not associated with site or with fever. Moreover, 3 samples were positive for other *Rickettsia* species.

Virological tests results were available for 1470 plasma and 1473 throat swab samples. Of the plasma samples, 80/1470 (5.4%) were found positive for Dengue virus type 2 (44/80, 55.0%), type 1 (22/80, 27.5%), type 4 (8/80, 10.0%) and type 3 (6/80, 7.5%). The overall prevalence was not significantly different between sites, but more frequent in febrile patients (75/1190, 6.3%) than in non-febrile individuals (5/280, 1.8%, p = 0.01, OR = 3.7, 95% CI: 1.5–9.3, AFe = 73%). The prevalence of type 2 and type 4 was highest in Ou Chra and Soun Komar HC in Pailin province, respectively. The temporal distribution of the dengue cases clearly showed an annual epidemic peaking between May and October (Figure S3).

Both Influenza A (87/1473, 5.9%) and B serotypes (26/1473, 1.8%) were detected in the throat swabs. The overall prevalence was significantly different between sites: 11.3% in Ou Chra HC, 5.5% in Soun Komar HC and 3.4% in Snoul HC (p<0.01) and between groups (106/1191, 8.9% case group *vs.* 7/282, 2.5% in control group, p = 0.001). Influenza A cases were more frequent in febrile patients (83/1193, 7.0%) than in non-febrile individuals (4/280, 1.4%, p = 0.01, OR = 5.2, 95% CI: 1.9–14.4, AFe = 81%). As observed with Dengue, the temporal distribution of Influenza cases clearly showed a seasonal emergence between September and November (Figure S4).

Among 1128 blood cultures collected from febrile patients, only 9/1128 samples (0.8%) containing pathogenic bacteria were considered as evidence of community acquired septicemia (CAS): *S. pneumoniae* (n = 1), *E. coli* (n = 1), *E. cloacae* (n = 5), *S. typhi* (n = 1) and *S. paratyphi* (n = 1). In 2 cases (*E. cloacae* and *S. paratyphi*) was associated with *P. vivax* infection. Other positive bacteria growths (98/1128) identifying as *Staphylococcus non-aureus*, *Corynebacteria* spp., *Pseudomonas fluorescens* and *Pseudomonas putida* were considered as contamination. These results were immediately reported back to the health center and all patients were provided the appropriate antimicrobial treatment.

The distribution and the proportion of pathogens found in samples from febrile patients enrolled in 3 sites are presented in Table 3.

Co-infections

A substantial proportion of co-infections (more than one pathogen detected by PCR) was observed in this study. *O. tsutsugamushi* was present as the only pathogen in 31 samples and in co-infection with other pathogens in 28 cases (n = 19, *P. falciparum* and *P. vivax;* n = 7, Leptospira; n = 1, Dengue virus and n = 1, *E. cloaceae*). Dengue virus was also frequently observed in co-infections (32/56, 57%), especially with malaria parasites (n = 27, *P. falciparum* and *P. vivax*). Similarly, Influenza virus was also frequently detected in co-infections (42/114, 37%), especially with malaria parasites (n = 32, *P. falciparum* and *P. vivax*). Other co-infections included *Leptospira* (n = 6), *O. tsutsugamushi* (n = 1), Dengue virus (n = 1), *E. cloacae* (n = 1) and *Rickettsia* (n = 1).

C-Reactive Protein (CRP) Quantitative Detection

Quantitative detection of CRP was performed on 1475 plasma samples. The results are presented in Table 4. Significant differences in median were observed between febrile patients and non-febrile individuals (25.7 mg/l *vs.* 1.4 mg/l, p<0.01). The lowest median CRP concentrations were observed in viral infections (Dengue = 8.2 mg/l and Influenza = 9.6 mg/l) being

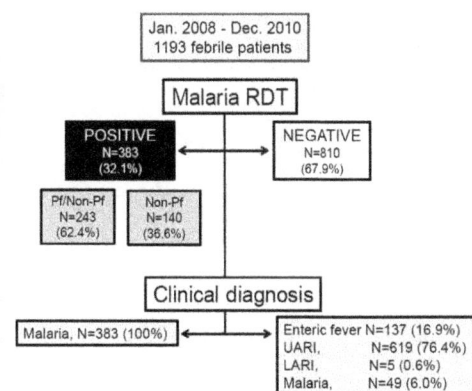

Figure 2. Diagnoses for febrile patients in the study sites, with use of malaria RDT and clinical symptoms.

Table 2. Prevalences of the detected pathogens in the cases and controls study population and attributable fractions among cases, Cambodia, January 2008–December 2010.

Detected pathogen	Total (N = 1,475)		Cases (n = 1,193)		Controls (n = 282)		p-value	OR (95% CI)	p-value	Attributable fraction among cases (AFe)
	N	%	N	%	N	%				
Plasmodium spp.	754	51.1	676	56.7	78	27.7	<0.01	3.4 (2.6–4.5)	<0.01	70%
P. vivax	389	26.4	359	30.1	30	10.6	<0.01	3.6 (2.4–5.4)	<0.01	72%
P. falciparum	306	20.7	277	23.2	29	10.3	<0.01	2.6 (1.7–4.0)	<0.01	61%
P. vivax + falciparum	56	3.8	39	3.3	17	6.0	0.07	n/a	n/a	n/a
P. ovale	1	0.1	0	0.0	1	0.4	n/a	n/a	n/a	n/a
P. knowlesi	2	0.1	1	0.1	1	0.4	n/a	n/a	n/a	n/a
Pathogenic *Leptospira* spp.	140	9.5	112	9.4	28	9.9	0.42	n/a	n/a	n/a
L. interrogans	85	5.8	61	5.1	24	8.5	0.20	n/a	n/a	n/a
L. weilii	47	3.2	44	3.7	3	1.1	0.08	n/a	n/a	n/a
L. kmetyi	3	0.2	2	0.2	1	0.4	n/a	n/a	n/a	n/a
L. kirschnerii	1	0.1	1	0.1	0	0.0	n/a	n/a	n/a	n/a
L.santosaraii	1	0.1	1	0.1	0	0.0	n/a	n/a	n/a	n/a
L. genomospecies1	1	0.1	1	0.1	0	0.0	n/a	n/a	n/a	n/a
L. wolffii	1	0.1	1	0.1	0	0.0	n/a	n/a	n/a	n/a
L. noguchii	1	0.1	1	0.1	0	0.0	n/a	n/a	n/a	n/a
O. tsutsugamushi	54	3.7	47	3.9	7	2.5	0.48	n/a	n/a	n/a
Rickettsia spp.	3	0.2	2	0.2	1	0.4	n/a	n/a	n/a	n/a
Dengue virus 1–4	80	5.4	75	6.3	5	1.8	0.01	3.7 (1.5–9.3)	0.005	73%
Influenza A virus	87	5.9	83	7.0	4	1.4	0.01	5.2 (1.9–14.4)	0.001	81%
Influenza B virus	26	1.8	23	1.9	3	1.1	0.77	n/a	n/a	n/a
Cultured bacteria	9	0.8	9	0.8	0	-	n/a	n/a	n/a	n/a

n/a: Not calculated.

Table 3. The distribution and the proportion of pathogens found in samples from febrile patients enrolled in 3 sites, Cambodia 2008–2010.

Pathogens		Sampling sites			Total	
		Soun Kouma HC	Ou Chra HC	Snoul HC		
		N = 576	N = 450	N = 167	N = 1193	
no pathogen		148	146	25	319	26.7%
one pathogen	Plasmodium sp.	280	156	107	543	45.5%
	Influenza viruses	15	48	3	66	5.5%
	Leptospira	26	11	7	44	3.7%
	Dengue viruses	17	23	2	42	3.5%
	Orientia tsutsugamushi	12	12	1	25	2.1%
	Enterobacter cloacae	2	0	0	2	0.2%
	Escherichia coli	0	1	0	1	0.1%
	Pseudomonas fluorescens	1	0	0	1	0.1%
	Pseudomonas putida	1	0	0	1	0.1%
	Rickettsia	1	0	0	1	0.1%
	Streptococcus pneumoniae	0	1	0	1	0.1%
	Salmonella typhi	0	1	0	1	0.1%
two pathogens	Plasmodium sp. – Leptospira	29	15	8	52	4.4%
	Plasmodium sp. - Influenza viruses	16	10	3	29	2.4%
	Plasmodium sp. - Dengue viruses	14	8	6	28	2.3%
	Plasmodium sp. - O. tsutsugamushi	7	6	1	14	1.2%
	Plasmodium sp. - E. cloacae	1	0	0	1	0.1%
	Plasmodium sp. - S. paratyphi	0	0	1	1	0.1%
	Dengue viruses – Leptospira	0	1	1	2	0.2%
	Dengue viruses - Influenza viruses	0	1	0	1	0.1%
	E. cloacae - Influenza viruses	1	0	0	1	0.1%
	O. tsutsugamushi – Leptospira	0	1	1	2	0.2%
	O. tsutsugamushi - E. cloacae	1	0	0	1	0.1%
	Rickettsiae - Influenza viruses	0	1	0	1	0.1%
	Influenza viruses – Leptospira	1	4	0	5	0.4%
three pathogens	Plasmodium sp. - O. tsutsugamushi – Leptospira	2	1	0	3	0.3%
	Plasmodium sp. - Dengue viruses – Leptospira	0	0	1	1	0.1%
	Plasmodium sp. - Influenza viruses – Leptospira	0	2	0	2	0.2%
	Plasmodium sp. - O. tsutsugamushi - Dengue viruses	0	1	0	1	0.1%
	Plasmodium sp. - O. tsutsugamushi - Influenza viruses	1	0	0	1	0.1%

significantly different to CRP levels in patients with malaria (37.9 mg/l p<0.01) and scrub typhus (26.4 p<0.006). Median CRP concentration was intermediate in febrile patients where no pathogen was detected (6.3 mg/l) or with multiple infections (16.2 mg/l). The sensitivity, specificity, positive predictive (PPV) and negative predictive values (NPV) of CRP>5 mg/ml for bacterial mono-infection versus viral infections were 87.8% (CI95%: 78.2–94.3%), 30.8% (CI95%: 22.3–40.5%), 46.8% (CI95%: 38.3–55.4%) and 78.6% (CI95%: 63.2–89.7%), respectively. The interactive dot diagram analysis indicating the cut-off point with the best separation (minimal false negative and false positive results) was set up at 21.3 mg/L with 52.5% of sensitivity and 84.3% of specificity.

Discussion

The diagnosis of non-malaria febrile illness in resource-limited rural areas remains challenging [29]. One of the main findings of this study was the observation that whilst the clinical management of malaria is reportedly working well in Cambodia, the majority of malaria-RDT negative febrile patients did not receive an appropriate diagnosis and treatment. Clinical diagnosis together, with the RDTs performed in the field, succeeded in identifying

Table 4. CRP levels in different patient subgroups.

Patient subgroup	N	Median CRP concentration	IQR	Range
Global	1475	17.7 mg/L	3.3–53.3 mg/L	0.1–389 mg/L
Febrile patients	1193	25.7 mg/L	7.6–69.5 mg/L	0.2–389 mg/L
Non-febrile individuals	282	1.4 mg/L	1.0–5.0 mg/L	0.2–236 mg/L
Malaria	612	37.9 mg/L	8.9–86.3 mg/L	0.3–366 mg/L
Dengue virus	44	8.2 mg/L	3.0–15.5 mg/L	1.0–75.5 mg/L
Influenza virus	71	9.6 mg/L	3.6–15.8 mg/L	0.2–68.1 mg/L
Leptospirosis	63	19.2 mg/L,	1.4–62.8 mg/L	0.5–284 mg/L
Scrub typhus	31	26.4 mg/L	6.3–78.9 mg/L	1.0–244 mg/L
Febrile patients where no pathogen was detected	487	6.3 mg/L	1.4–28.6 mg/L	0.1–376 mg/L
Multiple infections	167	16.2 mg/L	5.3–44.7 mg/L	0.2–389 mg/L

and appropriately treating 56.6% (383/676) of the malaria cases. However, even when RDTs are currently the most important tool available in peripheral health centers to diagnose malaria especially caused by *P. falciparum* (243/316, 76.9%), an important proportion of low-density malaria infections is still missed as demonstrated by PCR in this study. Most of the RDT-negative febrile cases were carrying malaria parasites that were detected by PCR but not by RDT (314/810, 38.7%, mainly *P. vivax*; 188/314, 60%). Although it is not clear if those low-density malaria infections are actually the cause of fever in those patients (AFe among malaria case 70%), these results emphasize the need for more sensitive diagnostic tools for detection and treatment of all infections to target elimination. We observed that most of the RDT-negative cases were clinically diagnosed as UARI and treated apparently indiscriminately with antimicrobial drugs (mainly AMX). Only 14% of them received an effective treatment against the pathogen identified by PCR. These findings underline the need of specific diagnostic tools and clinical training of the health center staff for the effective management of febrile patients and rational use of antimicrobials. Leptospirosis was frequently observed in people with AUFI, regardless the clinical status (case and control groups). This could be due to the recruitment of controls among family members or other accompanying persons, who had been exposed to the same risk-factors as the patients. The high prevalence of leptospirosis detected in this study was consistent with previous reports from similar settings in Thailand, Lao PDR [9,10,12], and Cambodia [5]. This underlines the importance of this disease in the region. However, the high frequency observed in the asymptomatic/non-febrile group is new. The awareness about leptospirosis needs to be raised and further research on its epidemiology, clinical symptoms and outcomes in Cambodia, including its significance in afebrile people, should be undertaken. Furthermore, suitable diagnostic tools for leptospirosis should be made available in peripheral health services. Since no serological tests were applied, no information on the serovar could be obtained.

A high frequency of dengue fever was observed in our sampled population, mostly adult and rural, while dengue is known to be more common in urban settings and young children [11]. These results underline the importance of awareness by health center staff to be able to distinguish viral infections and be aware of their possible complications. Dengue and influenza infections had annual epidemic waves, implying that at the corresponding time of the year, HC staff should consider these viral diseases as important differential diagnoses for malaria. Both viral infections

were also associated with a significantly lower CRP-level compared to malaria or bacterial infections. CRP could be a helpful tool to distinguish viral infections as cause of NMFI in the future however further studies to define more accurate thresholds are required.

Co-infections were also frequent in this study (~14%). Most frequently, these included malaria parasites (*P. falciparum* and *P. vivax*) and a second non-malarial pathogen such as *Leptospira* spp., *Rickettsia* spp., *O. tsutsugamushi* or dengue virus. Reports of malaria co-infections with other pathogens such as HIV or helminthes are numerous especially from sub-Saharan Africa. In Southeast Asia, however, reports of co-infections in malaria patients remain rare. Malaria in Southeast Asia is often associated with outdoor occupations including logging, mining and agriculture, activities that also expose people at risk for leptospirosis, rickettsiosis and scrub typhus. In many cases of malaria co-infections, *P. vivax* was the most frequent species found by PCR (very at low density of infection). These cases could be interpreted as chronic asymptomatic infections with *P. vivax* plus a simultaneous acute infection with another pathogen. Unfortunately nothing is known about the interactions of these pathogens in co-infections so far, but it can be assumed that multiple infections complicate malaria and may lead to failure to respond to treatment [30]. The awareness of the possibility of co-infections should be raised and physicians should be suspicious of it in malaria cases with poor treatment response or atypical manifestations. Additional tests to improve guidance for antimicrobial therapy are needed. In their absence, empirical treatment with doxycycline could be a valid therapeutic option [31].

Although a broad test battery was applied for the detection of pathogens causing fever, it was not possible to detect a causative agent in ~27% of febrile patients. A variety of other pathogens come into consideration as cause of fever, not all of which were evaluated here. For example, HIV infections, viral hepatitis and tuberculosis were not evaluated due to ethical approval conditions but are likely to contribute to the overall burden of NMFI. Japanese Encephalitis Virus (JEV) was also a possible cause, especially in cases of prolonged fever or additional signs of meningitis. However convalescent serum samples were not available for additional testing. A combined *Flavivirus* MAC-ELISA (JE–Dengue IgM Combo ELISA; Panbio Diagnostics, Australia) was run on 10 samples of patients with a history of more than 5 days of fever and 2 had a positive result for JEV and 3 samples were positive for dengue virus. Another viral disease of interest to evaluate in the future is Chikungunya virus infection, of which several outbreaks were reported from Thailand in 2008 and 2009 [32]. Further possible causes of NMFI include viral infections by Epstein-Barr-virus, Hepatitis A, Hepatitis E, and Coxsackie virus, and other bacterial infections such as Q-fever, brucellosis and melioidosis.

The clinical evaluation of the subjects recruited for this study has not revealed any predictor symptoms or specific risk factors to differentiate between the different causes of NMFI. The evaluation of CRP-levels, as the only biological marker for infection in this study, did show an informative value for the presence of any infection (versus no pathogen identified), as well as for the cause of the infection (viral vs. bacterial). However, this correlation is still weak to be used to assign a definite diagnosis and guide treatment decisions. Accessory information such as a full blood cell count and other biomarkers could provide additional useful diagnostic clues that may help to refine decision-making.

This first NMFI study conducted in Cambodia provides highly valuable information for the planning and design of further investigations. Further studies where district hospitals and HCs are compared for disease burden and diagnosis of severe infections should also be considered. Seasonality of fever cases as demonstrated in this study should also be considered to target resources and increase cost-effectiveness. Paired serum samples should be collected from all patients to define previous or recent exposure to pathogens and guide epidemiological studies. Based on the results of this study, future studies should also collect data on: (i) regional disease burden and seasonality of infectious diseases, (ii) clinical condition of patients and severity of disease (case fatality rates with and without treatment), and (iii) availability and level of health care facilities and services. Studies should assess disease burden and laboratory gaps across each level of health care. To develop effective clinical guidelines it is imperative to involve physicians, nurses and other health care professionals from various levels of health care as well as health policy makers [29]. Intervention packages have to be in line with the current clinical management efforts and the Ministry of Health's planning for human resources, facility upgrades and laboratory strengthening.

Acknowledgments

We thank all patients, all field staff in HCs and all participating staff at CNM Cambodia, the Ministry of Health Cambodia and the Institut Pasteur du Cambodge (Departments of Molecular Epidemiology, Virology and Bacteriology).

Author Contributions

Conceived and designed the experiments: TCM SS FA IJG EMC RA FvS DB DM. Performed the experiments: TCM SS SK NK EF PB BG DM. Analyzed the data: TCM SS NK PB BG IJG EMC FvS DB DM. Wrote the paper: TCM IJG EMC FvS DB DM.

References

1. Dondorp AM, Nosten F, Yi P, Das D, Phyo AP, et al. (2009) Artemisinin resistance in *Plasmodium falciparum* malaria. N Engl J Med 361: 455–467.
2. National Centre for Parasitology (2011) National Strategic Plan for Malaria Elimination (2011–2025). Phnom Penh: Ministry of Health, Cambodia.
3. National Centre for Parasitology (2001) Annual Progress Report. Phnom Penh: Ministry of Health, Cambodia.
4. World Health Organization. Global Malaria Programme (2010) World Malaria Report 2010. Geneva: World Health Organization.
5. Beaute J, Vong S (2010) Cost and disease burden of dengue in Cambodia. BMC Public Health 10: 521.
6. Berlioz-Arthaud A, Guillard B, Goarant C, Hem S (2010) Hospital-based active surveillance of human leptospirosis in Cambodia. Bull Soc Pathol Exot 103: 111–118.
7. Berman SJ, Irving GS, Kundin WD, Gunning JJ, Watten RH (1973) Epidemiology of the acute fevers of unknown origin in South Vietnam: effect of laboratory support upon clinical diagnosis. Am J Trop Med Hyg 22: 796–801.
8. Blair PJ, Wierzba TF, Touch S, Vonthanak S, Xu X, et al. (2010) Influenza epidemiology and characterization of influenza viruses in patients seeking treatment for acute fever in Cambodia. Epidemiol Infect 138: 199–209.
9. Chhour YM, Ruble G, Hong R, Minn K, Kdan Y, et al. (2002) Hospital-based diagnosis of hemorrhagic fever, encephalitis, and hepatitis in Cambodian children. Emerg Infect Dis 8: 485–489.
10. Ellis RD, Fukuda MM, McDaniel P, Welch K, Nisalak A, et al. (2006) Causes of fever in adults on the Thai-Myanmar border. Am J Trop Med Hyg 74: 108–113.
11. Huy R, Buchy P, Conan A, Ngan C, Ong S, et al. (2010) National dengue surveillance in Cambodia 1980–2008: epidemiological and virological trends and the impact of vector control. Bull World Health Organ 88: 650–657.
12. Laras K, Cao BV, Bounlu K, Nguyen TK, Olson JG, et al. (2002) The importance of leptospirosis in Southeast Asia. Am J Trop Med Hyg 67: 278–286.
13. Leelarasamee A, Chupaprawan C, Chenchittikul M, Udompanthurat S (2004) Etiologies of acute undifferentiated febrile illness in Thailand. J Med Assoc Thai 87: 464–472.
14. Mardy S, Ly S, Heng S, Vong S, Huch C, et al. (2009) Influenza activity in Cambodia during 2006–2008. BMC Infect Dis 9: 168.
15. McGready R, Ashley EA, Wuthiekanun V, Tan SO, Pimanpanarak M, et al. (2010) Arthropod borne disease: the leading cause of fever in pregnancy on the Thai-Burmese border. PLoS Negl Trop Dis 4: e888.
16. Phongmany S, Rolain JM, Phetsouvanh R, Blacksell SD, Soukkhaseum V, et al. (2006) Rickettsial infections and fever, Vientiane, Laos. Emerg Infect Dis 12: 256–262.
17. Pradutkanchana J, Pradutkanchana S, Kemapanmanus M, Wuthipum N, Silpapojakul K (2003) The etiology of acute pyrexia of unknown origin in children after a flood. Southeast Asian J Trop Med Public Health 34: 175–178.
18. Sreng B, Touch S, Sovann L, Heng S, Rathmony H, et al. (2010) A description of influenza-like illness (ILI) sentinel surveillance in Cambodia, 2006–2008. Southeast Asian J Trop Med Public Health 41: 97–104.
19. Sripanidkulchai R, Lumbiganon P (2005) Etiology of obscure fever in children at a university hospital in northeast Thailand. Southeast Asian J Trop Med Public Health 36: 1243–1246.
20. Suttinont C, Losuwanaluk K, Niwatayakul K, Hoontrakul S, Intaranongpai W, et al. (2006) Causes of acute, undifferentiated, febrile illness in rural Thailand: results of a prospective observational study. Ann Trop Med Parasitol 100: 363–370.
21. Syhavong B, Rasachack B, Smythe L, Rolain JM, Roque-Afonso AM, et al. (2010) The infective causes of hepatitis and jaundice amongst hospitalised patients in Vientiane, Laos. Trans R Soc Trop Med Hyg 104: 475–483.
22. Steenkeste N, Incardona S, Chy S, Duval L, Ekala MT, et al. (2009) Towards high-throughput molecular detection of *Plasmodium*: new approaches and molecular markers. Malar J 8: 86.
23. Merien F, Portnoi D, Bourhy P, Charavay F, Berlioz-Arthaud A, et al. (2005) A rapid and quantitative method for the detection of Leptospira species in human leptospirosis. FEMS Microbiol Lett 249: 139–147.
24. Paris DH, Blacksell SD, Stenos J, Graves SR, Unsworth NB, et al. (2008) Real-time multiplex PCR assay for detection and differentiation of rickettsiae and orientiae. Trans R Soc Trop Med Hyg 102: 186–193.
25. Vong S, Khieu V, Glass O, Ly S, Duong V, et al. (2010) Dengue incidence in urban and rural Cambodia: results from population-based active fever surveillance, 2006–2008. PLoS Negl Trop Dis 4: e903.

26. Bellau-Pujol S, Vabret A, Legrand L, Dina J, Gouarin S, et al. (2005) Development of three multiplex RT-PCR assays for the detection of 12 respiratory RNA viruses. J Virol Methods 126: 53–63.

27. Buecher C, Mardy S, Wang W, Duong V, Vong S, et al. (2010) Use of a multiplex PCR/RT-PCR approach to assess the viral causes of influenza-like illnesses in Cambodia during three consecutive dry seasons. J Med Virol 82: 1762–1772.

28. National Centre for Parasitology (2004) National Treatment Guideline for Malaria. Phnom Penh: Ministry of Health, Cambodia.

29. Crump JA, Gove S, Parry CM (2011) Management of adolescents and adults with febrile illness in resource limited areas. Bmj 343: d4847.

30. Singhsilarak T, Phongtananant S, Jenjittikul M, Watt G, Tangpakdee N, et al. (2006) Possible acute coinfections in Thai malaria patients. Southeast Asian J Trop Med Public Health 37: 1–4.

31. Mayxay M, Castonguay-Vanier J, Chansamouth V, Dubot-Pérès A, Paris DH, et al. (2013) Causes of non-malarial fever in Laos: a prospective study. Lancet Glob Health 1: e46–e54.

32. Pongsiri P, Auksornkitti V, Theamboonlers A, Luplertlop N, Rianthavorn P, et al. (2010) Entire genome characterization of Chikungunya virus from the 2008–2009 outbreaks in Thailand. Trop Biomed 27: 167–176.

8

Differential Susceptibility of Two Field *Aedes aegypti* Populations to a Low Infectious Dose of Dengue Virus

Arissara Pongsiri[1], Alongkot Ponlawat[1], Butsaya Thaisomboonsuk[2], Richard G. Jarman[2¤], Thomas W. Scott[3,4], Louis Lambrechts[5*]

1 Department of Entomology, Armed Forces Research Institute of Medical Sciences, Bangkok, Thailand, 2 Department of Virology, Armed Forces Research Institute of Medical Sciences, Bangkok, Thailand, 3 Department of Entomology and Nematology, University of California Davis, Davis, California, United States of America, 4 Fogarty International Center, National Institutes of Health, Bethesda, Maryland, United States of America, 5 Insect-Virus Interactions Group, Department of Genomes and Genetics, Institut Pasteur – Centre National de la Recherche Scientifique, Unité de Recherche Associée 3012, Paris, France

Abstract

Background: The infectious dose required to infect mosquito vectors when they take a blood meal from a viremic person is a critical parameter underlying the probability of dengue virus (DENV) transmission. Because experimental vector competence studies typically examine the proportion of mosquitoes that become infected at intermediate or high DENV infectious doses in the blood meal, the minimum blood meal titer required to infect mosquitoes is poorly documented. Understanding the factors influencing the lower infectiousness threshold is epidemiologically significant because it determines the transmission potential of humans with a low DENV viremia, possibly including inapparent infections, and during the onset and resolution of the viremic period of acutely infected individuals.

Methodology/Principal Findings: We compared the susceptibility of two field-derived *Aedes aegypti* populations from Kamphaeng Phet, Thailand when they were orally exposed to low titers of six DENV-2 isolates derived from the serum of naturally infected humans living in the same region. The infectious dose, time-point post-blood feeding, viral isolate and mosquito population, were significant predictors of the proportion of mosquitoes that became infected. Importantly, the dose-response profile differed significantly between the two *Ae. aegypti* populations. Although both mosquito populations had a similar 50% oral infectious dose (OID_{50}), the slope of the dose-response was shallower in one population, resulting in a markedly higher susceptibility at low blood meal titers.

Conclusions/Significance: Our results indicate that mosquitoes in nature vary in their infectious dose-response to DENV. Thus, different mosquito populations have a differential ability to acquire DENV infection at low viremia levels. Future studies on human-to-mosquito DENV transmission should not be limited to OID_{50} values, but rather they should be expanded to account for the shape of the dose-response profile across a range of virus titers.

Editor: Lark L. Coffey, University of California Davis, United States of America

Funding: This study was primarily supported by grant R01 GM083224 from the United States National Institutes of Health and by the United States Military Infectious Diseases Research Program. L.L. received funding from the French Agence Nationale de la Recherche (grant ANR-09-RPDOC-007-01) and from the French Government's Investissement d'Avenir program, Laboratoire d'Excellence Integrative Biology of Emerging Infectious Diseases (grant ANR-10-LABX-62-IBEID). T.W.S. received support from the Research and Policy for Infectious Disease Dynamics program of the Science and Technology Directorate, Department of Homeland Security, and Fogarty International Center, United States National Institutes of Health. The funders had no role in study design, data collection and analysis, decision to publish, or preparation of the manuscript.

Competing Interests: The authors have declared that no competing interests exist.

* E-mail: louis.lambrechts@pasteur.fr

¤ Current address: Viral Diseases Branch, Walter Reed Army Institute of Research, Silver Spring, Maryland, United States of America

Introduction

Recent estimations bring to almost 400 million the number of human dengue virus (DENV) infections that occur worldwide each year, of which about three quarters are expected to be clinically inapparent [1]. Dengue is a self-limiting infection caused by RNA viruses of the genus *Flavivirus* that are transmitted among humans by mosquitoes [2]. DENV include four serotypes (DENV-1, -2, -3 and -4) that are phylogenetically closely related, but antigenically distinct. The principal mosquito vector species of DENV worldwide is *Aedes aegypti*, although *Ae. albopictus* has occasionally been implicated in relatively small-scale dengue outbreaks [3].

Currently, there is no licensed vaccine or commercially available therapeutic for dengue. Disease prevention relies on the control of mosquito vector populations. Transmission occurs when a mosquito bites a human during their viremic period, which typically lasts 4–5 days [4–6]. On average, the probability of DENV transmission from symptomatic humans to mosquitoes follows the kinetics of viremia [7], from as soon as two days before the onset of fever to the day following defervescence [8].

One critical parameter underlying a successful human-to-mosquito DENV transmission event is the magnitude of human viremia required to infect mosquitoes. It is well established that the proportion of infected mosquitoes is positively associated with the virus dose ingested in artificial blood meals [9,10]. The dose-response of mosquitoes generally follows a sigmoid relationship with 0% infection below a lower threshold and 100% infection above an upper threshold. A recent study documented the dose-response of *Ae. aegypti* fed directly on the blood from clinically ill, naturally infected humans in Vietnam [7]. Analysis of the proportion of infected mosquitoes as a function of human plasma viremia confirmed the sigmoid shape of the mosquito dose-response. There was no or little transmission below 10^3 viral RNA copies/ml of plasma, and close to 100% transmission above 10^9 viral RNA copies/ml. Estimates for the 50% oral infectious dose (OID_{50}), defined as the virus concentration resulting in 50% infected mosquitoes, ranged from $10^{6.29}$ to $10^{7.52}$ viral RNA copies/ml of plasma [7]. Interestingly, the OID_{50} differed among serotypes, indicating that viral factors influence the shape of the mosquito dose-response.

Most vector competence studies use blood meal titers that are in the higher part of the mosquito dose-response to DENV (e.g., [11–14]). In other words, virus titers in blood meals are typically around or greater than the OID_{50}. The lower part of the dose-response (i.e., mosquito infection rates <50%) has generally not been examined, perhaps because vector-virus interaction studies need to maximize the number of infected mosquitoes. Gaining a better understanding of the lower part of the dose-response to DENV is epidemiologically important for at least three reasons. First, epidemic DENV transmission is not always associated with high human viremias [15,16]. Second, even when peak viremia is high, there are periods of low viremia during the onset and resolution of the viremic period that may contribute to human-to-mosquito DENV transmission. Third, understanding infectiousness to mosquitoes at low viremia levels is important to quantify the potential contribution of people with mild or clinically inapparent infections to overall DENV transmission. Inapparent and mild DENV infections are assumed to be associated with lower viremia levels by extrapolating the positive relationship observed between viremia and disease severity in symptomatic human cases [7,17–19]. The contribution of mild human infections to DENV transmission may be epidemiologically underappreciated because they have not been studied and they tend to outnumber the more severe infections that make up the bulk of the cases detected and studied by public health systems [1,20,21].

Here, we investigated the susceptibility of two field-derived *Ae. aegypti* populations that were orally exposed to low infectious doses of six low-passage DENV-2 isolates obtained from human serum samples. All experiments were carried out using the first laboratory-reared generation of mosquitoes derived from wild *Ae. aegypti* collected in Na Bo Kham (NB) and Nakhon Chum (NC), two villages located approximately 25 km apart in Kamphaeng Phet Province, Thailand. Our results indicate that dose-response differed between the two mosquito populations, with one population being more susceptible to DENV infection at low infectious doses despite a similar OID_{50}.

Materials and Methods

Mosquitoes

Wild *Ae. aegypti* immatures (larvae and pupae) were collected from a variety of artificial containers in several households in Na Bo Kham (NB) and Nakhon Chum (NC) sub-districts, Muang district, Kamphaeng Phet Province, Thailand during December 2011 (experiment 1) and August 2012 (experiment 2). F_0 adults were allowed to emerge in the laboratory, mate randomly, and feed on defibrinated sheep blood (National Laboratory Animal

Center, Mahidol University, Nakhon Pathom, Thailand) through a membrane feeding system. F_1 eggs were collected on paper towel lining oviposition cups and stored under high humidity. Prior to the experiments, they were hatched synchronously by placing them under low pressure for 30 min. Larvae were reared in $24 \times 34 \times 9$ cm plastic trays filled with 2.0 liters of dechlorinated tap water at a density of approximately 200 first instars per tray and fed a standard diet of approximately 1.0 g of fish food pellets (C.P. Hi Pro, Perfect Companion Group Co. Ltd, Bangkok, Thailand) per tray. After emergence, F_1 adults were housed in plastic $30 \times 30 \times 30$ cm cages (Megaview Science Education Service Co. Ltd, Taichung, Taiwan) with permanent access to 10% sucrose. They were maintained under insectary conditions at $28 \pm 1°C$, 80% humidity, and with a 12:12 hour light:dark cycle.

Virus isolates

Six DENV-2 isolates (designated as 29, 50, 51, 54, 66, and 67) were derived from serum samples obtained between July and September 2010 from people with acute dengue infections in Nakhon Chum (isolates 29, 50, 51), Sa Kaeo (isolate 54) and Na Bo Kham (isolates 66, 67). These villages are located 25–35 km apart in Muang district, Kamphaeng Phet Province, Thailand. The serum samples were obtained as part of larger geographic cluster investigations initiated from 'index' cases admitted to the Kamphaeng Phet Provincial Hospital with DENV infections confirmed by RT-PCR. The study site and cluster investigation methodology have been described previously [22]. Virus isolation and identification was performed according to published methods [23]. Phylogenetic analysis based on their complete envelope gene sequence assigned the viruses to the Asian genotype II of DENV-2 (data not shown). Each isolate was passaged four times in *Ae. albopictus* cells (C6/36, ATCC CRL-1660) prior to its use in experimental infections of mosquitoes.

Ethics statement

The study protocol was approved by the Institutional Review Boards of the Thai Ministry of Public Health, Walter Reed Army Institute of Research, and University of California at Davis. Written informed consent was obtained from study participants and/or parents of participants; assent was obtained from persons more than seven years of age.

Oral challenge

Experimental infections were conducted as previously described [24]. Briefly, two sets of two-day-old confluent cultures of C6/36 cells in 25 cm² flasks (approximately 10^7 cells/flask) were inoculated with 1.0 ml of stock virus per flask and incubated at 35°C. Supernatant was harvested five days post-inoculation to prepare the infectious blood meal. The artificial blood meal consisted of 1:1 mix of defibrinated sheep blood (National Laboratory Animal Center, Mahidol University, Nakhon Pathom, Thailand) and virus suspension. Three infectious doses were prepared by using the viral supernatant undiluted, diluted 0.5 and diluted 0.1 in RPMI 1640 medium with 5% heat-inactivated fetal bovine serum (HIFBS). Four- to seven-day-old *Ae. aegypti* F_1 females deprived of sucrose and water for 24 hours were offered an infectious blood meal for 30 min through pieces of desalted porcine intestine stretched over water-jacketed glass feeders maintained at 37°C. Samples of the blood meals were saved for subsequent titration by plaque assay. After blood feeding, mosquitoes were briefly sedated with CO_2 from dry ice and fully engorged females were transferred to clean paper cups. Unfed or partially fed females were discarded. Engorged females were maintained under standard insectary conditions, as described above, and provided cotton soaked with 10% sucrose *ad libitum*.

Susceptibility

Infection of *Ae. aegypti* midguts by the six DENV-2 isolates was assessed for the three infectious doses at 7 and 14 days post-blood feeding based on the proportion of infected mosquitoes determined by plaque assay. Upon harvest, mosquito bodies were kept individually in 1.0 ml of mosquito diluent (MD), consisting of RPMI 1640 medium with 10% HIFBS with 100 units/ml penicillin and 100 μg/ml streptomycin. Samples were stored at $-70°C$ before processing. They were quickly thawed in a water bath at $35±2°C$ and homogenized in a mixer mill (Qiagen, Hilden, Germany) at 24 cycles/sec for 2 min. Plaque assay was performed in rhesus monkey kidney cells (LLC-MK$_2$, ATCC CCL-7) as previously described [25]. Briefly, the homogenized samples were passed individually through a 0.22 μm syringe filter unit and 0.5 and 0.1 dilutions were prepared in MD. The samples were placed in an ice bath and 100 μl/well were inoculated into a monolayer of LLC-MK$_2$ cells in 24-well plates. The virus was adsorbed for 1 hour at room temperature (20–28°C) on a rocker platform. The inoculum was removed and 0.5 ml/well of a first overlay of medium was added. The cells were incubated for 5 days at $35±1°C$ in a $5±0.5\%$ CO$_2$ incubator. The cells were stained with a second overlay of medium containing 4% neutral red (Sigma, St. Louis, USA). Plaques were counted and plaque forming units (PFU)/ml were calculated.

Data analysis

The study was run in two separate experiments that involved two different sets of DENV isolates and used populations of *Ae. aegypti* that were sampled from the same locations, but on different dates. The isolate and population effects, therefore, were nested within the effect of the experiment. The proportion of mosquitoes that became infected following the infectious blood meal was analyzed with a multifactorial logistic regression that included the effects of experiment, time-point post-blood feeding, infectious dose (log$_{10}$-transformed), mosquito population, viral isolate, and their interactions up to the second-order. An initial analysis with third-order interactions showed that none of the third-order terms had a significant effect. In the models, each mosquito was represented by a single binary value (0 = uninfected; 1 = infected) so that individual variation was accounted for. Estimates of odds ratios and their standard errors were obtained with a separate logistic fit of infection status as a function of infectious dose for each combination of time-point, isolate and population. The same logistic fit was used to derive OID$_{50}$ and OID$_{10}$ values and their 95% confidence intervals. All analyses were performed with the software JMP v10.0.2.

Results

A total of 769 *Ae. aegypti* females were examined for DENV infection by plaque assay, of which 363 (47.2%) were tested at 7 days post-blood feeding (pbf), and 406 (52.8%) at 14 days pbf. The two mosquito populations (referred to as NB and NC here after) were exposed to dilutions of six DENV-2 isolates (experiment 1: isolates 29, 54, 66 and 67; experiment 2: isolates 50 and 51). Among isolates, infectious doses were distributed from $10^{3.74}$ to $10^{5.74}$ PFU/ml in each blood meal (median $10^{4.74}$ PFU/ml). Each combination of mosquito population, virus isolate, and infectious dose was represented by 6–37 mosquitoes (median 19.5). Distribution of sample sizes is given in Table S1. One dose was

missing for pairs 54-NB and 67-NB at 7 and 14 days pbf, respectively.

Overall, 76 (20.9%) of the mosquitoes had detectable infections at 7 days pbf, and 129 (31.8%) at 14 days pbf. The difference in the proportion of infected mosquitoes between the two time-points was statistically significant (Table 1). The average viral titer in infected bodies (across infectious doses) was $10^{2.41}$ PFU/ml at 7 days pbf versus $10^{3.02}$ PFU/ml at 14 days pbf. The strongest effect influencing the proportion of mosquitoes that became infected following the infectious blood meal was infectious dose (Table 1). In general, the percentage of infected mosquitoes strongly increased with increasing dose (Fig. 1). In addition, there was a statistically significant interaction between the mosquito population and the virus isolate (Table 1), indicating that infection probability was partly determined by the specific pairing of mosquito and virus strains. There was no evidence for a differential effect of mosquito-virus pairs from the same or a different geographical location.

There was also a highly significant effect of the interaction between the infectious dose and the mosquito population (Table 1). This effect reflected a different shape of the dose-response profile between the two mosquito populations. Across isolates, the dose-response of the NC population was the typical sigmoid relationship with a steep exponential phase. The NB population displayed a shallower dose-response (Fig. 1). The difference was more obvious at 14 (Fig. 1B) than 7 days pbf (Fig. 1A).

The difference in the overall shape of the dose-response between the two mosquito populations was further analyzed with various metrics derived from the logistic fits of the data. The 50% oral infectious dose (OID$_{50}$) varied among virus isolates, but was almost identical between the two mosquito populations both at 7 (Fig. 2A) and 14 days pbf (Fig. 2D). For most isolates, however, the 10% oral infectious dose (OID$_{10}$) estimates were lower at 14 days pbf for the NB population compared to the NC population (Fig. 2E), supporting the conclusion that the NB population is more susceptible than the NC population to low doses of DENV. This difference was not apparent at 7 days pbf (Fig. 2B). Likewise, the odds ratio of the prevalence-dose relationship was always higher for the NC population at 14 (Fig. 2F), but not 7 days pbf (Fig. 2C). In this case, the odds ratio describes the relative increase in prevalence for a one-unit increase in infectious dose. Higher odds ratio reflect the stronger correlation (i.e., steeper sigmoid) between the proportion of infected mosquitoes and the blood meal titer for the NC population than for the NB population.

Discussion

We carried out experimental infections of mosquitoes at the lower part of their dose-response to DENV. A recent estimate of DENV-2 OID$_{50}$ measured 12 days after the infectious blood meal in *Ae. aegypti* was $10^{6.29}$ viral RNA copies/ml of plasma [7]. Based on their calibration of the quantitative RT-PCR assay used to measure plasma viremia levels, Nguyen *et al.* [7] estimated that $10^{6.29}$ DENV-2 genome copies/ml were equivalent to $10^{4.43}$ PFU/ml of plasma. Blood meal titers in our experiments ranged from $10^{3.74}$ to $10^{5.74}$ PFU/ml of blood, thus bracketing the previously reported OID$_{50}$ value for DENV-2. Accordingly, we observed an infection prevalence ranging from 0% to 75% among population-isolate-dose combinations (Fig. 1). We chose to use plaque assay rather than a more sensitive quantitative RT-PCR assay because viral RNA concentration does not directly translate into infectious titer [26]. Fourteen days after the infectious blood meal, virus in the bodies of mosquitoes with an established DENV

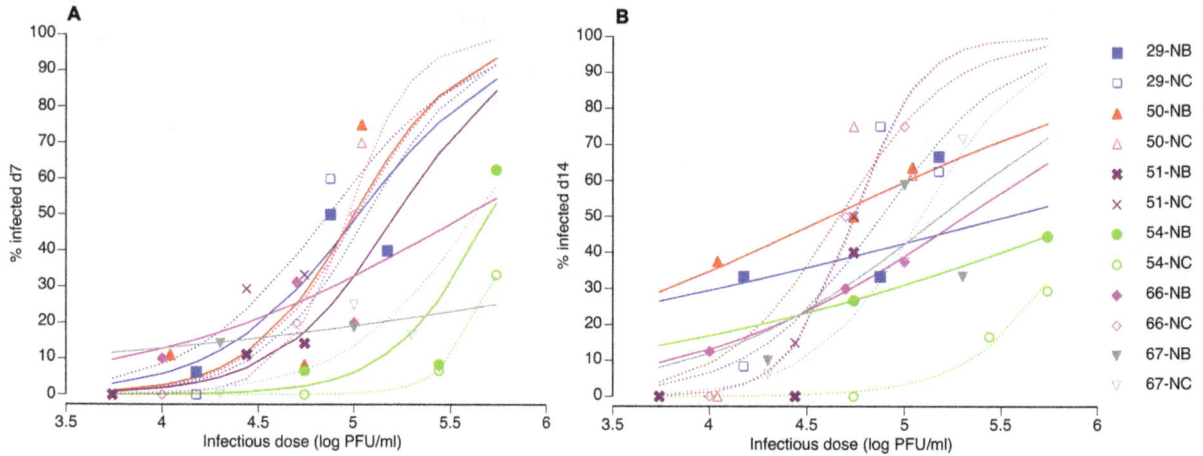

Figure 1. Logistic fits of the observed dose-responses. The percentage of mosquitoes found virus-positive 7 days (**A**) and 14 days (**B**) after oral challenge is shown as a function of the blood meal titer for all combinations of two *Ae. aegypti* populations (NB = Na Bo Kham; NC = Nakhon Chum) and six DENV-2 virus isolates (experiment 1: isolates 29, 54, 66 and 67; experiment 2: isolates 50 and 51). Symbols represent empirical data and lines are logistic fits of the data. Solid symbols and lines correspond to the NB population; Open symbols and dashed lines represent the NC population. Note that the logistic fit of the 51-NB pair at day 14 was omitted from the figure because parameter estimates were unstable.

infection is expected to have reached infectious titers largely exceeding the plaque assay detection threshold (10 PFU/ml).

Our results support the idea that wild type *Ae. aegypti* vary in their infectious dose-response to oral DENV challenge. Because environmental conditions were controlled in our experiments, we interpret phenotypic differences observed between NB and NC populations as genetic. A previous study reported that *Ae. aegypti* populations sampled within 25 km of each other in Thailand, including the Kamphaeng Phet area, were genetically differentiated [27]. Elucidating the genetic factors responsible for the higher susceptibility of the NB population at a low infectious dose compared to the NC population may provide greater insight into the genetic basis of vector competence. Although there was considerable variation in infection prevalence among the six low-passage DENV-2 isolates (OID$_{50}$ values ranged from $10^{4.61}$ to $10^{6.02}$ PFU/ml at 14 days pbf), we observed that the overall shape

of the dose-response profile of both *Ae. aegypti* populations was consistent across isolates. In particular, odds ratios of the prevalence-dose relationship estimated at 14 days pbf were always higher for the NC population than for the NB population (Fig. 2F), as illustrated by the steeper slope of the central part of the sigmoid relationship. This indicates that the overall shape of the dose-response is an intrinsic feature of the mosquito population that transcends specific interactions that have been reported to occur between mosquito and virus genotypes [28].

We examined only two *Ae. aegypti* populations and a limited set of DENV-2 isolates of the Asian genotype II. Additional studies are necessary to determine whether our conclusions can be extrapolated to other mosquito populations and virus genotypes. Here, we provide proof-of-principle that variation in dose-response may exist among mosquito populations and should be considered in the design of future studies. Although individual

Table 1. Multifactorial logistic regression of infection status.

Source	df	L-R χ^2	*P*-value
Experiment	1	12.3	**0.0005**
Time-point	1	11.5	**0.0007**
Experiment*Time-point	1	0.92	0.3386
Dose	1	61.3	**<0.0001**
Experiment*Dose	1	1.06	0.3041
Time-point*Dose	1	2.62	0.1054
Isolate [within Experiment]	4	22.5	**0.0002**
Population [within Experiment]	2	9.51	**0.0086**
Isolate*Time-point [within Experiment]	4	5.55	0.2352
Isolate*Population [within Experiment]	4	17.2	**0.0018**
Isolate*Dose [within Experiment]	4	2.18	0.7026
Population*Time-point [within Experiment]	2	0.90	0.6390
Population*Dose [within Experiment]	2	11.8	**0.0027**

Significant *P*-values (<0.05) are in bold. df: degrees of freedom; L-R: likelihood ratio.

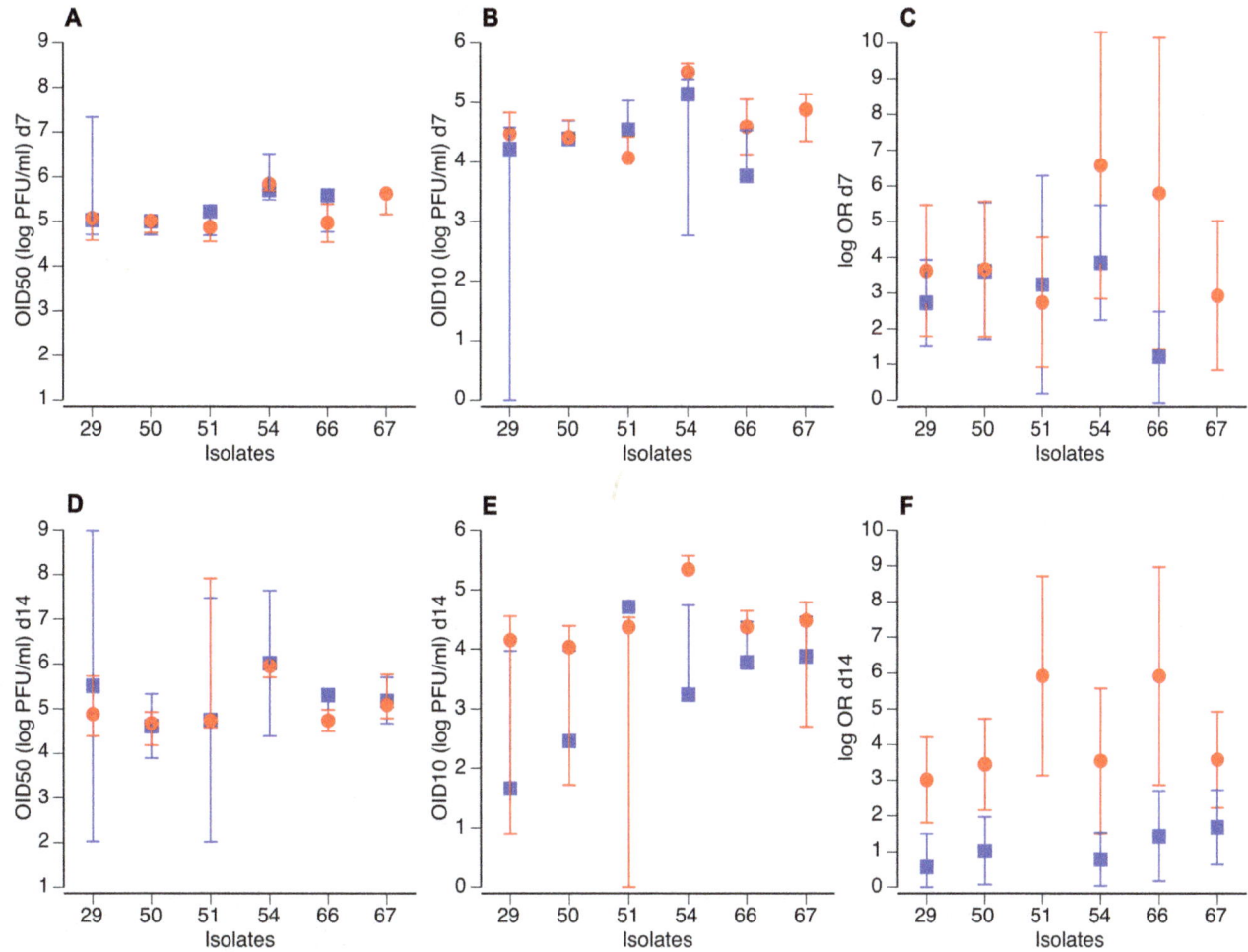

Figure 2. Dose-responses differ between the two *Ae. aegypti* populations. For both *Ae. aegypti* populations (blue squares: Na Bo Kham [NB]; red circles: Nakhon Chum [NC]), OID_{50} values (**A**, **D**), OID_{10} values (**B**, **E**) and estimated odds ratios (**C**, **F**) are shown for each of the six DENV-2 virus isolates. Upper panels (**A–C**) correspond to 7 days and lower panels (**D–F**) to 14 days after the infectious blood meal. Vertical bars indicate 95% confidence intervals of the OID values and standard errors of the odds ratios. Missing error bars mean that they could not be reliably estimated.

dose-responses curves of some population-isolate pairs lacked accuracy because of relatively small sample sizes (Table S1), the interaction between mosquito population and infectious dose was statistically significant across population-isolate pairs. In other words, the overall effect was robustly supported by larger sample sizes than those obtained for each population-isolate pair.

Differences in the ability of vector populations to acquire DENV infection at low blood meal titers may help to explain some puzzling aspects of dengue epidemiology. For example, this process may have contributed to rare instances of epidemic DENV transmission associated with low viremia in humans [15,16]. Variation in the ability of mosquito populations to acquire DENV infection at low viremia levels also may result in heterogeneities in the potential contribution of people with mild dengue infections to overall DENV transmission. Assuming that inapparent/mild DENV infections are associated with lower viremias [7,17–19], their epidemiological significance may depend on the local mosquito population with which they interact.

A caveat of our study is that we focused on mosquito infection prevalence and did not consider virus dissemination from the midgut to other tissues and, thus, the potential for transmission (i.e., vector competence). Because the blood meal titers were

relatively low, the numbers of mosquitoes that developed a disseminated infection in head tissues (data not shown) were too small for a meaningful analysis. Infection of the mosquito midgut is a critical prerequisite for transmission via mosquito bite [29]. Whether our conclusions hold for actual mosquito-to-human DENV transmission requires additional investigation. When possible, in future studies we recommend that investigators try to move away from artificial mosquito feedings methods by including more natural conditions of DENV transmission [30]. A recent study conducted in Vietnam [7] has set a higher standard for human-to-mosquito transmission experiments and highlighted the shortcomings of artificial blood meals. For example, DENV-reactive antibody levels in human plasma samples were negatively correlated with the probability of virus transmission by mosquitoes, independently of viremia level [7]. Such immunological factors are not accounted for in artificial infectious blood meals.

One important implication of our results is that a single summary metric, such as the OID_{50}, is not sufficient to describe the complexity of mosquito-virus interactions that underlies mosquito susceptibility to DENV infection and, perhaps, mosquito-to-virus interactions in general. Indeed, *Ae. aegypti* populations in NB and NC had similar OID_{50} values, yet their susceptibilities to

DENV at a low infectious dose were significantly different. We recommend, therefore, that in the future investigators studying human-to-mosquito DENV transmission consider the entire infectious dose-response profile.

Supporting Information

Table S1 Sample sizes. For each combination of mosquito population, virus isolate and infectious dose, the number of individual mosquitoes assayed (N) is indicated.

Acknowledgments

We acknowledge the invaluable contributions of the clinical, laboratory, and entomological personnel of AFRIMS and Kamphaeng Phet AFRIMS Virology Research Unit (KAVRU). We thank Thanyalak Fansiri for technical advice. We are grateful to Robert Gibbons, Stefan Fernandez, Timothy Endy, Anthony Schuster and three anonymous reviewers for their insights. The opinions or assertions contained herein are the private views of the authors and are not to be construed as reflecting the official views of the United States Army, Royal Thai Army, or the United States Department of Defense.

Author Contributions

Conceived and designed the experiments: A. Pongsiri A. Ponlawat BT RGJ TWS LL. Performed the experiments: A. Pongsiri BT. Analyzed the data: LL. Wrote the paper: TWS LL.

References

1. Bhatt S, Gething PW, Brady OJ, Messina JP, Farlow AW, et al. (2013) The global distribution and burden of dengue. Nature 496: 504–507.
2. Simmons CP, Farrar JJ, Nguyen VV, Wills B (2012) Dengue. N Engl J Med 366: 1423–1432.
3. Lambrechts L, Scott TW, Gubler DJ (2010) Consequences of the expanding global distribution of *Aedes albopictus* for dengue virus transmission. PLoS Negl Trop Dis 4: e646.
4. Gubler DJ, Suharyono W, Tan R, Abidin M, Sie A (1981) Viraemia in patients with naturally acquired dengue infection. Bull World Health Organ 59: 623–630.
5. Siler JF, Hall MW, Hitchens AP (1926) Dengue: its history, epidemiology, mechanism of transmission, etiology, clinical manifestations, immunity, and prevention. Philippine J Sci 29: 1–302.
6. Simmons JS, St. John JH, Reynolds FHK (1931) Experimental studies of dengue. Philippine J Sci 44: 1–247.
7. Nguyen N, Thi Hue Kien D, Tuan T, Quyen N, Tran C, et al. (2013) Host and viral features of human dengue cases shape the population of infected and infectious *Aedes aegypti* mosquitoes. Proc Natl Acad Sci U S A 110: 9072–9077.
8. Nishiura H, Halstead SB (2007) Natural history of dengue virus (DENV)-1 and DENV-4 infections: reanalysis of classic studies. J Infect Dis 195: 1007–1013.
9. Bennett KE, Olson KE, de Lourdes Munoz M, Fernandez-Salas I, Farfan-Ale JA, et al. (2002) Variation in vector competence for dengue 2 virus among 24 collections of *Aedes aegypti* from Mexico and the United States. Am J Trop Med Hyg 67: 85–92.
10. Vazeille-Falcoz M, Mousson L, Rodhain F, Chungue E, Failloux AB (1999) Variation in oral susceptibility to dengue type 2 virus of populations of *Aedes aegypti* from the islands of Tahiti and Moorea, French Polynesia. Am J Trop Med Hyg 60: 292–299.
11. Armstrong PM, Rico-Hesse R (2001) Differential susceptibility of *Aedes aegypti* to infection by the American and Southeast Asian genotypes of dengue type 2 virus. Vector Borne Zoonotic Dis 1: 159–168.
12. Gubler DJ, Nalim S, Tan R, Saipan H, Sulianti Saroso J (1979) Variation in susceptibility to oral infection with dengue viruses among geographic strains of *Aedes aegypti*. Am J Trop Med Hyg 28: 1045–1052.
13. Hanley KA, Nelson JT, Schirtzinger EE, Whitehead SS, Hanson CT (2008) Superior infectivity for mosquito vectors contributes to competitive displacement among strains of dengue virus. BMC Ecol 8: 1.
14. Sanchez-Vargas I, Scott JC, Poole-Smith BK, Franz AW, Barbosa-Solomieu V, et al. (2009) Dengue virus type 2 infections of *Aedes aegypti* are modulated by the mosquito's RNA interference pathway. PLoS Pathog 5: e1000299.
15. Gubler DJ, Reed D, Rosen L, Hitchcock JR, Jr. (1978) Epidemiologic, clinical, and virologic observations on dengue in the Kingdom of Tonga. Am J Trop Med Hyg 27: 581–589.
16. Gubler DJ, Suharyono W, Lubis I, Eram S, Gunarso S (1981) Epidemic dengue 3 in central Java, associated with low viremia in man. Am J Trop Med Hyg 30: 1094–1099.
17. Libraty DH, Endy TP, Houng HS, Green S, Kalayanarooj S, et al. (2002) Differing influences of virus burden and immune activation on disease severity in secondary dengue-3 virus infections. J Infect Dis 185: 1213–1221.
18. Murgue B, Roche C, Chungue E, Deparis X (2000) Prospective study of the duration and magnitude of viraemia in children hospitalised during the 1996–1997 dengue-2 outbreak in French Polynesia. J Med Virol 60: 432–438.
19. Vaughn DW, Green S, Kalayanarooj S, Innis BL, Nimmannitya S, et al. (2000) Dengue viremia titer, antibody response pattern, and virus serotype correlate with disease severity. J Infect Dis 181: 2–9.
20. Endy TP, Anderson KB, Nisalak A, Yoon IK, Green S, et al. (2011) Determinants of inapparent and symptomatic dengue infection in a prospective study of primary school children in Kamphaeng Phet, Thailand. PLoS Negl Trop Dis 5: e975.
21. Yoon IK, Rothman AL, Tannitisupawong D, Srikiatkhachorn A, Jarman RG, et al. (2012) Underrecognized mildly symptomatic viremic dengue virus infections in rural thai schools and villages. J Infect Dis 206: 389–398.
22. Mammen MP, Pimgate C, Koenraadt CJ, Rothman AL, Aldstadt J, et al. (2008) Spatial and temporal clustering of dengue virus transmission in Thai villages. PLoS Med 5: e205.
23. Klungthong C, Gibbons RV, Thaisomboonsuk B, Nisalak A, Kalayanarooj S, et al. (2007) Dengue virus detection using whole blood for reverse transcriptase PCR and virus isolation. J Clin Microbiol 45: 2480–2485.
24. Lambrechts L, Fansiri T, Pongsiri A, Thaisomboonsuk B, Klungthong C, et al. (2012) Dengue-1 virus clade replacement in Thailand associated with enhanced mosquito transmission. J Virol 86: 1853–1861.
25. Thomas SJ, Nisalak A, Anderson KB, Libraty DH, Kalayanarooj S, et al. (2009) Dengue plaque reduction neutralization test (PRNT) in primary and secondary dengue virus infections: How alterations in assay conditions impact performance. Am J Trop Med Hyg 81: 825–833.
26. Choy MM, Ellis BR, Ellis EM, Gubler DJ (2013) Comparison of the mosquito inoculation technique and quantitative real time polymerase chain reaction to measure dengue virus concentration. Am J Trop Med Hyg 89: 1001–1005.
27. Bosio CF, Harrington LC, Jones JW, Sithiprasasna R, Norris DE, et al. (2005) Genetic structure of *Aedes aegypti* populations in Thailand using mitochondrial DNA. Am J Trop Med Hyg 72: 434–442.
28. Fansiri T, Fontaine A, Diancourt L, Caro V, Thaisomboonsuk B, et al. (2013) Genetic mapping of specific interactions between *Aedes aegypti* mosquitoes and dengue viruses. PLoS Genet 9: e1003621.
29. Black WC, Bennett KE, Gorrochotegui-Escalante N, Barillas-Mury CV, Fernandez-Salas I, et al. (2002) Flavivirus susceptibility in *Aedes aegypti*. Arch Med Res 33: 379–388.
30. Lambrechts L, Failloux AB (2012) Vector biology prospects in dengue research. Mem Inst Oswaldo Cruz 107: 1080–1082.

9

Performance of Simplexa Dengue Molecular Assay Compared to Conventional and SYBR Green RT-PCR for Detection of Dengue Infection in Indonesia

R. Tedjo Sasmono[1][*][⑨], Aryati Aryati[2][⑨], Puspa Wardhani[2], Benediktus Yohan[1], Hidayat Trimarsanto[1,3], Sukmal Fahri[4], Tri Y. Setianingsih[1], Febrina Meutiawati[1]

1 Eijkman Institute for Molecular Biology, Jakarta, Indonesia, **2** Clinical Pathology Department, School of Medicine and Institute of Tropical Disease, Airlangga University, Surabaya, Indonesia, **3** Agency for the Assessment and Application of Technology, Jakarta, Indonesia, **4** Health Polytechnic, Jambi Provincial Health Office, Kotabaru, Jambi, Indonesia and Graduate School in Medicine, Diponegoro University, Semarang, Indonesia

Abstract

Diagnostic tests based on detection of dengue virus (DENV) genome are available with varying sensitivities and specificities. The Simplexa Dengue assay (Focus Diagnostics) is a newly developed real-time RT-PCR method designed to detect and serotype DENV simultaneously. To assess the performance of the Simplexa Dengue assay, we performed comparison with conventional RT-PCR and SYBR Green real-time RT-PCR on patients sera isolated from eight cities across Indonesia, a dengue endemic country. A total of 184 sera that were confirmed using NS1 and/or IgM and IgG ELISA were examined. Using conventional and SYBR Green real-time RT-PCR, we detected DENV in 53 (28.8%) and 81 (44.0%) out of 184 sera, respectively. When the Simplexa Dengue assay was employed, the detection rate was increased to 76.6% (141 out of 184 samples). When tested in 40 sera that were confirmed by virus isolation as the gold standard, the conventional RT-PCR yielded 95% sensitivity while the sensitivity of SYBR Green real-time RT-PCR and Simplexa Dengue assay reached 97.5% and 100%, respectively. The specificities of all methods were 100% when tested in 43 non-dengue illness and 20 healthy human samples. Altogether, our data showed the higher detection rate of Simplexa Dengue compared to conventional and SYBR Green real-time RT-PCR in field/surveillance setting. In conclusion, Simplexa Dengue offers rapid and accurate detection and typing of dengue infection and is suitable for both routine diagnostic and surveillance.

Editor: Kwok H. Chan, University of Hong Kong, Hong Kong

Funding: This study was funded by SINAS 2012 grant from the Ministry of Research and Technology of the Republic of Indonesia and PHKI grant from the Ministry of Education of the Republic of Indonesia. The funders had no role in study design, data collection and analysis, decision to publish, or preparation of the manuscript.

Competing Interests: The authors have declared that no competing interests exist.

* Email: sasmono@eijkman.go.id

⑨ These authors contributed equally to this work.

Introduction

Dengue is the most important arthropod-borne viral infection of humans with a large global burden. There are an estimated 50 million infections per year occurring across approximately 100 countries in tropical and sub-tropical regions in the world with potential for wider distribution. The disease affects approximately 2.5 billion people living in Southeast Asia, the Pacific, and the Americas [1,2]. Dengue disease causes varying clinical manifestations ranging from an undifferentiated fever (Dengue Fever, DF) to the more severe forms of the disease including Dengue Hemorrhagic Fever (DHF) and Dengue Shock Syndrome (DSS) [3].

Dengue disease is caused by dengue virus (DENV), a member of Flaviviridae family, with a substantial genetic diversity shown by the presence of four serotypes (DENV-1, -2, -3, and -4) and multiple genotypes (or subtypes) within each serotype [4,5]. DENV is transmitted through a human-mosquito cycle with the aid of *Aedes aegypti* and *Ae. albopictus* mosquito vectors. The genome consists of single-stranded positive-sense RNA which encodes three structural (C, prM/M, E) and seven non-structural proteins (NS1, NS2A, NS2B, NS3, NS4A, NS4B, NS5) [1].

Laboratory confirmation of dengue is important since the broad spectrum of clinical presentations causes the difficulties in making an accurate diagnosis. The available dengue diagnostic tools employ the detection of dengue virus, viral antigen, dengue genome/RNA, and/or serology [6]. Serological detection is useful and is currently the most widely-used dengue diagnostic [6,7] for dengue detection after 1 week of the fever [8], but it cannot be used earlier than 3–5 days after fever or for discriminating serotypes [9].

The molecular detection of DENV RNA genome is an alternative to the serological detection of the virus infection. This method offers a sensitive, rapid and simple mean for clinical diagnosis, and has been widely used in DENV research, including entomological surveillance and molecular epidemiological studies, dengue pathogenesis, antiviral drug and vaccine studies [7]. Because of their sensitivity, molecular techniques have gradually replaced traditional virus isolation method as the new standard for DENV detection in acute-phase serum samples [10]. Common methods in DENV nucleic acid detection include reverse-transcription and polymerase chain reaction (RT-PCR), one step or nested PCR, nucleic acid sequence-based amplification (NASBA), and real-time RT-PCR [10,11].

Among the many available strategies for RT-PCR DENV detection, a two-step RT-PCR method developed by Lanciotti et al. [12] has been widely used. This method offers simple detection and typing of dengue viruses, especially in laboratory with limited resources. It utilizes consensus PCR primers that amplify the C and prM genes of dengue viruses. The D1 and D2 primers used in the first run of RT-PCR rapidly detect DENV genome, while the 4 serotype-specific primers TS1, TS2, TS3, and TS4 in the second run are used for serotyping by analyzing the unique sizes of the amplicons for each serotype [12]. This method is proven to be more sensitive than other available conventional RT-PCR methods [13].

A fluorescent-based real-time RT-PCR methods for dengue detection have been used increasingly and have better sensitivity and specificity compared to conventional RT-PCR [11]. One of the methods offers a cost-effective assay using the SYBR Green dye [14]. This method utilizes pan-dengue primers to detect all serotypes of DENV and was proven to be more sensitive than other methods [15].

Other methods of real-time based RT-PCR are also available and have been evaluated for their performance [16,17].

A new generation of real-time RT-PCR for the detection and serotyping of dengue has been developed recently. The Simplexa Dengue (Focus Diagnostics) assay employs bi-functional fluorescent probe-primers and reverse primers to amplify NS5, NS3, NS5, and capsid genes of DENV. This new method has been successfully used for dengue detection both in human and mosquito vectors [18,19]. Because of the limited information on performance of this method, we sought to determine the usefulness of this method in detecting dengue infection on patients recruited during our surveillance in eight cities in Indonesia. Comparison with the conventional RT-PCR and SYBR Green real-time RT-PCR was performed on antigen/serologically and virus isolation-confirmed dengue patients' sera.

Materials and Methods

Ethics statement

Ethical clearances were obtained from Medical Research Ethics Committees of Airlangga University, Surabaya and Diponegoro University, Semarang, Indonesia. Samples from dengue patients were included in the study upon obtaining written informed consents from adult patients. For minors/children participants, written informed consents were sought from their parent/legal guardians.

Sample collection and serological tests

A total of 184 dengue-positive clinical samples used in this study were collected from hospitals and health centers in eight provincial capital cities across Indonesian archipelago, namely Jakarta, Surabaya, Semarang, Medan, Denpasar, Kendari, Jayapura and Samarinda in 2010–2012. All samples were collected during acute phase, typically within the first five days of illness. Detection of DENV NS1 antigen was performed using Panbio Dengue Early ELISA (Alere, Brisbane, Australia), according to manufacturer's instructions. To complement NS1 detection, the Panbio Dengue Duo IgM & IgG Capture ELISA (Alere) was also performed on all samples and used to determine the infection status (primary or secondary infection) according to manufacturer's protocol. Briefly, the positive IgM result (>11 of Panbio Units) is indicative of active

primary or secondary infection. IgG positive result (>22 Panbio Units) is indicative of active secondary infection. Primary infection was determined by positive IgM (>11 Panbio Units) and negative IgG (<22 Panbio Units) while secondary infection was determined by positive IgG (>22 Panbio Units) which may be accompanied by elevated IgM levels. For virus isolation, sera which were confirmed positive by NS1 ELISA were then cultured. Of those, 40 samples were successfully virus-isolated and E gene-sequenced. These samples were used as the gold standard for comparison of conventional RT-PCR, SYBR Green real-time RT-PCR, and Simplexa Dengue for method evaluation. A total of 43 sera from patients diagnosed as having non-dengue infection, i.e. typhoid (n = 24), leptospirosis (n = 1), measles (n = 1), pertussis (n = 1), malaria (n = 15) and bacterial septicemia (n = 1) confirmed by clinical and laboratory tests, were used as non-dengue cases control. Twenty healthy human samples were also included to test the specificity of the assays. The number of sample for dengue (n = 184) and non-dengue (n = 63) used in this study exceeded the required minimum sample size estimated by Conner's formula for McNemar's test in paired study design [20]. Assuming that the RT-PCR method has 75% sensitivity and 100% specificity versus the estimated 90% sensitivity and 85% specificity of Simplexa assay, with a 5% alpha and 20% beta errors, the minimum sample sizes for dengue and non-dengue are n = 102 and n = 49, respectively.

RNA extraction

Strict controls on RNA extraction and PCR preparation/reaction procedures were employed to prevent cross-contamination between samples, in which activities were performed in separate areas/containments and using separate sets of equipment. For RT-PCR activity, reagent preparation and PCR amplification were performed in areas dedicated for each activity. All experiments were conducted in a GCLP-certified laboratory under the UK-Research Quality Association scheme [21] that ensures the compliance with Good Clinical Laboratory Practice.

Viral RNAs were extracted from serum samples using QIAamp Viral RNA Mini Kits (Qiagen, Hilden, Germany) or MagNA Pure LC Total Nucleic Acid Isolation Kit (Roche, Mannheim, Germany) performed in an automated MagNA Pure LC 2.0 Instrument (Roche) according to manufacturers' instructions. Because of the limited volume of sera available, we were not able to extract all samples using both extraction methods. Extraction using the QIAamp Viral RNA Mini kit was performed for 134 samples, while extraction using MagNA Pure LC was performed for 50 samples. To ensure the uniformity of RNA samples between two methods of extraction employed, the same RNA sample from each dengue patient was assayed using conventional RT-PCR, SYBR Green real-time RT-PCR, and the Simplexa Dengue assay.

Conventional RT-PCR

DENV nucleic acid detection and serotyping using conventional RT-PCR was done according to the two step protocol previously described by Lanciotti, et al [12], with modification according to Harris, et al. [22]. Dengue viral RNAs extracted as described above were reverse-transcribed into cDNA using Superscript III reverse transcriptase (RT) (Invitrogen-Life Technologies, Carlsbad, CA). Subsequently, cDNA was amplified using Taq DNA polymerase (Roche). The detection of DENV was facilitated by amplification of 511 bp PCR product which was then used as template for the DENV serotyping. The four dengue serotypes were distinguished by PCR product size upon electrophoresis of PCR products on 2% agarose gels.

SYBR Green real-time RT-PCR using generic pan-dengue primers

Real-time RT-PCR assay was established according to the cost-effective real-time RT-PCR protocol to screen for dengue virus [14]. The assay uses generic pan-dengue primers targeting 3′-untranslated region conserved for all serotypes of DENV. The primer sequences were as follows: pan-dengue F (5′-TTGAG-TAAACYRTGCTGCCTGTAGCTC-3′) and pan-dengue R (5′-GAGACAGCAGGATCTCTGGTCTYTC-3′). The one-step RT-PCR assay was performed using Superscript III Platinum SYBR Green One-Step qRT-PCR Kit (Invitrogen-Life Technologies), according to manufacturer's recommendation. The reaction was prepared in a 96-well plate format, using 5 μl of RNA template and 200 nM of each primer in a final volume of 20 μl. The 5-carboxy-X-rhodamine (ROX) reference dye was used to normalize the fluorescent reporter signal according to manufacturer's instruction. The reactions were allowed to run on an ABI 7500 real-time PCR machine (Applied Biosystems, Foster City, CA). Thermal cycle settings consist of a 10 minutes reverse transcription step at 50°C, followed by 5 minutes of *Taq* polymerase activation at 95°C, 40 cycles of 15 seconds denaturation step at 95°C and 45 seconds of annealing and extension steps at 60°C, continued with default melting curve analysis step. The fluorescence emitted was captured at the annealing and extension step of each cycle at 530 nm. Cycle threshold (Ct) value was determined as the cycle where the fluorescence of a sample increases to a level higher than the background fluorescence. No-template controls (NTCs) and dengue-positive RNAs extracted from DENV-1 WestPac, DENV-2 NGC, DENV-3 H87, and DENV-4 H241 were included in each assay run as controls. The melting temperature (Tm) of each PCR amplification product was checked to verify the correct products. Reactions with a high Ct value or ambiguous Tm value were analyzed by gel electrophoresis on a 2% agarose gel to confirm the presence of correct amplicon size. On this study, this method was used only for dengue detection and not for DENV serotyping.

Simultaneous DENV detection and serotyping using Simplexa Dengue

The same RNA samples were also subjected to dengue detection and serotyping using the Simplexa Dengue assay (Focus Diagnostics, Cypress, CA, USA). The assay is a real-time RT-PCR that discriminates DENV-1 and -4 in one reaction, and DENV-2 and -3 in another reaction. Bi-functional Scorpion-based fluorescent probe-primers together with reverse primers were used in this method to amplify NS5, NS3, NS5, and capsid genes of DENV-1, DENV-2, DENV-3, and DENV-4, respectively. An RNA internal control (RNA IC) is used to monitor the RNA extraction process and to detect RT-PCR inhibition. Briefly, two reaction mixes (1 & 4 and 2 & 3) were prepared according to manufacturer's instructions. The mixes consist of serotype-specific primers mixes, *Taq* Polymerase, and RT enzyme. Five microliters of the reaction mixes were added into designated wells of Universal Disc (3M-Focus Diagnostics) followed by the addition of 5 μl RNA samples, Molecular Control (MC, consisted of inactivated dengue virus serotypes -1, -2, -3, and -4), and No Template Control (NTC). Each sample was tested using serotype 1 & 4 and 2 & 3 reaction mixes in different spokes. Following the sample addition step, wells were sealed and the disc was then inserted into the 3M Integrated Cycler real-time RT-PCR instrument (3M-Focus Diagnostics). Samples were run using pre-programmed conditions set by the manufacturer. Data collection and analysis were performed using Integrated Cycler Studio Software version 4.2. The criteria for valid detection i.e. the positive detection of MC, negative detection of NTC, and the presence of RNA IC amplification curve in negative samples. Samples were considered positive for DENV infection when the Ct value of each serotype was ≤40.0, and ≠ 0. Representative of Simplexa Dengue amplification curves of samples positive for dengue are shown in Figure 1.

Virus isolation and Envelope gene sequencing

Virus isolation was performed by inoculation of NS1-positive serum samples into C6/36 (*Aedes albopictus*, mid gut) cell line culture [23]. Briefly, a monolayer of cells in T25 flask (Corning, NY, USA) was inoculated with 200 μl of sera in 2 ml of 1X RPMI medium supplemented with 2% of Fetal Bovine Serum (FBS), 2 mM of l-glutamine, 100 U/ml of Penicillin, and 100 μg/ml of Streptomycin (all from Gibco-Life Technologies). Flasks were incubated for 1 hour at 28°C to allow virus attachment. Following the incubation period, inoculation medium was discarded and the medium was replenished with 3 ml of fresh medium. Infected cells were incubated at 28°C for up to 14 days. The presence of virus was confirmed by Envelope gene sequencing, which was performed on DENV RNA extracted from the tissue culture supernatant using method as described previously [19]. Briefly, extracted RNAs were reverse-transcribed into cDNA using Superscript III RT (Invitrogen-Life Technologies). The resulted cDNAs were then used as templates for PCR amplification of the Envelope gene (1,485 nt in length) using *Pfu* Turbo Polymerase (Stratagene-Agilent Technologies, La Jolla, CA, USA). The PCR products were then subjected to sequencing reaction using BigDye Dideoxy Terminator sequencing kits v3.1 (Applied Biosystems) using six overlapping primers described previously [24]. Using this method, we successfully obtained complete sequences of Envelope genes from 40 serum samples (data not shown).

Data and statistical analysis

All statistical analyses were performed using R statistical software (http://www.r-project.org). To assess the significance of the different results of Simplexa Dengue against the other two methods, we applied McNemar's test on 2×2 contingency tables derived from the results of each detection method. To assess the significance of infection status and extraction method as factors that might contribute to the performance of each detection method, Wald statistics test on the logistic regression model as implemented in *anova* function of *rms* library from R statistical software was performed [25,26]. The baseline logistic regression model was *prediction ~ infection status+extraction method*.

Results

Detection rate of Simplexa Dengue compared to conventional RT-PCR and SYBR Green real-time RT-PCR

DENV genome detections were performed in all samples. When tested by conventional RT-PCR method, 53 (28.8%) samples were positive for dengue infection. The SYBR Green real-time RT-PCR detected 81 (44.0%) of dengue-positive samples. Using the same set of samples, Simplexa Dengue detection was employed and demonstrated a significantly increased detection rate in which 141 (76.6%) out of 184 samples were positive for the presence of dengue RNA (Table 1). In all conventional RT-PCR-positive samples (n = 53), one sample was detected as negative by Simplexa Dengue (Positive Percent Agreement = 98.1% (52/53)). In all SYBR Green RT-PCR-positive samples (n = 81), two samples were detected as negative by Simplexa Dengue (Positive Percent Agreement = 97.5% (79/81)).

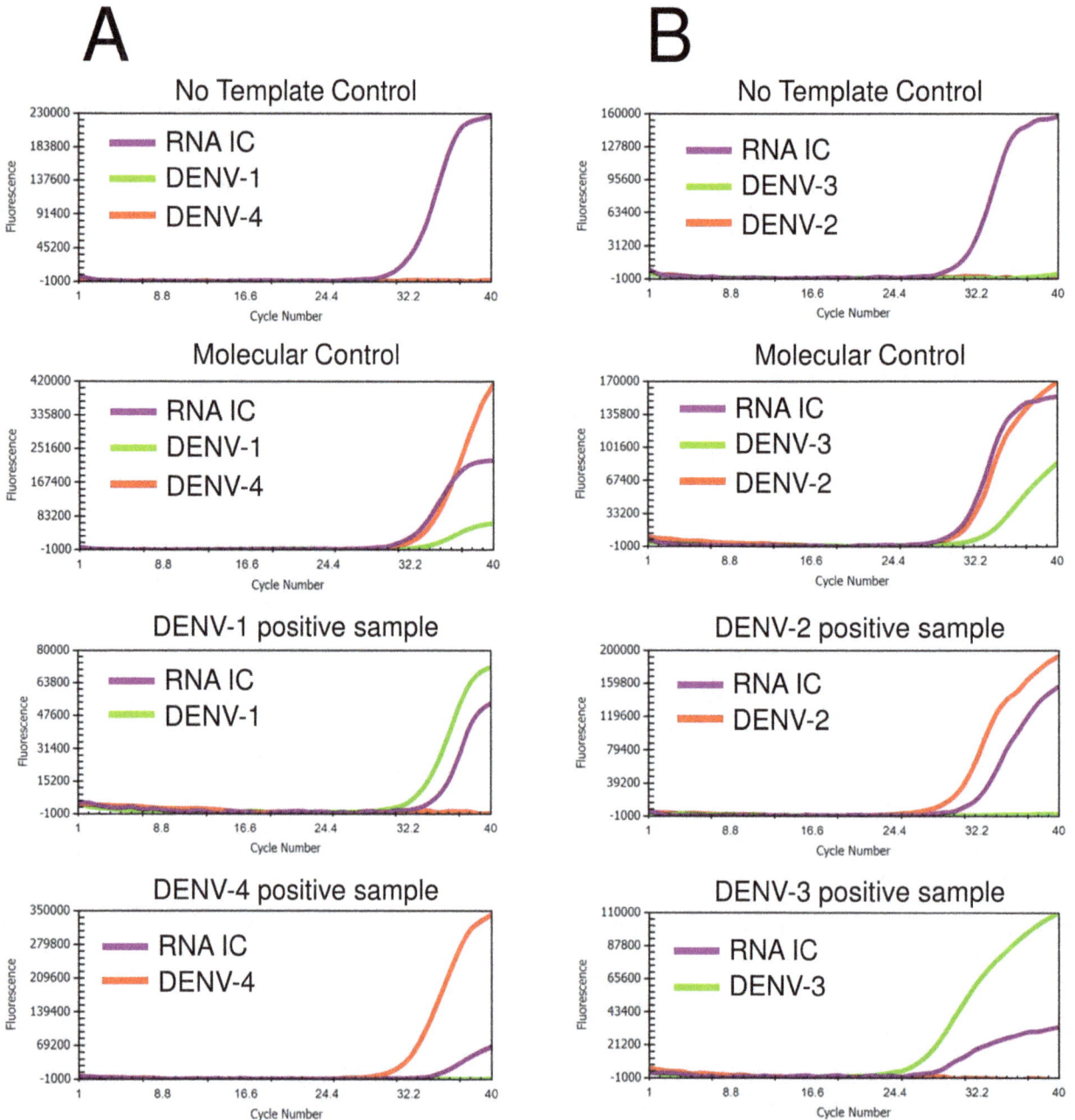

Figure 1. Representative of Simplexa Dengue real-time RT-PCR amplification curves of dengue detection. Detection reactions were separated in two tubes, i.e. DENV-1 and DENV-4 (A) and DENV-2 and DENV-3 (B). Assessment of results were based on the value of controls, which include the Molecular control (MC), RNA internal control (RNA IC) for extraction, and no-template control (NTC).

Virus isolation is currently the gold/reference standard for dengue detection [10]. To further evaluate the sensitivity of the assays against gold standard, all samples that were positive for NS1 ELISA assay were subjected to virus isolation using the C6/36 cell line and the presence of DENV was confirmed by sequencing of the whole Envelope gene. A total of 40 samples were positive by this method. We then correlated the detection results by conventional RT-PCR, SYBR Green real-time RT-PCR, and Simplexa Dengue assays with the positivity of the gold standard. Of 40 samples confirmed by virus isolation and sequencing, conventional RT-PCR successfully detected 38 samples (sensitivity = 95%), while SYBR Green real-time RT-PCR detected 39

samples (sensitivity = 97.5%) and Simplexa Dengue detected all samples as positive (sensitivity = 100%) (Table 1).

When dengue detections were performed using all evaluated methods in 43 confirmed non-dengue cases and 20 healthy human samples, no dengue virus was detected, which indicated that the specificities of conventional RT-PCR, SYBR Green real-time RT-PCR, and Simplexa Dengue were 100% (Table 2). For all methods, we obtained PPV (positive predictive value) = 1 as there were no false positive result. The negative predictive value (NPV) of RT-PCR, SYBR GREEN real time RT-PCR and Simplexa Dengue were 0.32, 0.38 and 0.59, respectively.

Table 1. Sensitivity of conventional RT-PCR, SYBR Green real-time RT-PCR, and Simplexa Dengue on dengue clinical samples from Indonesia.

Dengue detection	No. of sera tested	No. of positive tests	Sensitivity (%)	95% CI
On sera confirmed with virus isolation				
a. Conventional RT-PCR	40	38	95.0	83.1–99.4
b. SYBR Green real-time RT-PCR	40	39	97.5	86.8–99.9
c. Simplexa Dengue	40	40	100.0	91.2–100.0
On sera confirmed with serology/antigen detection				
a. Conventional RT-PCR	184	53	28.8	22.4–35.9
b. SYBR Green real-time RT-PCR	184	81	44.0	36.7–51.5
c. Simplexa Dengue	184	141	76.6	69.8–82.5

CI: confidence interval.

Performance of the DENV detection methods in relation with the DENV serotypes

To determine how much higher was the sensitivity of Simplexa with respect to each of DENV serotypes, we compared the detection rate of each DENV serotypes for both the conventional RT-PCR and the Simplexa Dengue assays. As shown in Table 3, the detection rate of Simplexa Dengue was higher than that of conventional RT-PCR for all serotypes, except for DENV-3 which had similar detection rate. We did not assess the performance of the SYBR Green real-time RT-PCR in relation with the DENV serotypes because this method was only used for dengue detection and not for serotyping.

The presence of concurrent infection of multiple DENV serotypes have been reported in several studies [27–31]. In our study, using conventional RT-PCR, we detected four (7.5%) out of 53 RT-PCR-positive samples with mixed infections. When we used the Simplexa Dengue assay, eight out of 141 Simplexa Dengue-positive samples (5.7%) were detected as mixed/concurrent infections (Table 3).

Performance of the DENV detection methods in relation with infection status and RNA extraction methods

In the sample collection used in this study, we determined the infection status of 184 patients based on IgM and IgG ELISA values. A total of 127 (69.0%) samples were secondary infection, while the rest (57 samples or 31.0%) were primary infection. All

three methods detected more positive samples on primary infection samples compared to secondary infection (Table 4). When comparing the detection rates of the evaluated methods against each other, the Simplexa Dengue significantly detected more positive samples in both primary and secondary infection samples compared to other two methods (Table 4).

In this study, we employed two different RNA extraction methods namely the QIAamp Viral RNA Mini Kit (Qiagen) and automated Magna Pure LC (Roche). On RNAs extracted using the above methods, the Simplexa Dengue exhibited significantly higher detection rate (79% and 70%) compared to both conventional RT-PCR (30% and 24%) and SYBR Green real-time RT-PCR (49% and 30%) on samples extracted using QIAamp Viral RNA Mini Kit and automated Magna Pure LC RNA extraction platforms, respectively (Table 4).

To assess whether the infection status and RNA extraction methods affected the detection rate of each evaluated method, we performed ANOVA with logistic regression on the detection results against the two factors as covariates (Table 5). The results indicated that the detection rate of Simplexa Dengue appeared to be not affected by any of those two factors.

Discussion

Molecular diagnosis of dengue is gradually replacing the traditional method of virus isolation as the gold standard test for viral detection [10,22,32]. Various molecular methods are

Table 2. Specificity of conventional RT-PCR, SYBR Green real-time RT-PCR, and Simplexa Dengue on non-dengue illness and healthy human samples.

Dengue detection	No. of sera tested	No. of negative tests	Specificity (%)	95% CI
On sera of confirmed non-dengue illness				
a. Conventional RT-PCR	43	43	100	89.79–100
b. SYBR Green real-time RT-PCR	43	43	100	89.79–100
c. Simplexa Dengue	43	43	100	89.79–100
On sera of normal healthy donors				
a. Conventional RT-PCR	20	20	100	79.95–100
b. SYBR Green real-time RT-PCR	20	20	100	79.95–100
c. Simplexa Dengue	20	20	100	79.95–100

CI: confidence interval.

Table 3. DENV serotype positive detection rate ratio of Simplexa Dengue compared to conventional RT-PCR.

Serotype	Conventional RT-PCR		Simplexa		Positive Detection Rate Ratio[a]
	N	%	N	%	
DENV-1	25	47.2	76	53.9	3.04
DENV-2	6	11.3	14	10.0	2.33
DENV-3	10	18.9	11	7.8	1.1
DENV-4	8	15.1	32	22.6	4
Mix	4	7.5	8	5.7	2
Total	53	100	141	100	2.66

[a]Positive detection rate ratio was calculated as N $_{Simplexa}$ ÷ N $_{Conventional\ RT-PCR}$.

available either as commercial kits or as in-house developed methods with variable sensitivity [10,11,17]. In this study, we evaluated the performance of a newly developed real-time RT-PCR detection method in clinical samples. During our molecular surveillance study, samples were previously screened using NS1 and/or IgM and IgG ELISA detection, in which a total of 184 samples were positive for dengue. Using these clinical samples, we assessed the performance of a newly-developed and commercially available Simplexa Dengue assay by comparing the detection rate with two other methods, namely the conventional RT-PCR based on method by Lanciotti et al. [12] and SYBR Green real-time RT-PCR using pan-dengue primers [14]. Using the conventional RT-PCR, we detected DENV in 28.8% of samples (Table 1). The use of SYBR Green real-time RT-PCR increased the detection rate into 44.0%. We then employed the newly developed Simplexa Dengue real-time RT-PCR and obtained a higher detection rate (76.6%). Our evaluation of those three detection methods was further continued using gold standards consisted of sera that were confirmed by virus isolation and Envelope gene sequencing. As expected, detection of DENV genome in sera that were confirmed using the above gold standard yielded higher sensitivity, in which the conventional RT-PCR reached 90%; the SYBR Green real-time RT-PCR reached 97.5%, while Simplexa Dengue reached 100% (Table 1). The specificities of all methods were 100% when tested in 43 non-dengue and 20 healthy human samples (Table 2). Altogether, these findings demonstrated better performance of the Simplexa Dengue assay than that of the conventional RT-PCR and SYBR Green real-time RT-PCR for detection of DENV in the field/surveillance setting.

In our study, one of the clear advantages of using Simplexa Dengue was the higher detection rate compared to conventional and SYBR Green real-time RT-PCR. The higher detection rate of Simplexa Dengue compared to conventional RT-PCR is as expected, since fluorescent-based real-time RT-PCR generally has a better sensitivity than the conventional RT-PCR [11]. Currently, many laboratories in Indonesia are still routinely using conventional RT-PCR method for dengue detection and serotyping, in part because of its simplicity, easy to perform, and does not require expensive equipment. In our laboratory, when this method was used, typically only about 20–30% of dengue-suspected samples collected were positive for DENV genome (Sasmono et al., unpublished). Simplexa Dengue presented almost a three-fold increase in the number of DENV-positive samples (in this study reached 76.6%) and also serotyped them simultaneously. This high detection rate will be very useful in epidemiologic surveillance, especially in Indonesia where data on DENV serotype distribution is scarce. Moreover, this method offers rapid

detection in which results can be obtained within one hour, compared to conventional RT-PCR which requires about two to three hours for the results.

The lower detection rates of conventional and SYBR Green real-time RT-PCR might be attributed to the primers used in those two methods. The conventional RT-PCR method was developed more than two decades ago. The DENV possesses high rate of mutation due to the lack of proof-reading RNA polymerase which is typical of other RNA viruses [33]. The mutations that occurred in the DENV genomes may cause nucleotide mismatches with the primers used in the PCR detection. The primers used in conventional RT-PCR method [12] have been modified to increase the sensitivity [22,34]. To assess the identity of the original conventional RT-PCR primers [12] with the DENV genome sequences, we aligned the nucleotide sequence of D1 and D2 primers, which are located in the Capsid-prM genes, with 86 DENV genomes of all serotypes from Indonesia and other countries. We observed 21 different patterns of mismatches (Table S1A). The mismatches were also occurred in one nucleotide position corresponds to modified D1 primer described previously [34]. For the SYBR Green real-time RT-PCR, alignment was also performed on primers located in the 3'UTR region [14], in which 9 mismatch patterns were observed in the forward pan-dengue primer (Table S1B). Altogether, these nucleotide mismatches, which can reduce the efficiency of the primers to bind their genomic target sequences, may underlie the lower sensitivity of both conventional RT-PCR and SYBR Green real-time RT-PCR compared to Simplexa Dengue assay. We were not able to align the Simplexa Dengue primers with the DENV genomes as the primer sequences were not publicly available. Based on the manufacturer's information, the binding sites of the Simplexa Dengue primers were in the NS5, NS3, NS5, and capsid genes for DENV-1, DENV-2, DENV-3, and DENV-4, respectively.

To assess the performance of Simplexa Dengue in detecting different DENV serotypes in clinical samples, we analyzed our serotype data and linked them with the detection rates. We observed higher positive detection rate ratios of Simplexa Dengue for all serotypes, except for DENV-3 which was quite similar with the conventional RT-PCR detection rate (Table 3). A study by Tricou et al. [35] described the serotype-specific viremia kinetics and NS1 levels in dengue patients, in which DENV-1 exhibited a relatively higher viremia than DENV-2. The different viremia levels of particular DENV serotypes may have implications in the sensitivity of dengue molecular assays. We were not sure whether DENV-3 strains in our study indeed possessed higher viremia levels compared to other DENV, which might account for similar detection rates of both conventional RT-PCR and Simplexa

Table 4. Detection rates of evaluated methods in relation with infection status and RNA extraction methods.

Parameter	Conventional		SYBR Green		Simplexa		p^a	p^b
	N	%	N	%	N	%		
Infection status								
Primary (n = 57)	24	42.1	30	52.6	47	82.5	<0.01	<0.01
Secondary (n = 127)	29	22.8	51	40.2	94	74.0	<0.01	<0.01
RNA extraction method								
QIAamp Viral RNA (n = 134)	41	30.6	66	49.3	106	79.1	<0.01	<0.01
MagNA Pure LC (n = 50)	12	24.0	15	30.0	35	70.0	<0.01	<0.01

[a]McNemar's Chi-squared test for comparison between conventional RT-PCR and Simplexa.
[b]McNemar's Chi-squared test for comparison between SYBR Green RT-PCR and Simplexa.

Table 5. The significance of infection status and extraction method on the performance of DENV detection method.

Parameters	df	Conventional		SYBR Green		Simplexa	
		χ^2	*p*-value	χ^2	*p*-value	χ^2	*p*-value
Infection status	1	7.16	**0.0075**	2.86	0.091	1.69	0.1939
Extraction method	1	1.00	0.3175	5.70	**0.0169**	1.82	0.1768

p-value was calculated using Wald statistics on baseline logistic regression model: *detection ~ extraction method+infection status*, where detection corresponds to the results of conventional RT-PCR, SYBR Green RT-PCR, and Simplexa. *p*-value <0.05 was considered as significant. df: degree of freedom.

Dengue. Measurement of viremia levels in patients infected by DENV would be beneficial to confirm this. The higher detection rate of Simplexa Dengue suggested that the method has lower detection limit than conventional RT-PCR but this need to be confirmed using a Limit of Detection study for all four serotypes.

We observed a higher detection rate of DENV-4 identified by the Simplexa Dengue assay than conventional RT-PCR (Table 3). Currently, we are not sure why the Simplexa Dengue assay is more sensitive for DENV-4 than conventional RT-PCR. It is possible that the conventional RT-PCR primers by Lanciotti et al. [12] did not match with the currently circulating virus strains and thus decreased sensitivity for detecting DENV-4. Indeed, we observed one nucleotide mismatch in the forward primer and two-to four nucleotide mismatches in the reverse primers compared to the genome sequences of eight Indonesian DENV-4 strains (unpublished results). However, when new primers were generated and used to re-PCR the RT-PCR-negative DENV-4 samples, the detection rate was not increased.

In our study, using conventional RT-PCR we detected four concurrent infections with more than one dengue serotype (Table 3). The Simplexa Dengue detected eight samples as concurrent infections. Concurrent infections of multiple dengue serotypes have been reported in Indonesia, Mexico, and Puerto Rico [36] as well as other countries [29,31,37,38]. During epidemics in those countries, DENV concurrent infections were detected in about 5.5% of the samples [36]. In our study, a little higher percentage of concurrent infection was observed and most of them involved infection of DENV-1. This phenomenon was possible because during the surveillance period (2010–2012), DENV-1 was prominent in many Indonesian cities studied. For example, we observed the predominance of DENV-1 (35.5%) in Semarang city [19], and similar predominance was also observed in other eight cities (Sasmono et al., manuscript in preparation). The proportion of DENV serotypes in samples used in this study also clearly demonstrated the predominance of DENV-1 (Table 3). We were able to confirm the presence of concurrent/multiple DENV serotypes infection in two samples using virus isolation and Envelope gene sequencing, including determining the genotypes of the infecting viruses (data not shown). The possibility of cross-contamination generating the detection of concurrent infections cannot be ruled out. However, in our study, we employed strict measures to prevent cross-contamination by processing the samples in dedicated containments/rooms and using separate equipment for each step of the extraction and amplification (single directional flow system). Furthermore, our laboratory also followed the quality assurance program that was necessary for laboratories that performed and offered services for diagnosis for dengue [6]. Overall, our data suggest the presence of concurrent DENV infections in hyperendemic region such as Indonesia, in which all DENV serotypes are currently circulating.

Our data showed that not all samples that were antigenically or serologically positive for dengue were positive by all RT-PCR methods evaluated, although the samples were collected in the early stage of the disease. This is understandable since serological tests are generally more sensitive than the RT-PCR. Previous studies have described the difficulty of virus detection in the presence of neutralizing antibody [39], which is one of the characteristics of secondary infection. Our sample collection was dominated by secondary infection (69.0%). Therefore, the lower detection rates of RT-PCR compared to serological tests was likely. Our detection methods also exhibited higher detection rates in primary infection compared to secondary infection (Table 4). This is in accordance with previous studies that observed higher levels of viremia in primary versus secondary infection and earlier

and faster clearance of viremia in secondary infection [35,40]. The high levels of viremia in primary infection facilitated the higher sensitivity of the assays in detecting DENV RNA genome.

In terms of the DENV RNA extraction method, we compared two extraction protocols. The first was manual extraction using the affinity column produced by Qiagen (QIAamp Viral RNA Mini Kit) and the second one was automated extraction using the MagNA Pure LC (Roche) extraction systems. Using both methods, Simplexa Dengue had higher detection rate compared to both SYBR Green and conventional RT-PCR (Table 4). Although the proportion of the positively detected samples appeared to be higher in QIAamp compared to MagNA Pure extracted samples, RNA extraction methods were not a factor that influenced Simplexa Dengue detection rate (Table 5). This finding also supports previous report about the comparability of Qiagen and MagNA Pure extraction methods on the yield and purity of the extraction products [41]. The use of an automated extraction method will be beneficial especially when processing a large number of samples, for example in outbreak settings, although the disadvantage will be the need to provide expensive equipment. In term of consumables/reagents cost effectiveness, we observed that the cost of automated RNA extraction per sample is similar to manual extraction (data not shown). For Simplexa Dengue usage, this finding suggests the compatibility of this new DENV detection method with RNA obtained from either manual or automated extraction.

The Simplexa Dengue method employs the use of an internal control (IC) to monitor the validity of the nucleic acid extraction, a positive molecular control (MC) and no template control (NTC). The assay combines reverse transcription and PCR detection in single reaction which greatly decreases the test's duration (performed within one hour) and the risks of contamination. Furthermore, this method applies automated amplification and data analysis processes as well as using assay's specific and dedicated reagents. Altogether, these features minimize the involvement of humans during the detection process which reduces the possibility of human errors. Combined with an automated nucleic acid extraction system, which is also rapid and minimizes the human involvement during extraction process, these methods will be suitable for dengue detection in various settings such as epidemiological surveillance, clinical management, dengue research, and vaccine trials. Of particular interest, the dengue vaccine clinical trials require the confirmation of dengue cases in vaccinated individuals to determine the vaccine efficacy and for the early detection of vaccine-escape mutants [11]. The high sensitivity and specificity of Simplexa Dengue for dengue detection will be beneficial for rapid and accurate diagnosis of dengue infection in various settings.

Supporting Information

Table S1 A. Alignment of conventional RT-PCR primers based on Lanciotti et al (1992) with DENV genome sequences from Indonesia and other countries; B. Alignment of Pan-dengue RT-PCR primer based on Lai et al (2007) with DENV genome sequences from Indonesia and other countries; C. GenBank accession number of DENV genomes used in primer alignments.

Acknowledgments

We would like to thank Sanofi Pasteur SA for the donation of MagNA Pure LC Nucleic Acid Extraction and Simplexa Dengue assay systems. We thank Drs D. Syafruddin and P.B. Asih for sharing the malaria-confirmed sera.

Author Contributions

Conceived and designed the experiments: RTS AA. Performed the experiments: RTS AA PW BY SF TYS FM. Analyzed the data: RTS AA BY HT. Contributed reagents/materials/analysis tools: RTS AA PW SF. Wrote the paper: RTS BY HT.

References

1. Guzman MG, Halstead SB, Artsob H, Buchy P, Farrar J, et al. (2010) Dengue: a continuing global threat. Nat Rev Microbiol 8: S7–16. doi:10.1038/nrmicro2460.
2. Simmons CP, Farrar JJ, Nguyen van VC, Wills B (2012) Dengue. N Engl J Med 366: 1423–1432. doi:10.1056/NEJMra1110265.
3. Martina BEE, Koraka P, Osterhaus ADME (2009) Dengue virus pathogenesis: an integrated view: 564–581.
4. Holmes EC, Burch SS (2000) The causes and consequences of genetic variation in dengue virus. Trends Microbiol 8: 74–77.
5. Holmes EC, Twiddy SS (2003) The origin, emergence and evolutionary genetics of dengue virus. Infect Genet Evol 3: 19–28.
6. Peeling RW, Artsob H, Pelegrino JL, Buchy P, Cardosa MJ, et al. (2010) Evaluation of diagnostic tests: dengue. Nat Rev Microbiol 8: S30–38.
7. Guzmán MG, Kourí G (2004) Dengue diagnosis, advances and challenges. Int J Infect Dis 8: 69–80.
8. Cuzzubbo AJ, Vaughn DW, Nisalak A, Solomon T, Kalayanarooj S, et al. (2000) Comparison of PanBio Dengue Duo IgM and IgG capture ELISA and venture technologies dengue IgM and IgG dot blot. J Clin Virol 16: 135–144.
9. De Oliveira Poersch C, Pavoni DP, Queiroz MH, de Borba L, Goldenberg S, et al. (2005) Dengue virus infections: comparison of methods for diagnosing the acute disease. J Clin Virol 32: 272–277. doi:10.1016/j.jcv.2004.08.008.
10. Shu P-Y, Huang J-H (2004) Current advances in dengue diagnosis. Clin Diagn Lab Immunol 11: 642–650. doi:10.1128/CDLI.11.4.642-650.2004.
11. Tang KF, Ooi EE (2012) Diagnosis of dengue: an update. Expert Rev Anti Infect Ther 10: 895–907. doi:10.1586/eri.12.76.
12. Lanciotti RS, Calisher CH, Gubler DJ, Chang GJ, Vorndam AV (1992) Rapid detection and typing of dengue viruses from clinical samples by using reverse transcriptase-polymerase chain reaction. J Clin Microbiol 30: 545–551.
13. Raengsakulrach B, Nisalak A, Maneekarn N, Yenchitsomanus P-T, Limsomwong C, et al. (2002) Comparison of four reverse transcription-polymerase chain reaction procedures for the detection of dengue virus in clinical specimens. J Virol Methods 105: 219–232.
14. Lai Y-L, Chung Y-K, Tan H-C, Yap H-F, Yap G, et al. (2007) Cost-effective real-time reverse transcriptase PCR (RT-PCR) to screen for Dengue virus followed by rapid single-tube multiplex RT-PCR for serotyping of the virus. J Clin Microbiol 45: 935–941. doi:10.1128/JCM.01258-06.
15. Waggoner JJ, Abeynayake J, Sahoo MK, Gresh L, Tellez Y, et al. (2013) Development of an internally controlled real-time reverse transcriptase PCR assay for pan-dengue virus detection and comparison of four molecular dengue virus detection assays. J Clin Microbiol 51: 2172–2181. doi:10.1128/JCM.00548-13.
16. Domingo C, Niedrig M, Teichmann A, Kaiser M, Rumer L, et al. (2010) 2nd International external quality control assessment for the molecular diagnosis of dengue infections. PLoS Negl Trop Dis 4. doi:10.1371/journal.pntd.0000833.
17. Hue KDT, Tuan TV, Thi HTN, Bich CTN, Anh HHL, et al. (2011) Validation of an internally controlled one-step real-time multiplex RT-PCR assay for the detection and quantitation of dengue virus RNA in plasma. J Virol Methods 177: 168–173. doi:10.1016/j.jviromet.2011.08.002.
18. Castro MG de, Nogueira RMR, Filippis AMB de, Ferreira AA, Lima M da RQ, et al. (2012) Dengue virus type 4 in Niterói, Rio de Janeiro: the role of molecular techniques in laboratory diagnosis and entomological surveillance. Mem Inst Oswaldo Cruz 107: 940–945.
19. Fahri S, Yohan B, Trimarsanto H, Sayono S, Hadisaputro S, et al. (2013) Molecular Surveillance of Dengue in Semarang, Indonesia Revealed the Circulation of an Old Genotype of Dengue Virus Serotype-1. PLoS Negl Trop Dis 7: e2354. doi:10.1371/journal.pntd.0002354.
20. Obuchowski NA (1998) Sample size calculations in studies of test accuracy. Stat Methods Med Res 7: 371–392.
21. Grant V, Stiles T (2012) Good Clinical Laboratory Practice (GCLP): An international quality system for laboratories which undertake the analysis of samples from clinical trials. Research Quality Association (RQA), Ipswich, UK.
22. Harris E, Roberts TG, Smith L, Selle J, Kramer LD, et al. (1998) Typing of dengue viruses in clinical specimens and mosquitoes by single-tube multiplex reverse transcriptase PCR. J Clin Microbiol 36: 2634–2639.
23. Igarashi A (1979) Characteristics of Aedes albopictus cells persistently infected with dengue viruses. Nature 280: 690–691.
24. Ong SH, Yip JT, Chen YL, Liu W, Harun S, et al. (2008) Periodic re-emergence of endemic strains with strong epidemic potential-a proposed explanation for the 2004 Indonesian dengue epidemic. Infect Genet Evol 8: 191–204.
25. Harrell F (2013) rms: Regression Modeling Strategies. Available: http://cran.r-project.org/package = rms.
26. Harrell F (2001) Regression Modeling Strategies with Application to Linear Models, Logistic Regression, and Survival Analysis. Springer New York.
27. Figueiredo RMP de, Naveca FG, Oliveira CM, Bastos M de S, Mourão MPG, et al. (2011) Co-infection of Dengue virus by serotypes 3 and 4 in patients from Amazonas, Brazil. Rev Inst Med Trop Sao Paulo 53: 321–323.
28. Dos Santos CLS, Bastos MAA, Sallum MAM, Rocco IM (2003) Molecular characterization of dengue viruses type 1 and 2 isolated from a concurrent human infection. Rev Inst Med Trop Sao Paulo 45: 11–16.
29. Wenming P, Man Y, Baochang F, Yongqiang D, Tao J, et al. (2005) Simultaneous infection with dengue 2 and 3 viruses in a Chinese patient return from Sri Lanka. J Clin Virol 32: 194–198. doi:10.1016/j.jcv.2004.04.010.
30. Gubler DJ, Kuno G, Sather GE, Waterman SH (1985) A case of natural concurrent human infection with two dengue viruses. Am J Trop Med Hyg 34: 170–173.
31. Laille M, Deubel V, Sainte-Marie FF (1991) Demonstration of concurrent dengue 1 and dengue 3 infection in six patients by the polymerase chain reaction. J Med Virol 34: 51–54.
32. Henchal EA, Polo SL, Vorndam V, Yaemsiri C, Innis BL, et al. (1991) Sensitivity and specificity of a universal primer set for the rapid diagnosis of dengue virus infections by polymerase chain reaction and nucleic acid hybridization. Am J Trop Med Hyg 45: 418–428.
33. Chen R, Vasilakis N (2011) Dengue–quo tu et quo vadis? Viruses 3: 1562–1608. doi:10.3390/v3091562.
34. Chien L-J, Liao T-L, Shu P-Y, Huang J-H, Gubler DJ, et al. (2006) Development of real-time reverse transcriptase PCR assays to detect and serotype dengue viruses. J Clin Microbiol 44: 1295–1304. doi:10.1128/JCM.44.4.1295-1304.2006.
35. Tricou V, Minh NN, Farrar J, Tran HT, Simmons CP (2011) Kinetics of viremia and NS1 antigenemia are shaped by immune status and virus serotype in adults with dengue. PLoS Negl Trop Dis 5: e1309. doi:10.1371/journal.pntd.0001309.
36. Loroño-Pino MA, Cropp CB, Farfán JA, Vorndam AV, Rodríguez-Angulo EM, et al. (1999) Common occurrence of concurrent infections by multiple dengue virus serotypes. Am J Trop Med Hyg 61: 725–730.
37. Araújo FM de C, Nogueira RMR, de Araújo JMG, Ramalho ILC, Roriz MLF de S, et al. (2006) Concurrent infection with dengue virus type-2 and DENV-3 in a patient from Ceará, Brazil. Mem Inst Oswaldo Cruz 101: 925–928.
38. Chinnawirotpisan P, Mammen MP Jr, Nisalak A, Thaisomboonsuk B, Narupiti S, et al. (2008) Detection of concurrent infection with multiple dengue virus serotypes in Thai children by ELISA and nested RT-PCR assay. Arch Virol 153: 2225–2232. doi:10.1007/s00705-008-0249-9.
39. Chan SY, Kautner IM, Lam SK (1994) The influence of antibody levels in dengue diagnosis by polymerase chain reaction. J Virol Methods 49: 315–322.
40. Duyen HTL, Ngoc TV, Ha DT, Hang VTT, Kieu NTT, et al. (2011) Kinetics of plasma viremia and soluble nonstructural protein 1 concentrations in dengue: differential effects according to serotype and immune status. J Infect Dis 203: 1292–1300. doi:10.1093/infdis/jir014.
41. Beránek M, Voborníková J, Hypiusová V, Palička V (2005) MagNA Pure System for DNA Extraction from Whole Blood Clinical Verification of Pre-Analytical Phase of DNA Testing. Klin Biochem Metab 13: 10–13.

.

10

Genome-Wide Analysis of Codon Usage and Influencing Factors in Chikungunya Viruses

Azeem Mehmood Butt[1]9, Izza Nasrullah[2]9, Yigang Tong[3]*

1 Centre of Excellence in Molecular Biology (CEMB), University of the Punjab, Lahore, Pakistan, 2 Department of Biochemistry, Faculty of Biological Sciences, Quaid-i-Azam University, Islamabad, Pakistan, 3 State Key Laboratory of Pathogen and Biosecurity, Beijing Institute of Microbiology and Epidemiology, Beijing, People's Republic of China

Abstract

Chikungunya virus (CHIKV) is an arthropod-borne virus of the family *Togaviridae* that is transmitted to humans by *Aedes* spp. mosquitoes. Its genome comprises a 12 kb single-strand positive-sense RNA. In the present study, we report the patterns of synonymous codon usage in 141 CHIKV genomes by calculating several codon usage indices and applying multivariate statistical methods. Relative synonymous codon usage (RSCU) analysis showed that the preferred synonymous codons were G/C and A-ended. A comparative analysis of RSCU between CHIKV and its hosts showed that codon usage patterns of CHIKV are a mixture of coincidence and antagonism. Similarity index analysis showed that the overall codon usage patterns of CHIKV have been strongly influenced by *Pan troglodytes* and *Aedes albopictus* during evolution. The overall codon usage bias was low in CHIKV genomes, as inferred from the analysis of effective number of codons (ENC) and codon adaptation index (CAI). Our data suggested that although mutation pressure dominates codon usage in CHIKV, patterns of codon usage in CHIKV are also under the influence of natural selection from its hosts and geography. To the best of our knowledge, this is first report describing codon usage analysis in CHIKV genomes. The findings from this study are expected to increase our understanding of factors involved in viral evolution, and fitness towards hosts and the environment.

Editor: Fausto Baldanti, Fondazione IRCCS Policlinico San Matteo, Italy

Funding: This research was supported by grants from the National Hi-Tech Research and Development (863) Program of China (No. 2012AA022-003), China Mega-Project on Major Drug Development (No. 2011ZX09401-023), and China Mega-Project on Infectious Disease Prevention (No. 2013ZX10004-605, No. 2013ZX10004-607, No. 2013ZX10004-217, and No. 2011ZX10004-001). The funders had no role in study design, data collection and analysis, decision to publish, or preparation of the manuscript.

Competing Interests: The authors have declared that no competing interests exist.

* E-mail: tong62035@gmail.com

9 These authors contributed equally to this work.

Introduction

Chikungunya virus (CHIKV), a member of the genus *alphavirus* of the family *Togaviridae*, is a small (60–70 nm), enveloped, single-strand positive-sense RNA virus. The genome is approximately 12 kb in size and comprises two open reading frames (ORFs) encoding non-structural and structural proteins, respectively [1]. The CHIKV genome is arranged in the order of 5-'cap-nsP1-nsP2-nsP3-nsP4-(junction region)-C-E3-E2-6K-E1-poly(A)-3' [1]. Since the first isolation of CHIKV from a febrile individual in Tanzania in 1953 [2], CHIKV has caused several outbreaks in Asia, Africa, and Indian Ocean islands, emerging as a serious public health concern [3–6]. CHIKV infection is characterized by abrupt onset of high fever, headache, rashes, arthralgia and myalgia. The typical clinical sign of the disease is poly-arthralgia, which is a very painful condition affecting joints and may persist for several months to years in some cases [7]. Being an arthropod-borne virus, the mode of transmission is the mosquitoes of the *Aedes* spp. It is generally accepted that CHIKV originated from Africa, where it is primarily maintained in a yellow fever-like zoonotic sylvatic cycle and depends upon non-human primates and arboreal, peridomestic mosquitoes as reservoir hosts. However, the spread of CHIKV in Asia and urban endemics are associated with a dengue-like "human-mosquito-human" direct transmission cycle, where *A. aegypti* and *A. albopuctus* serve as primary transmission vectors and humans serve as hosts [7–9].

The genetic code comprises 64 codons that can be divided into 20 groups, where each group consists of one to six codons, and each group corresponds to each of the standard amino acids. Alternative codons within the same group coding for the same amino acid are often termed 'synonymous' codons, although their corresponding tRNAs might differ in their relative abundance in cells and in the speed by which they are recognized by the ribosome. This redundancy of the genetic code, in which most of the amino acids can be translated by more than one codon, represents a key step in modulating the efficiency and accuracy of protein production, while maintaining the same amino acid sequence of the protein. On the other hand, the synonymous codons are not chosen randomly both within and between genomes, which is referred to as codon usage bias [10,11]. This phenomenon of synonymous codon usage bias has been studied in a wide range of organisms, from prokaryotes to eukaryotes and viruses [12–17]. Studies on codon usage have determined several factors that could influence codon usage patterns, including mutational pressure, natural or translational selection, secondary protein structure, replication and selective transcription, hydrophobicity and hydrophilicity of the protein and the external environment. Among these, the major factors responsible for codon usage variation among different organisms are considered to be compositional constraints under mutational pressure and natural selection [12,18–20].

Previous studies on codon usage in different viruses have highlighted mutational pressure as the major factor in shaping codon usage patterns compared with natural selection [12,21–23]; however, as our understanding of codon usage increases, it appears that although mutational pressure is still a major driving force, it is certainly not the only one when considering different types of RNA and DNA viruses [24–27]. Considering their comparatively small genome size and other viral features, such as dependence on host's machinery for key process including replication, protein synthesis and transmission in comparison with prokaryotic and eukaryotic genomes, the interplay of codon usage among viruses and their hosts is expected to affect overall viral survival, fitness, evasion from host's immune system and evolution [15,28]. Therefore, knowledge of the codon usage in viruses can not only reveal information about molecular evolution, but also improve our understanding of the regulation of viral genes expression and aid vaccine design, where the efficient expression of viral proteins may be required to generate immunity. In the present study, we report the detailed codon usage data and analysis of various factors shaping the codon usage patterns in CHIKV genomes.

Results and Discussion

Nucleotide Composition Analysis of CHIKV Genomes

Codon usage bias, or preference for one type of codon over another, can be influenced greatly by the overall nucleotide composition of genomes [21]. Therefore, we first analyzed the nucleotide composition of coding sequences from CHIKV genomes. As shown in Table 1, the mean A% (28.91) was the highest, followed by similar composition of G% (25.75) and C% (25.19), with the U% being the lowest (20.16). The mean GC and AU compositions were 50.91% and 49.06% respectively. This appears to suggests there might be equal or almost equal distribution of A, U, G, and C nucleotides among codons of CHIKVs, with potentially more preference towards A-ended codons followed by G/C-ended codons. However, a clearer picture of overall nucleotide composition that could influence the codon usage preference in CHIKV genomes emerged from the analysis of the nucleotide composition of the third position of codons (A_3, U_3, G_3, C_3) and of GC_1, $GC_{1,2}$, GC_3 and AU_3 (Table 1). The mean C_3 and G_3 were the highest, followed by A_3 and U_3. The GC_3 values ranged from 54.9% to 57.2%, with a mean of 55.86% and a standard deviation (SD) 0.40 compared with that of AU_3, whose values ranged from 42.8% to 45.1%, with a mean of 44.14% and an SD of 0.41. The GC_1 ranged from 50.6% to 53.8%, with a mean of 53.56% and an SD 0.27. The $GC_{1,2}$ values ranged from 48.2% to 48.7%, with an average of 48.45% and an SD of 0.07. Therefore, from the initial nucleotide composition analysis, it is expected that G/C-ended codons might be preferred over A/U-ended codons in CHIKV genomes.

Relative Synonymous Codon Usage (RSCU) Analysis of CHIKV

To determine the patterns of synonymous codon usage and to what extent G/C-ended codons might be preferred, we performed RSCU analysis and calculated the RSCU values. Among the 18 most abundantly used codons in CHIKV genomes, eleven (UUC, CUG, AUC, GUG, CCG, UAC, UGC, CAC, CAG, AAC and GAC) were G/C-ended (C-ended: 7; G-ended: 4) and the remaining seven (ACA, GCA, UCA, AGA, AAA, GAA, GGA)

were A-ended codons; none of the preferred codons were U-ended (Figure 1A and Table 2). From RSCU analysis, we observed that CHIKV exhibits comparatively higher codon usage bias towards G/C- and less towards A-ended codons. However, it is also interesting to note that the mean GC% and AU% values are very similar (Table 1), yet the G/C- ending codons were used in a comparatively biased manner, indicating that the G/C content at the third position of the codons influenced the shaping of the overall synonymous codons usage patterns. The overall general trend of the 59 synonymous codon usages was also relatively consistent among different genotypes of CHIKV, indicating that the evolutionary processes of the three genotypes of CHIKV are restricted by the synonymous codon usage pattern to some extent (Figure 1B and Table 2). Furthermore, analysis of over- and under-represented codons showed that codons with an RSCU>1.6 are infrequently observed in CHIKV genomes. The RSCU values of the majority of preferred and non-preferred codons fell between 0.6 and 1.6. We further divided the RSCU data into three groups; (A) codons with RSCU<0.6 (under-represented), (B) codons with RSCU values between 0.6 and 1.6 (unbiased/randomly represented), and (C) codons with RSCU values >1.6 (over-represented). Among 59 codons, only CUG (Leu) and AGA (Arg) had an RSCU>1.6. However, the under-represented codons (RSCU<0.6), were identified as follows: CUU, CUC for Leu, GUU for Val, and CGU, CGG for Arg. The remaining 52 codons had RSCU values between 0.6–1.6 (Figure 1 and Table 2). These findings suggested that despite being an RNA virus with a high mutation rate in its lifecycle, CHIKV has evolved to form a relatively stable genetic composition at some specific levels of synonymous codon usage. This was further confirmed by ENC and CAI analysis as discussed in coming sections. Combining nucleotide composition and RSCU analysis, we deduced that the selection for preferred codons has been mostly influenced by compositional constraints, which also accounts for the presence of mutational pressure. However, we suspect that the compositional constraints may not be the sole factor associated with codon usage patterns in CHIKV, because although the overall RSCU values could reveal the codon usage pattern for the genomes, it may hide the codon usage variation among different genes in a genome [29].

Codon Usage Bias among CHIKV

To quantify the extent of variation in codon usage among different genomes of CHIKV arising from different geographical regions and genotypes, the ENC values for each genome were calculated. The ENC values among CHIKV genomes ranged from 54.55 to 56.41, with a mean of 55.56 and an SD of 0.34 (Table 1). An average value of 55.56 (ENC>40) represents stable ENC values and indicates a relatively conserved genomic composition among different CHIKV genomes. In general, there is an inverse relationship between ENC and gene expression; i.e., a lower ENC value indicates a higher codon usage preference and higher gene expression and vice versa [30]. Our results show that the overall codon usage bias and gene expression among different CHIKV genomes is lower, slightly biased and would be mainly affected by the base composition. Previous studies on codon usage analysis among other RNA viruses, such as bovine viral diarrhea virus (ENC: 50.91) [22], classical swine fever virus (ENC = 51.7) [17] and HCV (ENC = 52.62) [31], have also reported lower codon usage bias. The same is also true in the case of arthropod-borne RNA viruses, including West Nile virus (ENC: 53.81) [15] and dengue virus (DENV) (ENC: 49.70: DENV-1; 48.78: DENV-2; 49.52: DENV-3; and 50.81: DENV-4) [14]. A possible explanation for the weak codon bias of RNA viruses is that it

Table 1. Nucleotide composition analysis of CHIKV genomes (%).

No	A	U	G	C	A₃	U₃	G₃	C₃	AU	GC	GC₁	GC₂	AU₃	GC₃	GC₁₂	ENC
1	29.0	19.9	25.7	25.4	27.1	16.7	26.8	29.3	48.9	51.1	53.7	43.5	43.8	56.2	48.6	55.13
2	28.9	20.0	25.7	25.4	27.0	16.7	26.9	29.3	48.9	51.1	53.7	43.3	43.7	56.3	48.5	55.11
3	28.9	20.3	25.9	24.9	26.7	17.7	27.4	28.2	49.2	50.8	53.5	43.3	44.4	55.6	48.4	55.66
4	28.9	19.9	25.8	25.4	26.7	16.9	27.2	29.2	48.8	51.2	53.8	43.4	43.6	56.4	48.6	55.09
5	28.9	20.1	25.7	25.3	27.0	17.2	27.0	28.9	49.0	51.0	53.7	43.4	44.2	55.9	48.6	55.54
6	29.0	20.1	25.7	25.3	27.2	16.9	26.7	29.2	49.1	51.0	53.7	43.4	44.1	55.9	48.6	55.33
7	28.8	20.4	25.9	24.9	26.6	17.9	27.4	28.1	49.2	50.8	53.5	43.3	44.5	55.5	48.4	55.95
8	28.8	20.4	25.9	24.9	26.6	17.9	27.4	28.1	49.2	50.8	53.5	43.3	44.5	55.5	48.4	55.94
9	28.8	20.4	25.9	24.9	26.6	17.9	27.3	28.1	49.2	50.8	53.5	43.4	44.5	55.5	48.5	55.91
10	28.7	20.1	25.9	25.2	26.0	17.2	27.8	28.9	48.8	51.2	53.4	43.4	43.2	56.7	48.4	54.93
11	28.7	20.1	25.9	25.3	26.2	17.0	27.7	29.1	48.8	51.2	53.4	43.4	43.2	56.8	48.4	54.81
12	28.7	20.2	25.9	25.2	26.2	17.3	27.7	28.8	48.9	51.1	53.4	43.4	43.5	56.5	48.4	54.97
13	28.9	20.4	25.8	24.9	26.8	18.0	27.3	28.0	49.3	50.7	53.5	43.3	44.8	55.2	48.4	55.88
14	28.9	20.4	25.8	24.9	26.8	18.0	27.2	28.0	49.3	50.7	53.5	43.3	44.8	55.2	48.4	55.84
15	28.8	20.5	25.9	24.8	26.6	18.2	27.5	27.7	49.3	50.6	53.5	43.2	44.8	55.3	48.4	56.09
16	29.0	20.0	25.7	25.4	27.1	16.9	26.8	29.1	49.0	51.0	53.7	43.4	44.0	55.9	48.6	55.24
17	28.8	20.5	25.9	24.8	26.6	18.1	27.6	27.7	49.3	50.7	53.5	43.3	44.7	55.3	48.4	56.04
18	29.0	20.2	25.7	25.1	27.0	17.5	26.9	28.6	49.2	50.8	53.6	43.4	44.5	55.5	48.5	55.52
19	28.7	20.1	25.9	25.3	26.2	17.1	27.7	29.1	48.8	51.2	53.4	43.4	43.3	56.7	48.4	54.92
20	28.7	20.0	26.0	25.3	26.1	17.0	27.8	29.2	48.7	51.3	53.4	43.5	43.1	56.9	48.5	54.66
21	28.9	20.2	25.7	25.2	26.2	17.1	27.6	29.1	49.1	51.2	53.4	43.5	43.3	56.7	48.5	54.85
22	29.0	20.1	25.7	25.3	27.0	17.3	27.0	28.8	49.1	50.9	53.6	43.5	44.3	55.8	48.6	55.53
23	28.8	20.5	25.9	24.8	26.7	18.1	27.5	27.8	49.3	50.7	53.4	43.3	44.8	55.3	48.4	56.08
24	28.7	20.1	25.9	25.4	26.0	17.1	27.7	29.2	48.8	51.3	53.5	43.4	43.1	56.9	48.5	54.80
25	29.1	20.0	25.6	25.3	27.2	17.2	26.7	28.9	49.1	50.9	53.6	43.5	44.4	55.6	48.6	55.48
26	28.8	20.5	25.9	24.8	26.6	18.2	27.4	27.7	49.3	50.6	53.5	43.3	44.8	55.1	48.4	56.11
27	28.8	20.5	25.9	24.8	26.6	18.1	27.5	27.8	49.3	50.7	53.5	43.2	44.7	55.3	48.4	56.02
28	28.9	20.5	25.9	24.8	26.7	18.1	27.5	27.8	49.4	50.7	53.5	43.2	44.8	55.3	48.4	56.02
29	29.1	20.0	25.6	25.3	27.4	16.9	26.7	29.1	49.1	50.9	53.7	43.4	44.3	55.8	48.6	55.08
30	28.9	20.0	25.7	25.3	27.0	16.9	26.9	29.2	48.9	51.0	53.5	43.4	43.9	56.2	48.5	55.32
31	28.8	20.5	25.9	24.8	26.5	18.2	27.6	27.7	49.3	50.7	53.4	43.4	44.7	55.3	48.4	56.15
32	28.7	20.0	26.0	25.4	25.9	16.9	27.9	29.3	48.7	51.3	53.4	43.4	42.8	57.2	48.4	54.57
33	28.6	20.0	26.0	25.3	26.0	17.0	27.8	29.2	48.6	51.3	53.6	43.4	43.0	57.0	48.5	54.56
34	28.8	20.6	25.9	24.7	26.6	18.4	27.5	27.5	49.4	50.6	53.5	43.3	45.0	55.0	48.4	56.26
35	28.8	20.6	25.9	24.7	26.6	18.3	27.6	27.5	49.4	50.6	53.4	43.3	44.9	55.1	48.4	56.22
36	28.8	20.6	25.9	24.7	26.6	18.3	27.5	27.6	49.4	50.6	53.4	43.3	44.9	55.1	48.4	56.28
37	29.0	20.1	25.7	25.3	26.9	17.3	27.0	28.8	49.1	50.9	53.6	43.4	44.2	55.7	48.5	55.55
38	28.7	20.1	25.9	25.2	26.1	17.2	27.7	29.0	48.8	51.1	53.4	43.3	43.3	56.7	48.4	54.55
39	29.0	20.0	25.7	25.3	26.9	17.1	27.0	29.1	49.0	51.0	53.6	43.3	44.0	56.0	48.5	55.45
40	29.0	20.0	25.7	25.3	26.9	17.1	27.0	29.1	49.0	51.0	53.6	43.3	44.0	56.0	48.5	55.45
41	28.9	20.1	25.7	25.3	26.4	16.8	27.1	29.7	49.0	51.4	53.8	43.7	43.2	56.8	48.8	55.44
42	28.8	19.7	25.9	25.6	26.7	18.4	27.4	27.5	48.5	50.5	53.4	43.3	45.1	54.9	48.4	56.25
43	28.8	20.7	25.9	24.6	26.9	17.2	26.9	29.0	49.5	50.9	53.6	43.3	44.1	55.9	48.5	55.51
44	29.0	20.1	25.7	25.3	26.7	18.4	27.3	27.5	49.1	50.5	53.4	43.3	45.1	54.9	48.4	56.28
45	28.8	20.7	25.9	24.6	26.7	18.4	27.4	27.5	49.5	50.6	53.5	43.3	45.1	54.9	48.4	56.23
46	28.8	20.7	25.9	24.6	26.8	17.2	27.0	29.0	49.5	51.0	53.6	43.3	44.0	56.0	48.5	55.49
47	29.0	20.1	25.7	25.3	26.9	17.2	26.9	28.9	49.1	50.9	53.6	43.3	44.1	55.9	48.5	55.53
48	29.0	20.1	25.7	25.3	27.0	17.1	26.9	29.0	49.1	51.0	53.7	43.3	44.1	55.9	48.5	55.42
49	29.0	20.0	25.7	25.3	26.8	17.2	27.0	29.0	49.0	50.9	53.6	43.3	44.0	55.9	48.5	55.46
50	29.0	20.0	25.7	25.3	26.9	17.1	27.0	29.1	49.0	51.0	53.6	43.3	44.0	56.0	48.5	55.46

Table 1. Cont.

No	A	U	G	C	A$_3$	U$_3$	G$_3$	C$_3$	AU	GC	GC$_1$	GC$_2$	AU$_3$	GC$_3$	GC$_{12}$	ENC
51	28.9	20.1	25.7	25.3	26.8	17.2	27.0	29.0	49.0	51.0	53.6	43.3	44.0	56.0	48.5	55.46
52	29.0	20.1	25.7	25.3	26.8	17.2	27.0	29.0	49.1	50.9	53.6	43.3	44.0	55.9	48.5	55.51
53	29.0	20.1	25.7	25.3	26.9	17.1	27.0	29.0	49.1	51.0	53.6	43.4	44.0	56.0	48.5	55.44
54	29.0	20.1	25.7	25.3	26.8	17.2	27.0	29.0	49.1	51.0	53.6	43.3	44.0	56.0	48.5	55.47
55	28.9	20.1	25.7	25.3	26.9	17.2	26.9	29.0	49.0	50.9	53.5	43.3	44.1	55.9	48.4	55.46
56	29.0	20.1	25.7	25.3	26.8	17.2	27.0	28.9	49.1	51.0	53.6	43.4	44.0	55.9	48.5	55.53
57	28.9	20.1	25.7	25.3	26.9	17.2	27.0	28.9	49.0	50.9	53.6	43.3	44.1	55.9	48.5	55.52
58	29.0	20.1	25.7	25.3	26.9	17.2	26.9	29.0	49.1	51.0	53.6	43.3	44.1	55.9	48.5	55.43
59	29.0	20.1	25.7	25.3	26.9	17.3	27.0	28.9	49.1	50.9	53.6	43.3	44.2	55.9	48.5	55.53
60	29.0	20.1	25.7	25.3	26.9	17.3	27.0	28.9	49.1	50.9	53.7	43.2	44.2	55.8	48.5	55.54
61	29.0	20.1	25.7	25.3	26.9	17.3	26.9	28.9	49.1	50.9	53.6	43.2	44.2	55.8	48.4	55.49
62	29.0	20.1	25.7	25.3	26.8	17.1	27.0	29.0	49.1	51.0	53.6	43.3	43.9	56.0	48.5	55.44
63	29.0	20.0	25.7	25.3	26.9	17.0	27.0	29.1	49.0	51.0	53.6	43.3	43.9	56.1	48.5	55.45
64	29.0	20.1	25.7	25.3	26.8	17.2	27.0	29.0	49.1	50.9	53.6	43.3	44.0	56.0	48.5	55.50
65	29.0	20.1	25.7	25.3	26.9	17.2	26.9	29.0	49.1	51.0	53.6	43.3	44.1	55.9	48.5	55.50
66	29.0	20.1	25.7	25.3	26.9	17.2	27.0	29.0	49.1	50.9	53.6	43.3	44.1	55.9	48.5	55.49
67	28.7	20.1	25.9	25.3	26.9	17.1	26.9	29.1	48.8	51.0	53.6	43.4	44.0	56.0	48.5	55.49
68	29.0	20.1	25.7	25.3	26.8	17.2	27.0	29.0	49.1	51.0	53.6	43.3	44.0	56.0	48.5	55.50
69	29.0	20.1	25.7	25.3	26.9	17.2	26.9	29.0	49.1	50.9	53.5	43.3	44.1	55.9	48.4	55.52
70	29.1	20.0	25.9	25.0	27.1	16.9	27.1	28.9	49.1	50.9	53.7	43.2	44.0	56.0	48.5	55.11
71	28.7	20.6	26.0	24.7	26.9	17.2	27.0	28.9	49.3	50.9	53.6	43.3	44.1	55.9	48.5	55.42
72	29.0	20.1	25.6	25.2	26.6	18.3	27.5	27.7	49.1	50.6	53.4	43.4	44.9	55.1	48.4	56.28
73	29.0	20.1	25.7	25.3	26.9	17.2	27.0	28.9	49.1	50.9	53.6	43.3	44.1	55.9	48.5	55.57
74	29.0	20.1	25.7	25.2	26.9	17.2	27.0	28.9	49.1	51.0	53.6	43.3	44.1	55.9	48.5	55.55
75	29.0	20.1	25.7	25.3	26.9	17.3	27.0	28.9	49.1	50.9	53.6	43.3	44.2	55.8	48.5	55.55
76	29.0	20.1	25.7	25.3	26.9	17.2	26.9	28.9	49.1	50.9	53.6	43.2	44.1	55.9	48.4	55.49
77	29.0	20.1	25.7	25.2	26.8	17.3	27.0	28.9	49.1	51.0	53.7	43.4	44.1	55.9	48.6	55.61
78	28.9	20.1	25.7	25.3	26.9	17.2	27.0	29.0	49.0	51.0	53.7	43.4	44.1	56.0	48.6	55.58
79	29.0	20.1	25.7	25.2	26.9	17.3	27.0	28.9	49.1	50.9	53.6	43.3	44.2	55.9	48.5	55.58
80	28.9	20.1	25.7	25.2	26.9	17.3	27.0	28.9	49.0	50.9	53.5	43.4	44.2	55.9	48.5	55.55
81	28.9	20.1	25.7	25.3	26.8	17.2	27.0	29.0	49.0	51.0	53.6	43.3	44.0	56.0	48.5	55.55
82	28.9	20.1	25.7	25.3	26.8	17.2	27.0	29.0	49.0	50.9	53.6	43.3	44.0	56.0	48.5	55.51
83	29.0	20.1	25.6	25.2	27.0	17.3	26.8	28.9	49.1	50.8	53.5	43.3	44.3	55.7	48.4	55.63
84	29.0	20.1	25.7	25.2	26.8	17.3	27.0	28.8	49.1	50.9	53.6	43.3	44.1	55.9	48.5	55.60
85	28.9	20.1	25.7	25.3	26.9	17.3	27.0	28.9	49.0	50.9	53.6	43.3	44.2	55.8	48.5	55.48
86	28.9	20.1	25.7	25.3	26.8	17.3	27.0	28.8	49.0	50.9	53.6	43.3	44.1	55.8	48.5	55.61
87	29.0	20.1	25.7	25.3	26.8	17.2	27.0	29.0	49.1	50.9	53.6	43.3	44.0	56.0	48.5	55.51
88	28.9	20.1	25.7	25.2	27.0	17.2	26.8	29.0	49.0	50.9	53.6	43.3	44.2	55.8	48.5	55.53
89	29.0	20.1	25.6	25.3	26.8	17.3	27.0	28.9	49.1	50.9	53.6	43.3	44.1	56.0	48.5	55.58
90	29.0	20.1	25.6	25.3	26.9	17.2	27.0	29.0	49.1	50.9	53.6	43.2	44.1	55.9	48.4	55.38
91	29.0	20.1	25.6	25.3	27.0	17.3	26.8	28.9	49.1	50.9	53.6	43.3	44.3	55.8	48.5	55.54
92	29.0	20.1	25.7	25.3	27.0	17.2	26.9	29.0	49.1	50.9	53.6	43.3	44.2	55.8	48.5	55.53
93	29.0	20.1	25.7	25.3	26.9	17.2	27.0	29.0	49.1	50.9	53.6	43.2	44.1	56.0	48.4	55.44
94	29.0	20.1	25.7	25.3	26.9	17.2	27.0	28.9	49.1	50.9	53.6	43.2	44.1	55.9	48.4	55.42
95	28.9	20.1	25.7	25.2	26.8	17.3	27.0	28.9	49.0	50.9	53.6	43.3	44.1	55.9	48.5	55.59
96	29.0	20.1	25.7	25.2	26.9	17.2	27.0	29.0	49.1	50.9	53.6	43.3	44.1	55.9	48.5	55.43
97	29.0	20.1	25.7	25.3	26.8	17.3	27.0	28.9	49.1	50.9	53.5	43.3	44.1	55.9	48.4	55.57
98	28.9	20.2	25.7	25.2	26.9	17.2	27.0	29.0	49.1	50.9	53.6	43.2	44.1	56.0	48.4	55.42
99	29.0	20.1	25.7	25.3	26.8	17.3	27.0	28.9	49.1	50.9	53.6	43.3	44.1	55.9	48.5	55.59
100	28.9	20.2	25.7	25.2	27.0	17.2	26.9	29.0	49.1	50.9	53.6	43.3	44.2	55.9	48.5	55.41

Table 1. Cont.

No	A	U	G	C	A_3	U_3	G_3	C_3	AU	GC	GC_1	GC_2	AU_3	GC_3	GC_{12}	ENC
101	29.0	20.1	25.7	25.3	26.7	17.3	27.1	28.9	49.1	50.9	53.6	43.3	44.0	56.0	48.5	55.56
102	29.0	20.1	25.7	25.3	26.8	17.3	27.0	28.9	49.1	50.9	53.5	43.2	44.1	56.0	48.4	55.59
103	29.0	20.1	25.7	25.3	26.8	17.3	27.0	28.9	49.1	50.9	53.6	43.3	44.1	55.9	48.5	55.63
104	28.9	20.1	25.7	25.2	26.8	17.3	27.0	28.9	49.0	51.0	53.6	43.3	44.1	55.9	48.5	55.58
105	28.9	20.1	25.7	25.3	26.8	17.2	27.0	29.0	49.0	51.0	53.7	43.4	44.0	56.0	48.6	55.56
106	28.9	20.1	25.7	25.2	26.8	17.3	27.0	28.8	49.0	50.9	53.6	43.3	44.1	55.8	48.5	55.60
107	28.9	20.1	25.7	25.2	26.8	17.3	27.0	28.9	49.0	50.9	53.6	43.3	44.1	55.9	48.5	55.63
108	28.9	20.1	25.7	25.3	26.8	17.3	27.0	28.9	49.0	50.9	53.6	43.3	44.1	55.9	48.5	55.65
109	28.9	20.1	25.7	25.2	26.8	17.3	27.0	28.9	49.0	50.9	53.6	43.3	44.1	55.9	48.5	55.65
110	28.9	20.1	25.7	25.2	26.8	17.3	27.0	28.9	49.0	50.9	53.6	43.3	44.1	55.9	48.5	55.63
111	28.9	20.1	25.7	25.2	26.8	17.3	27.0	28.9	49.0	50.9	53.6	43.3	44.1	55.9	48.5	55.66
112	28.9	20.1	25.7	25.2	26.8	17.3	27.0	28.8	49.0	50.9	53.6	43.3	44.1	55.8	48.5	55.67
113	28.9	20.1	25.7	25.2	26.8	17.3	27.0	28.9	49.0	50.9	53.6	43.3	44.1	55.8	48.5	55.63
114	28.9	20.1	25.7	25.2	26.8	17.2	27.0	28.9	49.0	50.9	53.6	43.3	44.0	56.0	48.5	55.58
115	29.0	20.2	25.6	25.2	26.9	17.4	26.9	28.8	49.2	50.8	53.5	43.3	44.3	55.7	48.4	55.62
116	29.0	20.1	25.6	25.2	27.0	17.3	26.8	28.9	49.1	50.9	53.6	43.3	44.3	55.7	48.5	55.59
117	28.9	20.1	25.7	25.2	26.3	17.0	27.2	29.5	49.0	51.4	53.8	43.7	43.3	56.7	48.8	55.49
118	28.8	19.8	25.9	25.5	26.8	17.4	27.0	28.8	48.6	50.9	53.6	43.3	44.2	55.8	48.5	55.63
119	28.9	20.1	25.7	25.3	26.8	17.3	27.0	28.9	49.0	50.9	53.6	43.3	44.1	55.9	48.5	55.59
120	28.9	20.1	25.7	25.2	26.8	17.3	27.0	28.8	49.0	50.9	53.6	43.4	44.1	55.8	48.5	55.63
121	28.9	20.2	25.7	25.2	26.8	17.4	27.0	28.8	49.1	50.9	53.5	43.3	44.2	55.8	48.4	55.66
122	28.9	20.2	25.7	25.2	26.8	17.5	27.0	28.7	49.1	50.9	53.6	43.3	44.3	55.7	48.5	55.79
123	28.9	20.1	25.7	25.2	26.8	17.4	27.1	28.8	49.0	50.9	53.6	43.4	44.2	55.9	48.5	55.55
124	28.9	20.2	25.7	25.2	26.7	17.5	27.1	28.8	49.1	50.9	53.6	43.3	44.2	55.9	48.5	55.84
125	28.9	20.1	25.7	25.2	26.8	17.3	27.1	28.8	49.0	51.0	53.6	43.3	44.1	56.0	48.5	55.55
126	28.9	20.1	25.7	25.2	26.8	17.4	27.0	28.8	49.0	50.9	53.6	43.3	44.2	55.8	48.5	55.77
127	28.9	20.1	25.7	25.2	26.8	17.3	27.0	28.9	49.0	50.9	53.7	43.3	44.1	55.9	48.5	55.68
128	28.9	20.2	25.7	25.2	26.8	17.4	27.0	28.8	49.1	50.9	53.6	43.4	44.2	55.8	48.5	55.54
129	29.0	20.1	25.7	25.3	27.1	16.9	26.9	29.1	49.1	50.9	53.4	43.3	44.0	56.0	48.4	55.28
130	28.7	20.6	26	24.7	26.5	18.3	27.6	27.6	49.3	50.7	53.5	43.3	44.8	55.2	48.4	56.19
131	28.9	20.1	25.7	25.2	26.9	17.4	27.0	28.8	49.0	50.9	53.7	43.3	44.3	55.7	48.5	55.60
132	28.9	20.1	25.7	25.2	26.9	17.3	27.0	28.8	49.0	50.9	53.7	43.3	44.2	55.8	48.5	55.60
133	28.9	20.1	25.7	25.2	26.9	17.3	27.0	28.8	49.0	50.9	53.7	43.3	44.2	55.8	48.5	55.60
134	28.9	20.1	25.7	25.3	26.9	17.3	27.0	28.8	49.0	50.9	53.7	43.3	44.2	55.8	48.5	55.59
135	28.9	20.1	25.7	25.3	26.9	17.3	27.0	28.8	49.0	50.9	53.7	43.3	44.2	55.8	48.5	55.59
136	28.9	20.1	25.7	25.2	26.9	17.3	27.0	28.8	49.0	50.9	53.7	43.3	44.2	55.8	48.5	55.61
137	28.9	20.1	25.7	25.2	26.9	17.3	27.0	28.8	49.0	50.9	53.7	43.3	44.2	55.8	48.5	55.61
138	28.8	20.6	26.0	24.7	26.6	18.2	27.5	27.7	49.4	50.6	53.3	43.2	44.8	55.3	48.3	56.41
139	28.8	20.6	26.0	24.7	26.5	18.2	27.6	27.7	49.4	50.6	50.6	50.6	44.7	55.3	48.3	56.41
140	29.0	20.1	25.9	25.3	27.0	17.1	26.8	29.1	49.1	51.0	53.6	43.4	44.1	55.9	48.5	55.39
141	28.9	20.0	25.7	25.3	27.3	17.0	26.7	29.0	48.9	50.9	53.7	43.3	44.3	55.7	48.5	55.25
Mean	28.91	20.16	25.75	25.19	26.78	17.36	27.10	28.76	49.07	50.91	53.56	43.38	44.14	55.86	48.45	55.56
SD	0.10	0.18	0.10	0.20	0.25	0.39	0.27	0.47	0.16	0.16	0.27	0.62	0.41	0.40	0.07	0.34

SD: Standard deviation.

might be advantageous for efficient replication in host cells, with potentially distinct codon preferences [21].

The codon adaptation index (CAI) is often used as measure of level of gene expression and to assess the adaptation of viral genes to their hosts. Highly expressed genes exhibit a strong bias for particular codons in many bacteria and small eukaryotes. In comparison to the ENC, which is another way of calculating codon usage bias and measures deviation from a uniform bias (null hypothesis), CAI measures the deviation of a given protein coding gene sequence with respect to a reference set of genes [32]. Here,

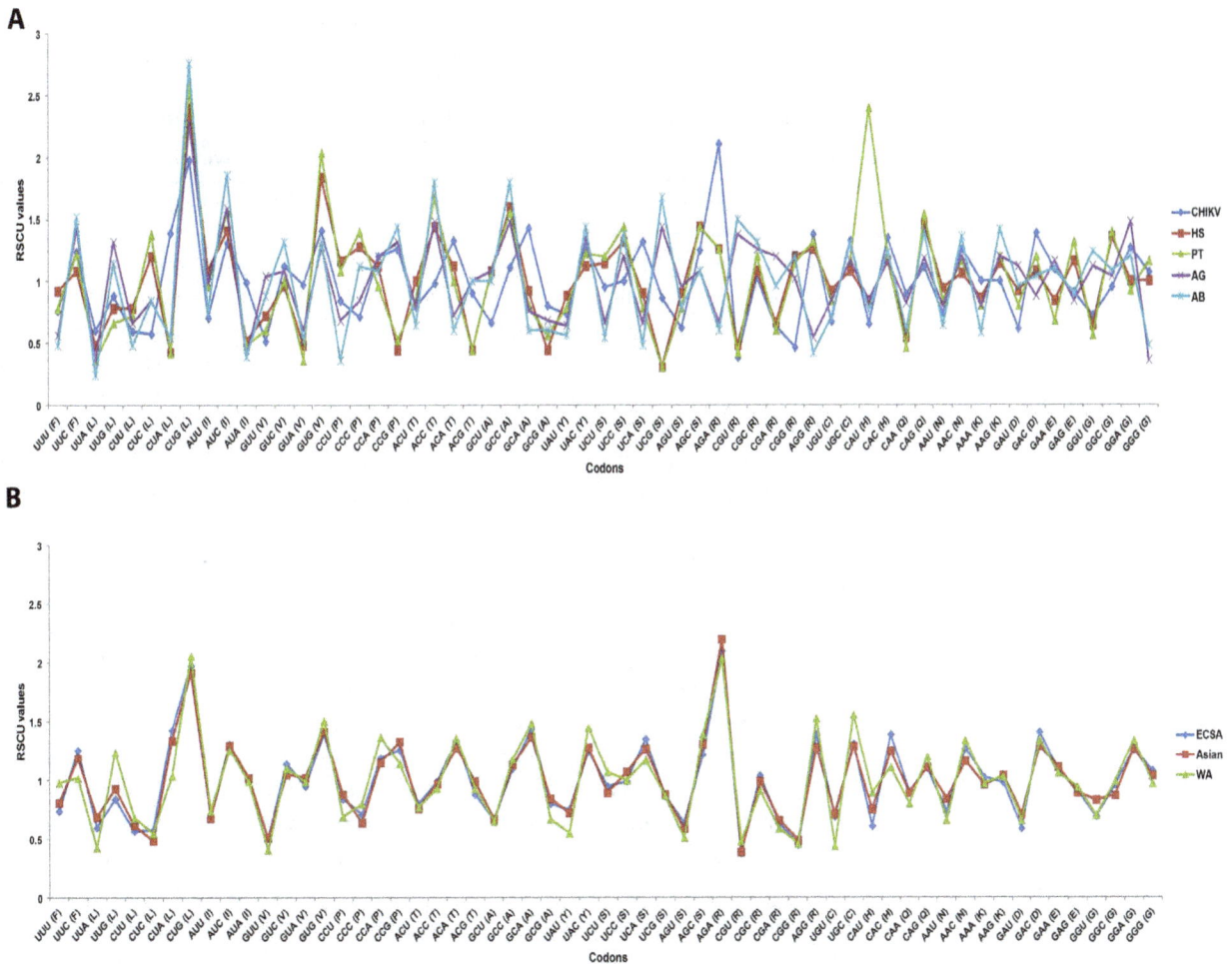

Figure 1. Comparative analysis of relative synonymous codon usage (RSCU) patterns. (**A**) between chikungunya virus (CHIKV), *Homo sapiens* (HS), *Pan troglodytes* (PT) and *Aedes aegypti* (AG) and *Aedes albopictus* (AB). (**B**) between east central south African (ECSA), Asian and West African (WA) genotypes of CHIKV.

we calculated the CAI values of coding sequences from CHIKV genomes. The CAI values ranged from 0.21 to 0.22, with a mean value of 0.22 and an SD of 0.001 (data not shown). The mean CAI value was low, indicating low codon usage bias and expression levels, which agreed with the ENC analysis.

Relationship between Codon Usage Patterns of CHIKV and its Hosts

Being parasitic organisms, it can be expected that the codon usage patterns of viruses would be affected by its hosts to some extent [33]. For instance, the codon usage pattern of poliovirus is reported to be mostly coincident with that of its host [34], while the codon usage pattern of hepatitis A was reported to be antagonistic to that of its host [35]. We therefore computed and compared the codon usage of CHIKV with its two hosts (*Homo sapiens* and *Pan troglodytes*), and transmission vectors (*A. aegypti* and *A. albopictus*). The results showed that the codon usage patterns of CHIKV were a mixture of coincidence and antagonism to its hosts and vectors (Table 2). In detail, the preferred codons for 12 out of 18 amino acids were common between CHIKV and *H. sapiens*. This included UUC (Phe), CUG (Leu), AUC (Ile), GUG (Val),

UAC (Tyr), AGA (Arg), UGC (Cys), CAC (His), CAG (Gln), AAC (Asn), AAG (Lys) and GAC (Asp). Furthermore, all common preferred codons between CHIKV and *H. sapiens* were G/C-ended (C-ended: 7; G-ended: 4), with exception of an A-ended preferred codon for amino acid Arg. Similarly, preferred codons for 10 out of 18 amino acids were common between CHIKV and *P. troglodytes*. In case of the two transmission vectors, 10 out of 18 preferred codons were common among both mosquito species and CHIKV. It is also interesting to note that, except for amino acid Arg, the remaining 10 highly preferred codons were same among CHIKV, *H. sapiens*, *A. aegypti* and *A. albopictus*. Moreover, the preferred codon usage profiles of *A. aegypti* and *A. albopictus* were also very similar: 16 out of 18 preferred codons were common between, with exceptions for the preferred codons for Asp and Gly (Table 2). These results indicated that selection pressures from hosts and vectors have influenced the codon usage pattern of CHIKV and the possible fitness of the virus to adjust among its dynamic range of hosts and vectors. A mixture of coincidence and antagonism has also been reported previously in the case of HCV [31] and enterovirus 71 [13]. It was suggested that the coincident portions of codon usage among viruses and their hosts could enable the corresponding amino acids to be translated efficiently,

Table 2. The synonymous codon usage patterns of CHIKV, its hosts and transmission vectors.

AA	Codon	RSCU CHIKV Overall	ECSA	Asian	WA	Hosts & Vectors HS	PT	AG	AB	AA	Codon	RSCU CHIKV Overall	ECSA	Asian	WA	Hosts & Vectors HS	PT	AG	AB
Phe[b,c]	UUU	0.76	0.74	0.81	0.98	0.92	0.78	0.56	0.48	Ser[a,c]	UCU	0.95	0.95	0.89	1.07	1.14	1.20	0.66	0.54
	UUC	**1.24**	**1.26**	**1.19**	**1.02**	**1.08**	**1.22**	**1.44**	**1.52**		UCC	1.00	0.99	1.07	1.00	1.32	1.44	1.20	1.38
Leu[b,d]	UUA	0.60	0.60	0.69	0.43	0.48	0.36	0.36	0.24		**UCA**	**1.32**	1.35	1.27	1.17	0.90	0.78	0.66	0.48
	UUG	0.88	0.84	0.93	1.24	0.78	0.66	1.32	1.14		UCG	0.86	0.86	0.88	0.87	0.30	0.30	**1.44**	**1.68**
	CUU	0.59	0.57	0.62	0.68	0.78	0.72	0.66	0.48		AGU	0.62	0.64	0.59	0.51	0.90	0.78	0.96	0.78
	CUC	0.57	0.58	0.49	0.55	1.20	1.38	0.84	0.84		AGC	1.25	1.22	**1.31**	**1.39**	**1.44**	**1.44**	1.08	1.08
	CUA	1.39	1.43	1.34	1.04	0.42	0.42	0.54	0.54	Arg[a,c]	**AGA**	**2.11**	**2.10**	**2.20**	**2.04**	**1.26**	**1.26**	0.66	0.60
	CUG	**1.98**	**1.98**	**1.92**	**2.06**	**2.40**	**2.58**	**2.28**	**2.76**		CGU	0.38	0.38	0.39	0.48	0.48	0.42	**1.38**	**1.50**
Ile[b,c]	AUU	0.70	0.70	0.68	0.74	1.08	0.96	0.99	0.75		CGC	1.03	1.04	0.99	0.91	1.08	1.20	1.26	1.32
	AUC	**1.31**	**1.31**	**1.30**	**1.26**	**1.41**	**1.56**	**1.59**	**1.86**		CGA	0.63	0.63	0.66	0.59	0.66	0.60	1.20	0.96
	AUA	0.99	0.99	1.02	0.99	0.51	0.48	0.39	0.39		CGG	0.46	0.45	0.49	0.46	1.20	1.14	1.02	1.20
Val[b,c]	GUU	0.51	0.51	0.51	0.41	0.72	0.60	1.04	0.88		AGG	1.38	1.39	1.28	1.53	1.26	**1.32**	0.54	0.42
	GUC	1.12	1.14	1.05	1.10	0.96	1.00	1.08	1.32	Cys[b,c]	UGU	0.67	0.69	0.71	0.44	0.92	0.84	0.84	0.70
	GUA	0.97	0.95	1.02	0.99	0.48	0.36	0.60	0.52		**UGC**	**1.33**	**1.31**	**1.29**	**1.56**	**1.08**	**1.16**	**1.16**	**1.30**
	GUG	**1.41**	**1.40**	**1.42**	**1.51**	**1.84**	**2.04**	**1.28**	**1.32**	His[b,c]	CAU	0.65	0.61	0.75	0.89	0.84	**2.40**	0.84	0.76
Pro[b,d]	CCU	0.84	0.84	0.88	0.69	1.16	1.08	0.68	0.36		**CAC**	**1.35**	**1.39**	**1.25**	**1.11**	**1.16**	1.20	**1.16**	**1.24**
	CCC	0.71	0.71	0.64	0.80	**1.28**	**1.40**	0.84	1.12	Gln[b,c]	CAA	0.89	0.90	0.89	0.80	0.54	0.46	0.82	0.60
	CCA	1.20	1.19	1.15	**1.37**	1.12	0.96	1.20	1.08		**CAG**	**1.11**	**1.10**	**1.11**	**1.20**	**1.46**	**1.54**	**1.18**	**1.40**
	CCG	**1.26**	**1.26**	**1.33**	1.14	0.44	0.52	**1.32**	**1.44**	Asn[b,c]	AAU	0.74	0.73	0.84	0.66	0.94	0.84	0.80	0.64
Thr[a,c]	ACU	0.79	0.80	0.76	0.77	1.00	0.84	0.80	0.64		**AAC**	**1.26**	**1.27**	**1.16**	**1.34**	**1.06**	**1.16**	**1.20**	**1.36**
	ACC	0.98	0.99	0.97	0.93	**1.44**	**1.68**	**1.48**	**1.80**	Lys[a,d]	AAA	1.00	**1.02**	0.96	0.97	0.86	0.80	0.80	0.58
	ACA	**1.33**	**1.34**	**1.28**	**1.36**	1.12	1.00	0.72	0.60		**AAG**	**1.00**	0.98	**1.04**	**1.03**	**1.14**	**1.20**	**1.20**	**1.42**
	ACG	0.90	0.88	0.99	0.93	0.44	0.44	1.00	1.00	Asp[b,c]	GAU	0.61	0.59	0.71	0.66	0.92	0.80	**1.12**	0.96
Ala[a,c]	GCU	0.66	0.66	0.67	0.65	1.08	1.08	1.08	1.00		**GAC**	**1.39**	**1.41**	**1.29**	**1.34**	**1.08**	**1.20**	0.88	**1.04**
	GCC	1.11	1.10	1.13	1.18	**1.60**	**1.56**	**1.48**	**1.80**	Glu[a,d]	**GAA**	**1.09**	1.09	1.11	1.06	0.84	0.68	**1.16**	**1.10**
	GCA	**1.43**	**1.44**	**1.37**	**1.49**	0.92	0.80	0.76	0.60		GAG	0.91	0.91	0.89	0.94	**1.16**	**1.32**	0.84	0.90
	GCG	0.80	0.80	0.84	0.67	0.44	0.56	0.68	0.60	Gly[a,c]	GGU	0.72	0.69	0.83	0.70	0.64	0.56	1.12	**1.24**
Tyr[b,c]	UAU	0.73	0.75	0.72	0.55	0.88	0.78	0.64	0.56		GGC	0.95	0.96	0.87	0.99	**1.36**	**1.40**	1.04	1.08
	UAC	**1.27**	**1.25**	**1.28**	**1.45**	**1.12**	**1.22**	**1.36**	**1.44**		**GGA**	**1.27**	**1.26**	**1.27**	**1.34**	1.00	0.92	**1.48**	1.20
											GGG	1.07	1.08	1.04	0.97	1.00	1.16	0.36	0.48

AA: amino acid, HS: *H. sapiens*, AG: *A. aegypti*, AB: *A. albopictus*, PT: *P. troglodytes*. Preferred codons of CHIKV, *H. sapiens*, *A. aegypti*, *A. albopictus* and *P. troglodytes* are shown in bold.
[a]Amino acids with A/U-ended preferred codons in CHIKV.
[b]Amino acids with G/C-ended preferred codons in CHIKV.
[c]Amino acids with A/U-ended preferred codons in CHIKV.
[d]Amino acids with G/C-ended preferred codons in CHIKV.

while the antagonistic portions of codon usage may enable viral proteins to be folded properly, although the translation efficiency of the corresponding amino acids might decrease [31].

Although the comparative analysis of individual RSCU values as given above is frequently employed as a method of estimating the effect of synonymous codons usage of the hosts on that of specific viruses, it has its limitations in revealing the effect of the overall codon usage of the hosts on the formation of codon usage patterns of the viruses. Therefore, we took advantage of a method proposed recently that estimates the similarity degree of the overall codon usage patterns comprehensively between viruses and their hosts by treating the 59 synonymous codons as 59 different spatial vectors. The advantage of this formula, as reported by the authors

in the case of dengue viruses, is that the comparative overall codon usage takes the place of the direct estimation of each synonymous codon usage; thus, the new method avoids the situation that the variations of 59 synonymous codon usage confuse the correct estimation of the effect of the host on the virus for codon usage [36]. The similarity index $D(A,B)$ was therefore calculated for each genotype of CHIKV in relation to its hosts and vectors. The similarity index was found to be highest for *A. albopictus vs.* CHIKV group followed by *P. troglodytes vs.* CHIKV, *A. aegypti vs.* CHIKV and lowest in the case of *H. sapiens vs.* CHIKV (Figure 2), indicating that the effect of *A. albopictus* and *P. troglodytes* on the formation of the overall codon usage patterns of CHIKV is relatively higher than that of the *A. aegypti* and *H. sapiens*. Secondly,

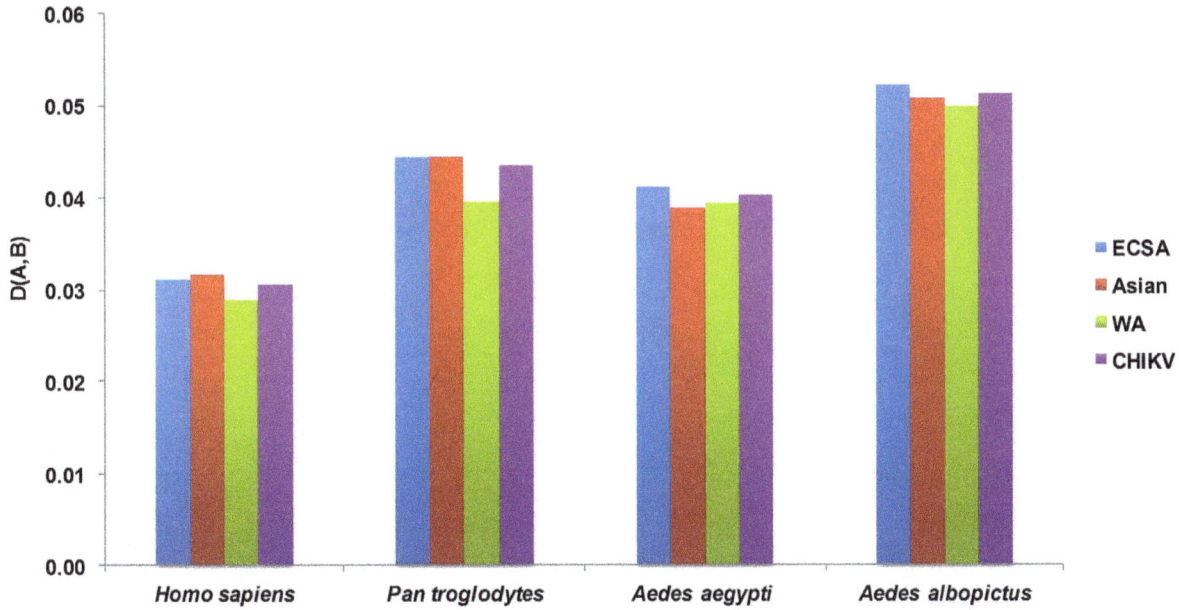

Figure 2. The similarity index analysis of the codon usage between CHIKV, its hosts and transmission vectors.

we computed the effect of transmission vectors on the formation of the overall codon usage patterns of three genotypes of CHIKV. *A. aegypti* had the strongest effect on the east central south African (ECSA) genotype, followed by West African (WA) and Asian genotypes. In the case of *A. albopictus*, the strongest effect was noted on the ECSA genotype, followed by Asian and WA genotypes. As for the effects of the two primates on the formation of the overall

codon usage of CHIKV, the strongest effect of *H. sapiens* was on the Asian genotype, closely followed by the ECSA and WA genotypes. By contrast, *P. troglodytes* had its strongest and equal effect on ECSA and Asian genotypes, followed by WA genotype (Figure 2). Therefore, from the similarity index analysis, we observed that selection pressure from hosts and vectors have contributed to shaping the molecular evolution of CHIKV at the

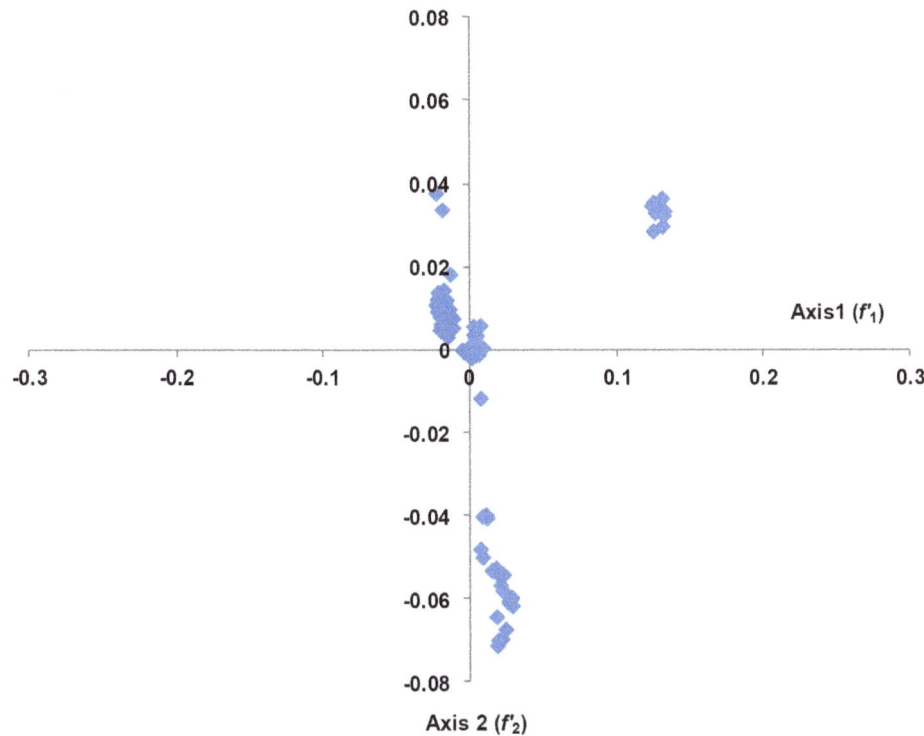

Figure 3. Correspondence analysis of codon usage patterns in CHIKV genomes.

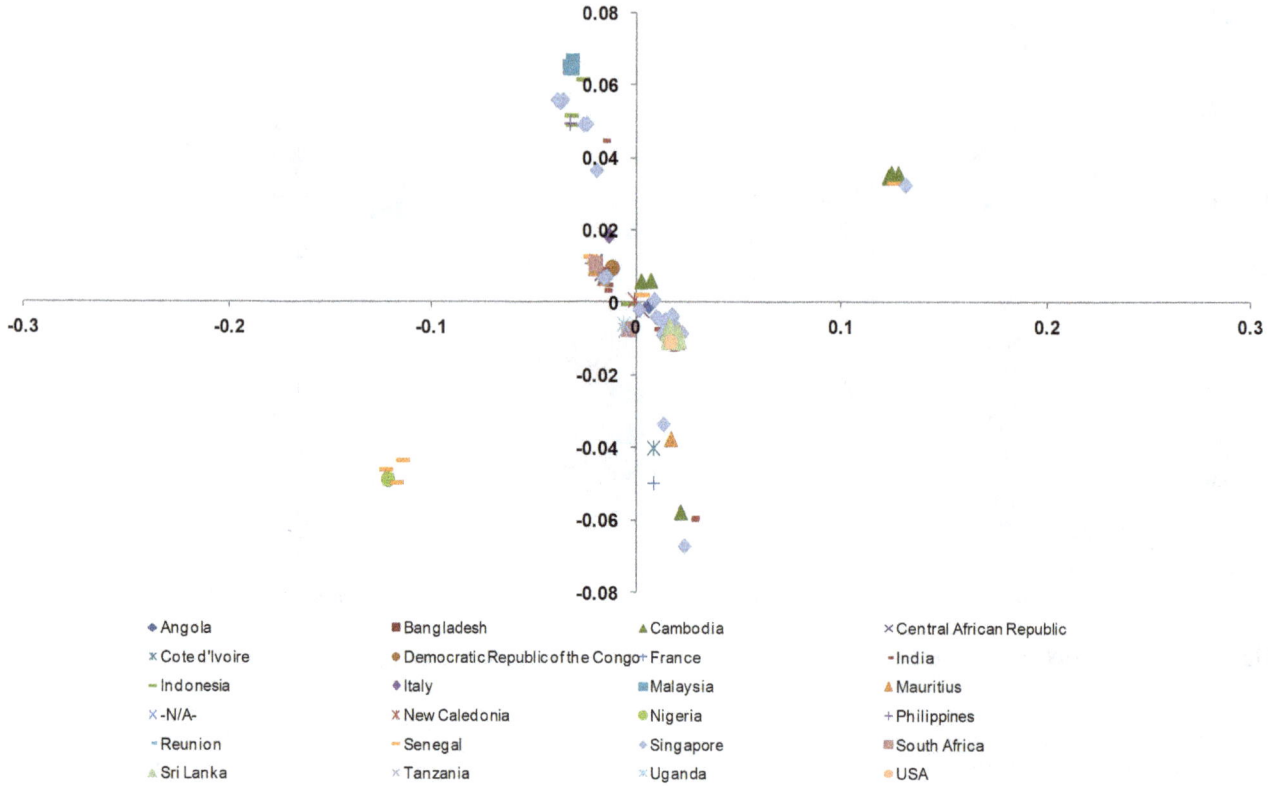

Figure 4. Correspondence analysis of codon usage patterns in CHIKV genomes based on region of isolation.

level of codon usage. The effect of the hosts was unevenly distributed among different genotypes, potentially indicating different evolutionary rates of CHIKV isolates. The calculation

of the effects of primates and transmission vectors on the overall codon usage patterns of CHIKV showed that *P. troglodytes* and *A. albopictus* dominate the effects of *H. sapiens* and *A. aegypti*,

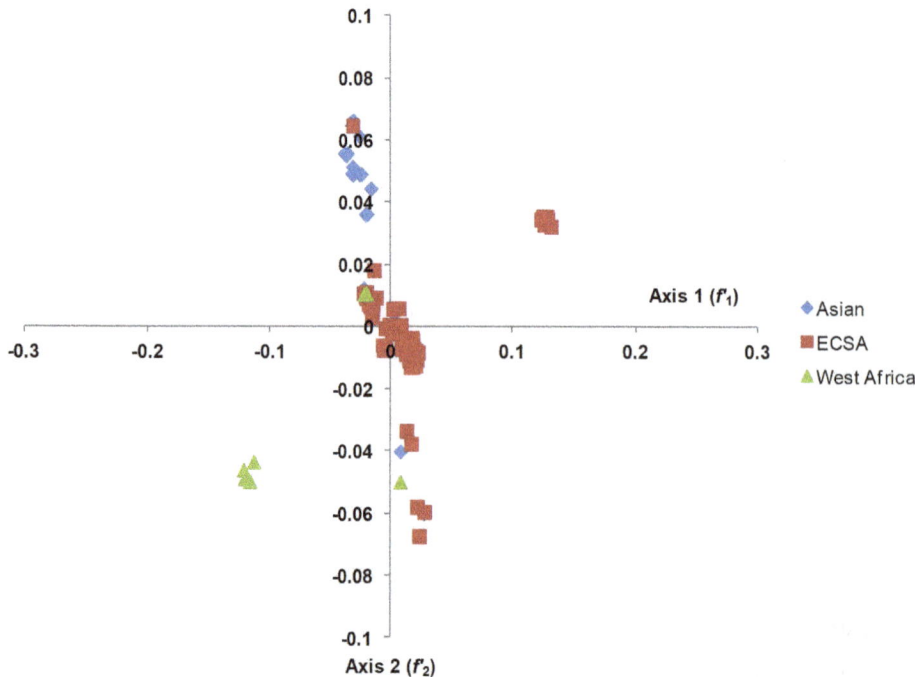

Figure 5. Correspondence analysis of codon usage patterns in CHIKV genomes based on virus genotypes.

respectively, on the formation of the overall codon usage patterns of CHIKV (Figure 2). The stronger effect of *P. troglodytes* than *H. sapiens* could also be attributed to the maintenance of CHIKV in a yellow fever-like zoonotic sylvatic cycle and its dependence upon non-human primates as reservoir hosts [7,9]. Moreover, the similarity index of codon usage was also the highest between CHIKV and *A. albopictus*, as compared with *A. aegypti*, *P. troglodytes* and *H. sapiens*. The successful human-to-human transmission of CHIKV depends on *Aedes* mosquitoes [7,9]; therefore, the stronger effect of *A. albopictus* on all three genotypes of CHIKV suggests that this vector might be a more efficient reservoir for viral replication and transmission compared with *A. aegypti*. These results are in agreement with recent studies showing more efficient dissemination and transmission of CHIKV by *A. albopictus*, which contribute to its ongoing re-emergence in a series of large-scale epidemics [37,38].

Trends of Codon Usage Variation in CHIKV

Correspondence Analysis (COA). Codon usage is multivariate by its very nature; therefore, it is necessary to analyze the data using multivariate statistical techniques, such as COA [39]. Therefore, to determine the trends in codon usage variation among different CHIKV genomes, we performed COA on the RSCU values, which were examined as a single dataset based on the RSCU value of each coding region (Figure 3). The first principal axis (f'_1) accounted for 53.57% of the total variation, and the next three axes $(f'_2–f'_4)$ accounted for 25.16%, 7.62%, and 2.06% of the total variation in synonymous codon usage, respectively. For further analysis, plots were reconstructed based on different geographical locations (Figure 4) and genotypes of CHIKV isolates (Figure 5). As expected the CHIKV isolates belonging to ECSA genotype were distributed across all planes of axes. When these plots were accessed on regional basis, it was found that different genotypes are circulating in single country. This analysis showed that the three different genotypes of CHIKV might have common ancestor. This further implies that the geographical diversity and associated factors, such as presence of favorable transmission vectors, climate features, host range and susceptibility, have also contributed to shaping the molecular evolution and codon usage in CHIKV, even though it appears to be less influential than mutational pressure (based on the current analysis).

Effect of mutational pressure in shaping the codon usage patterns in CHIKV. Mutational pressure and natural selection are considered the two major factors that shape codon usage patterns [40]. A general mutational pressure, which affects the whole genome, would certainly account for the majority of the codon usage among certain RNA viruses [21]. To determine the extent of the influence of these two factors on CHIKV codon usage, we performed correlation analysis between different nucleotide constraints. A complex correlation was observed among different nucleotide constraints (Table 3). $U_3\%$ had a significant positive correlation with U% ($r=0.621$, $P<0.01$) and G% ($r=0.185$, $P<0.05$), whereas it had significant negative correlations with C% ($r=-0.606$, $P<0.01$) A% ($r=-0.278$, $P<0.01$) and GC% ($r=-0.806$, $P<0.01$). $C_3\%$ had significant positive correlation with C% ($r=0.621$, $P<0.01$), A ($r=0.261$, $P<0.01$) and GC% ($r=0.798$, $P<0.01$), and negative correlations with U% ($r=-0.5877$, $P<0.01$) and G% ($r=-0.217$, $P<0.01$). $A_3\%$ had positive correlations with A ($r=0.625$, $P<0.01$), C% ($r=0.327$, $P<0.01$) and negative correlations with U% ($r=-0.373$, $P<0.01$) and G% ($r=-0.576$, $P<0.01$), whereas no correlation was observed between $A_3\%$ and the GC%. $G_3\%$ was positively correlated with G% ($r=0.658$, $P<0.01$) U% ($r=0.354$, $P<0.01$),

and negatively correlated with C% ($r=-0.377$, $P<0.01$) and A% ($r=-0.610$, $P<0.01$); the correlation with the GC% was non-significant. In the case of $GC_3\%$, positive correlation was noted with C% ($r=0.498$, $P<0.01$) and GC% ($r=0.852$, $P<0.01$), and negative correlation with U% ($r=-0.480$, $P<0.01$); the correlation with G% was non-significant. Finally the GC and GC_{12} were also compared with GC_3 and a highly significant positive correlations ($r=0.28$, $P<0.01$; GC_{12} versus GC_3) ($r=0.85$, $P<0.01$; GC versus GC_3) was observed as shown in Figure 6A and 6B respectively. Furthermore, a significant negative correlation between GC_3 and ENC values was also observed ($r=-0.756$, $P<0.01$). This analysis collectively indicates that mutational pressure is most likely responsible for the patterns of nucleotide composition and, therefore, codon usage patterns, because the effects were present at all codon positions.

In addition to correlation analysis, linear regression analysis was also performed to determine correlations between the first two principle axes $(f'_1$ and $f'_2)$ and nucleotide constraints of CHIKV genomes. Again, several significant correlations were observed between the two principle axes and nucleotide contents (Table 4). f'_1 showed a significantly positive correlation with $U_3\%$ ($r=0.31$, $P<0.01$), $G_3\%$ ($r=0.58$, $P<0.01$), U% ($r=0.25$, $P<0.01$) and C% ($r=0.51$, $P<0.01$); however, it showed significantly negative correlations with A% ($r=-0.54$, $P<0.01$), G% ($r=-0.29$, $P<0.01$), $A_3\%$ ($r=-0.50$, $P<0.01$), C_3 ($r=-0.35$, $P<0.01$), GC_3 ($r=-0.24$, $P<0.01$; Figure 7A) and GC% ($r=-0.21$, $P<0.01$). In the case of f_2, $A_3\%$, $G_3\%$ and C% had non-significant correlations. f'_2 axis showed significantly positive correlations with C_3 ($r=0.69$, $P<0.01$), $GC_3\%$ ($r=0.74$, $P<0.01$; Figure 7B), GC% ($r=0.64$, $P<0.01$), A% ($r=0.17$, $P<0.05$) and G% ($r=0.39$, $P<0.01$) whereas, negative correlations with $U_3\%$ ($r=-0.66$, $P<0.01$), and U% ($r=-0.34$, $P<0.01$) (Table 4). Our analysis shows that mutational pressure has played a major role in shaping the dynamics of codon usage patterns within CHIKV genomes.

Correlation analysis between ENC and GC_3 values. A plot of ENC versus GC_3 (Nc plot) is widely used to study codon usage variation among genes in different organisms. It has been postulated that an ENC-plot of genes, whose codon choice is constrained only by a G_3+C_3 mutational bias, will lie on or just below the continuous curve of the predicted ENC values [30]. Although, the nucleotide composition correlation analysis showed that codon usage in CHIKV genomes is mainly caused by compositional constraints or mutational pressure, we were interested to determine the possible influence of other factors, such as natural selection. Therefore, we constructed a corresponding relation distribution plot between the ENC and GC_3 values. As

Table 3. Summary of correlation analysis between nucleotide constraints in CHIKV genomes.

	$A_3\%$	$U_3\%$	$C_3\%$	$G_3\%$	$GC_3\%$
A%	0.625**	−0.278**	0.261**	−0.610**	0.090^{NS}
U%	−0.373**	0.621**	−0.587**	0.354**	−0.480**
C%	0.327**	−0.606**	0.621**	−0.377**	0.498**
G%	−0.576**	0.185*	−0.217**	0.658**	−0.080^{NS}
GC%	0.103^{NS}	−0.806**	0.798**	−0.153^{NS}	0.852**

The numbers in the each column represents correlation coefficient "r" values, which are calculated in each correlation analysis.
NS: non-significant ($P>0.05$).
*represents $0.01<P<0.05$.
**represents $P<0.01$.

A

B

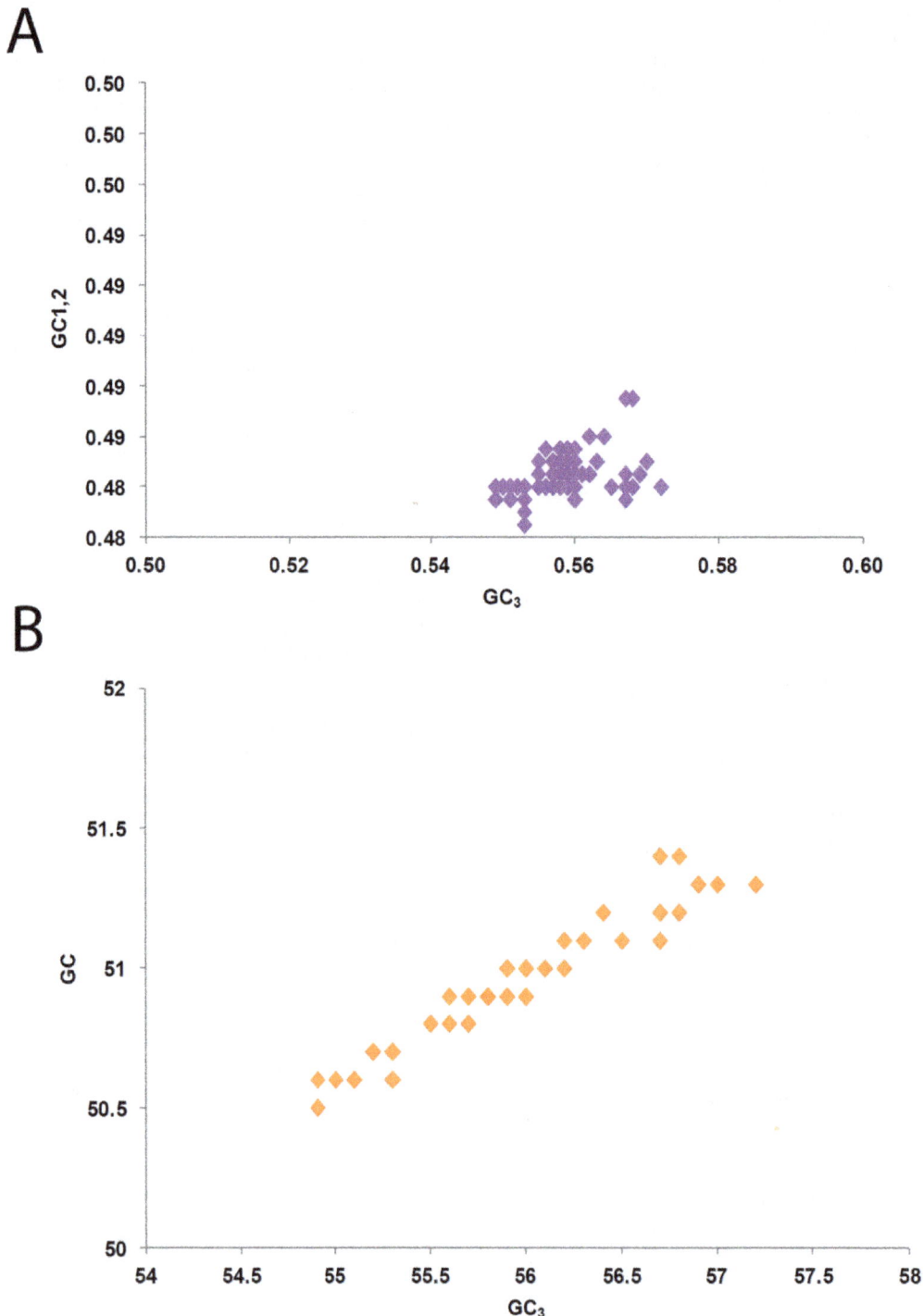

Figure 6. Correlation analysis. (A) $GC_{1,2}$ with that at GC_3, (B) GC with that at GC_3.

shown in Figure 8, all points aggregated closely towards the right side under the expected ENC curve, indicating that, apart from mutation pressure, the codon usage patterns have also been influenced by other factors to some extent.

Relationship between dinucleotide and codon usage patterns in CHIKV. It has been suggested that dinucleotide bias can affect overall codon usage bias in several organisms, including DNA and RNA viruses [41–43]. To study the possible effect of dinucleotides on codon usage in CHIKV genomes, we calculated the relative abundances of the 16 dinucleotides from the coding sequences of CHIKV. The occurrences of dinucleotides were not randomly distributed, and no dinucleotides were present at the expected frequencies (Table 5). Under-representation of CpG dinucleotides in different RNA and DNA viruses has been reported [41]. In the case of CHIKV, the relative abundance of CpG showed deviation from the "normal range" (mean ±

Table 4. Summary of correlation between the first two principle axes and nucleotide constraints in CHIKV genomes.

Composition (%)	f_1 (53.57%)	f_2 (25.16%)
A_3	−0.50**	−0.97[NS]
U_3	0.310**	−0.659**
C_3	−0.35**	0.69**
G_3	0.58**	−0.134[NS]
GC_3	−0.24**	0.740**
GC	−0.21*	0.640**
A	−0.54**	0.174*
U	0.25**	−0.340**
G	−0.29**	0.390**
C	0.517**	−0.126[NS]

The numbers in the each column represents correlation coefficient "r" values, which are calculated in each correlation analysis.
NS: non-significant ($P>0.05$).
*represents $0.01<P<0.05$.
**represents $P<0.01$.

SD = 0.808±0.016) and was under-represented. Interestingly, GpC dinucleotides also deviated from the normal range and were instead slightly over-represented (mean ± SD = 1.001±0.007) (Table 5). The RSCU values of the eight codons containing CpG (CCG, GCG, UCG, ACG, CGC, CGG, CGU, and CGA) and the six codons containing GpC (GCU, GCC, GCA, UGC, AGC, GGC) were also analyzed to determine the possible effects of CpG and GpC representations on codon usage bias. In the case of CpG-containing codons, all codons were under-represented (RSCU<1.6) and were not preferred codons for their respective amino acid, except for CCG (RSCU = 1.26), a preferred codon for proline (Table 2). On the other hand, despite slight over-representation of the GpC dinucleotide, all GpC-containing codons were also under-represented (RSCU<1.6) and were not preferred codons for their respective amino acids, with two exceptions; GCA (Ala, RSCU = 1.43) and UGC (Cys, RSCU = 1.33) (Table 2). It has been proposed that CpG deficiency in pathogens is associated with the immunostimulatory properties of unmethylated CpGs, which are recognized by the host's innate immune system as a pathogen signature [28]. Recognition of umethylated CpGs by Toll like receptor 9 (TLR9), a type of intracellular pattern recognition receptor (PRR), leads to activation of several immune response pathways [44]. The vertebrate immune system relies on unmethylated CpG recognition in DNA molecules as a signature of infection, and CpG under-representation in RNA viruses is exclusively observed in vertebrate viruses; therefore, it is reasonable to suggest that a TLR9-like mechanism exists in the vertebrate immune system that recognizes CpGs when in an RNA context (such as in the genomes of RNA viruses) and triggers immune responses [45].

Compared with differential (over- and under-) representation of CpGs in different organisms, UpA under-representation also exists in several organisms, including vertebrates, invertebrates, plants and prokaryotes [41]. The presence of TpA in two out of three canonical stop codons and in transcriptional regulatory motifs (e.g., the TATA box sequence) is believed to be responsible for its under-representation. Therefore, UpA under-representation is expected to reduce the risk of nonsense mutations and minimizes improper transcription [43,46]. In the case of CHIKV, the relative abundance of UpA also deviated from the "normal range" (mean ± SD = 0.859±0.022) and was under-represented, similarly to CpG. The six codons containing UpA (UUA, CUA, GUA, UAU, UAC and AUA) were also under-represented (RSCU<1.6) and were not preferred codons for their respective amino acids. The CpA (mean ± SD = 1.125±0.017) and UpG (mean ± SD = 1.275±0.022) dinucleotides were over-represented compared with the rest of the 14 dinucleotide pairs (Table 5). Similarly, the eight codons containing CpA (UCA, CCA, ACA, GCA, CAA, CAG, CAU and CAC) and five codons containing UpG (UUG, CUG, GUG, UGU and UGC) were also over-represented compared with the rest of the codons for their respective amino acids and a majority of them were also preferential codons for their respective amino acids, based on RSCU analysis (Table 2). Over-representation of CpA and UpG in different organisms has been observed and is regarded as a consequence of the under-representation of CpG dinucleotides. One possible explanation is that methylated cytosines are prone to mutate into thymines through spontaneous deamination, resulting in the dinucleotide TpG and the subsequent presence of a CpA on the opposite strand after DNA replication [47]. However, this theory cannot explain under-representation of CpGs in RNA viruses. Moreover, under-representation of CpGs has also been observed in several vertebrate viruses, where it is independent of their genomic composition and replication cycles. Recently, two studies performed large-scale dinucleotide analyses in different viruses and suggested that the CpG usage of +ssRNA viruses is affected greatly by their hosts. As a result, most +ssRNA viruses mimic their hosts' CpG usage and the existence of an RNA dinucleotide recognition system, probably linked to the innate immune system of the host, has also been proposed [41,48].

Finally, the relative abundance of dinucleotides was also correlated with the first two principal axes. Among the 16 dinucleotides, 11 significantly (positive and negative) correlated with the first axis and 16 significantly (positive and negative) correlated with the second axis (Table 5). These observations indicated that the composition of dinucleotides determines the variation in synonymous codon usage. Therefore, from the present dinucleotide composition analysis, it is evident that selection pressure associated with (i) maintenance of efficient replication and transmission cycles among multiple hosts, and (ii) evolution of escape mechanisms to evade from the host antiviral responses, have contributed to shaping the overall synonymous codon usage in CHIKV.

Effect of natural selection in shaping the codon usage patterns in CHIKV. It has been suggested that if synonymous codon usage bias is affected by mutational pressure alone, then the frequency of nucleotides A and U/T should be equal to that of C and G at the synonymous codon third position [26]. However, in case of CHIKV genomes, variations in nucleotide base compositions were noted (Table 1), indicating that other factors, such as natural selection, could also influence overall synonymous codon usage bias. As the role of natural selection is also evident from previous codon usage analysis studies in several viruses [25,26,49], we were interested to determine to what extent natural selection might be involved in the codon usage patterns of CHIKV. For this purpose, we computed the GRAVY and aromaticity (ARO) values for each CHIKV isolate (Table S1) and a linear regression analysis was performed between GRAVY, ARO and the f'_1, f'_2, ENC, GC and GC_3 values. The analysis results showed that the GRAVY values were not significant for f'_1 and were highly significant for f'_2, ENC, GC_3 and GC. In the case of ARO, an opposite trend was observed: ARO values were significantly negatively correlated with f'_1 and correlations with f'_2, ENC, GC_3 and GC were not significant (Table 6). These results indicated that, although natural

A

B

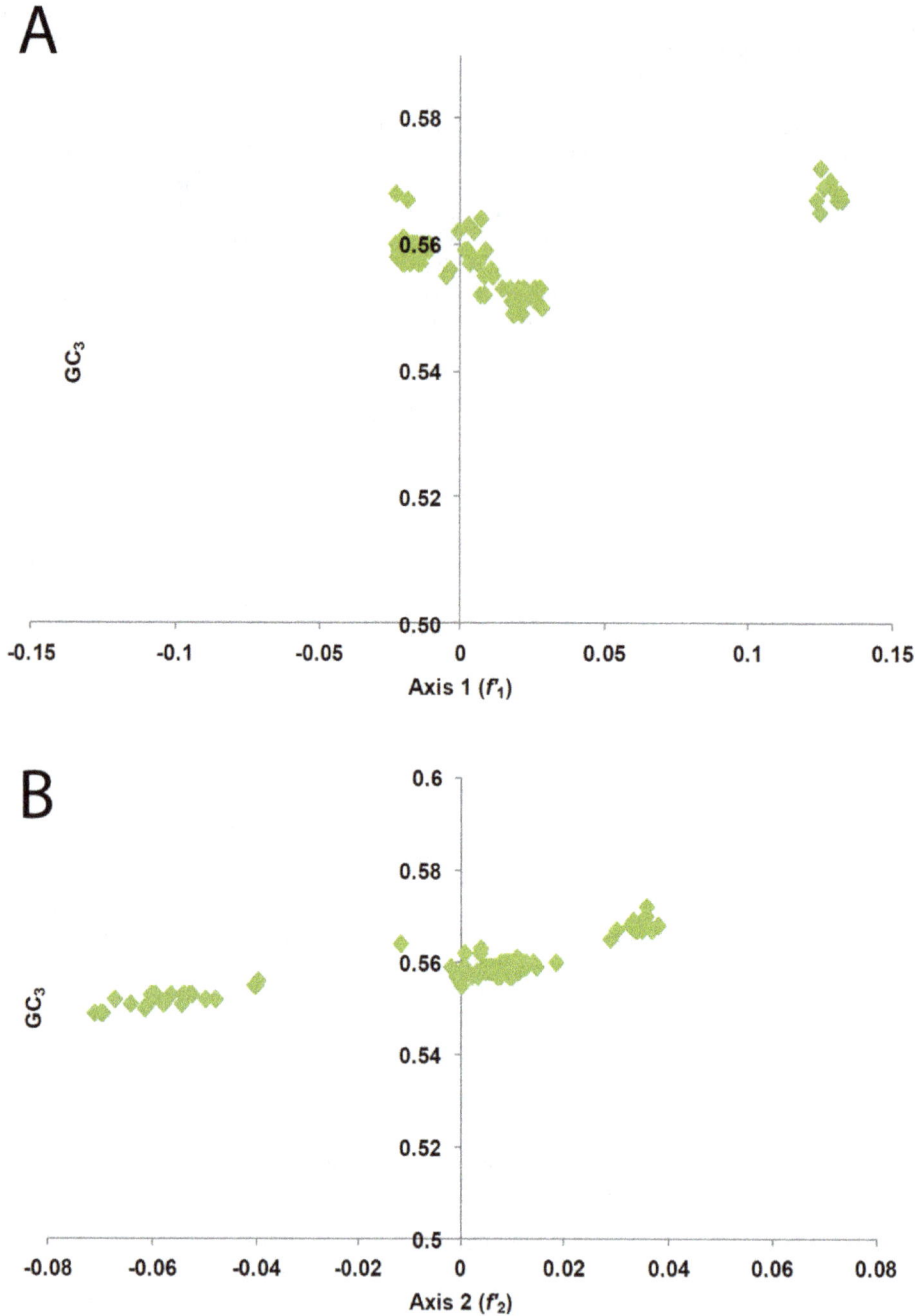

Figure 7. Correlation between the first axis (A) and second axis (B) values of COA and GC$_3$ values.

selection has influenced codon usage of CHIKV genomes to some extent, it is much weaker compared with mutational pressure.

Conclusions

Taken together, our analysis showed that overall codon usage bias in CHIKV is slightly biased, and the major factor that has contributed to shaping codon usage pressure is mutational pressure. In addition, contributions of other factors, including hosts, geography, dinucleotides composition and natural selection, are also evident from our analysis. Our data suggested that codon usage in CHIKV is undergoing an evolutionary process, probably reflecting a dynamic process of mutation and natural selection to

re-adapt its codon usage to different environments and hosts. To the best our knowledge, this is first report of codon usage analysis in CHIKV and is expected to deepen our understanding of the mechanisms contributing towards codon usage and evolution of CHIKV.

Materials and Methods

Sequences

The complete genome sequences of 141 CHIKV isolates (in FASTA format) were obtained from the National Center for Biotechnology (NCBI) GenBank database (http://www.ncbi.nlm.

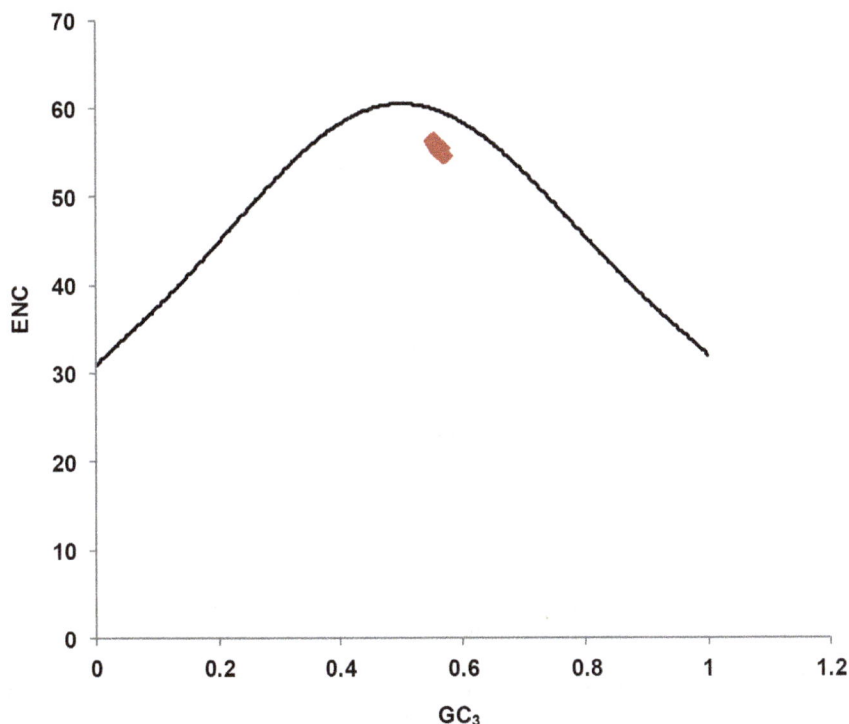

Figure 8. The relationship between the effective number of codons (ENC) values and the GC content at the third synonymous codon position (GC₃). The curve indicates the expected codon usage if GC compositional constraints alone account for codon usage bias.

nih.gov). The accession numbers and other detailed information of the selected CHIKVs' genomes, such as isolation date, isolation place, host and genome size were also retrieved (Table 7).

Compositional Analysis

The following compositional properties were calculated for the CHIKV genomes; (i) the overall frequency of occurrence of the nucleotides (A %, C %, U/T %, and G %); (ii) the frequency of each nucleotide at the third site of the synonymous codons ($A_{3\%}$, $C_{3\%}$, $U_{3\%}$ and $G_{3\%}$); (iii) the frequencies of occurrence of nucleotides G+C at the first (GC_1), second (GC_2), and third synonymous codon positions (GC_3); (iv) the mean frequencies of nucleotide G+C at the first and the second position ($GC_{1,2}$); and (v) the overall GC and AU content. The codons AUG and UGG are

Table 5. Summary of correlation analysis between the first two principal axes and relative abundance of dinucleotides in CHIKV genomes.

	UU	UC	UA	UG	CU	CC	CA	CG
Mean ± SD	0.954±0.030	0.935±0.020	0.859±0.022	1.275±0.022	1.082±0.026	0.979±0.017	1.125±0.017	0.808±0.016
Range	0.886–1.082	0.862–0.964	0.784–0.934	1.214–1.329	1.022–1.107	0.946–1.025	1.058–1.172	0.781–0.856
Axis 1	r 0.755**	−0.664**	0.213*	−0.071^NS	−0.724**	0.612**	−0.262**	0.236**
	P0.000	0.000	0.011	0.403	0.000	0.000	0.002	0.005
Axis 2	r −0.357**	0.233**	−0.665**	0.429**	0.418**	−0.305**	0.611**	−0.548**
	P0.000	0.005	0.000	0.000	0.000	0.000	0.000	0.000
	AU	AC	AA	AG	GU	GC	GA	GG
Mean ± SD	0.929±0.015	1.055±0.014	0.987±.0078	1.024±0.006	1.054±0.014	1.001±0.007	1.012±0.009	0.931±0.010
Range	0.884–0.987	0.998–1.097	0.963–1.008	1.009–1.037	1.007–1.117	0.965–1.020	0.996–1.037	0.900–0.954
Axis 1	r 0.145^NS	0.39^NS	−0.387**	0.236**	0.80^NS	−0.009^NS	0.698**	−0.366**
	P0.086	0.645	0.000	0.005	0.345	0.919	0.000	0.000
Axis 2	r −0.601**	−0.381**	0.221**	−0.404**	−0.508**	0.279**	−0.288**	0.168*
	P0.000	0.000	0.009	0.000	0.000	0.001	0.001	0.047

NS: non-significant (P>0.05).
*represents 0.01<P<0.05.
**represents P<0.01.

Table 6. Correlation analysis among GRAVY, ARO, ENC, GC$_3$, GC and the first two principle axes.

		f_1 (53.57%)	f_2 (25.16%)	ENC	GC$_3$	GC
GRAVY	r	0.118^{NS}	−0.558**	0.420**	−0.529**	−0.568**
	P	0.164	0.000	0.003	0.000	0.000
ARO	r	0.169*	−0.149^{NS}	0.081^{NS}	0.026^{NS}	−0.021^{NS}
	P	0.045	0.077	0.340	0.758	0.803

ARO: Aromaticity.
NS: non-significant ($P>0.05$).
*represents $0.01<P<0.05$.
**represents $P<0.01$.

the only codons for Met and Trp, respectively, and the termination codons UAA, UAG and UGA do not encode any amino acids. Therefore, these five codons are expected not to exhibit any usage bias and were therefore excluded from the analysis.

RSCU Analysis

The RSCU values for all the coding sequences of CHIKV genomes were calculated to determine the characteristics of synonymous codon usage without the confounding influence of amino acid composition and the size of coding sequence of different gene samples, following a previously described method [18]. The RSCU index was calculated as follows:

$$RSCU = \frac{gij}{\sum\limits_{j}^{ni} gij} ni$$

where gij is the observed number of the ith codon for the jth amino acid which has n_i kinds of synonymous codons. RSCU values represent the ratio between the observed usage frequency of one codon in a gene sample and the expected usage frequency in the synonymous codon family given that all codons for the particular amino acid are used equally. The synonymous codons with RSCU values >1.0 have positive codon usage bias and were defined as abundant codons, while those with RSCU values <1.0 have negative codon usage bias and were defined as less-abundant codons. When the RSCU values is 1.0, it means there is no codon usage bias for that amino acid and the codons are chosen equally or randomly [50]. Moreover, the synonymous codons with RSCU values >1.6 and <0.6 were treated as over-represented and under-represented codons, respectively [23].

Influence of Overall Codon Usage of the Hosts on that of CHIKV

For the comparative analysis of codon usage between CHIKVs and its vectors and hosts; codon usage data for two transmission vectors (*A. aegypti*, *A. albopictus*), and hosts (*H. sapiens*, *P. troglodytes*) were obtained from the codon usage database (http://www.kazusa.or.jp/codon/) [51]. Zhou et al. proposed a method recently to determine the potential impact of the overall codon usage patterns of the hosts in the formation of the overall codon usage of viruses [36]. Here, we applied the same approach in case of CHIKV and the similarity index $D(A,B)$ was calculated as follows:

$$R(A,B) = \frac{\sum\limits_{i=1}^{59} ai \times bi}{\sqrt{\sum\limits_{i=1}^{59} ai^2 \times bi^2}}$$

$$D(A,B) = \frac{1 - R(A,B)}{2}$$

where $R(A,B)$ is defined as a cosine value of an included angle between A and B spatial vectors representing the degree of similarity between CHIKV and a specific host at the aspect of the overall codon usage pattern, a_i is defined as the RSCU value for a specific codon among 59 synonymous codons of CHIKV coding sequence, b_i is termed as the RSCU value for the same codon of the host. $D(A,B)$ represents the potential effect of the overall codon usage of the host on that of CHIKV, and its value ranges from zero to 1.0 [36].

Measures of Relative Dinucleotides Abundance

The relative abundance of dinucleotides in the coding regions of CHIKV genomes was calculated using a previously described method [43]. A comparison of actual and expected dinucleotide frequencies of the 16 dinucleotides in coding regions of the CHIKV was also undertaken. The odds ratio was calculated using the following formula:

$$P_{xy} = \frac{f_{xy}}{f_y f_x}$$

where f_x denotes the frequency of the nucleotide X, f_y denotes the frequency of the nucleotide Y, $f_y f_x$ the expected frequency of the dinucleotide XY and f_{xy} the frequency of the dinucleotide XY, etc,. for each dinucleotide were calculated. As a conservative criterion, for $P_{xy}>1.23$ (or <0.78), the XY pair is considered to be over-represented (or under-represented) in terms of relative abundance compared with a random association of mononucleotides.

CAI Analysis

The CAI is used as a quantitative method of predicting the expression level of a gene based on its codon sequence. The CAI value ranges from 0 to 1. The most frequent codons simply have the highest relative adaptiveness values, and sequences with higher CAIs are preferred over those with lower CAIs [32].

ENC Analysis

The ENC is used to quantify the absolute codon usage bias of the gene (s) of interest, irrespective of gene length and the number of amino acids [30]. In this study, this measure was calculated to evaluate the degree of codon usage bias exhibited by the coding sequences of CHIKVs. The ENC values ranged from 20 for a gene showing extreme codon usage bias using only one of the possible synonymous codons for the corresponding amino acid, to 61 for a gene showing no bias using all possible synonymous codons equally for the corresponding amino acid. The larger the extent of codon preference in a gene, the smaller the ENC value is. It is also generally accepted that genes have a significant codon bias when the ENC value is less than or equal to 35 [30,52]. The ENC was calculated using the following formula:

$$ENC = 2 + \frac{9}{\overline{F_2}} + \frac{1}{\overline{F_3}} + \frac{5}{\overline{F_4}} + \frac{3}{\overline{F_6}},$$

Table 7. Demographics of CHIKV genomes analyzed in present study.

No	Strain Name	GenBank Accession	Length (bp)	Year	Host	Country	Genotype
1	Ross low-psg	HM045811	11775	1953	Human	Tanzania	ECSA
2	Vereeniging	HM045792	11836	1956	Human	South Africa	ECSA
3	TH35	HM045810	11986	1958	Human	Thailand	Asian
4	LSFS	HM045809	11753	1960	Human	DRC	ECSA
5	Angola M2022	HM045823	11754	1962	–	Angola	ECSA
6	A301	HM045821	11823	1963	Bat	Senegal	ECSA
7	Gibbs 63–263	HM045813	11976	1963	Human	India	Asian
8	I-634029	HM045803	11897	1963	Human	India	Asian
9	IND-63-WB1	EF027140	11784	1963	–	India	Asian
10	IbH35	HM045786	11844	1964	Human	Nigeria	WA
11	PM2951	HM045785	11844	1966	Mosquito	Senegal	WA
12	SH 3013	HM045816	11823	1966	Human	Senegal	WA
13	PO731460	HM045788	11988	1973	Human	India	Asian
14	IND-73-MH5	EF027141	11805	1973	–	India	Asian
15	1455–75	HM045814	11939	1975	Human	Thailand	Asian
16	AR 18211	HM045805	11686	1976	Mosquito	South Africa	ECSA
17	3412–78	HM045808	11968	1978	Human	Thailand	Asian
18	HB78	HM045822	11753	1978	Human	CAR	ECSA
19	ArD 30237	HM045815	11823	1979	Mosquito	Senegal	WA
20	ArA 2657	HM045818	11823	1981	Mosquito	Cote d'Ivoire	WA
21	IPD/A SH 2807	HM045804	11847	–	Human	Senegal	WA
22	UgAg4155	HM045812	11774	1982	Human	Uganda	ECSA
23	JKT23574	HM045791	11992	1983	Human	Indonesia	Asian
24	37997	AY726732	11881	1983	Mosquito	Senegal	WA
25	DakAr B 16878	HM045784	11772	1984	Mosquito	CAR	ECSA
26	RSU1	HM045797	11979	1985	Human	Indonesia	Asian
27	Hu/85/NR/001	HM045800	11897	1985	Human	Philippines	Asian
28	PhH15483	HM045790	11907	1985	Human	Philippines	Asian
29	ALSA-1	HM045806	11768	1986	–	India	ECSA
30	CAR256	HM045793	11767	–	–	CAR	ECSA
31	6441–88	HM045789	11855	1988	Human	Thailand	Asian
32	ArD 93229	HM045819	11860	1993	Mosquito	Senegal	WA
33	ArA 30548	HM045820	11817	1993	Mosquito	Cote d'Ivoire	WA
34	CO392-95	HM045796	11979	1995	Human	Thailand	Asian
35	SV0444-95	HM045787	11968	1995	Human	Thailand	Asian
36	K0146-95	HM045802	11975	1995	–	Thailand	Asian
37	IND-00-MH4	EF027139	11814	2000	Human	India	ECSA
38	HD 180760	HM045817	11832	2005	Human	Senegal	WA
39	IMTSSA6424C	FR717337	11559	2005	Human	France	ECSA
40	IMTSSA6424S	FR717336	11559	2005	Human	France	ECSA
41	BNI-CHIKV_899	FJ959103	11832	2006	Human	Mauritius	ECSA
42	MY019IMR/06/BP	EU703761	12028	2006	Human	Malaysia	Asian
43	DHS4263-Calif AB	HM045794	11774	2006	Human	USA	ECSA
44	MY003IMR/06/BP	EU703760	12028	2006	Human	Malaysia	Asian
45	MY002IMR/06/BP	EU703759	12028	2006	Human	Malaysia	Asian
46	DRDE-06	EF210157	11774	2006	Human	India	ECSA
47	0611aTw	FJ807896	11811	2006	Human	Singapore	ECSA
48	TM25	EU564334	11772	2006	Human	Mauritius	ECSA
49	IND-KA51	FJ000068	11812	2006	Human	India	ECSA
50	IND-MH51	FJ000067	11812	2006	Human	India	ECSA

Table 7. Cont.

No	Strain Name	GenBank Accession	Length (bp)	Year	Host	Country	Genotype
51	IND-GJ52	FJ000062	11812	2006	Human	India	ECSA
52	IND-GJ53	FJ000065	11813	2006	Human	India	ECSA
53	IND-KR51	FJ000066	11812	2006	Human	India	ECSA
54	IND-GJ51	FJ000064	11807	2006	Human	India	ECSA
55	IND-06-Guj	JF274082	11829	2006	Human	India	ECSA
56	IND-KA52	FJ000063	11812	2006	Human	India	ECSA
57	RGCB05/KL06	GQ428211	11764	2006	Human	India	ECSA
58	RGCB03/KL06	GQ428210	11764	2006	Human	India	ECSA
59	CHIK31	EU564335	11810	2006	Human	India	ECSA
60	SL10571	AB455494	11829	2006	Human	–	ECSA
61	SL11131	AB455493	11829	2006	Human	–	ECSA
62	IND-06-KA15	EF027135	11729	2006	Human	India	ECSA
63	D570/06	EF012359	11806	2006	–	Mauritius	ECSA
64	IND-06-RJ1	EF027137	11767	2006	–	India	ECSA
65	IND-06-AP3	EF027134	11779	2006	Human	India	ECSA
66	IND-06-TN1	EF027138	11750	2006	Human	India	ECSA
67	LR2006_OPY1	DQ443544	11840	2006	Human	Reunion	ECSA
68	IND-06-MH2	EF027136	11800	2006	Human	India	ECSA
69	SL-CR 3	HM045799	11758	2007	Human	Sri Lanka	ECSA
70	ITA07-RA1	EU244823	11788	2007	–	Italy	ECSA
71	SL-CK1	HM045801	11766	2007	Human	Sri Lanka	ECSA
72	0706aTw	FJ807897	12013	2007	Human	Indonesia	Asian
73	LKRGCH1507	FJ445428	11717	2007	Human	Sri Lanka	ECSA
74	IND-KR52	FJ000069	11812	2007	Human	India	ECSA
75	DRDE-07	EU372006	11774	2007	Human	India	ECSA
76	LKMTCH2707	FJ445427	11717	2007	Human	Sri Lanka	ECSA
77	RGCB80/KL07	GQ428212	11764	2007	Human	India	ECSA
78	RGCB120/KL07	GQ428213	11764	2007	Human	India	ECSA
79	0810aTw	FJ807898	11811	2008	Human	Bangladesh	ECSA
80	SD08Pan	GU199351	11793	2008	Human	China	ECSA
81	0810bTw	FJ807899	11811	2008	Human	Malaysia	ECSA
82	SGEHICHS277108	FJ445510	11800	2008	Human	Singapore	ECSA
83	SVUKDP-08	JN558835	11733	2008	Human	India	ECSA
84	FD080178	GU199352	11677	2008	Human	China	ECSA
85	FD080008	GU199350	11687	2008	Human	China	ECSA
86	FD080231	GU199353	11687	2008	Human	China	ECSA
87	SGEHICHD13508	FJ445511	11719	2008	Human	Singapore	ECSA
88	LK(PB)CH5808	FJ513637	11710	2008	Human	Sri Lanka	ECSA
89	LK(PB)CH3008	FJ513632	11693	2008	Human	Sri Lanka	ECSA
90	LK(PB)CH1608	FJ513629	11716	2008	Human	Sri Lanka	ECSA
91	LK(PB)CH5308	FJ513635	11726	2008	Human	Sri Lanka	ECSA
92	LK(PB)chik6008	GU013529	11718	2008	Human	Sri Lanka	ECSA
93	LK(PB)CH1008	FJ513628	11722	2008	Human	Sri Lanka	ECSA
94	LK(PB)chik3408	GU013528	11715	2008	Human	Sri Lanka	ECSA
95	LK(EH)CH6708	FJ513654	11717	2008	Human	Sri Lanka	ECSA
96	LK(EH)CH7708	FJ513657	11696	2008	Human	Sri Lanka	ECSA
97	LK(EH)CH4408	FJ513645	11714	2008	Human	Sri Lanka	ECSA
98	LK(EH)CH20108	FJ513679	11717	2008	Human	Sri Lanka	ECSA
99	LK(EH)CH18608	FJ513675	11716	2008	Human	Sri Lanka	ECSA
100	LK(EH)chik19708	GU013530	11714	2008	Human	Sri Lanka	ECSA

Table 7. Cont.

No	Strain Name	GenBank Accession	Length (bp)	Year	Host	Country	Genotype
101	LKEHCH13908	FJ445426	11717	2008	Human	Sri Lanka	ECSA
102	LK(EH)CH17708	FJ513673	11710	2008	Human	Sri Lanka	ECSA
103	SGEHICHT077808	FJ445484	11790	2008	Human	Singapore	ECSA
104	RGCB356/KL08	GQ428215	11764	2008	Human	India	ECSA
105	RGCB355/KL08	GQ428214	11764	2008	Human	India	ECSA
106	SGEHICHS422308	FJ445432	11722	2008	Human	Singapore	ECSA
107	SGEHICHS421708	FJ445431	11722	2008	Human	Singapore	ECSA
108	SGEHICHD93508	FJ445430	11722	2008	Human	Singapore	ECSA
109	SGEHICHD96808	FJ445463	11729	2008	Human	Singapore	ECSA
110	SGEHICHS424108	FJ445443	11714	2008	Human	Singapore	ECSA
111	SGEHICHS422808	FJ445433	11729	2008	Human	Singapore	ECSA
112	SGEHICHS425208	FJ445445	11719	2008	Human	Singapore	ECSA
113	SGEHICHD122508	FJ445502	11717	2008	Human	Singapore	ECSA
114	CU-Chik10	GU301780	11811	2008	Human	Thailand	ECSA
115	SVUCTR-09	JN558834	11733	2009	Human	India	ECSA
116	SVUKDP-09	JN558836	11733	2009	Human	India	ECSA
117	CU-Chik661	GQ905863	11752	2009	Human	Thailand	ECSA
118	CU-Chik683	GU301781	11811	2009	Human	Thailand	ECSA
119	CU-Chik_OBF	GU908223	11670	2009	Mosquito	Thailand	ECSA
120	CU-Chik009	GU301779	11811	2009	Human	Thailand	ECSA
121	NL10/152	KC862329	11836	2010	Human	Indonesia	ECSA
122	GD05/2010	JX088705	11811	2010	Human	China	ECSA
123	GZ0991	JQ065890	11684	2010	Human	China	ECSA
124	GD113	HQ846357	11720	2010	Human	China	ECSA
125	GD139	HQ846358	11730	2010	Human	China	ECSA
126	GD115	HQ846356	11746	2010	Human	China	ECSA
127	GD134	HQ846359	11725	2010	Human	China	ECSA
128	GZ1029	JQ065891	11687	2010	Human	China	ECSA
129	CHI2010	JQ067624	11724	2010	Human	China	ECSA
130	NC/2011-568	HE806461	11621	2011	Human	New Caledonia	ECSA
131	V0603310_KH11_BTB	JQ861260	11743	2011	Human	Cambodia	ECSA
132	V1024311_KH11_PVH	JQ861256	11754	2011	Human	Cambodia	ECSA
133	V1024308_KH11_PVH	JQ861254	11750	2011	Human	Cambodia	ECSA
134	V1024314_KH11_PVH	JQ861258	11733	2011	Human	Cambodia	ECSA
135	V1024306_KH11_PVH	JQ861253	11745	2011	Human	Cambodia	ECSA
136	V1024310_KH11_PVH	JQ861255	11736	2011	Human	Cambodia	ECSA
137	V1024313_KH11_PVH	JQ861257	11755	2011	Human	Cambodia	ECSA
138	CHIKV-JC2012	KC488650	11889	2012	Human	China	Asian
139	Chik-sy	KF318729	12017	2012	Human	China	Asian
140	Wuerzburg	EU037962	11805	–	Human	Mauritius	ECSA
141	S27-African prototype	AF369024	11826	–	Human	–	ECSA

Dashes (−) indicates data not available. East Central South African, ECSA; Democratic Republic of Congo, DRC; Central African Republic, CAR; West African; WA.

Where $\overline{F_k}$ (k = 2,3,4,6) is the mean of F_k values for the k-fold degenerate amino acids, which is estimated using the formula as follows:

$$F_k = \frac{nS-1}{n-1},$$

where n is the total number of occurrences of the codons for that amino acid and

$$S = \sum_{i=1}^{k} \left(\frac{n_i}{n}\right)^2,$$

where n_i is the total number of occurrences of the i th codon for that amino acid. Genes, whose codon choice is constrained only by a mutation bias, will lie on or just below the curve of the expected ENC values. Therefore, for elucidating the relationship between GC_3 and ENC values, the expected ENC values for different GC_3 were calculated as follows:

$$ENC^{\mathrm{expected}} = 2 + s + \frac{29}{s^2 + (1 - s^2)}$$

where s represents the given GC_3% value [30].

COA of Codon Usage

COA is a multivariate statistical method that is used to explore the relationships between variables and samples. In the present study, COA was used to analyze the major trends in codon usage patterns among CHIKVs coding sequences. COA involves a mathematical procedure that transforms some correlated variable (RSCU values) into a smaller number of uncorrelated variables called principal components. To minimize the effect of amino acid composition on codon usage, each coding sequence was represented as a 59 dimensional vector, and each dimension corresponded to the RSCU value of each sense codon, which only included several synonymous codons for a particular amino acid, excluding the codons AUG, UGG and the three stop codons.

Correlation Analysis

Correlation analysis was carried out to identify the relationship between nucleotide composition and synonymous codon usage patterns of CHIKV. This analysis was implemented based on the Spearman's rank correlation analysis. All statistical processes were carried out using the statistical software SPSS 16.0 for windows.

Supporting Information

Table S1 Hydrophobicity (GRAVY) and aromaticity (ARO) indices in CHIKV genomes.

Author Contributions

Conceived and designed the experiments: AMB YT. Performed the experiments: AMB IN. Analyzed the data: AMB IN YT. Contributed reagents/materials/analysis tools: AMB IN YT. Wrote the paper: AMB IN.

References

1. Strauss JH, Strauss EG (1994) The alphaviruses: gene expression, replication, and evolution. Microbiol Rev 58: 491–562.
2. Robinson MC (1955) An epidemic of virus disease in Southern Province, Tanganyika Territory, in 1952–53. I. Clinical features. Trans R Soc Trop Med Hyg 49: 28–32.
3. Schuffenecker I, Iteman I, Michault A, Murri S, Frangeul L, et al. (2006) Genome microevolution of chikungunya viruses causing the Indian Ocean outbreak. PLoS Med 3: e263.
4. Powers AM, Brault AC, Tesh RB, Weaver SC (2000) Re-emergence of Chikungunya and O'nyong-nyong viruses: evidence for distinct geographical lineages and distant evolutionary relationships. J Gen Virol 81: 471–479.
5. Kumar NP, Joseph R, Kamaraj T, Jambulingam P (2008) A226V mutation in virus during the 2007 chikungunya outbreak in Kerala, India. J Gen Virol 89: 1945–1948.
6. Theamboonlers A, Rianthavorn P, Praianantathavorn K, Wuttirattanakowit N, Poovorawan Y (2009) Clinical and molecular characterization of chikungunya virus in South Thailand. Jpn J Infect Dis 62: 303–305.
7. Jupp PG, McIntosh BM (1988) Chikungunya disease. In: Monath TP, editor. The Arboviruses: Epidemiology and Ecology. Boca Raton (Florida): CRC Press. 137–157.
8. Powers AM, Logue CH (2007) Changing patterns of chikungunya virus: re-emergence of a zoonotic arbovirus. J Gen Virol 88: 2363–2377.
9. Pialoux G, Gauzere BA, Jaureguiberry S, Strobel M (2007) Chikungunya, an epidemic arbovirosis. Lancet Infect Dis 7: 319–327.
10. Grantham R, Gautier C, Gouy M, Mercier R, Pave A (1980) Codon catalog usage and the genome hypothesis. Nucleic Acids Res 8: r49–r62.
11. Marin A, Bertranpetit J, Oliver JL, Medina JR (1989) Variation in G+C-content and codon choice: differences among synonymous codon groups in vertebrate genes. Nucleic Acids Res 17: 6181–6189.
12. Gu W, Zhou T, Ma J, Sun X, Lu Z (2004) Analysis of synonymous codon usage in SARS Coronavirus and other viruses in the Nidovirales. Virus Res 101: 155–161.
13. Liu YS, Zhou JH, Chen HT, Ma LN, Pejsak Z, et al. (2011) The characteristics of the synonymous codon usage in enterovirus 71 virus and the effects of host on the virus in codon usage pattern. Infect Genet Evol 11: 1168–1173.
14. Ma JJ, Zhao F, Zhang J, Zhou JH, Ma LN, et al. (2013) Analysis of Synonymous Codon Usage in Dengue Viruses. Journal of Animal and Veterinary Advances 12: 88–98.
15. Moratorio G, Iriarte A, Moreno P, Musto H, Cristina J (2013) A detailed comparative analysis on the overall codon usage patterns in West Nile virus. Infect Genet Evol 14: 396–400.
16. Sharp PM, Cowe E, Higgins DG, Shields DC, Wolfe KH, et al. (1988) Codon usage patterns in Escherichia coli, Bacillus subtilis, Saccharomyces cerevisiae, Schizosaccharomyces pombe, Drosophila melanogaster and Homo sapiens; a review of the considerable within-species diversity. Nucleic Acids Res 16: 8207–8211.
17. Tao P, Dai L, Luo M, Tang F, Tien P, et al. (2009) Analysis of synonymous codon usage in classical swine fever virus. Virus Genes 38: 104–112.
18. Sharp PM, Li WH (1986) Codon usage in regulatory genes in Escherichia coli does not reflect selection for 'rare' codons. Nucleic Acids Res 14: 7737–7749.
19. Duret L, Mouchiroud D (1999) Expression pattern and, surprisingly, gene length shape codon usage in Caenorhabditis, Drosophila, and Arabidopsis. Proc Natl Acad Sci U S A 96: 4482–4487.
20. Van der Linden MG, de Farias ST (2006) Correlation between codon usage and thermostability. Extremophiles 10: 479–481.
21. Jenkins GM, Holmes EC (2003) The extent of codon usage bias in human RNA viruses and its evolutionary origin. Virus Res 92: 1–7.
22. Wang M, Zhang J, Zhou JH, Chen HT, Ma LN, et al. (2011) Analysis of codon usage in bovine viral diarrhea virus. Arch Virol 156: 153–160.
23. Wong EH, Smith DK, Rabadan R, Peiris M, Poon LL (2010) Codon usage bias and the evolution of influenza A viruses. Codon Usage Biases of Influenza Virus. BMC Evol Biol 10: 253.
24. Chen Y (2013) A comparison of synonymous codon usage bias patterns in DNA and RNA virus genomes: quantifying the relative importance of mutational pressure and natural selection. Biomed Res Int 2013: 406342.
25. Shi SL, Jiang YR, Liu YQ, Xia RX, Qin L (2013) Selective pressure dominates the synonymous codon usage in parvoviridae. Virus Genes 46: 10–19.
26. Zhang Z, Dai W, Wang Y, Lu C, Fan H (2013) Analysis of synonymous codon usage patterns in torque teno sus virus 1 (TTSuV1). Arch Virol 158: 145–154.
27. Zhang Z, Dai W, Dai D (2013) Synonymous Codon Usage in TTSuV2: Analysis and Comparison with TTSuV1. PLoS ONE 8: e81469.
28. Shackelton LA, Parrish CR, Holmes EC (2006) Evolutionary basis of codon usage and nucleotide composition bias in vertebrate DNA viruses. J Mol Evol 62: 551–563.
29. Hassan S, Mahalingam V, Kumar V (2009) Synonymous codon usage analysis of thirty two mycobacteriophage genomes. Adv Bioinformatics: 316936.
30. Wright F (1990) The 'effective number of codons' used in a gene. Gene 87: 23–29.
31. Hu JS, Wang QQ, Zhang J, Chen HT, Xu ZW, et al. (2011) The characteristic of codon usage pattern and its evolution of hepatitis C virus. Infect Genet Evol 11: 2098–2102.
32. Sharp PM, Li WH (1987) The codon Adaptation Index–a measure of directional synonymous codon usage bias, and its potential applications. Nucleic Acids Res 15: 1281–1295.
33. Zhou JH, Wang H, Huang LF, Naylor M, Clifford P (2005) Heterogeneity in codon usages of sobemovirus genes. Arch Virol 150: 1591–1605.
34. Mueller S, Papamichail D, Coleman JR, Skiena S, Wimmer E (2006) Reduction of the rate of poliovirus protein synthesis through large-scale codon deoptimization causes attenuation of viral virulence by lowering specific infectivity. J Virol 80: 9687–9696.
35. Sanchez G, Bosch A, Pinto RM (2003) Genome variability and capsid structural constraints of hepatitis a virus. J Virol 77: 452–459.
36. Zhou JH, Zhang J, Sun DJ, Ma Q, Chen HT, et al. (2013) The distribution of synonymous codon choice in the translation initiation region of dengue virus. PLoS One 8: e77239.
37. Tsetsarkin KA, Weaver SC (2011) Sequential adaptive mutations enhance efficient vector switching by Chikungunya virus and its epidemic emergence. PLoS Pathog 7: e1002412.
38. Tsetsarkin KA, Vanlandingham DL, McGee CE, Higgs S (2007) A single mutation in chikungunya virus affects vector specificity and epidemic potential. PLoS Pathog 3: e201.

39. Greenacre M (1984) Theory and Applications of Correspondence Analysis: Academic Pr. 364 p.
40. Tatarinova TV, Alexandrov NN, Bouck JB, Feldmann KA (2010) GC3 biology in corn, rice, sorghum and other grasses. BMC Genomics 11: 308.
41. Cheng X, Virk N, Chen W, Ji S, Ji S, et al. (2013) CpG usage in RNA viruses: data and hypotheses. PLoS One 8: e74109.
42. Chiusano ML, Alvarez-Valin F, Di Giulio M, D'Onofrio G, Ammirato G, et al. (2000) Second codon positions of genes and the secondary structures of proteins. Relationships and implications for the origin of the genetic code. Gene 261: 63–69.
43. Karlin S, Burge C (1995) Dinucleotide relative abundance extremes: a genomic signature. Trends Genet 11: 283–290.
44. Dorn A, Kippenberger S (2008) Clinical application of CpG-, non-CpG-, and antisense oligodeoxynucleotides as immunomodulators. Curr Opin Mol Ther 10: 10–20.
45. Lobo FP, Mota BE, Pena SD, Azevedo V, Macedo AM, et al. (2009) Virus-host coevolution: common patterns of nucleotide motif usage in Flaviviridae and their hosts. PLoS One 4: e6282.

46. Karlin S, Mrazek J (1997) Compositional differences within and between eukaryotic genomes. Proc Natl Acad Sci U S A 94: 10227–10232.
47. Bird AP (1980) DNA methylation and the frequency of CpG in animal DNA. Nucleic Acids Res 8: 1499–1504.
48. Greenbaum BD, Levine AJ, Bhanot G, Rabadan R (2008) Patterns of evolution and host gene mimicry in influenza and other RNA viruses. PLoS Pathog 4: e1000079.
49. Barrett JW, Sun Y, Nazarian SH, Belsito TA, Brunetti CR, et al. (2006) Optimization of codon usage of poxvirus genes allows for improved transient expression in mammalian cells. Virus Genes 33: 15–26.
50. Sharp PM, Li WH (1986) An evolutionary perspective on synonymous codon usage in unicellular organisms. J Mol Evol 24: 28–38.
51. Nakamura Y, Gojobori T, Ikemura T (2000) Codon usage tabulated from international DNA sequence databases: status for the year 2000. Nucleic Acids Res 28: 292.
52. Comeron JM, Aguade M (1998) An evaluation of measures of synonymous codon usage bias. J Mol Evol 47: 268–274.

11

The Microbial Detection Array for Detection of Emerging Viruses in Clinical Samples - A Useful Panmicrobial Diagnostic Tool

Maiken W. Rosenstierne[1]*, Kevin S. McLoughlin[2], Majken Lindholm Olesen[1], Anna Papa[3], Shea N. Gardner[2], Olivier Engler[4], Sebastien Plumet[5], Ali Mirazimi[6,7,8], Manfred Weidmann[9], Matthias Niedrig[10], Anders Fomsgaard[1,11], Lena Erlandsson[1]

1 Department of Microbiological Diagnostics and Virology, Statens Serum Institut, Copenhagen, Denmark, 2 Global Security, Lawrence Livermore National Laboratory, Livermore, California, United States of America, 3 Department of Microbiology, Aristotle University of Thessaloniki, Thessaloniki, Greece, 4 Spiez Laboratory, Federal Office for Civil Protection, Spiez, Switzerland, 5 Virology department, French Army Forces Biomedical Institute (IRBA), Marseille, France, 6 Swedish Institute for Communicable Disease Control, Solna, Sweden, 7 National Veterinary Institute (SVA), Uppsala, Sweden, 8 Department of Clinical and Experimental Medicine, Linköping University, Linköping, Sweden, 9 Institute of Aquaculture, University of Stirling, Stirling, United Kingdom, 10 Centre for Biosafety, Robert Koch-Institute, Berlin, Germany, 11 Institute of Clinical Research, University of Southern Denmark, Odense, Denmark

Abstract

Emerging viruses are usually endemic to tropical and sub-tropical regions of the world, but increased global travel, climate change and changes in lifestyle are believed to contribute to the spread of these viruses into new regions. Many of these viruses cause similar disease symptoms as other emerging viruses or common infections, making these unexpected pathogens difficult to diagnose. Broad-spectrum pathogen detection microarrays containing probes for all sequenced viruses and bacteria can provide rapid identification of viruses, guiding decisions about treatment and appropriate case management. We report a modified Whole Transcriptome Amplification (WTA) method that increases unbiased amplification, particular of RNA viruses. Using this modified WTA method, we tested the specificity and sensitivity of the Lawrence Livermore Microbial Detection Array (LLMDA) against a wide range of emerging viruses present in both non-clinical and clinical samples using two different microarray data analysis methods.

Editor: Charles Y. Chiu, University of California, San Francisco, United States of America

Funding: The authors have no funding or support to report.

Competing Interests: The authors have declared that no competing interests exist.

* Email: MWR@ssi.dk

Introduction

Emerging viruses may be defined as viruses that are newly discovered or have the potential to increase in incidence or geographical range. Some important emerging viruses cause severe acute syndromes such as viral haemorrhagic fevers or encephalitides. They are endemic to tropical and sub-tropical regions. The majority are RNA viruses, from the *Arenaviridae, Bunyaviridae, Filoviridae, Flaviviridae* and *Togaviridae* virus families, but some are from DNA virus families such as *Poxviridae*. Their survival often depends on a vertebrate or arthropod host (non-human primates, bats, birds, rodents, ticks, sandflies or mosquitoes) [1–4]. They are usually restricted to geographical areas where the host species lives. Human cases occur through zoonosis, often resulting in life-threatening diseases with high mortality rates [3]. Knowledge of some of these viruses is limited, and originates exclusively from case reports and animal models. Some of them were first described during surveillance of veterinary diseases, e.g. Usutu virus, and only later became implicated in human clinical cases [5,6].

Due to increased global travel, lifestyle changes and climate change, the risk of importing rare, exotic and emerging diseases to Europe has increased [3]. Some areas in Europe already maintain environmental conditions favourable to these pathogens, e.g. hantavirus [7], Crimean-Congo haemorrhagic fever virus (CCHFV) [8] and West Nile virus (WNV) [9]. Travellers visiting endemic areas are a potential source for spreading these diseases, which manifest as febrile illness coinciding with the peak of viral shedding and consequent risk of transmission. Disease symptoms may be nonspecific and similar to those of other common diseases, making them clinically difficult to recognize and diagnose [10]. There is a demand for rapid and accurate identification of the virus to initiate specific treatment, if available, as well as appropriate case management such as isolation and contact tracking [10,11]. The use of real-time PCR has been critical for case management and epidemiological investigation, complementing serological diagnostic tools [12]. However, a PCR assay can only detect the presence of a specific virus, or a small group of viruses, and real-time PCR multiplexing is limited by overlapping fluorophore emission spectra and available detection channels in real-time PCR cyclers [13].

Several metagenomic approaches, such as microarrays [14–16], resequencing microarrays [17] and next generation sequencing [18], have been shown to be promising new tools for broad-spectrum diagnosis of common viral infections [19–21], arboviral diseases [22] and tropical febrile illnesses [23,24]. These methods all have the ability to simultaneously test for the presence of thousands of viruses in a single assay and thereby remove the need for a specific clinical hypothesis regarding a suspected pathogen.

The Lawrence Livermore Microbial Detection Array (LLMDA) is a high density oligonucleotide microarray that contains probes for all sequenced viruses and bacteria [14]. It has been used to detect a wide range of viruses in both clinical samples [19,25] and vaccine products [26]. In this study we report a modified Whole Transcriptome Amplification (WTA) protocol that increases the unbiased amplification of viruses, especially RNA viruses. Using this method we show that the version 2 of the LLMDA (LLMDAv2) is sensitive and specific to a wide range of emerging viruses and successfully identifies emerging virus present in clinical samples. In addition we compare the simpler SSI-developed data analysis method with the more sophisticated CLiMax software developed especially for LLMDA arrays.

Materials and Methods

Ethics Statement

Exemption for review by the ethical committee system and informed consent was given by the Committee on Biomedical Research Ethics-Capital region in accordance with Danish law on assay development projects.

Data Availability Statement

All authors comply with the data availability policy.

Virus from Non-clinical Samples

Within the European Network for Diagnostics of Imported Viral Diseases (ENIVD) we gathered a wide range of emerging viruses, as inactivated culture supernatants or as purified viral DNA or RNA (Table 1). Viruses were inactivated by heat and/or gamma-irradiation, or by suspension in an RNA-extraction reagent (TRIzol, Life Technologies; TriFast, Peqlab; AVL buffer, Qiagen) [27]. The majority of viruses were grown in Vero E6 cell-cultures (kidney epithelial cell line derived from African green gonkey) (ATCC CRL-1586), but poliovirus (PV) was grown in L20B cells (a murine recombinant cell line) [28]. We also used six control samples from the QCMD EQA programme for 2010 and 2013 (WNV10-01, WNV10-07, WNV13-01, WNV13-10, WNV13-11 and DENV13-01). The WNV13-01 sample contained West Nile virus (WNV) at a concentration of 1.0×10^7 copies/ml and the DENV13-01 sample contained Dengue virus (DENV) type 1 at a concentration of 1.0×10^6 copies/ml. The WNV10-01 and WNV13-10 samples contained a mixture of flaviviruses (DENV type 1, 2 and 4, and Japanese encephalitis virus (JEV)). The WNV10-07 and WNV13-11 samples contained a mixture of DENV type 3, tick-borne encephalitis virus (TBEV) and yellow fever virus (YFV), each at a concentration of 1.0×10^6 copies/ml.

Virus from Clinical Samples

We used clinical samples received for routine diagnostic analysis at Statens Serum Institut (SSI), Copenhagen, Denmark (Danish National reference laboratory (ISO 17025; 2005)), from the CCH Fever Project bio-bank at the Swedish Institute for Communicable Disease Control (Sweden), and from the Department of Microbiology, Aristotle University of Thessaloniki (Greece). The samples were (Table 2): i) One parapoxvirus-positive skin lesion (blister) sample from the hands of a shepherd; ii) One Chikungunya virus-positive serum sample from a traveller hospitalized for Dengue-like symptoms (high fever, joint pain, rash) after visiting Thailand; iii) Eight DENV-positive serum samples from travellers experiencing

mosquito bites in the jungle of Thailand, iv) One CCHFV-positive serum sample (from the CCH Fever program); v) One sandfly fever Toscana virus-positive cerebrospinal fluid (CSF) sample from a traveller hospitalized with meningitis after visiting Toscana, Italy; vi) Six WNV-positive urine samples from patients hospitalized with West Nile fever (two of them with encephalitis). In addition, we used six hepatitis C virus (HCV)-positive serum samples and five HCV-positive plasma samples. One of the HCV-positive serum samples had a known viral concentration (1.2×10^6 IU/ml) determined by standardisation against the WHO control. As negative controls we used virus-negative clinical samples (urine, CSF and serum).

Purification of Samples

As previously described [19] we centrifuged 230 µl of sample at 17,000 g for 10 min, filtered the supernatant through a 0.22 µm Spin-X spin filter (Costar) and treated it with DNase (Invitrogen or New England Biolabs) for 30 min-1 ½ h. The viral nucleic acid (NA) was extracted using the PureLink Viral RNA/DNA kit (Invitrogen), without the addition of carrier RNA. All samples were treated with this protocol with the exception of the QCMD panel samples, CSF, urine, and plasma samples, which were not DNase treated. Virus-positive supernatants suspended in RNA-extraction reagent were purified according to the manufacturer's instructions (TRIzol, Life Technologies; TriFast, Peqlab; AVL buffer, Qiagen). The resulting RNA was further purified using the QIAamp RNA viral Mini kit (Qiagen). The extracted viral NA was eluted with 30–50 µl DNase/RNase-free water, and stored at − 20°C or immediately used.

Reverse Transcription

Reverse transcription (RT) on purified viral RNA was performed with three different methods: i) The P-N6/SSIII method, which uses the Superscript III Reverse Transcription kit (Invitrogen), combined with 5′-phosphorylated random hexamers (P-N$_6$) (Eurofins MWG Operon). Briefly, 11–12 µl viral RNA was mixed with 1 µl 10 mM dNTP mix and 1 µl 250 ng/µl P-N$_6$, incubated at 85°C for 5 min, and cooled on ice. Next, 4 µl 5x first strand buffer, 1 µl 0.1 M DTT, 1 µl RNaseOUT (40 U/µl) (optional) and 1 µl Superscript III RT enzyme (200 U/µl) was added, and the sample mixed and incubated at 25°C for 10 min, 42°C for 60 min and 95°C for 5 min. ii) The RT-reaction included in the WTA kit (Qiagen), which uses T-Script reverse transcriptase combined with random and oligo-dT primers. RT was performed according to the manufacturer's instructions. iii) The VILO method, which uses a cDNA Synthesis kit (Invitrogen) containing Superscript III reverse transcriptase combined with random primers. The method was performed as previously described [19,29]. The samples were stored at −20°C or immediately used.

Whole Transcriptome Amplification

For viral RNA amplification we used the WTA method [29] with the QuantiTect WTA kit (Qiagen), except for the reverse transcription step that was replaced by one of the three RT methods described above. We also modified the protocol by performing amplification at 30°C for 2–8 h. We purified Repli-g amplified DNA according to the supplementary protocol, using the QIAamp DNA Mini Kit (Qiagen), and validated its purity and concentration using a NanoDrop spectrophotometer (Thermo Scientific). The DNA was stored at −80°C or immediately used. To avoid contamination between samples, we adopted precautions normally used during routine viral diagnostic PCR analysis at SSI,

Table 1. Microarray detection range on WT-amplified samples.

Sample type	Sample	Conc[a]	Volume[b]	RT-reaction[c]	Before WTA[c]	After WTA[a]	ΔC_t*	Fold increase[+]	Microarray detection
SN	RVFV-6	3.3×10^6	1	3.6×10^5	1.8×10^5	3.4×10^9	20–19	34	na
	RVFV-5	3.3×10^5		3.6×10^4	1.8×10^4	3.2×10^9	22–19	154	na
	RVFV-4	3.3×10^4		3.6×10^3	1.8×10^3	8.7×10^8	26–21	474	+
	RVFV-3	3.3×10^3		360	180	4.1×10^8	29–22	2.7×10^3	+
	RVFV-2	330		36	18	1.7×10^5	34–34	25	ND
WNV13-01	WNV-7	1.2×10^7	0.6	2.9×10^6	1.4×10^5	4.3×10^8	20–14	1.7×10^3	na
	WNV-6	1.2×10^6		2.9×10^5	1.4×10^4	6.3×10^6	24–22	122	+
	WNV-5	1.2×10^5		2.9×10^4	1.4×10^4	1.8×10^9	30–25	1.1×10^3	+
	WNV-4	1.2×10^4		2.9×10^3	1.4×10^3	6.7×10^{10}	36–17	9.9×10^6	+
	WNV-3	1.2×10^3		290	140	1.6×10^6	41–38	185	+[95]
	WNV-2	120		29	14	4.3×10^5	42–41	34	ND
WNV13-10[§]	JEV-6[§]	1.0×10^6	0.6	2.4×10^5	1.2×10^5	3.0×10^8	20–17	320	+
	JEV-5[§]	1.0×10^5		2.4×10^4	1.2×10^4	4.1×10^6	23–25	10	+
	JEV-4[§]	1.0×10^4		2.4×10^3	1.2×10^3	1.5×10^6	28–27	52	+
	JEV-3[§]	1.0×10^3		240	120	1.0×10^4	33–36	4	ND
WNV13-11[#]	TBEV-6[#]	1.0×10^6	0.6	2.4×10^5	1.2×10^5	3.6×10^6	23–28	1	+
	TBEV-5[#]	1.0×10^5		2.4×10^4	1.2×10^4	ND	28–ND	-	+
	TBEV-4[#]	1.0×10^4		2.4×10^3	1.2×10^3	3.4×10^4	33–37	1	+
	TBEV-3[#]	1.0×10^3		240	120	2.1×10^4	37–38	7	ND
	YFV-6	1.0×10^6		2.4×10^5	1.2×10^5	7.5×10^5	27–34	0,1	+
	YFV-5	1.0×10^5		2.4×10^4	1.2×10^4	ND	31–ND	–	+
	YFV-4	1.0×10^4		2.4×10^3	1.2×10^3	ND	36–ND	–	ND
	YFV-3	1.0×10^3		240	120	ND	ND	–	ND
DENV13-01	DENV-6	1.0×10^6	0.6	2.4×10^5	1.2×10^5	8.4×10^9	28–19	1.3×10^4	+
	DENV-5	1.0×10^5		2.4×10^4	1.2×10^4	7.8×10^8	31–23	8.4×10^3	+
	DENV-4	1.0×10^4		2.4×10^3	1.2×10^3	1.1×10^5	35–39	2	+
	DENV-3	1.0×10^3		240	120	3.1×10^5	40–37	247	ND

Table 1. Cont.

Sample type	Sample	Conc[a]	Volume[b]	RT-reaction[c]	Before WTA[c]	After WTA[a]	ΔC_t*	Fold increase[+]	Microarray detection
Serum	HCV-6	1.2×10^6	1	2.9×10^5	1.4×10^5	3.8×10^8	26-14	1.3×10^5	na
	HCV-5	1.2×10^5		2.9×10^4	1.4×10^4	5.1×10^8	29-13	1.3×10^6	+
	HCV-4	1.2×10^4		2.9×10^3	1.4×10^3	1.1×10^{11}	33-15	6.4×10^6	+
	HCV-3	1.2×10^3		290	140	7.5×10^7	36-26	3.0×10^4	+
	HCV-2	120		29	14	4.4×10^5	39-33	1.4×10^3	ND

NOTE. Conc, Concentration; SN, supernatant; RVFV, Rift-Valley fever virus; WNV13-01, sample from QCMD EQA WNV panel 13-01; WNV, West Nile virus; JEV, Japanese encephalitis virus; TBEV, tick borne encephalitis virus; DENV13-01, sample from QCMD EQA DENV panel 13-01; DENV, Dengue virus; HCV, hepatitis C virus; ND, not detected; na, not analysed.

[S]WNV13-10 contain additional viruses (DENV-1, DENV-2 and DENV-4).

[#]WNV13-11 contain addition viruses (YFV, DENV-3).

[95]results obtained using a 95 percentile threshold.

[a]copies/ml (HCV; IU/ml).

[b]ml (volume of sample for purification).

[c]Number of copies into reaction.

*Difference in C_t-value in real-time PCR before and after WT amplification.

[+]Fold increase after WT amplification, calculated from ΔC_t combined with dilution factors for each sample.

where extraction, amplification and analyses are physically separated and negative samples are included in all steps.

Quantification and Confirmation by Real-time PCR

The technique used for routine diagnostic virus analysis at SSI is quality-assured real-time PCR (ISO 17025; 2005, SSI). To confirm presence of virus in the samples and quantify the virus before and after WTA, we performed virus-specific real-time PCR. We used in-house assays for DENV, WNV, orthopoxvirus, parapoxvirus, Usutu virus, Hantaan virus, Toscana virus, BK virus (BKV) and rotavirus A; and previously published assays for JC virus (JCV) [30], cowpox and monkeypox viruses [31], Chikungunya virus [32], Eastern equine encephalitis virus (EEEV) [33], JEV [34], TBEV [35], YFV [36], Lassa virus and CCHFV [37], Dobrava-Belgrade virus (DOBV) [38], Puumala virus [39], Rift Valley fever virus (RVFV) [36] and Marburg virus [40]. PCR was performed using an Mx3005P (Stratagene) thermal cycler. We calculated the fold difference in concentration from the ΔC_t obtained from real-time PCR before and after WTA, combined with dilution factors. Here we made the assumption that 1 cycle change in C_t-value was equivalent to a doubling of target DNA. We estimated the sample concentrations of the HCV-positive, DENV-positive and WNV-positive clinical samples by performing a series of 10-fold dilutions of the HCV-positive serum sample $(1.2\times10^6$ IU/ml), the DENV13-01 QCMD sample $(1.0\times10^6$ copies/ml) and the WNV13-01 QCMD sample $(1.0\times10^7$ copies/ml), under the assumption that no viral NA was lost during purification.

Microarray Analysis

We analysed samples with the LLMDAv2 microarray, developed at the Lawrence Livermore National Laboratory (LLNL), USA and described elsewhere [14,19,41]. The LLMDAv2 contains 388,000 oligonucleotides probes designed from all sequenced viruses and bacteria [14]. Labelling and microarray hybridization was performed according to manufacturer protocols (Gene expression analysis, Roche NimbleGen) with the exception that 8 µg, instead of 2 µg, of labelled material was used for hybridization. Microarray data was analysed using a simple Excel-based data analysis method developed at SSI (SSI analysis) as described previously [19]. Since the SSI analysis is not optimized for bacteria, any bacterial hits were excluded from the results. Non-human, non-zoonotic pathogens were also excluded since they are assumed to be clinically irrelevant in a diagnostic setting. Additional data analyses were performed on the samples using the CLiMax software developed at LLNL and described elsewhere [14,41].

Microarray data were submitted to the Gene Expression Omnibus (GEO) database http://ncbi.nlm.nih.gov/geo/with the accession number GSE55576. All microarray data used in this study are MIAME compliant.

Results

A Modified WTA Protocol Using 5′-Phosphorylated Random Primers for cDNA Synthesis

To enable successful microarray identification of virus in clinical samples, we have previously used the Phi29 polymerase-based WTA method (Qiagen) [19,29]. The WTA protocol includes three sequential reactions: a reverse transcription reaction to generate cDNA, ligation of cDNA fragments into large linear chains, and amplification by the Phi29 polymerase [29]. To assure an efficient ligation, we replaced the included RT reaction with Superscript III and 5′-phosphorylated random hexamers (P-N$_6$) hereafter

Table 2. Microarray results on non-clinical samples using two different data analysis methods.

Group*	Genus	Virus	Sample	Detected virus SSI analysis	Detected virus CliMax analysis
dsDNA	Orthopoxvirus	Cowpox	pur. DNA	**Cowpox virus**, Variola virus, Monkeypox virus, Vaccinia virus, HERV	**Cowpox virus**, Variola minor virus^, BEV, HERV
		Monkeypox	Pur. DNA	**Monkeypox virus,** Variola virus, Cowpox virus, Vaccinia virus, HERV	**Monkeypox virus**, Variola minor virus^, BEV, HERV
(+) ssRNA	Alphavirus	EEEV	SN	**EEEV**, HERV	**EEEV**, BEV, HERV, SRV-1^
	Flavivirus	Usutu	pur. RNA	**Usutu virus**, HERV, JEV	**Usutu virus**, BEV, HERV
		WNV	pur. RNA	**WNV**, HERV	**WNV,** BEV, HERV
		JEV, DENV-2, DENV-1, DENV-4	WNV10-01	**JEV, DENV-2, DENV-1, DENV-4**	**JEV, DENV-2, DENV-1, DENV-4**, DENV-3, BVDV-1^, RV-A, PRV-C
		TBE, DENV-3, YF	WNV10-07	**TBEV, DENV-3, YFV**, DENV-1, DENV-2, OHFV, HERV	**TBEV, DENV-3, YFV**, DENV-2, SV5, RV-A, PRV-C
	Enterovirus	PV-1, PV-2	SN	**PV-1, PV-2**, PV-3	**PV-1, PV-2**, MuLV, SV40, MDEV, MMTV
(−) ssRNA	Arenavirus	Lassa	SN	**Lassa virus**	**Lassa virus**
	Hantavirus	DOBV	SN	**DOBV**	**DOBV**
		Hantaan	SN	**Hantaan virus**	**Hantaan virus**, MRV-3, MRV-1, MuLV
		Puumala	SN	**Puumala virus**, HERV	**Puumala virus**, BEV, HERV, BVDV-1^
		Seoul	SN	**Seoul virus**, HERV	**Seoul virus**
		Sin Nombre	SN	**Sin Nombre**virus, HERV	**Sin Nombre virus**, BEV, HERV, SRV-1
	Nairovirus	CCHF	SN	**CCHFV**, HERV	**CCHFV**, HERV, BEV
	Phlebovirus	RVF	SN	**RVFV**, HERV	**RVFV**, CCHFV, SV5, BEV, HERV
		Naples	SN	**Naples virus**	**Naples virus**, BVDV-1
		Sicilian	SN	**Sicilian virus**	**Sicilian virus**
		Toscana	SN	**Toscana virus**, HERV	**Toscana virus**, BEV, HERV, SRV-1
	Ebolavirus	Ebola Zaire	SN	**Ebola Zaire virus**, HERV	**Ebola Zaire virus**, HERV, BEV, SRV-1
	Marburgvirus	Marburg	SN	**Marburg virus**, HERV	**Marburg virus,** HERV, BEV, RVFV^

NOTE. EEEV, Eastern equine encephalitis virus; WNV, West Nile virus; CCHFV, Crimean-Congo haemorrhagic fever virus; RVFV, Rift-Valley fever virus; TBEV, Tick borne encephalitis virus; OHFV, Omsk hemoratic fever virus; YFV, yellow fever virus; PV, poliovirus; HERV, human endogenous retrovirus; JEV, Japanese encephalitis virus; DENV, Dengue virus; DOBV, Dobrava-Belgrade virus; RV-A, rotavirus A; PRV-C, porcine rotavirus C; BEV, baboon endogenous virus; SRV-1, simian retrovirus 1; MuLV, murine leukemia virus; SV40, simian virus 40; MDEV, *mus dunni* endogeneous virus; MMTV, mouse mammary tumour virus; MRV, mammalian orthoreovirus; BVDV, bovine viral diarrhea virus; SV5, simian virus 5; pur. DNA, purified DNA; SN, cell culture supernatant; pur. RNA, purified RNA; WNV10-01, sample from QCMD EQA WNV panel 10-01; WNV10-07, sample from QCMD EQA WNV panel 10-07 Bold represents correctly identified virus.
^Viruses with fragmented alignment plots.
*Viruses are grouped based on nucleic acid content, according to the Baltimore Classification.

called P-N6/SSIII. This was done in order to phosphorylate the 5′-end of the cDNA fragments so that new phosphodiester bonds could be formed during the ligation step [42,43]. We compared this method to the manufacturers RT reaction (T-Script using random and oligo-dT primers) and to RT using Superscript VILO cDNA kit [19,29]. Prior to RT and amplification, samples were pre-treated according to a previously described protocol [19]. The different RT protocols were tested in parallel on 10-fold serial dilutions of an HCV-positive serum sample (1.2×10^6 IU/ml) (Figure 1A), on two supernatants containing the hantaviruses Puumala virus and DOBV, respectively (Figure 1B), and on 10 HCV-positive clinical samples with varying viral concentrations (Figure 1C–1D). For all samples tested, whole transcriptome (WT) amplification of cDNA generated by P-N6/SSIII was more efficient than VILO or T-Script. Therefore, the P-N6/SSIII RT-reaction was used for all further WT amplifications.

WT Amplification of Emerging Virus in Non-clinical Samples

WT amplification using the P-N6/SSIII RT-method was tested for its ability to amplify emerging viruses. Due to difficulty in getting access to clinical samples positive for a diverse set of emerging viruses, we initially tested the method on a wide range of virus-positive cell culture supernatants (SN), purified viral NA or QCMD panel samples (Table S1). The WT amplification was analysed using virus specific real-time PCRs before and after amplification (Table S1 and Figure 2). For all samples tested, amplification of the emerging virus was observed (Figure 2A). For EEEV (Alphavirus), Usutu virus (Flavivirus), WNV (Flavivirus), PV (Enterovirus), Hantaan virus (Hantavirus), RVFV (Phlebovirus) and Toscana virus (Phlebovirus) the amplification was relatively small with a fold increase between 25–500 (Table S1 and Figure 2A). However, for other samples much larger fold increases were observed, such as JEV (Flavivirus) with a fold increase of 1.5×10^6, DOBV (Hantavirus) with a fold increase of 4.5×10^6 and Puumala virus (Hantavirus) with a fold increase of 1.4×10^4 (Table S1 and Figure 2A). When we examined the relationship between amplification (fold increase) and viral content (C_t-values before WT amplification) (Figure 2B), we observed a significant correlation between WT amplification and viral content. Samples containing a high viral content were amplified to a lesser extent than samples containing a lower viral content, which could reflect that for samples with a high concentration of NA, primers and nucleotides are depleted quickly, resulting in a lower WT amplification.

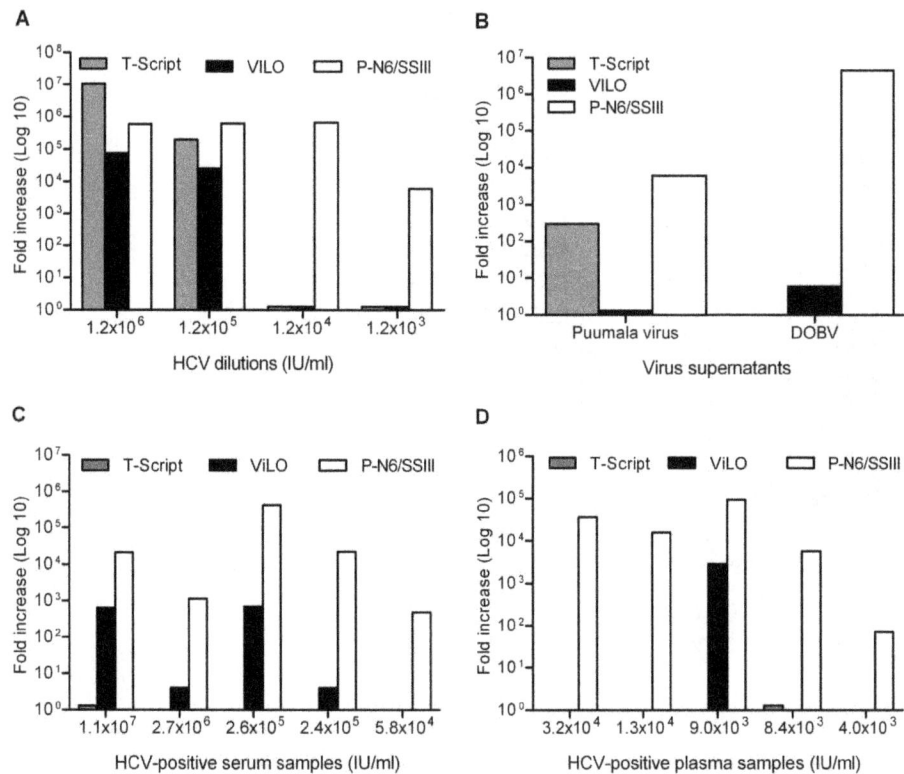

Figure 1. Improved WT amplification when using 5′-phosphorylated random hexamers in RT-reaction. Comparison of three different RT-reactions in the Whole Transcriptome Amplification (WTA) protocol. Purified viral RNA was amplified by WTA using VILO, T-Script or P-N6/SSIII RT-reaction. Virus-specific real-time PCR was performed before and after the amplification step, and fold increase was calculated using ΔC_t-values and dilution factors for each sample tested. (A) WTA-protocols tested with a 10-fold serial dilution of an HCV-positive serum sample with known concentration. (B) WTA-protocols tested with two different virus-positive cell culture supernatants, Puumala virus and Dobrava-Belgrade virus (DOBV), respectively. (C) WTA-protocols tested with five HCV-positive serum samples with estimated concentration (IU/ml). (D) WTA-protocols tested with five HCV-positive plasma samples with estimated concentration (IU/ml).

To investigate whether the presence of several viruses in a sample would interfere with WT amplification, we tested two QCMD panels of samples (WNV10-01 and -07) containing mixtures of four and three different flaviviruses, respectively, each at a concentration of 1.0×10^6 copies/ml (Table S1 and Figure 2A). All seven flaviviruses were WT amplified; however DENV-1 was amplified to a lower degree than to the other DENV subtypes or flaviviruses (Figure 2A). This most likely reflect a difference in the sensitivity of the Dengue subtype-specific primers used to analyse the WT amplification rather than virus subtype-specific variation in the WT amplification. In summary, the modified WT amplification method was able to amplify emerging viruses in 21 different non-clinical samples.

Microarray Detection Range

To test the sensitivity of the previously described LLMDA microarray [14,19,26] for RNA viruses, we performed microarray analysis on a 10-fold dilution series of a HCV-positive serum sample (1.2×10^6 IU/ml), a RVFV-positive supernatant (3.3×10^6 copies/ml), a WNV-positive QCMD panel sample (WNV13-01) (1.2×10^7 copies/ml), a DENV-positive QCMD panel sample (DENV13-01) (1.0×10^6 copies/ml) and two QCMD panel samples (WNV13-10 and WNV13-11) containing mixtures of JEV, DENV-1, DENV-2, DENV-4 and YFV, DENV-3, TBEV respectively (1.0×10^6 copies/ml) (Table 1). Dilutions ranging from 10^6 to 10^2 copies/ml were WT amplified, labelled and hybridised to the LLMDAv2 microarray. Microarray analysis was performed using the SSI [19] and CLiMax data analysis methods [14,41] (data not shown).

For the HCV, RVFV and WNV samples, dilutions of 10^6 to 10^3 copies/ml yielded sufficient viral material for successful identification by the LLMDAv2, while dilutions of 10^2 copies/ml were not detected by the microarray (Table 1). Dilutions of 10^2 copies/ml will theoretically result in an input of 24 copies to the RT-reaction and 12 copies to the WTA-reaction. Analyses of the viral concentrations after WT amplification of the non-detectable 10^2 copies/ml dilutions showed that RVFV, HCV and WNV were amplified to 1.7×10^5, 4.3×10^5 and 4.4×10^5 copies/ml, respectively (Table 1).

The detection limit for DENV, JEV and TBEV was 10^4 copies/ml (Table 1) and the detection limit for YFV was higher (10^5 copies/ml) than the rest of the flaviviruses analysed. The WNV13-11 sample was documented as containing YFV, DENV-3 and TBEV, each at 1.0×10^6 copies/ml; however, analysis of the C_t-values of YFV and TBEV before amplification showed a higher value for YFV ($C_t = 27$) compared to TBEV ($C_t = 23$) (Table 1), which could indicate a lower viral content of YFV in the WNV13-11 sample than was documented. Analysis of the viral concentration after WT amplification of the non-detectable 10^3 copies/ml dilutions showed that DENV, JEV and TBEV were amplified to 3.1×10^5, 1.0×10^4 and 2.1×10^4 copies/ml, respectively (Table 1). From this we conclude that at least 10^3 copies/ml is needed for a successful amplification with the modified WTA method and at least 10^5 copies/ml is needed after WT amplification in order to

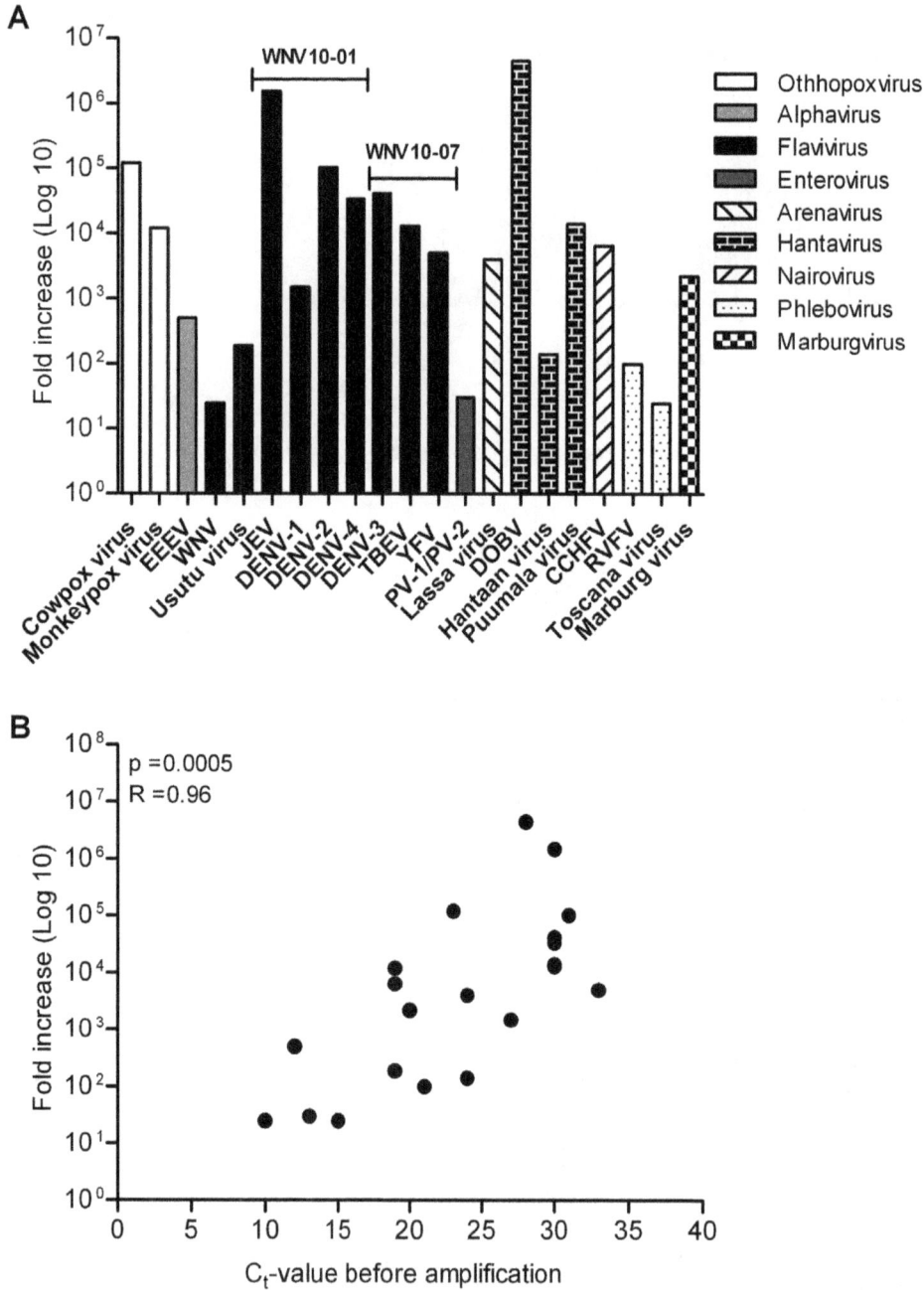

Figure 2. Modified WT amplification of non-clinical samples containing emerging virus. Purified viral RNA from a wide range of virus-positive cell culture supernatants (SN) or QCMD panel samples was amplified by WTA using the P-N6/SSIII RT-reaction. Virus-specific real-time PCR was performed before and after the amplification step, and fold increase was calculated using ΔC_t-values and dilution factors for each sample tested. (A) Fold increase of WT-amplified emerging viruses belonging to different virus genera. The two QCMD panel samples (WNV10-01 and WNV10-07) containing mixtures of different flaviviruses are highlighted. (B) The correlation between fold increase in WT amplification and viral sample content (C_t before WT amplification).

reliably identify viruses with the LLMDAv2. This concentration is equivalent to 0.17 femtomolar, demonstrating exquisite sensitivity of the LLMDAv2 platform.

Microarray Detection of Emerging Virus in Non-clinical Samples

The LLMDA microarray [14,19,26] was tested for its ability to correctly identify a wide range of virus-positive cell culture supernatants (SN), purified viral NA or QCMD panel samples

containing emerging viruses (Table 2). The WT amplified samples previously described (Table S1) were labelled and hybridised to the LLMDAv2 microarray. Microarray analysis was performed using the SSI [19] and CLiMax data analysis methods [14,41].

In all 21 samples analysed, both methods identified the correct virus (Table 2). In more than half of the samples, human endogenous retroviruses (HERV) were also found (Table 2), consistent with the presence of human host DNA. The CLiMax method identified additional retroviruses such as baboon endogenous virus

A

Log-odds

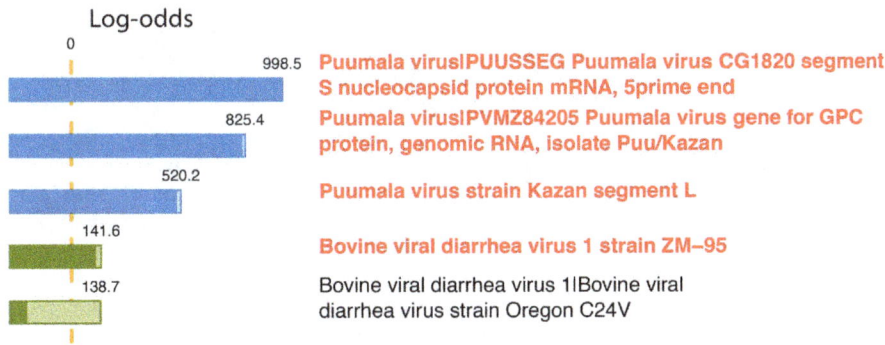

998.5 Puumala virus|PUUSSEG Puumala virus CG1820 segment S nucleocapsid protein mRNA, 5prime end

825.4 Puumala virus|PVMZ84205 Puumala virus gene for GPC protein, genomic RNA, isolate Puu/Kazan

520.2 Puumala virus strain Kazan segment L

141.6 Bovine viral diarrhea virus 1 strain ZM–95

138.7 Bovine viral diarrhea virus 1|Bovine viral diarrhea virus strain Oregon C24V

B

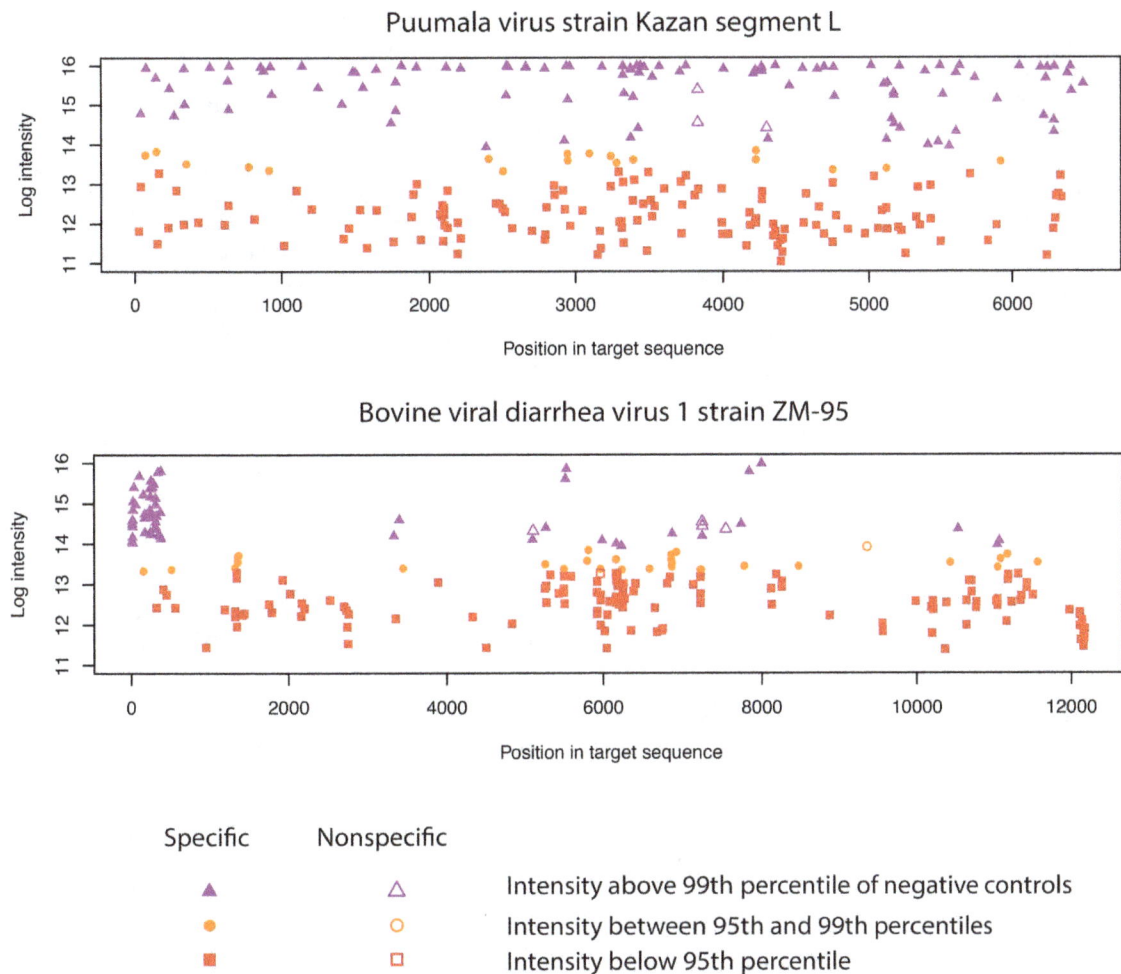

Figure 3. CLiMax analysis detects Puumala virus in a non-clinical sample. The results of microarray analyses of WT-amplified viral DNA-samples, using CLiMax analysis. (A) Log-odds scores for a Puumala virus-positive sample. The lighter and darker-coloured portions of the bars represent the unconditional and conditional log-odds scores, respectively. The conditional log-odds scores shows the contribution from a target that cannot be explained by another, more likely target above it, while the unconditional score illustrates that some very similar targets share a number of probes. (B) Target sequence-probe alignment plots for segment L of the Puumala virus genome and for BVDV-1, showing probe intensity vs probe position in the viral genome. Plot symbol and color indicates positive (>99th percentile), negative (<95th percentile), or equivocal hybridisation signals; hollow symbols indicate probes found to hybridise non-specifically. The pattern seen for BVDV-1, in which positive probes are restricted to a few narrow genome regions, is a typical cross-hybridisation result.

(BEV), simian retrovirus 1 (SRV-1), *Mus dunni* endogeneous virus (MDEV), murine leukemia virus (MuLV) and mouse mammary tumour virus (MMTV). These additional viruses were not identified by the SSI method because non-human, non-zoonotic pathogens were considered clinically irrelevant and excluded in the SSI data analysis.

For four of the samples (cowpox virus, monkeypox virus, PV-1/PV-2 and Usutu virus), the SSI method had difficulties in distinguishing between different genus-members and subtypes. In the Usutu virus sample (Flavivirus), the SSI method identified both Usutu virus and JEV, another Flavivirus species, as being present, while the CliMax analysis correctly identified Usutu virus only. In the PV sample, the CLiMax analysis correctly identified PV-1 and PV-2, while the SSI analysis made an additional false-positive detection of PV subtype 3 (Table 2). In the samples of cowpox virus and monkeypox virus, both methods identified additional members of the *Orthopoxviridae* family as present. The SSI analysis identified both samples as mixtures of cowpox, monkeypox, vaccinia and variola viruses, while the CliMax analysis identified the correct cowpox or monkeypox virus together with the variola minor virus (Table 2), which belongs to the same genus. Detailed examination of the probes with positive signals (greater than the 99th percentile of the negative control intensities) showed that all such probes with alignments to the variola minor virus genome had strong matches in the cowpox and monkeypox genomes; so that the identification of variola minor virus in the CliMax analysis in these samples is most likely due to cross-hybridization of these probes.

For five samples (Hantaan virus, Puumala virus, RVFV, Naples virus and Marburg virus) the CLiMax analysis identified additional viruses that were not observed using the SSI analysis (Table 2). To better understand the source of these additional predictions, we used the CliMax software to generate sequence-probe alignment plots, where the intensity of each probe is plotted against its alignment position in the viral genome. These plots clarify whether identification of a virus is based on presence of the whole genome or may be due to cross-hybridization from probes matching sub-regions of other genomes present in the sample. For example, the sequence-probe alignment plots for the Puumala virus sample show the positive probes to be uniformly distributed across all three Puumala virus genome segments, indicating the presence of the whole viral genome (Figure 3B, top). Probe hits for the bovine viral diarrhea virus 1 (BVDV-1) genome show a different pattern, landing in only a narrow region suggesting nonspecific- or cross-hybridisation (Figure 3B, bottom). We refer to this pattern as a fragmented alignment plot.

We observed a similar fragmented alignment pattern for RVFV segment S in the Marburg sample, indicating non-specific cross-hybridisation (data not shown). In contrast, we obtained uniform positive probe distributions for mammalian orthoreovirus 1 and 3 (MRV) genomes in the Hantaan virus sample, for CCHFV and Simian virus 5 (SV5) genomes in the RVFV sample, and for BVDV-1 in the Naples virus sample, indicating that these complete viral genomes were truly present (data not shown). CCHFV specific PCR could not confirm the presence of CCHFV in the RVFV sample (data not shown). The other additional findings were all considered clinically irrelevant and therefore not further investigated by PCR.

The presence of several viruses in a sample did not interfere with identification, as can be seen by the microarray analysis of the two panels of samples (WNV10-01 and -07) containing mixtures of different flaviviruses (Table 2). Microarray analysis correctly identified all four viruses present in WNV10-01 and all three viruses present in WNV10-07 (Table 2). However, the individual

DENV subtypes were difficult to distinguish completely. In the WNV10-10 sample the CLiMax analysis identified DENV type 3, and in the WNV10-07 sample both analysis methods detected DENV type 1 and 2. These extra DENV findings were later confirmed as false-positives by Dengue subtype-specific PCR (data not shown). In addition, the SSI analysis of the WNV10-07 sample identified Omsk haemorrhagic fever virus (OHFV), which also belongs to the Flavivirus genus [44]. This finding was not observed using the CLiMax analysis and hence not checked by PCR. The CLiMax analysis also found HERV, rotavirus A and porcine rotavirus C in both samples as well as BVDV-1 in WNV10-01 and SV5 in WNV10-07. The presence of rotavirus A was confirmed by rotavirus A-specific PCR (data not shown). BVDV, SV5 and porcine rotavirus C were considered clinically irrelevant and therefore not confirmed by PCR.

In summary, the LLMDAv2 correctly identified single and multiple viruses present in non-clinical samples with a very low level of false positive signals. The CLiMax analysis method identified every virus present in the samples whereas the simpler SSI analysis method only identified clinically relevant human pathogens.

Microarray Detection of Emerging Viruses in Clinical Samples

We tested the LLMDAv2 microarray on 18 clinical samples previously identified as positive by real-time PCR for emerging viruses. The correct virus was identified in 17 samples using both the SSI (Table 3) and CLiMax analyses (data not shown). The sample identified only as a parapoxvirus was determined to be Orf virus, a member of the Parapoxvirus genus. Seven of the eight DENV-positive samples were clearly determined by the microarray analysis to be positive for DENV type 2, DENV type 1 or DENV type 3. DENV type 4 was not identified in any of the clinical samples. Additional DENV subtypes were detected in four of the samples, but at very low probe signal intensities compared to the correct DENV subtype probe signal (Figure 4A+4B). These were confirmed as negative by Dengue subtype-specific PCR (data not shown). One DENV-positive sample was also positive for hepatitis GB virus C (GBV-C). One DENV-positive sample was not identified by the microarray. Six urine samples were positive for WNV and two of these samples were identified as having additional viruses (Table 3). One WNV sample was also positive for the polyomaviruses JCV and BKV (Figure 4C), which later were confirmed as present by PCR (data not shown). Another WNV sample was positive for JEV (Figure 4D), but this finding could not be confirmed by PCR (data not shown). In addition, the microarray detected HERV in almost all samples, consistent with the presence of human DNA, and the common Torque Teno virus (TTV) [19,23,45] in the CCHFV and two DENV samples. Virus-negative urine, CSF and serum were also analysed and confirmed to be negative for virus (Table 3), except for HERV found in the CSF sample. In summary, the LLMDAv2 correctly identified emerging viruses present in 17 of the 18 clinical samples analysed. The only sample not identified was a DENV-positive sample, in which the viral concentration was determined to be below the detection limit, as described below.

To assess viral concentration in clinical samples, we performed specific real-time PCR before and after WT amplification. We estimated the viral concentration of 6 WNV-positive urine samples and 6 DENV-positive serum samples by comparison to PCR results for the series of 10-fold dilutions of the QCMD panel WNV and DENV samples (Table 2 and Table 3). The WNV-positive urine samples were determined to have concentrations between 3.7×10^4 and 4.9×10^5 copies/ml before WTA and concentrations

Table 3. Microarray results on clinical samples containing emerging viruses.

Group[*]	Genus	Virus	Sample	Detected virus (SSI analysis)	ΔC_t[a]	Fold increase[b]	After WTA[c]	Sample conc[c]
dsDNA	Parapoxvirus	Parapox sp.	skin lesion	Orf[95]	45-23	3.6×10^6	ND	ND
(+) ssRNA	Alphavirus	Chikungunya	Serum	**Chikungunya virus**	30-24	3.5×10^4	ND	ND
	Flavivirus	DENV	Serum	**DENV-2**, DENV-4, DENV-3, DENV-1, HERV	23-ND	-	ND	ND
		DENV	Serum	**DENV-2**, HERV, TTV	29-ND	-	ND	ND
		DENV	Serum	**DENV-1, GBV-C,** DENV-3, DENV-4, DENV-2, JEV, HERV, TTV	24-8	1.5×10^6	2.5×10^{12}	1.8×10^7
		DENV	Serum	**DENV-3,** DENV-1, DENV-4, DENV-2, HERV	25-12	1.7×10^5	2.7×10^{11}	1.1×10^7
		DENV	Serum	**DENV-1**	26-13	2.4×10^5	1.6×10^{11}	5.1×10^6
		DENV	serum	**DENV-1**	31-16	8.5×10^5	2.8×10^{10}	3.2×10^5
		DENV	serum	**DENV-1,** DENV-3, DENV-4, DENV2, HERV	34-23	3.2×10^4	5.3×10^8	8.3×10^4
		DENV	serum	HERV	37-38	15	1.4×10^5	1.1×10^4
		WNV	urine	**WNV,** HERV	28-26	133	2.8×10^7	4.9×10^5
		WNV	urine	**WNV,** HERV, JCV, BKV	30-28	73	8.6×10^6	2.2×10^5
		WNV	urine	**WNV,** HERV	31-29	103	6.4×10^6	1.3×10^5
		WNV	urine	**WNV,** HERV	31-31	32	2.9×10^6	1.3×10^5
		WNV	urine	**WNV,** HERV	32-36	1	3.0×10^5	8.9×10^4
		WNV	urine	**WNV,** JEV, HERV	34-26	7.4×10^3	2.5×10^7	3.7×10^4
(-) ssRNA	Nairovirus	CCHFV	serum	**CCHFV,** HERV, TTV	ND	-	ND	ND
	Phlebovirus	Toscana	CSF	**Toscana virus,** HERV	31	25	-	2.4×10^3
-	-	Neg. ctrl	Urine	-	ND	-	-	-
-	-	Neg. ctrl	CSF	HERV	ND	-	-	-
-	-	Neg. ctrl	serum	-	ND	-	-	-

NOTE. Conc, Concentration; DENV; Dengue virus; WNV, West Nile virus; JCV, JC polyomavirus; BKV, BK polyomavirus; CCHFV, Crimean-Congo haemorrhagic fever virus; Neg. ctrl, Negative control; GBV-C, hepatitis GB virus C; JEV, Japanese encephalitis virus; CSF, Cerebrospinal fluid; HERV, human endogenous retrovirus; TTV, torque teno virus; ND, not determined. Bold represents correctly identified virus.
*Viruses are grouped based on nucleic acid content, according to the Baltimore Classification.
[95]results obtained using a 95 percentile threshold.
[a]Difference in C_t-value in real-time PCR before and after WT amplification.
[b]Fold increase after WT amplification, calculated from ΔC_t combined with dilution factors for each sample.
[c]Copies/ml (HCV; IU/ml).

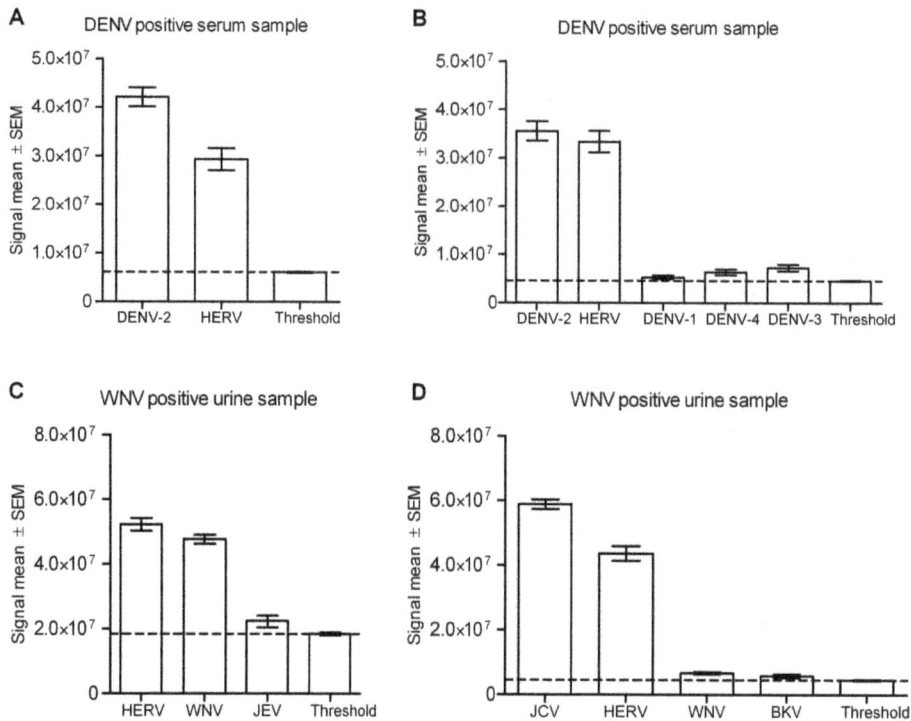

Figure 4. Microarray analysis correctly identifies emerging viruses in clinical samples. The results of microarray analysis of WT-amplified virus-positive clinical samples, using the SSI analysis method. Graphs show the signal mean for the probe intensities for each detected virus. The bar across the graph demonstrates the signal threshold at the 99th percentile of the random control intensities. (A) Microarray analysis of a Dengue-positive serum sample. (B) Microarray analysis of another Dengue-positive serum sample. (C) Microarray analysis of a WNV-positive urine sample. (D) Microarray analysis of another WNV-positive urine sample.

between 3.0×10^5 and 2.8×10^7 copies/ml after WT amplification (Table 3). These samples all had concentrations above the detection limit (10^3 copies/ml) determined for dilutions of the WNV-positive QCMD sample (WNV13-01) (Table 1). Analysis of the WT amplification showed that WNV from urine samples was not amplified as efficiently as WNV from the QCMD sample (Table 1 and Table 3), however the concentration after WTA was still above 10^5 copies/ml and hence detectable by the LLMDAv2.

The DENV-positive serum samples were determined to have concentrations between 1.1×10^4 and 1.8×10^7 copies/ml before WT amplification and between 1.4×10^5 and 2.5×10^{12} copies/ml after WTA (Table 3). The DENV-positive sample which was not detected by the microarray had an estimated concentration of 1.1×10^4 copies/ml, which was near the pre-amplification detection limit seen for dilutions of the QCMD DENV sample (10^4 copies/ml) (Table 1 and Table 3); and a concentration after WTA of 1.4×10^5 copies/ml, which is near the post-WTA limit of detection (10^5 copies/ml). This sample was also near the limit of detection with real-time PCR, with a C_t value of 37 before amplification. In summary, 11 out of 12 clinical samples analysed had viral concentrations above the detection limit of the LLMDAv2.

Discussion

The disease symptoms for emerging viruses are often similar to those of other more common viruses, posing a diagnostic challenge to clinicians unfamiliar with the novel organism. In the case of emerging viruses it is crucial for patient treatment and for containment of a potential epidemic to quickly identify the correct virus. We demonstrate the ability of the LLMDAv2 array

combined with a modified WTA protocol to correctly identify 29 different emerging viruses in both clinical and non-clinical samples. Previously we have also shown that LLMDAv2 can detect a broad range of common viruses in clinical samples [19]. We show a sensitivity of 10^3–10^4 copies/ml for different emerging RNA viruses, which is in the range of clinical relevance, but not as sensitive as specific real-time PCR. However, the use of PCR requires a specific hypothesis as to the causative agent, which is not the case with the LLMDA array. We use a modified random WTA method to amplify the RNA virus and show at least 10^5 copies/ml of amplified material is needed in order to have a successful identification by the LLMDAv2. This is equivalent to the recently published data that show detection of 10^5 copies of vaccinia virus DNA without any amplification prior to hybridization to the 4x72K version of the LLMDA [46].

The samples used in this study to measure sensitivity were all dilutions of viral samples or supernatants and do not represent clinical samples containing low viral concentrations. Therefore, further experiments to investigate clinical sensitivity are warranted. Previous reports have shown high clinical sensitivity (86–97%) and specificity (98–99%) of another microarray, the Virochip [15], when it was applied to samples from different respiratory virus infections that were confirmed by specific PCR [20,21]. In our study, we correctly identified emerging viruses in 17 out of 18 clinical samples that were positive by specific PCR, corresponding to a clinical sensitivity of 94%. However, this study must be considered preliminary due to its small size. We are currently comparing the LLMDAv2 against standard diagnostic real-time PCR tests for a wide range of viruses and clinical sample materials. However, our ability to compare diagnostic assays for emerging viruses is limited due to the relatively small number of clinical samples received at SSI containing these viruses.

Overall, the LLMDAv2 demonstrates high specificity and sensitivity with few false positives. The majority of additional hits found by the microarray data analysis are retroviruses normally found in mammalian genomes (HERV, BEV, MDEV, MuLV and MMTV). They are clinically irrelevant and most probably originate from host or cell culture DNA. The BEV identified in the Ebola virus, cowpox virus and monkeypox virus SN samples is not surprising, since cross-hybridization of endogenous retroviruses in African green monkey-derived Vero E6 cell cultures to the BEV probes has been previously reported [26]. The MDEV, MuLV and MMTV identified in the poliovirus sample are consistent with the fact that PV is cultured in mouse-derived L20B cells. In a few samples (Usutu virus, cowpox virus, monkeypox virus, RVFV, Marburg virus, the WNV10-panel samples, one clinical DENV sample, and one clinical WNV sample), additional viruses were identified that predominantly belonged to the same family or genus as the correct virus. All of them were determined to be false positives by virus-specific PCR indicating a need to improve the specificity of the probes or the analysis methods. Both data analysis methods had difficulty in distinguishing between the four different DENV subtypes (Table 1 and Figure 3B). This was not surprising, since viral strain subtyping was not a goal of the LLMDAv2 design [14]. Nevertheless, our work shows that improvements to LLMDA probe specificity are needed to increase its value for diagnosis and outbreak detection.

The CLiMax software is numerically intensive and requires a large-memory LINUX server harbouring a library of probe-target binding probabilities that are the basis for pathogen identification [14,41]. The CLiMax analysis is sophisticated and powerful, providing a user-friendly web interface to a database that keeps track of requested analyses and their results. In addition to a list of probable viruses, the CLiMax software can generate a target sequence-probe alignment plot showing probe fluorescence intensities together with the location of probe hits across each viral genome detected. This can help to distinguish the presence of whole viral genomes from non-specific probe hits and cross-reactivity.

The analysis developed in-house at SSI processes microarray feature intensities produced by the NimbleScan software within a Microsoft Excel framework [19]. While the CLiMax analysis is designed for broad-spectrum detection of all microbial targets represented on the LLMDA, the Excel-based SSI analysis is more focused toward identification of human-infecting viral pathogens. The relative simplicity of the SSI analysis is attractive for a clinical diagnostic environment, since it requires less costly computing hardware, and provides a clearer diagnostic result for clinicians, because clinically irrelevant non-human and non-zoonotic pathogens are excluded from the analysis. The CLiMax software is a more sophisticated, precise tool for data analysis in a research environment. Its ability to identify microbial pathogens from all host species makes this analysis method ideal for analysis of special cases such as detection of novel zoonotic viruses and research purposes.

Acknowledgments

We thank Solvej Jensen, Birgit Knudsen, Bente Østergaard and Britt Christensen for expert technical help. We thank the CCH Fever Network supported by the European Commission under the Health Cooperation Work Program of the 7th Framework Program (no. 260427) for contributing with CCHFV-positive clinical samples. This work was performed in part under the auspices of the U.S. Department of Energy by Lawrence Livermore National Laboratory under Contract DE-AC52-07NA27344.

Author Contributions

Conceived and designed the experiments: MWR LE AF. Performed the experiments: MWR LE MLO. Analyzed the data: MWR LE MLO KM. Contributed reagents/materials/analysis tools: MWR KM AP OE SP AM MW MN SG. Wrote the paper: MWR LE KM SG. Copy-editing: SG KM.

References

1. Calzolari M, Gaibani P, Bellini R, Defilippo F, Pierro A, et al. (2012) Mosquito, bird and human surveillance of West Nile and Usutu viruses in Emilia-Romagna Region (Italy) in 2010. PLoS One 7: e38058. Available: http://www.pubmedcentral.nih.gov/articlerender.fcgi?artid=3364206&tool=pmcentrez&rendertype=abstract. Accessed 6 December 2013.

2. Heyman P, Cochez C, Hofhuis A, van der Giessen J, Sprong H, et al. (2010) A clear and present danger: tick-borne diseases in Europe. Expert Rev Anti Infect Ther 8: 33–50. doi:10.1586/eri.09.118.

3. Nichol ST, Arikawa J, Kawaoka Y (2000) Emerging viral diseases. Proc Natl Acad Sci U S A 97: 12411–12412. Available: http://www.pnas.org/content/97/23/12411.full. Accessed 28 February 2014.

4. Van der Poel WHM, Lina PHC, Kramps JA (2006) Public health awareness of emerging zoonotic viruses of bats: a European perspective. Vector Borne Zoonotic Dis 6: 315–324. doi:10.1089/vbz.2006.6.315.

5. Cavrini F, Gaibani P, Longo G, Pierro AM, Rossini G, et al. (2009) Usutu virus infection in a patient who underwent orthotropic liver transplantation, Italy, August-September 2009. Euro Surveill Bull Eur sur les Mal Transm Eur Commun Dis Bull 14: 1–2.

6. Pecorari M, Longo G, Gennari W, Grottola A, Sabbatini AMT, et al. (2009) First human case of Usutu virus neuro invasive infection, Italy, August - September 2009. Euro Surveill Bull Eur sur les Mal Transm Eur Commun Dis Bull 14: 9–10.

7. Heyman P, Ceianu CS, Christova I, Tordo N, Beersma M, et al. (2011) A five-year perspective on the situation of haemorrhagic fever with renal syndrome and status of the hantavirus reservoirs in Europe, 2005–2010. Eurosurveillance 16: 2005–2010.

8. Maltezou HC, Papa A (2010) Crimean-Congo hemorrhagic fever: risk for emergence of new endemic foci in Europe? Travel Med Infect Dis 8: 139–143. doi:10.1016/j.tmaid.2010.04.008.

9. Papa A (2012) West Nile virus infections in Greece: an update. Expert Rev Anti Infect Ther 10: 743–750. doi:10.1586/eri.12.59.

10. Whitehouse C a (2004) Crimean-Congo hemorrhagic fever. Antiviral Res 64: 145–160. doi:10.1016/j.antiviral.2004.08.001.

11. Tomashek KM, Gregory CJ, Sánchez AR, Bartek M a, Garcia Rivera EJ, et al. (2012) Dengue Deaths in Puerto Rico: Lessons Learned from the 2007 Epidemic. PLoS Negl Trop Dis 6: 1–9. doi:10.1371/journal.pntd.0001614.

12. Wang Y, Zhang X, Wei H (2011) Laboratory detection and diagnosis of filoviruses. Virol Sin 26: 73–80. doi:10.1007/s12250-011-3186-9.

13. Weidmann M, Armbruster K, Hufert FT (2008) Challenges in designing a Taqman-based multiplex assay for the simultaneous detection of Herpes simplex virus types 1 and 2 and Varicella-zoster virus. J Clin Virol 42: 326–334. doi:10.1016/j.jcv.2008.03.005.

14. Gardner SN, Jaing CJ, McLoughlin KS, Slezak TR (2010) A microbial detection array (MDA) for viral and bacterial detection. BMC Genomics 11: 668. doi:10.1186/1471-2164-11-668.

15. Wang D, Coscoy L, Zylberberg M, Avila PC, Boushey HA, et al. (2002) Microarray-based detection and genotyping of viral pathogens. Proc Natl Acad Sci U S A 99: 15687–15692. Available: http://www.pnas.org/content/99/24/15687.short. Accessed 27 January 2014.

16. Grubaugh ND, Petz LN, Melanson VR, McMenamy SS, Turell MJ, et al. (2013) Evaluation of a field-portable DNA microarray platform and nucleic acid amplification strategies for the detection of arboviruses, arthropods, and bloodmeals. Am J Trop Med Hyg 88: 245–253. Available: http://www.ncbi.nlm.nih.gov/pubmed/23249687. Accessed 29 November 2013.

17. Berthet N, Paulous S, Coffey LL, Frenkiel MP, Moltini I, et al. (2013) Resequencing microarray method for molecular diagnosis of human arboviral diseases. J Clin Virol 56: 238–243. Available: http://www.ncbi.nlm.nih.gov/pubmed/23219893. Accessed 6 December 2013.

18. Bexfield N, Kellam P (2011) Metagenomics and the molecular identification of novel viruses. Vet J 190: 191–198. Available: http://www.ncbi.nlm.nih.gov/pubmed/21111643. Accessed 21 November 2013.

19. Erlandsson L, Rosenstierne MW, McLoughlin K, Jaing C, Fomsgaard A (2011) The Microbial Detection Array Combined with Random Phi29-Amplification Used as a Diagnostic Tool for Virus Detection in Clinical Samples. PLoS One 6: e22631. doi:10.1371/journal.pone.0022631.

20. Kistler A, Avila PC, Rouskin S, Wang D, Ward T, et al. (2007) Pan-viral screening of respiratory tract infections in adults with and without asthma reveals unexpected human coronavirus and human rhinovirus diversity. J Infect Dis 196: 817–825. Available: http://www.ncbi.nlm.nih.gov/pubmed/17703411. Accessed 15 August 2013.

21. Chiu CY, Urisman A, Greenhow TL, Rouskin S, Yagi S, et al. (2008) Utility of DNA microarrays for detection of viruses in acute respiratory tract infections in children. J Pediatr 153: 76–83. doi:10.1016/j.jpeds.2007.12.035.

22. Grubaugh ND, McMenamy SS, Turell MJ, Lee JS (2013) Multi-gene detection and identification of mosquito-borne RNA viruses using an oligonucleotide microarray. PLoS Negl Trop Dis 7: e2349. Available: http://www.pubmedcentral.nih.gov/articlerender.fcgi?artid = 3744434&tool = pmcentrez&rendertype = abstract. Accessed 6 December 2013.

23. Yozwiak NL, Skewes-Cox P, Stenglein MD, Balmaseda A, Harris E, et al. (2012) Virus identification in unknown tropical febrile illness cases using deep sequencing. PLoS Negl Trop Dis 6: e1485. Available: http://www.pubmedcentral.nih.gov/articlerender.fcgi?artid = 3274504&tool = pmcentrez&rendertype = abstract. Accessed 11 November 2013.

24. Filippone C, Marianneau P, Murri S, Mollard N, Avsic-Zupanc T, et al. (2013) Molecular diagnostic and genetic characterization of highly pathogenic viruses: application during Crimean-Congo haemorrhagic fever virus outbreaks in Eastern Europe and the Middle East. Clin Microbiol Infect 19: E118–28. Available: http://www.pubmedcentral.nih.gov/articlerender.fcgi?artid = 3663000&tool = pmcentrez&rendertype = abstract.

25. Devault AM, McLoughlin K, Jaing C, Gardner S, Porter TM, et al. (2014) Ancient pathogen DNA in archaeological samples detected with a Microbial Detection Array. Sci Rep 4: 4245. Available: http://www.pubmedcentral.nih.gov/articlerender.fcgi?artid = 3945050&tool = pmcentrez&rendertype = abstract. Accessed 25 March 2014.

26. Victoria JG, Wang C, Jones MS, Jaing C, McLoughlin K, et al. (2010) Viral nucleic acids in live-attenuated vaccines: detection of minority variants and an adventitious virus. J Virol 84: 6033–6040. doi:10.1128/JVI.02690-09.

27. Blow JA, Dohm DJ, Negley DL, Mores CN (2004) Virus inactivation by nucleic acid extraction reagents. J Virol Methods 119: 195–198. doi:10.1016/j.jviromet.2004.03.015.

28. Wood DJ, Hull B (1999) L20B cells simplify culture of polioviruses from clinical samples. J Med Virol 58: 188–192. Available: http://www.ncbi.nlm.nih.gov/pubmed/10335869.

29. Berthet N, Reinhardt AK, Leclercq I, van Ooyen S, Batéjat C, et al. (2008) Phi29 polymerase based random amplification of viral RNA as an alternative to random RT-PCR. BMC Mol Biol 9: 77. Available: http://www.pubmedcentral.nih.gov/articlerender.fcgi?artid = 2535778&tool = pmcentrez&rendertype = abstract. Accessed 15 November 2013.

30. Ryschkewitsch C, Jensen P, Hou J, Fahle G, Fischer S, et al. (2004) Comparison of PCR-southern hybridization and quantitative real-time PCR for the detection of JC and BK viral nucleotide sequences in urine and cerebrospinal fluid. J Virol Methods 121: 217–221. Available: http://www.ncbi.nlm.nih.gov/pubmed/15381359. Accessed 15 August 2013.

31. Shchelkunov SN, Shcherbakov DN, Maksyutov R a, Gavrilova E V (2011) Species-specific identification of variola, monkeypox, cowpox, and vaccinia viruses by multiplex real-time PCR assay. J Virol Methods 175: 163–169. doi:10.1016/j.jviromet.2011.05.002.

32. Pastorino B, Bessaud M, Grandadam M, Murri S, Tolou HJ, et al. (2005) Development of a TaqMan RT-PCR assay without RNA extraction step for the detection and quantification of African Chikungunya viruses. J Virol Methods 124: 65–71. doi:10.1016/j.jviromet.2004.11.002.

33. Lambert AJ, Martin Da, Lanciotti RS (2003) Detection of North American eastern and western equine encephalitis viruses by nucleic acid amplification assays. J Clin Microbiol 41: 379–385. doi:10.1128/JCM.41.1.379.

34. Shirato K, Miyoshi H, Kariwa H, Takashima I (2005) Detection of West Nile virus and Japanese encephalitis virus using real-time PCR with a probe common to both viruses. J Virol Methods 126: 119–125. doi:10.1016/j.jviromet.2005.02.001.

35. Schwaiger M, Cassinotti P (2003) Development of a quantitative real-time RT-PCR assay with internal control for the laboratory detection of tick borne encephalitis virus (TBEV) RNA. J Clin Virol 27: 136–145. doi:10.1016/S1386-6532(02)00168-3.

36. Drosten C, Göttig S, Schilling S (2002) Rapid Detection and Quantification of Marburg Viruses, Lassa Virus, Crimean-Congo Hemorrhagic Fever Virus, Rift Valley Fever Virus, Dengue virus, and Yellow Fever Virus by Real-Time Reverse Transcription-PCR. J Clin Microbiol 40: 2323–2330. Available: http://jcm.asm.org/content/40/7/2323.short. Accessed 27 January 2014.

37. Weidmann M, Sall Aa, Manuguerra J-C, Koivogui L, Adjami A, et al. (2011) Quantitative analysis of particles, genomes and infectious particles in supernatants of haemorrhagic fever virus cell cultures. Virol J 8: 81. doi:10.1186/1743-422X-8-81.

38. Weidmann M, Schmidt P, Vackova M, Krivanec K, Munclinger P, et al. (2005) Identification of genetic evidence for dobrava virus spillover in rodents by nested reverse transcription (RT)-PCR and TaqMan RT-PCR. J Clin Microbiol 43: 808–812. doi:10.1128/JCM.43.2.808.

39. Kramski M, Meisel H, Klempa B, Krüger DH, Pauli G, et al. (2007) Detection and typing of human pathogenic hantaviruses by real-time reverse transcription-PCR and pyrosequencing. Clin Chem 53: 1899–1905. doi:10.1373/clinchem.2007.093245.

40. Weidmann M, Hufert FT, Sall Aa (2007) Viral load among patients infected with Marburgvirus in Angola. J Clin Virol 39: 65–66. doi:10.1016/j.jcv.2006.12.023.

41. McLoughlin KS (2011) Microarrays for pathogen detection and analysis. Brief Funct Genomics 10: 342–353. doi:10.1093/bfgp/elr027.

42. Karimi-Busheri F, Lee J, Tomkinson aE, Weinfeld M (1998) Repair of DNA strand gaps and nicks containing 3′-phosphate and 5′-hydroxyl termini by purified mammalian enzymes. Nucleic Acids Res 26: 4395–4400.

43. Ausubel FM, Brent R, Kingston RE, Moore DD, Seidman JG, et al. (2003) Current Protocols in Molecular Biology Vol. 1. 3.14.1-3.14.4. doi:10.1002/mrd.1080010210.

44. Růžek D, Yakimenko VV, Karan LS, Tkachev SE (2010) Omsk haemorrhagic fever. Lancet 376: 2104–2113. doi:10.1016/S0140-6736(10)61120-8.

45. Okamoto H (2009) History of discoveries and pathogenicity of TT viruses. Curr Top Microbiol Immunol 331: 1–20. doi:10.1002/rmv.524.

46. Thissen JB, McLoughlin K, Gardner S, Gu P, Mabery S, et al. (2014) Analysis of sensitivity and rapid hybridization of a multiplexed Microbial Detection Microarray. J Virol Methods 201: 73–78. Available: http://www.ncbi.nlm.nih.gov/pubmed/24602557. Accessed 3 April 2014.

12

Dengue Virus 2 American-Asian Genotype Identified during the 2006/2007 Outbreak in Piauí, Brazil Reveals a Caribbean Route of Introduction and Dissemination of Dengue Virus in Brazil

Leandra Barcelos Figueiredo[1], Tetsu Sakamoto[2], Luiz Felipe Leomil Coelho[3], Eliseu Soares de Oliveira Rocha[4], Marcela Menezes Gomes Cota[4], Gustavo Portela Ferreira[5], Jaquelline Germano de Oliveira[6], Erna Geessien Kroon[7]*

1 Departamento de Microbiologia, Universidade Federal de Minas Gerais, Belo Horizonte, Minas Gerais, Brazil, 2 Laboratório de Biodados, Universidade Federal de Minas Gerais, Belo Horizonte, Minas Gerais, Brazil, 3 Laboratório de Vacinas, Universidade Federal de Alfenas, Alfenas, Minas Gerais, Brazil, 4 Laboratório de Vírus, Universidade Federal de Minas Gerais, Belo Horizonte, Minas Gerais, Brazil, 5 Laboratório de Biotecnologia, Universidade Federal do Piauí, Parnaíba, Piauí, Brazil, 6 Laboratório de Imunologia Celular e Molecular, Fundação Oswaldo Cruz, Belo Horizonte, Minas Gerais, Brazil, 7 Laboratório de Vírus, Departamento de Microbiologia, Instituto de Ciências Biológicas, Universidade Federal de Minas Gerais, Belo Horizonte, Minas Gerais, Brazil

Abstract

Dengue virus (DENV) is the most widespread arthropod-borne virus, and the number and severity of outbreaks has increased worldwide in recent decades. Dengue is caused by DENV-1, DENV-2, DENV-3 and DENV-4 which are genetically distant. The species has been subdivided into genotypes based on phylogenetic studies. DENV-2, which was isolated from dengue fever patients during an outbreak in Piaui, Brazil in 2006/2007 was analyzed by sequencing the envelope (E) gene. The results indicated a high similarity among the isolated viruses, as well as to other DENV-2 from Brazil, Central America and South America. A phylogenetic and phylogeographic analysis based on DENV-2E gene sequences revealed that these viruses are grouped together with viruses of the American-Asian genotype in two distinct lineages. Our results demonstrate the co-circulation of two American-Asian genotype lineages in northeast Brazil. Moreover, we reveal that DENV-2 lineage 2 was detected in Piauí before it disseminated to other Brazilian states and South American countries, indicating the existence of a new dissemination route that has not been previously described.

Editor: Lisa F.P. Ng, Singapore Immunology Network, Agency for Science, Technology and Research (A*STAR), Singapore

Funding: This study was funded by Conselho Nacional de Desenvolvimento Científico e Tecnológico (CNPq), Coordenação de Aperfeiçoamento de Pessoal de Nível Superior (CAPES), Fundação de Amparo à Pesquisa do Estado de Minas Gerais (FAPEMIG), INCT and PRONEX-Dengue, Departamento de Ciência e Tecnologia do Ministério da Saúde (DECIT/MS). The funders had no role in study design, data collection and analysis, decision to publish, or preparation of the manuscript.

Competing Interests: The authors have declared that no competing interests exist.

* Email: ernagkroon@gmail.cozm

Introduction

Dengue is the most significant mosquito-borne viral disease that affects humans. Of all members of the *Flavivirus* genus, the *Dengue virus* (DENV) is responsible for the highest morbidity and mortality rates. DENV infection is endemic in more than 100 countries, with tens of millions of cases of dengue fever (DF) recorded per year, including up to 500,000 cases of dengue hemorrhagic fever/dengue shock syndrome (DHF/DSS), which require hospitalization for supportive treatment [1–2].

DENV is most commonly transmitted by the mosquito vector *Aedes aegypti*; however, it can also be transmitted by other members of the genus *Aedes*, including *Aedes albopictus*. The majority of infected humans is asymptomatic or develops DF, an acute febrile illness [3–5].

DENV belongs to the *Flavivirus* genus of the *Flaviviridae* family and has four genetically and antigenically distinct serotypes: DENV-1, DENV-2, DENV-3 and DENV-4. The virus is enveloped with a single-stranded, positive-sense RNA genome of approximately 11 kb containing a single open reading frame flanked by untranslated regions (5' and 3' UTRs) [6–7].

Phylogenetic and molecular analyses based on nucleic acid sequence data have been used to analyze the genetic variation of DENV, to characterize DENV serotypes and for epidemiological studies [8–11]. These approaches have revealed extensive variability among the DENVs, leading to the recognition of different genotypes within each species. Five DENV-2 genotypes have been described: Asian I (AS-I), Asian II (AS-II), American-Asian (AM/AS), Cosmopolitan (COS) and American (AM) [8,12–14]. In Brazil, DENV-2 was first identified in the state of Rio de Janeiro in 1990, and its introduction in Brazil resulted in several DF cases and the first severe forms of DHF as well as fatal cases of DSS [15–17]. This event was followed by a rapid spread of DENV-2 to other Brazilian states. [18–19]. An analysis of the envelope (E) gene of isolates from Rio de Janeiro and São Paulo collected during 2007–2008 and 2010 revealed that at least two lineages of the American-Asian genotype of DENV-2 have circulated in Brazil [20–22]. In addition, the virus that circulated in São Paulo in 2010 was closely related to the virus that circulated in Rio de Janeiro in 2007 and 2008 [21].

Piauí is located in the northeast region of Brazil; it has an area of 252,378 km^2 and a population of 3,118,360 (IBGE, 2010 [23]), and its northern region borders the Atlantic Ocean (Figure 1). It also borders the states of Maranhão (W), Ceará and Pernambuco (E) and Bahia and Tocantins (SW) [24]. According to the Ministry of Health, the first cases of dengue in the state of Piauí were reported in 1995, and in 2006, this state reported 4,759 cases of dengue. During 2006–2007, virological surveillance revealed that DENV-2 and DENV-3 were the most prevalent viruses in Piauí (data not published).

In the present study, we focused on the molecular epidemiology of DENV-2 isolates with different clinical manifestations from the outbreak in Piauí in 2006/2007 using Bayesian phylogeographic methods. Our phylogenetic analyses demonstrated the co-circulation of two different lineages of the DENV-2 American-Asian genotype in the state of Piauí during this outbreak, making this study the first report of co-circulation of different DENV-2 lineages in the same outbreak. Furthermore, by applying a spatiotemporal dynamics analysis, we suggest a new route of introduction of DENV-2 in Brazil.

Methods

Ethics Statement

This study was approved by the Committee of Ethics in Research of the Universidade Federal de Minas Gerais (number 415/04) and the blood collected was approved to be used in the research as unlinked anonymous samples.

Epidemiological Study and Clinical Samples

To study the epidemiological profile of dengue, 4,564 serum samples were collected from patients suspected of having febrile dengue who reported to health community centers distributed throughout the state of Piauí (northeast Brazil) during 2006/2007.

Serum was collected six days after symptom onset and sent to the Central Laboratory to confirm DENV infection via detection of specific IgM. Dengue cases were classified according to criteria established by the World Health Organization [1]. Demographic data (sex, age and location) were obtained from the standard notification form for dengue. Abiotic factors (pluviosity and average temperature) were obtained from the Agrometeorology Monitoring System of the Food and Animal Ministry (http://www.agritempo.gov.br).

Serum samples were obtained from a select subgroup of 46 patients in the acute phase without any type of hemorrhagic manifestation. The samples were collected six days after the osymptom onset, and stored at −70°C until use in viral isolation procedures and reverse transcription polymerase chain reactions (RT-PCR).

Detection of dengue IgM antibodies by ELISA

All sera were tested using the Dengue IgM Capture ELISA kit (Panbio, Australia) following the manufacturer's instructions.

Viral isolation in cell cultures

*Aedes albopictus*C6/36 cells were propagated in LeibovitzL15 medium (Gibco, USA) supplemented with 10% fetal calf serum (Cultilab, Brazil) at 28°C [25–26]. For virus isolation, a 50 μl serum sample was incubated with C6/36 cells supplemented with 2% fetal calf serum. Each sample was passaged at least three times. Infected C6/36 cells showing typical cytopathic effects were harvested, and the cell culture supernatants were used for viral RNA extraction. Uninfected cells used as controls were treated similarly, although the serum was omitted and replaced by medium. The cells inoculated with serum samples that did not show cytopathic effects even after the fifth passage were considered negative.

RNA extraction and RT-PCR

The QIAampViral RNA kit (Qiagen, USA) was used to extract viral RNA from the cell culture supernatants. Extracted RNA was

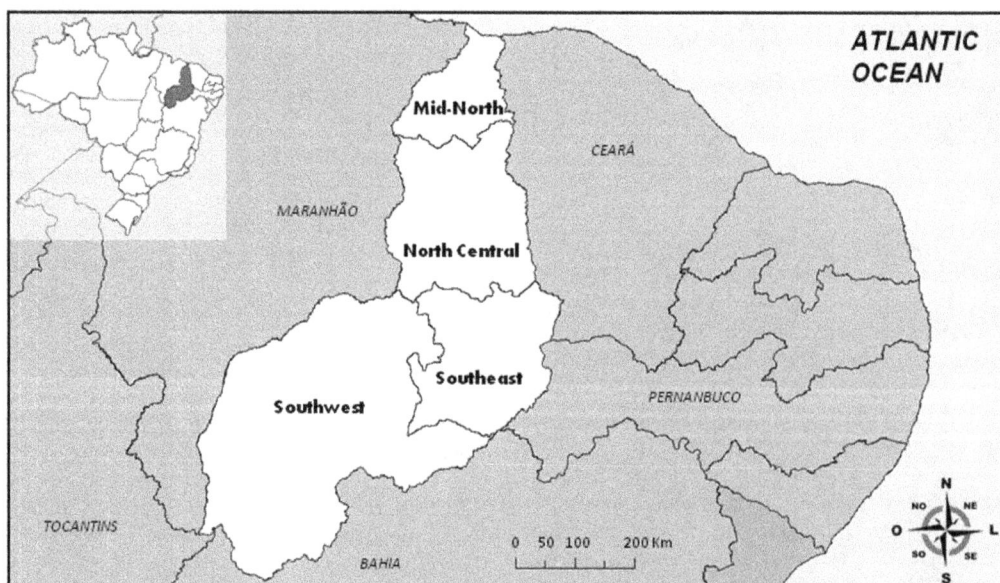

Figure 1. Geographic location of Piauí and its meso-regions. The state of Piauí is located in northeastern Brazil and is divided into the Mid-North, North Central, Southeast and Southwest regions. The state capital, Teresina, is indicated with an arrow on the map.

stored at $-70°C$ or immediately subjected to (RT-PCR. Virus in the cell cultures was directly detected and identified by RT-PCR according to a method developed by Lanciotti and colleagues [27] using primers specific for the C-prM gene. Target viral RNA was converted to cDNA using Moloney murine leukemia virus (M-MLV) reverse transcriptase (Promega, Corp., Madison, WI) and the consensus downstream primer D2. The cDNA was then amplified by PCR using *Taq* polymerase (Promega, Corp., Madison, WI) and consensus D1 and D2 primers. For the sequencing of isolates determined to be positive for DENV-2, specific primers for the E gene DNA that are able to detect all DENV-2 isolates were used. The primers designed to amplify a 945 bp fragment and a 651 bp fragment were D2 1EF (5'-GCTGTCGCTCCTTCAATG-3'), D2 2ER (5'-TTC TGC TAT TTC CTT CAC-3'), D2 3EF (5'-GTTCACGGGACATCTCAA -3)' and D2 4ER (5'-GTTCTTTATTTTTCCAGC- 3'). The amplification was carried out in a thermal cycler (Eppendorf Mastercycler-gradient 96-well,USA) as follows: 30 cycles at 95°C for 45 seconds, 60°C for 45 seconds, and 72°C for 120 seconds, followed by a final incubation at 72°C for 10 minutes. The PCR products were fractionated by agarose gel electrophoresis, stained with SYBR Safe DNA gel stain (Invitrogen, USA) and visualized under an UV transilluminator.

Nucleotide sequencing

The nucleotide sequence of the E gene was determined in eight isolates that were identified as DENV-2 by RT-PCR. The PCR-amplified E gene DNA was purified (QIAquick PCR purification kit-Qiagen, USA) and used directly in sequencing reactions. Each DNA sample was sequenced at least five times in both orientations (MegaBACE sequencer, GE Healthcare, USA). All sequences generated in this work were deposited in GenBank (http://www.ncbi.nlm.nih.gov), and their respective accession numbers are provided in Table 1.

Evolutionary analyses

To determine the evolutionary relationship of DENV-2 isolated from the state of Piauí with other isolates described in previous studies, we performed an analysis based on the Maximum Likelihood (ML) and Bayesian Inference (BI) methods.

DENV-2 E gene sequences deposited in the GenBank database were retrieved after a sequence similarity search using the BLAST algorithm [28]; the E genes obtained in this work were used as a query. A total of 43 samples were manually selected for further evolutionary analysis. All selected samples belong to the genotype American/Asian. From the same database, we also retrieved the E gene sequences of isolates representative of all five DENV-2 genotypes: American (3 sequences), Asian II (3 sequences), Asian I (5 sequences) and Cosmopolitan (10 sequences). All sequences used in this work are listed in Table S1 and are presented in the following format in all phylogenetic trees: gi number/country/ year of isolation. Samples from Brazil are identified as follows: gi number/city-state-BR/year of isolation. Retrieved nucleotide sequences, totalizing 64 sequences, were aligned with 8 DENV-2 E gene sequences from the state of Piauí using the software MUSCLE [29]. Selection of the best-fit nucleotide substitution model was performed using jModel Test [30]. Based on the Bayesian Information Criterion (BIC), the Tamura-Nei model with gamma correction (TN93+G) was the best-fit model and was used for phylogenetic tree reconstruction using ML and BI methods. Phylogenetic tree reconstruction using ML methods was performed using PhyML v.3.1 [31] with 100 bootstrap replicates. The final tree was then visualized in Fig Tree v. 1.4.0 [32].

To infer the time to the most recent common ancestor (TMRCA) and to trace the geographic flow of DENV-2 over time, we used the Markov Chain Monte Carlo algorithm implemented in the BEAST package [33–34].The *clocklikeness* of our DENV-2 datasets was examined using PATH-O-GEN software v.1.4 [35] using the ML tree generated by PhyMLas input [31]. This analysis revealed a high correlation coefficient (0.88) and R squared value (0.77), indicating that the data fit to a strict molecular clock model. The estimated mutation rate (slope rate) was 7.55E-4 substitution/site/year, which is in the range of the mutation rate for E genes of DENV-2 described in previous studies [36–37].

The date of isolation of each sample was used as a calibration point to estimate the divergence time in years. In addition, information about the specific location of each sample (Table S1) was assigned to each sequence, and a discrete phylogeographic analysis was performed. Runs were conducted using an extended Bayesian Skyline Plot coalescent model for 400,000,000 generations with sampling every 10,000 generations. The effective sample sizes (ESS) for each parameter sampled were examined using TRACER v.1.5 [38]. Posterior trees were summarized by discarding the first 10% of the sampled trees and choosing the Maximum Clade Credibility (MCC) tree from the remaining trees using TREEANNOTATOR v.1.7.5 [39]. The final tree was then visualized in Fig Tree v. 1.4.0 [32].

Table 1. Description of DENV-2 isolates from Piauí, Brazil.

Isolate	Disease	Sex[a]	AGE (YEARS)	Collection day	Passage [b] history	GenBank number
PI-55	FD	M	29	2	5th	KJ147102
PI-58	FD	M	40	-	5th	KJ147098
PI-59	FD	M	17	3	4th	KJ147100
PI-62	FD	F	30	3	4th	KJ147099
PI-74	FD	M	-	-	3rd	KJ147097
PI-82	FD	F	8	6	3rd	KJ147095
PI-83	FD	F	21	4	3rd	KJ147101
PI-111	FD	F	41	2	4th	KJ147096

[a]F is female and M is male.
[b]Number of passages in cell culture (C6/36 cell line) are shown.

Results

Epidemiological and laboratory findings showed a high number of serum samples that were positive for dengue virus by ELISA

Piauí is located in the northeast region of Brazil, and it is considered an area of high endemicity (Figure 1). A total of 4,564 samples were analyzed by ELISA: 1,742 (38.2%) were DENV IgM-positive and 2,822 (61.8%) were DENV IgM-negative. The highest number of suspected and ELISA positive serum samples were obtained in May and June, which is a period that was preceded by intense precipitation (Figure S1).The majority of IgM-positive dengue cases were women (1,080/62%). The most highly affected age group were individuals who were 16–30 years old, accounting for 29.4% (512 cases) of the IgM-positive samples, followed by those who were 31–45 years old, accounting for 26.2% (457 cases) of the IgM-positive samples (Table 2).

DENV-2 was isolated from eight of 46 acute-phase serum samples tested. The demographic and clinical information for these patients is summarized in Table 1. Microscopic examination of cells inoculated with serum from the patients showed a clearly visible cytopathic effect with changes in the monolayer, such as syncytial cell formation and cytoplasmic vacuoles, after the third passage.

Isolates from Piauí show a high level of identity with the American-Asian genotype of DENV-2

Pairwise alignment of the DENV-2 E gene sequences obtained in this work (1,344 nucleotides out of 1,485 nucleotides) showed percentages identities ranging from 96.2% to 99.9% for nucleotides (nt) and 98.4% to 100% for amino acids (aa) (Table S2). Lower identity values were found when the sequences were compared with the isolate PI-111 (KJ147096). Although the sample PI-111 is more distantly related to other samples from Piauí, when all these sequences were aligned and compared with several DENV-2 E gene sequences isolated worldwide (Table S2), all the samples showed a higher level of identity (96.06–99.93%) with isolates belonging to the American-Asian genotype. The genotype classification of samples from Piauí as American-Asian was further confirmed by phylogenetic analysis.

The dengue outbreak in the state of Piauí (2006/2007) involved the co-circulation of two DENV-2 lineages

A consensus ML tree and BI tree were built using the nucleotide sequences of DENV-2 E genes obtained in this work and those retrieved from the GenBank database (listed in Table S1). In this analysis, all five genotypes (American-Asian, American, Asian I, Asian II and Cosmopolitan) are represented. Both the ML tree (Figure S2) and BI tree (Figure 2) show that all sequenced samples from Piauí during the 2006/2007 outbreak clustered with the American-Asian genotype and other Brazilian DENV-2 isolates. However, samples from Piauí were separated in two different lineages, referred to as lineage 1 and lineage 2, with high posterior probability support in the branch (Figure 2). Lineage 1 is characterized to include older DENV2 isolates from various states of Brazil (1990–2003), whereas lineage 2 includes more recent Brazilian DENV-2 samples (2007–2010). Among samples from Piauí, one sample, PI-111 (Piauí/Brazil/2006) grouped in lineage 1, and the other seven isolates, PI-55, PI-58, PI-59, PI-62,PI-82, PI-83 (Piauí/Brazil/2006) and PI-74 (Piauí/Brazil/2007) clustered in lineage 2. The detection of samples from Piauí in both lineages is an evidence of a temporal co-circulation of two genetically distinct DENV-2 lineages in this state.

By comparing the amino acid sequences from DENV-2 American-Asian genotype lineages 1 and 2 with older DENV-2 samples of the American-Asian genotype in the phylogenetic tree (Jamaica/M20558/1983 and Puerto Rico/AY484607/1988) (Figure 3), we observed that samples from lineage 1 are characterized by one amino acid substitution D203E, whereas samples from lineage 2 have 5 amino acid substitutions: V129I, L131Q, I170T, M340T and I380V. Additionally, the isolate PI-111 from lineage 1, exhibited the H149N substitution, and the same amino acid was encountered in some samples from Asian I and Cosmopolitan genotypes. The F429S amino acid substitution is also observed in PI-74C, an isolate from lineage 2.

Introduction of the DENV-2 American-Asian genotype lineage 2 in Brazil occurred earlier than previously described

Phylogeographic analysis (Figure 2) from the same sequence dataset used for ML tree reconstruction estimated the time of introduction of both American-Asian DENV-2 lineages in Brazil. For lineage 1, coalescent analysis inferred that the MRCA of Brazilian samples originated from the state of Rio de Janeiro (modal state posterior probability = 99.65%) and had existed since 1989 (95% HPD = 1988–1990) (Figure 2, Node 1). Later, the virus spread to other Brazilian states, including Piauí. Introduction of this virus in Piauí was estimated to have occurred in 1997 (95% HPD = 1996–1998) (Figure 2, Node 2). In lineage 2, all samples

Table 2. Age and sex distribution of IgM-ELISA dengue positive patients from the 2006/2007 outbreak in Piauí, Brazil.

Age	Male		Female		Total	
	Number	%	Number	%	Number	%
0 a≤5	34	5,1	29	2,7	63	3,6
5 a15	105	15,9	116	10,7	221	12,7
16 a 30	192	29,0	320	29,6	512	29,4
31 a 45	155	23,4	302	28,0	457	26,2
46 a 60	83	12,5	192	17,8	275	15,8
>60	64	9,7	85	7,9	149	8,6
NI	29	4,4	36	3,3	65	3,7
Total	662	100	1080	100	1742	100

NI – not informed.

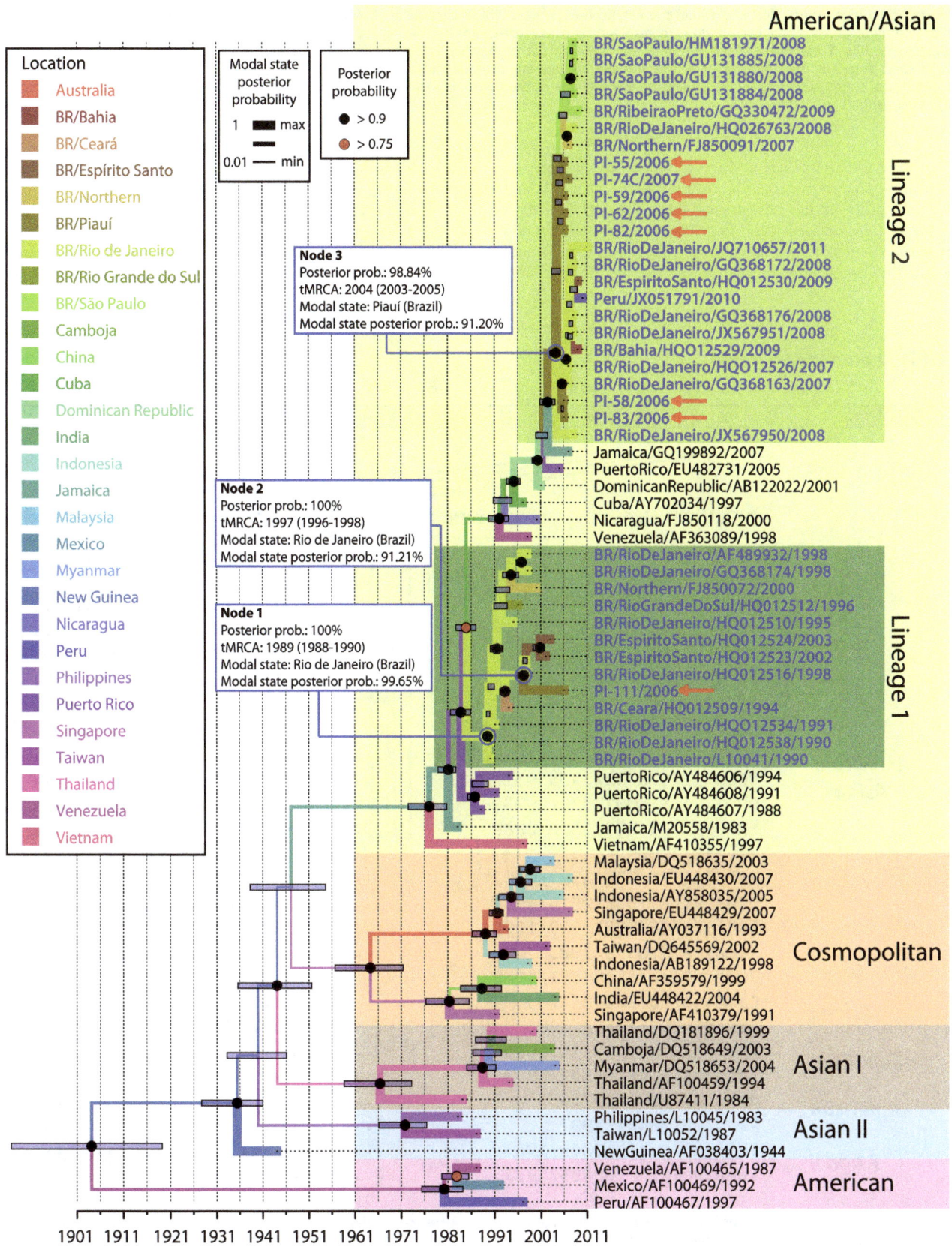

Figure 2. Evolutionary relationship between DENV-2 isolates from Piauí and the five genotypes of DENV-2. A maximum clade credibility (MCC) tree was selected after Bayesian inference analysis (strict molecular clock; TN93+G; 400,000,000 iterations) of 72 DENV-2 envelope sequences. The five DENV-2 genotypes (American-Asian, American, Asian I, Asian II and Cosmopolitan) are highlighted in different colors. Brazilian

isolates (bold blue letters) clustered within the American-Asian genotype and could be divided into two groups: lineage 1(dark green block) and lineage 2 (light green block). Each node is represented by colours black and red (●), which presented posterior probability value>0.9 and >0.75, respectively. Blue bars represent the extent of the 95% highest probability density (95% HPD) for each divergence time. The most probable geographic state for each internal node was inferred by discrete phylogeographic analysis. Different colors in the branch represent distinct geographical states according to the legend on the left side of the figure. Branch width is proportional to the probability value of the inferred ancestral geographical state.

from Piauí were positioned at the base of the branch (Figure 2). Coalescent analysis suggests that, in this lineage, the MRCA of Brazilian DENV-2 has existed since 2004 (95% HPD = 2003–2005) and was inferred to be from Piauí (modal state posterior probability = 91.20%). This virus most likely originated from a country in Central America, such as Jamaica, and later spread to

other Brazilian states and was introduced to other countries in South America, such as Peru.

To obtain more detail about the evolutionary history of both lineages of DENV-2 that were circulating in Piauí during 2006–2007, we re-analyzed the phylogeographic study of each lineage separately and included more E gene sequences retrieved from the

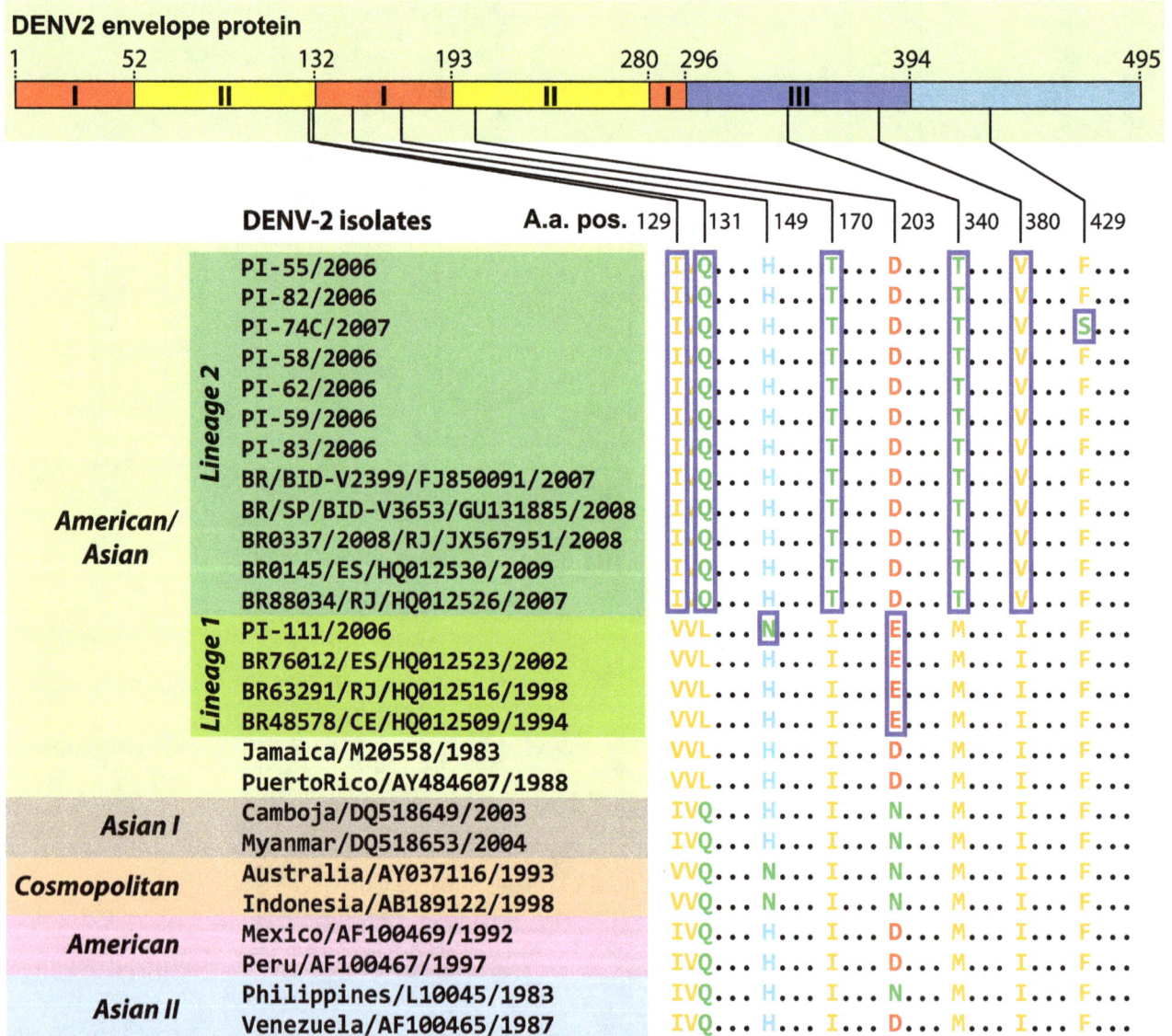

Figure 3. Amino acid polymorphisms in the envelope protein of the American/Asian DENV-2 genotype. (Top) A diagram of the DENV-2 envelope protein showing its three protein domains (I, II and III). (Bottom) A partial alignment of the envelope protein showing sites of amino acid polymorphism within the American-Asian genotype. Other DENV-2 genotypes (Asian I, Asian II, Cosmopolitan and American) are shown for comparison. Amino acid sites in blue boxes are those that most likely had underwent a non-synonymous mutation after the divergence of the two lineages because they differ from the two ancient American-Asian DENV-2 samples (Jamaica/M20558/1983 and Puerto Rico/AY484607/1988). Amino acids are colored according to their side chain charge (hydrophobic: yellow; polar: green; negatively charged: red; and positively charged: blue).

same BLAST search performed in the previous analysis. The ML and BI analysis steps were the same as those described previously in Methods. In BI analysis,we only reduced the number of runs to 200,000,000 generations since this number was sufficient to reach good ESS values for each parameter sampled (ESS >200). The best fit for the nucleotide substitution model for both lineage samples was TN93+G. *Clocklikeness* was determined using the ML trees as input. The correlation coefficient and substitution rate were 0.8729 and 6.68 95E-4 in lineage 1 samples and 0.8858and 6.8374E-4 in lineage 2 samples, respectively. The high correlation coefficient in both analyses demonstrates that both datasets fit to a strict molecular clock model. Phylogenetic trees generated from each lineage dataset using the ML method (data not shown) presented a topology similar to that of the respective phylogenetic trees generated using the BI method (Figure 4 and 5).

The addition of more samples in our phylogeographic analysis resulted in new values on the estimative of the time to MRCA and also revealed other evolutionary events relevant for describing the introduction and transmission of DENV-2 in Brazil. Discrete phylogeographic analysis detailing the lineage 1 (Figure 4) showed that the introduction of this lineage in Brazil most likely occurred in Rio de Janeiro in 1987 (95% HPD = 1985–1988; modal state posterior probability = 70.77%) (Figure 4, Node 1), two years earlier than estimated in the previous phylogeographic analysis (Figure 2, Node 1). The virus then spread to other Brazilian states, including Piauí, and it has been introduced to other countries in South America, such as Paraguay and Peru. Another distinctive aspect in this tree lies in the basal position of the lineage. We observe an early divergence between the isolates from Brazilian Southeast region (Rio de Janeiro and Espírito Santo states) and Northeast region (Pará, Ceará and Rio Grande do Norte states. The evolutionary history of PI-111 could not be clearly traced using phylogenetic analysis with the currently available DENV-2 samples in the GenBank database. However, the tree demonstrates that PI-111 is more related to a sample from Paraguay (Paraguay/EU045313/2005), and we can estimate that the introduction of DENV-2 in Piauí occurred in approximately 2003 (95% HPD = 2001–2004) (Figure 4, Node 2), four years later than estimated in the previous phylogeographic analysis (Figure 2, Node 2).

In the phylogenetic tree detailing the evolutionary history of lineage 2 (Figure 5), Brazilian samples shared the same MRCA with samples from Jamaica (GQ199892/2007, JF804034/2008 and AB545873/2007) and St. Vincent (JF968043/2010), which are inferred to have existed since 2003 (95% HPD = 2001–2005) (Figure 5, Node 1). In this tree, Brazilian isolates can be divided into two subgroups. One subgroup is represented by a unique early diverging sample from northern Brazil (BR/Northern/GQ199890/2008), referred as lineage 2b. The other group consists of all other Brazilian samples that have clustered together with isolates previously delineated as lineage 2, now referred as lineage 2a. In the later, isolates from Piauí (PI-55, PI-58, PI-59, PI-62, PI-74, PI-82 and PI-83) was also in basal position of the lineage. The MRCA of the samples from lineage 2a is estimated to have existed since 2004 (95% HPD = 2003–2005), as has been inferred in the previous analysis (Figure 2, Node 3), with a high modal state posterior probability of being from Piauí (93.39%) (Figure 5, Node 2). This suggests a dissemination route for this lineage in which DENV-2 passed through the state of Piauí before causing later outbreaks in other Brazilian states (Rio de Janeiro, São Paulo, Espírito Santo and Bahia) and also in other countries of South America (Peru, Paraguay and Bolivia).

Discussion

Various genomic regions of DENV have been used for molecular phylogenetic analyses [11–12,40–43], and the E gene appears to have epidemiologically relevant sequence information [11,41–42]. In this work, we have reconstructed the phylogeographic history of DENV-2 in Brazil, and for the first time, we have included samples from the state of Piauí collected during the 2006/2007 outbreak. Our study shows that all DENV-2 isolates obtained from this outbreak were grouped within the American-Asian genotype together with viruses from South and Central America, including those from the Caribbean islands and the southeastern states of Brazil (São Paulo and Rio de Janeiro) [44,20–22]. This genotype has been established as the major lineage of DENV-2 in Central and South America and has been described as a genotype with a high epidemiological impact due to its ability to spread and its potential to cause DHF [11].

The isolates from Piauí were separated into two different lineages (lineages 1 and 2), indicating temporal co-circulation of two genetically distinct DENV-2 lineages in this state. The co-circulation of more than one DENV-2 lineage has been described in Central and South America [44–45]. Among the six aa changes observed in the E protein between samples from lineages 1 and 2 three were non-conservative, while those at positions 129, 203 and 380 were conservative (Figure 3). Most aa substitutions found in our DENV-2 samples were observed in American-Asian genotype isolates and provide evidence of the Caribbean origin of Piauí samples, as do the genotype/lineage markers of the E gene from other Brazilian samples [46,45,20]. Notably, residue 131 in the E gene is located within a pH-dependent hinge region at the interface between domains I and II of the envelope protein. Mutations in this region may affect the pH threshold of fusion and the process of conformational change [47]. Only sample 74 had a serine (H), polar neutral, at position 429, while the other samples had phenylalanine (F), which is neutral and hydrophobic. This change increased the hydrophobicity of the protein. Because this change is located in domain III of the E protein, alterations in the binding of the virus to cell receptors may result.

The phylogeographic analysis presented here revealed that the American-Asian genotype DENV-2 was introduced into Brazil more than once since 1990, which agrees with previous studies [21–22]. The introduction of lineage 1 in Brazil was estimated to have occurred in 1987 (Figure 4, Node 2) in Rio de Janeiro after which this lineage disseminated to other Brazilian states, including Piauí. Lineage 1 was detected predominantly from 1990–2003. However, one isolate from Piauí that belongs to lineage 1 (PI-111/2006) was detected in 2006. Our detailed analysis reveals that more recent samples of this lineage were detected in other countries, such as Paraguay (Figure 4), which leads us to hypothesize that a new introduction event occurred in Brazil in 2003 (Figure 4, Node 2). It can also be speculated that this lineage was replaced by a more recent lineage of DENV-2 (lineage 2) in Piauí. The disproportion in the number of samples observed in each lineage (1 sample in lineage 1 and 7 samples in lineage 2) strengthens this assumption. Carrillo-Valenzo [48] also reported multiple introductions of viral lineages of various DENV serotypes in Mexico and frequent lineage replacement events.

A previous study suggested that lineage 2 could have been introduced into Brazil from the Caribbean islands via two parallel events: one in the southeast region in 2005 (Figure 5, lineage 2a) and another from the northern region (Figure 5, lineage 2b). This possibility was suggested because samples from both regions diverged early in the phylogeographic analysis [22]. Our results also demonstrate that these parallel events may have occurred.

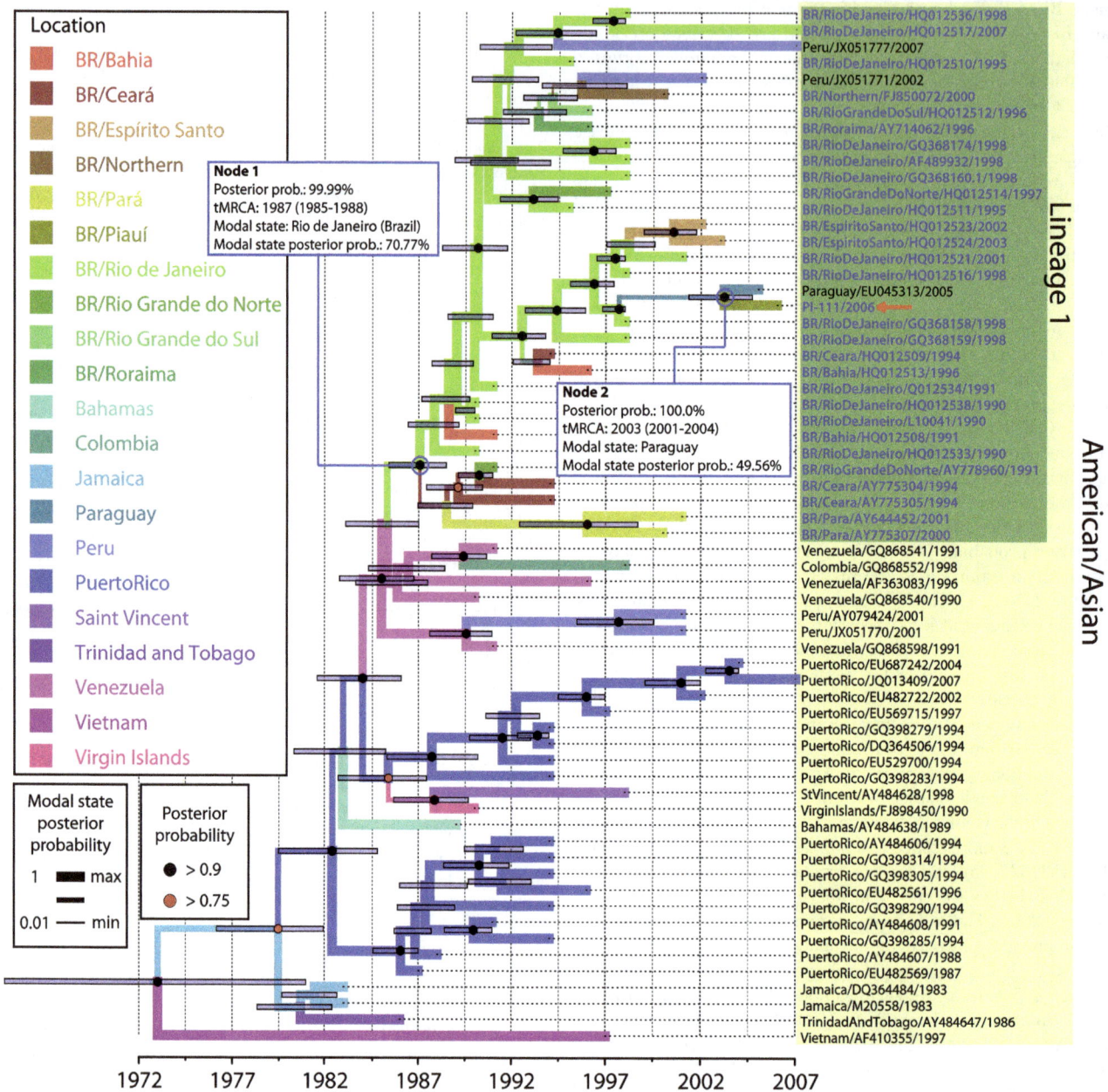

Figure 4. Bayesian coalescent and discrete phylogeographic analyses of Brazilian DENV-2 lineage 1 based on envelope nucleotide sequences. A maximum clade credibility tree was inferred by Bayesian inference analysis (strict molecular clock; TN93+G; 200,000,000 iterations) using 63 DENV-2 envelope sequences (summarized in Table S1) retrieved by a BLAST search against the entire GenBank database and using PI-111/2006 (indicated by a red arrow) as a query.PI-111/2006 is an isolate from the state of Piauí (Brazil) that clustered in Brazilian DENV-2 lineage 1. Nodes that presented posterior probability value of >0.9 and >0.75 are represented by black and red circle (●), respectively. Blue bars in each node represent the extent of the 95% highest probability density (95% HPD) for each divergence time. The most probable geographic state for each internal node was inferred by discrete phylogeographic analysis. Different colors in the branch represent distinct geographical states according to the legend on the left side of the figure. The branch width is proportional to the probability value of the inferred ancestral geographical state.

However, when we added sequences of isolates from the Piauí outbreak (2006/2007) into the phylogeographic analysis, those samples clustered together with samples from the southeast region (Figure 2 and lineage 2a). Moreover, the samples from Piauí were positioned at the base of the branch between the introduction of this lineage in Brazil and the first epidemic described in the southeast region, which occurred in the state of Rio de Janeiro during the years 2007–2008 [20]. Thus, there is a high probability

that DENV-2 entered through the state of Piauí, in 2006/2007 suggesting a new route of introduction and dissemination of this lineage in Brazil. This hypothesis was also suggested in the phylogeographic analysis of lineage 1 (Figure 4), since samples from the northeast region are situated in basal position of the lineage.

We suggested that from Piauí, this virus disseminated to other Brazilian states, such as Rio de Janeiro and São Paulo, and some

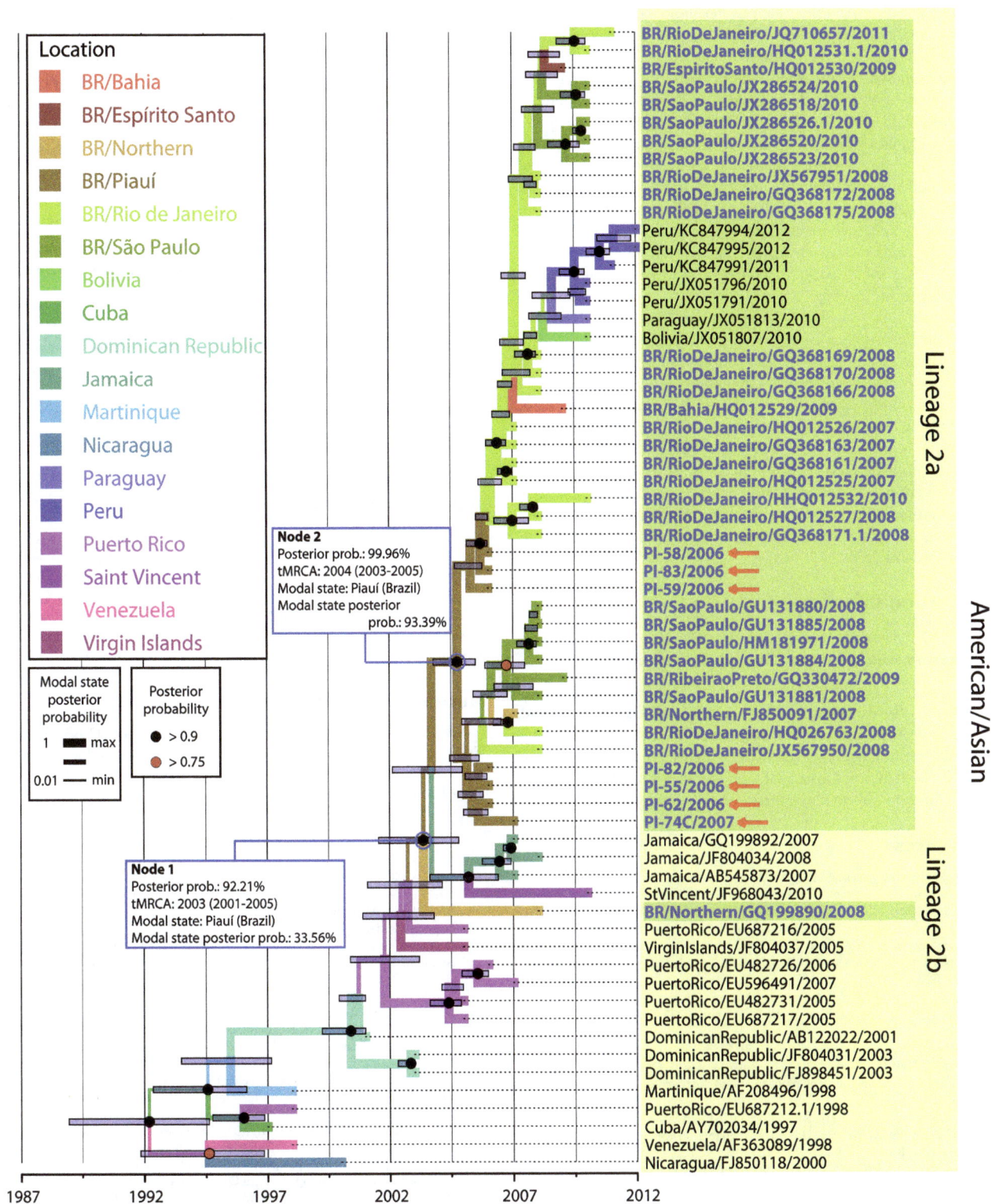

Figure 5. Bayesian coalescent and discrete phylogeographic analyses of Brazilian DENV-2 lineage 2 based on envelope nucleotide sequences. A maximum clade credibility tree was inferred by Bayesian inference analysis (strict molecular clock; TN93+G; 200,000,000 iterations). The 57 DENV-2 envelope sequences (summarized in Table S1) in the tree were retrieved using the BLASTn algorithm; envelope sequences from Piauí isolates (Brazil, indicated by red arrow) clustered in the Brazilian DENV-2 lineage 2 were used as a query. Brazilian isolates (in bold blue letters) weresubdivided into two subgroups that referred as lineage 2a and 2b, respectively. Nodes that presented posterior probability value of >0.9 and > 0.75 are represented by black and red circle (●), respectively. Different colors in the branch represent the different geographical states according to the legend on the left side of the figure. The branch width is proportional to the probability value of the inferred ancestral geographical state.

countries in South America, such as Peru and Bolivia. Moreover, our analysis demonstrates that outbreaks that occurred in other states, such as Rio de Janeiro and São Paulo (southeast region),originated from Piauí, supporting the idea that the introduction of this DENV-2 lineage in Brazil occurred before other outbreaks were described in Brazil (2007, 2008 and 2010). The state of Piauí is located in the northeast region and is near the Caribbean region, which could be considered the point of introduction and dissemination of a new DENV in Brazil. The close geographic proximity of the state of Piauí to the Caribbean region may explain the considerable influx of DENV-2 lineages across the northeastern Brazilian border. On the other hand, lineage 1 was most likely introduced through the southeastern Brazilian region [20–21].

In conclusion, our study demonstrates that all the DENV-2 isolated in Piauí during the 2006/2007 outbreak clustered within the American-Asian genotype and confirmed for the first time the occurrence of spatiotemporal co-circulation of two distinct lineages of DENV-2. Both lineages (lineage 1 and 2) identified in this work were most likely independently introduced into this state. The Caribbean islands are the main source of DENV-2 viruses in Brazil, and northeastern Brazil appears to be an important route of introduction and dissemination of this virus in the country. These findings can help us to further understand the complex phylogeographic history of dengue viruses and their evolution in dengue endemic regions.

Supporting Information

Figure S1 Average temporal distribution of precipitation and suspected or confirmed dengue cases.

Figure S2 Evolutionary relationships of DENV-2 based on the envelope nucleotide sequence. ML tree of 72 DENV-2 E genes including all five genotypes: American-Asian, American, Asian I, Asian II and Cosmopolitan. The taxon label is presented in the following format: country/GenBank accession number/

year. Samples from Brazil are identified as follows: BR-city-state/GenBank accession number/year of isolation (in bold blue letters). Isolates from Piauí/Brazil are indicated with a red arrow. Phylogenetic tree reconstruction using ML methods was performed using PhyML with the Tamura-Nei model with gamma correction (TN93+G) and a bootstrap test with 100 replicates. Bootstrap supporting values greater than 50 are shown at the nodes.

Table S1 GenBank accession numbers for DENV-2 sequences used in phylogenetic, phylogeographic and coalescent analyses, by country and year of isolation.

Table S2 Pairwise distance based on E gene nucleotide sequence among DENV-2 isolates from Piauí state and others viruses isolated worldwide. All values are in percentage of identity. Lower and higher values of identity are represented by red and green color respectively. Intermediate values are represented by yellow.

Acknowledgments

We would like to João R. dos Santos for their excellent technical and scientific assistance. We also thank Dr. Fabrício R. Santos laboratory (UFMG) where all sequencing were performed, José Miguel Ortega, associate professor at UFMG for their laboratory support, Paulo César P Ferreira, Cláudio A. Bonjardim, Giliane S.Trindade and Jônatas S.Abrahão for the collaboration and laboratory assistance. EGK is a CNPq fellow.

Author Contributions

Conceived and designed the experiments: EGK LBF LFLC ESOR GPF. Performed the experiments: LBF MMGC LFLC. Analyzed the data: LBF TS ESOR EGK. Contributed reagents/materials/analysis tools: EGK JGO LFLC. Wrote the paper: LBF TS EGK.

References

1. World Health Organization (2009) Dengue, guidelines for diagnosis, treatment, prevention and control. Available: http://whqlibdoc.who.int/publications/2009/9789241547871_eng.pdf. Accessed 20 September 2013.
2. Guzman MG, Halstead SB, Artsob H, Buchy P, Farrar J, et al. (2010) Dengue: a continuing global threat. Nat Rev Microbiol 8: 7–16.
3. Gubler DJ (1998) Dengue and Dengue Hemorrhagic Fever. Clin. Microbiol 11: 480–496.
4. Gubler DJ (2002) Epidemic Dengue/Dengue Hemorrhagic as a public health, social and economic problem in the 21 st. century. Trends Microbiol 10: 100–103.
5. Halstead SB (2007) Dengue. Lancet 370: 1644–1652.
6. Clyde K, Kyle JL, Harris E (2006) Recent advances in deciphering viral and host determinants of dengue virus replication and pathogenesis. J Virol 80: 11418–11431.
7. Lindenbach BD, Thiel HJ, Rice CM (2007) Flaviviridae: the viruses and their replication. In: Knipe DM, Howley PM, editors. Fields Virology. Philadelphia: Lippincott. Raven Publishers. 810–851.
8. Rico-Hesse R (1990) Molecular evolution and distribution of dengue viruses type 1 and 2 in nature. Virology 174: 479–493.
9. Rico-Hesse R, Harrison LM, Salas RA, Tovar D, Nisalak A, et al. (1997) Origins of Dengue type 2 viruses associated with increased pathogenicity in the Americas. Virology 230: 244–251.
10. Leitmeyer KC, Vaughn DW, Watts DM, Salas R, Villalobos I, et al. (1999) Dengue virus structural differences that correlate with pathogenicity. J Virol 73: 4738–4747.
11. Rico-Hesse R (2003) Microevolution and virulence of dengue viruses. Adv Virus Res 59: 315–341.
12. Twiddy SS, Woelk CH, Holmes EC (2002) Phylogenetic evidence for adaptive evolution of dengue viruses in nature. J Gen 83: 1679–1689.
13. Holmes E C, Twiddy SS (2003) The origin, emergence and evolutionary genetics of dengue virus. Infect Genet Evol 3: 19–28.
14. Wang WK, Lee CN, Kao CL, Lin YL, King CC (2000) Quantitative competitive reverse transcription.PCR for quantification of dengue virus RNA. J Clin Microbiol 38: 3306–3310.
15. Nogueira RMR, Miagostovich MP, Lampe E, Schatzmayr HG (1990) Isolation of dengue vírus type 2 in Rio de Janeiro. Mem Inst Oswaldo Cruz 85: 253.
16. Nogueira RMR, Miagostovich MP, Lampe E, Souza RW, Zagne SMO, et al.(1993) Dengue epidemic in the State of Rio de Janeiro, Brazil, 1990–1: co-circulation of dengue 1 and dengue 2 serotypes. Epidemiol Infect 111: 163–170.
17. De Simone TS, Nogueira RMR, Araújo ESM, Guimarães FR, Santos FB, et al. (2004). Dengue virus surveillance: the co.circulation of DENV.1, DENV.2 and DENV.3 in the State of Rio de Janeiro, Brazil. Trans R Soc Trop Med Hyg 98: 553–562.
18. Souza RV, Cunha RV, Miagostovich MP, Timbó MJ, Montenegro F, et al. (1995) An outbreak of dengue in the State of Ceará, Brazil. Mem Inst Oswaldo Cruz 90: 345–346.
19. Vasconcelos PFC, de Menezes DB, Melo LP, Pessoa ETF E, Rodrigues SG, et al. (1995) A large epidemic of dengue fever with dengue hemorrhagic cases in Ceara State, Brazil, 1994. Rev Inst Med Trop Sao Paulo 37: 253–255.
20. Oliveira M, Galvão Araujo J, Ferreira OJ, Ferreira D, Lima D, et al. (2010) Two lineages of dengue virus type 2, Brazil. Emerg Infect Dis 16: 576–578.
21. Romano CM, de Matos AM, Araujo ES, Villas-Boas LS, da Silva WC, et al. (2010) Characterization of Dengue virus type 2: new insights on the 2010 Brazilian epidemic. PloS one 5: e11811.
22. Drumond BP, Mondini A, Schmidt DJ, de Moraes RVB, Bosh I, et al. (2013) Circulation of different lineages of dengue virus 2, genotype american/asian in brazil: dynamics and molecular and phylogenetic characterization. Plos One, p. e59422.
23. Instituto Brasileiro de Geografia e Estatística. IBGE. Available: http://www.ibge.gov.br/estadosat/perfil.php. Accessed 18 November 2013.
24. De Castro JAF, De Andrade HM, Do Monte SJH, Da Silva AS, Gomes KCBL, et al. (2003) Dengue Viruses Activity in Piauí, Brazil. Mem Inst Oswaldo Cruz 98: 1021–1023.

25. Igarashi A (1978) Isolation of a Singh's *Aedes albopictus* cell clone sensitive to dengue and chikungunya viruses. J Gen Virol 40: 531–544.

26. Figueiredo LB, Cecílio AB, Ferreira GP, Drumond BP, Oliveira JG, et al. (2008) Dengue Virus 3 Genotype 1 Associated with Dengue Fever and Dengue Hemorrhagic Fever. Brazil. Emerg Infect Dis 14: 314–316.

27. Lanciotti RS, Calisher CH, Gubler DJ, Chang GJ, Vorndam AV (1992) Rapid detection and typing of dengue viruses from clinical samples by using reverse transcriptase polymerase chain reaction. J Clin Microbiol 30: 545–551.

28. Altschul SF, Madden TL, Schaffer AA, Zhang J, Zhang Z, et al. (1997) Gapped BLAST and PSI.BLAST: a new generation of protein database search programs. Nuclei Acids Research 25: 3389–3402.

29. Edgar RC (2004) MUSCLE: multiple sequence alignment with high accuracy and high throughput. Nucl Acids Res 32: 1792–1797.

30. Posada D (2011) jMODELTEST: phylogenetic model averaging. Available: http://darwin.uvigo.es/software/jmodeltest.html. Accessed 18 August 2013.

31. Guindon S, Dufayard JF, Lefort V, Anisimova M, Hordijk W, et al. (2010) New Algorithms and Methods to Estimate Maximum.Likelihood Phylogenies: Assessing the Performance of PhyML 3.0.SystBiol 59: 307–321.

32. Rambaut A (2006–2009) Tree Figure Drawing Tool Version 1.3.1. Available: http://tree.bio.ed.ac.uk/. Accessed 19 August 2013.

33. Drummond AJ, Rambaut A, Suchard MA (2002–2010) BEAST. Bayesian Evolutionary Analysis Sampling Trees Version v1.6.1. Available: http://beast. bio.ed.ac.uk. Accessed 19 August 2013.

34. Drummond AJ, Rambaut A, Xie W (2002–2010) BEAUTI. Bayesian Evolutionary Analysis Utility Version v1.6.1. Available: http://beast.bio.ed.ac. uk. Accessed 20 August 2013.

35. Rambaut A, Drummond AJ (2013) PATH-O-GEN software v.1.4. Available: (http://tree.bio.ed.ac.uk/software/pathogen. Accessed 20 August 2013.

36. Wang E, Ni H, Xu R, Barrett A T, Watowich SJ, et al. (2000). Evolutionary Relationships of Endemic/Epidemic and Sylvatic Dengue Viruses. J Virol 74: 3227–3234.

37. Zhang C, Mammen MPJ, Chinnawirotpisan P, Klungthong C, Rodpradit P, et al. (2006).Structure and age of genetic diversity of dengue virus type 2 in Thailand. J Gen Virol 87: 873–883.

38. Rambaut A, Drummond AJ (2003–2009) Tracer: MCMC Trace Analysis Tool Version v1.5.0. Available: http://beast.bio.ed.ac.uk/. Accessed 20 August 2013.

39. Rambaut A, Drummond AJ (2002–2010) TreeAnotator v1.6.1. Available: http://beast.bio.ed.ac.uk/. Accessed 20 August 2013.

40. Klungthon C, Putnak R, Mammem MP, Li T, Zhang C (2008) Molecular genotyping of dengue viruses by analysis of the sequence of individual genes. J Virol Methods 154: 175–181.

41. Wittke V, Robb TE, Thu HM, Nisalak A, Nimmannitya S, et al. (2002) Extinction and rapid emergence of strains of dengue 3 virus during an interepidemic period. Virology 301: 148–156.

42. Amarilla AA, De Almeida FT, Jorge DM, Alfonso HL, de Castro,Jorge LA, et al. (2009) Genetic diversity of the E protein of dengue type 3 virus.Virol J. 6: 1–13.

43. Costa RL, Voloch CM, Schrago CG (2012) Comparative evolutionary epidemiology of dengue virus serotypes. Infect Genet Evol 12: 309–314.

44. Anez G, Morales-Betoulle ME, Rios M (2011) Circulation of different lineages of dengue virus type 2 in Central America, their evolutionary time scale and selection pressure analysis. PLoSOne 6: e27459.

45. Méndez JA, Usme-Ciro JA, Domingo C, Rey GJ, Sánchez JA, et al. (2012) Phylogenetic reconstruction of dengue virus type 2 in Colombia. Virol J 9: 1–11.

46. Gardella-Garcia CE, Ramirez G, Espinosa JN, Cisneros A, Rojas FJ, et al. (2008) Specific genetic markers for detecting subtypes of dengue virus serotype.2 in isolates from the states of Oaxaca and Veracruz, Mexico. BMC Microbiol 8: 1–16.

47. Modis Y, Ogata S, Clements D, Harrison SC (2004) Structure of the dengue virus envelope protein after membrane fusion. Nature 427: 313–319.

48. Carrillo-Valenzo E, Danis-Lozano R, Velasco-Hernandez JX, Sanchez-Burgos G, Alpuche C, et al. (2010) Evolution of dengue virus in Mexico is characterized by frequent lineage replacement. Arch Virol 155: 1401–1412.

13

Low Levels of Antibody-Dependent Enhancement in Vitro Using Viruses and Plasma from Dengue Patients

Panjaporn Chaichana[1], Tamaki Okabayashi[1], Orapim Puiprom[1], Mikiko Sasayama[1], Tadahiro Sasaki[3,4], Akifumi Yamashita[3,4], Pongrama Ramasoota[2,4], Takeshi Kurosu[3,4], Kazuyoshi Ikuta[3,4]*

1 Mahidol-Osaka Center for Infectious Diseases (MOCID), Faculty of Tropical Medicine, Mahidol University, Bangkok, Thailand, 2 Center of Excellence for Antibody Research (CEAR), Faculty of Tropical Medicine, Mahidol University, Bangkok, Thailand, 3 Department of Virology, Research Institute for Microbial Diseases, Osaka University, Osaka, Japan, 4 JST/JICA, Science and Technology Research Partnership for Sustainable Development (SATREPS), Tokyo, Japan

Abstract

Background: The majority of dengue patients infected with any serotype of dengue virus (DENV) are asymptomatic, but the remainder may develop a wide spectrum of clinical symptoms, ranging from mild dengue fever (DF) to severe dengue hemorrhagic fever (DHF). Severe cases occur more often in patients who experience a secondary infection with a different virus serotype. A phenomenon called antibody-dependent enhancement (ADE) has been proposed to explain the onset of these severe cases, but the exact mechanism of ADE remains unclear.

Methodology/Principal Finding: Virus neutralization and ADE assays were performed using ultracentrifugation supernatants of acute-phase sera from patients with secondary infections or human monoclonal antibodies (HuMAbs) as anti-DENV antibodies. Virus sources included infectious serum-derived viruses from the ultracentrifugation precipitates, laboratory-culture adapted DENV, or recombinant DENVs derived from patient sera. In contrast to the high levels of ADE observed with laboratory virus strains, low ADE was observed with autologous patient-derived viruses, when patient sera were used to provide the antibody component in the ADE assays. Similar results were obtained using samples from DF and DHF patients. Recombinant-viruses derived from DHF patients showed only minor differences in neutralization and ADE activity in the presence of HuMAbs or plasma derived from the same DHF patient.

Conclusion/Significance: Serum or plasma taken from patients during the acute phase of a secondary infection showed high levels of ADE, but no neutralization activity, when assayed in the presence of laboratory-adapted virus strains. By contrast, serum or plasma from the same patient showed high levels of neutralization activity but failed to induce significant ADE when the assays were performed with autologous virus. These results demonstrate the significance of the virus source when measuring ADE. They also suggest that repeated passage of DENV in cell culture has endowed it with the capacity to induce high levels of ADE.

Editor: Alexander W. E. Franz, University of Missouri, United States of America

Funding: This work was supported by the program of the Japan Initiative for Global Research Network on Infectious Diseases (J-GRID) by the Ministry of Education, Cultures, Sports, Science and Technology of Japan; and the JST/JICA (SATREPS; 08080924), Japan. The funders had no role in study design, data collection and analysis, decision to publish, or preparation of the manuscript.

Competing Interests: The authors have declared that no competing interests exist.

* E-mail: ikuta@biken.osaka-u.ac.jp

Introduction

Dengue, a mosquito-borne infectious disease caused by four serotypes of dengue virus (DENV-1 to -4), is becoming more widespread in tropical and subtropical regions, posing an increasing global public health concern. DENV has a positive-sense, single-stranded RNA genome of approximately 11 kb that encodes a capsid protein (C), a pre-membrane protein (prM), and an envelope glycoprotein (E), in addition to seven nonstructural proteins, NS1, NS2A, NS2B, NS3, NS4A, NS4B, and NS5 [1].

Primary infection with any serotype of DENV establishes life-long immunity and protection against infection with the same serotype. However, the immune responses induced against one serotype of DENV do not protect against infection by other serotypes, allowing secondary infection with heterotypic DENV [2,3]. Epidemiologic studies suggest that acute cases of dengue

illness, including dengue hemorrhagic fever (DHF) and dengue shock syndrome (DSS), occur mostly among secondarily infected patients and cause severe symptoms [2,4-6]. A hypothetical mechanism for this phenomenon has been proposed, called antibody-dependent enhancement (ADE), in which one viral serotype can use pre-existing non-neutralizing anti-DENV antibodies induced by previous infection with a different serotype to gain entry to Fc receptor-positive macrophages [7]. This immune enhancement would be a major impediment to the development of dengue vaccines. Epidemiological studies show that most DENV infections are either asymptomatic or lead to uncomplicated dengue fever (DF) [8], even among patients secondarily infected with a heterotypic DENV serotype [9]. Symptomatic cases appear in only 1% to 5% of infections; however, such cases often result in DHF [3]. Thus, ADE might not always be responsible for severe symptoms in dengue patients. An epidemiological study of a large number of infants born to DENV-seropositive mothers showed that, although ADE could be detected, it did not correlate with the incidence of DF and DHF [10].

Immunohistochemical studies of DENV-infected human tissues identified macrophages in lung, spleen and lymph nodes as major targets of DENV infection [11,12]. Recent studies using quantitative RT-PCR and flow cytometry revealed the presence of positive strand DENV RNA and/or DENV antigens in a major cellular component of the peripheral blood mononuclear cell (PBMC) population, including monocytes, T/NK, B-cells and dendritic cells, with the highest amount found in B-cells [13–16]. Nonetheless viral RNA was equally distributed among different cell types in both DF and DHF patients, indicating that there was no preferential expansion of DENV in any particular cell type and, therefore, no role for anti-DENV antibodies in the expansion of discrete cell subsets.

Generally, in vitro ADE-related studies have used laboratory-adapted virus strains and murine and/or human monoclonal antibodies (MAbs) specific to viral surface proteins such as prM and E [17–23]. Recent clinical trials using a cocktail of yellow fever vaccine strains expressing both prM and E (prM-E) proteins derived from individual DENV serotypes (CYD-TDV; Sanofi Pasteur), demonstrated that no (or only minimal) ADE activity was induced in vitro when sera from vaccinated or control subjects were used at low dilutions [24,25]. This suggests that the mechanism of ADE in experimental in vitro systems is different from that during infections in patients.

Here, we examined virus neutralization and ADE in vitro using viruses and antibodies obtained directly from the sera of patients suffering from acute secondary DENV infection without any passage in cells. We found that virus neutralization and ADE activities differed greatly depending on whether the viruses were derived from patients or were laboratory-adapted strains.

Materials and Methods

Cells and viruses

Vero cells were cultured at $37°C$ in an atmosphere containing 5% CO_2 in minimum essential medium (MEM) (Sigma) supplemented with 10% fetal bovine serum (FBS; GIBCO BRL). C6/36 cells were cultured at $28°C$ (5% CO_2) in Leibovitz's L-15 medium (GIBCO BRL) supplemented with 10% FBS and 10% tryptose phosphate broth (Sigma). Both cell lines were kindly provided by Dr. Prida Malasit (Faculty of Medicine Siriraj Hospital, Mahidol University). Erythroleukemia-derived K562 cells (semi-adherence-type [a courtesy of Dr. Eiji Konishi, BIKEN Endowed Department of Dengue Vaccine Development, Mahidol University] and suspension-type [Research Institute for Microbial Diseases, Osaka University]), and THP-1 cells were maintained in RPMI-1640 medium (Hyclone) supplemented with 10% FBS at $37°C$ (5% CO_2). Suspension-type K562 cells were generally used in the ADE assays [10,25], whereas semi-adherent cells were used for virus titration assays (since their properties are more suited to the assay systems) [26].

All cell lines used in this study were originally purchased from American Type Culture Collection (ATCC), except semi-adherent K562 [26] and suspension THP-1 cells [23], where selective passages were established to obtain the desired sub-populations.

Laboratory strains of DENV-1 16007, DENV-2 16681, and DENV-3 16562 were propagated in Vero cells. These Southeast Asian genotype viruses were originally isolated from DHF patients in Thailand (DENV-1 and -2) and the Philippines (DENV-3) [27]. Recombinant DENVs and DENV-2 strain 16681 (control) were propagated in C6/36 cells.

Anti-DENV MAbs

Two hybridoma cell lines secreting anti-DENV human MAbs (HuMAbs), D30-3A1E2 and D30-1E7B8, were prepared by fusion of peripheral blood lymphocytes from a Thai DHF patient (D30) with a fusion partner cell, SPYMEG [28]. Hybridomas were cultured to confluency in DMEM supplemented with 10% FBS. The culture medium was then replaced with Hybridoma-SFM (serum-free medium, Life Technologies). HuMAb IgG_1 was purified from the serum-free culture fluid of hybridomas by using HiTrap Protein G HP Columns (GE Healthcare, UK) as previously described [23]. The IgG concentration was measured using the Pierce BCA Protein Assay kit (Thermo Scientific). Murine MAb against DENV E, named 4G2 [29], was used to detect foci in focus-forming immunoassays.

Serum samples from dengue patients

Blood samples were collected (without anticoagulant) from ten Thai dengue patients at the Hospital for Tropical Diseases (HTD), Faculty of Tropical Medicine, Mahidol University, Thailand. Samples were taken during the acute phase of infection (around 1 week after the onset of fever). In addition to clinical diagnosis, serum samples obtained from these patients were tested to confirm DENV infection using the in vitro immuno-chromatographic one step dengue NS1 antigen and IgM/IgG assay (SD BIOLINE Dengue Duo kit, SD, Kyonggi-do, Korea) according to the company's protocol.

DENV virions in patient sera were collected by ultracentrifugation at $77,000 \times g$ for 30 minutes at $4°C$ in a Beckman Coulter Optima TLX-Ultracentrifuge equipped with a TLA 100.3 rotor. Pellets containing DENV virions were suspended in MEM and kept at $-80°C$ until use. The supernatant containing anti-DENV antibodies were stored at $-80°C$ until further use.

Virus titration

Infectious titers of virus stocks were examined in focus-forming immunoassays in Vero cells [30] and K562 cells [26] and the results were expressed as focus-forming units (FFU). Briefly, monolayers of Vero cells or semi-adherent K562 cells grown in poly-L-lysine 96-well assay plate (BD Biosciences) were infected with DENV (serial 10-fold dilutions) and then incubated at $37°C$ (5% CO_2). After 24 hours (for K562 cells infected with DENV-2), 48 hours (for K562 cells infected with DENV-1 and DENV-3), or 72 hours (for Vero cells), infected cells were fixed and immunostained with murine DENV-specific MAb 4G2 followed by anti-mouse secondary antibody. Dark brown spots of infected cells were developed by adding substrates. Infected cells were then visualized under microscope. The number of foci per well was counted to calculate virus titers.

Reverse transcriptase-PCR (RT-PCR) for DENV serotyping

DENV serotypes in acute phase sera from dengue patients were determined by RT-PCR using primers specific for individual DENV serotypes, as previously described [31]. Briefly, viral RNA was extracted from serum samples using QIAmp viral RNA mini kit (QIAGEN) according to the manufacturer's instructions. RNA was used as a template for cDNA synthesis using the Superscript III RT kit (Invitrogen, Carlsbad, CA). The first PCR reaction was performed with Taq DNA polymerase (Takara, Kyoto, Japan) using primers DEUL and DEUR (Table 1). The resulting amplicon was then subjected to nested PCR using primer sets D1L/D1R, D2L/D2R, D3L/D3R, and D4L/D4R to detect different DENV serotypes (Table 1).

Table 1. List of primers used in the study.

Primer name	Primer sequence	Length (bp)	Reference
DEUL	5'-TGGCTGGTGCACAGACAATGGTT-3'	23	31
DEUR	5'-GCTGTGTCACCCAGAATGGCCAT-3	23	31
D1L	5'-GGGGCTTCAACATCCCAAGAG-3	21	31
D1R	5'-GCTTAGTTTCAAAGCTTTTTCAC-3'	23	31
D2L	5'-GCTTAGTTTCAAAGCTTTTTCAC-3	23	31
D2R	5'-CCGGCTCTACTCCTATGATG-3	20	31
D3L	5'-CAATGTGCTTGAATACCTTTGT-3	22	31
D3R	5'-GGACAGGCTCCTCCTTCTTG-3'	20	31
D4L	5'-GGACAACAGTGGTGAAAGTCA-3'	21	31
D4R	5'-GGTTACACTGTTGGTATTCTCA-3	22	31
prMFw	5'-AACATCTTGAAYAGGAGACGCAG-3'	23	This study
NS1Rv	5'-CCAGCTCACRACGCAACCRCTATC-3'	24	This study
prM-EFw	5'-ATCATTATGCTGATTCCAACAGTGATGG-3'	28	This study
prM-ERv	5'-CTATCGGCCTGCACCATGACTCCCAAATAC-3'	30	This study
pmwR05Fw	5'-GTGAGCTGGAAAAACAAAGAACTG-3'	24	This study
pmwR05Rv	5'-TTCAAGATGTTCAGCATCCTTCC-3'	23	This study

Preparation of anti-DENV antibodies from serum

Serum samples from dengue patients (HTDs) were ultracentrifuged at $77,000 \times$ g for 30 minutes at $4°C$, and the supernatants containing anti-DENV antibodies were stored at $-80°C$ until use [32]. IgM and IgG levels in the ultracentrifugation supernatants were determined using Dengue Virus IgM Capture DxSelect (OUS) and Dengue Virus IgG DxSelect (OUS), respectively, according to the manufacturer's instructions (Focus Diagnostics, Cypress, CA).

Generation of recombinant DENV cDNA clones

Viral RNA was extracted from the ultracentrifugation pellet of DHF patient (D30) acute-phase plasma using the QIAmp Viral RNA mini kit, as previously described [23]. To amplify the prM-E region of DENV, the viral RNA was subjected to RT-PCR using Primestar GXL DNA polymerase (Takara) and primers prMFw and NS1Rv (Table 1). The amplified product was cloned into the pCR4Blunt-TOPO vector (Invitrogen) and then transformed into competent *E. coli*. A total of 41 positive clones were selected for DNA sequencing at Macrogen Inc., Seoul, Korea. The nucleotide and amino acid sequences of the prM-E region were verified and aligned using BioEdit software. Subsequently, the prM-E encoding cDNA fragment of full-length infectious DENV-2 cDNA clone pmMW/R05-624 [30] was replaced by the corresponding cDNA fragments obtained from the individual clones (Figure 1). In brief, the prM-E region of the individual clones was amplified using primers prM-EFw and prM-ERv (Table 1). The pmMW/R05-624 plasmid was PCR amplified in parallel using the primers pmwR05Fw and pmwR05Rv (Table 1) to generate a linearized plasmid backbone lacking prM-E gene. Subsequently, the amplified products were subjected to In-Fusion reaction and then cloned into Stellar competent cells (Clontech). Resulting full-length cDNA clones were verified by sequencing. Plasmids with correct sequences were linearized and used as a template for RNA synthesis using the mMESSAGE mMACHINE kit (Ambion Inc, Austin, Tx). *In vitro*-transcribed viral RNA was transfected into C6/36 cells using Lipofectamine 2000 (Invitrogen). Supernatants from the transfected cells were collected and passaged once in C6/36 cells to produce recombinant virus stocks. Virus titers were determined in focus-forming immunoassays as described above and nucleotide sequences of the cloned prM-E regions were confirmed before further use.

Virus replication kinetics

Overnight cultures of C6/36 and Vero cells at 80% confluence were infected with the recombinant DENV or the DENV-2 16681 control virus at a multiplicity of infection (MOI) of 0.001. After incubating for 2 hours, the cells were washed and incubated for 5 days in medium supplemented with 2% FBS. The culture fluids were harvested daily for virus titration in focus-forming immunoassays in Vero cells, as described above.

For infection of suspension-type K562 cells, 50 μl of virus suspension were mixed with K562 cell pellets at MOI of 0.1. After incubating at $37°C$ for 2 hours, the virus was removed by centrifugation and infected cells were washed twice with RPMI-1640 medium. The cells were then incubated for a further 4 days in RPMI-1640 medium supplemented with 2% FBS. Supernatants were harvested daily for virus titration in Vero cells.

Virus neutralization and ADE assay

Heat-inactivated serum samples, D30-plasma, or purified HuMAbs were serially diluted 10-fold in RPMI-1640 medium and then mixed with virus solution at an MOI of 0.1 or 0.02. After incubating at $37°C$ (5% CO_2) for 30 minutes, virus-antibody mixtures were added to K562 cells and incubated under the same conditions for another 2 hours before transfer into 48-well microplates. Following cultivation of the infected K562 cells for 3 days in maintenance medium supplemented with 2% FBS, both the fluid and the floating cell fractions were harvested. The fluid fractions from low-speed centrifugation ($200 \times$ g for 5 minutes) were used for virus titration in focus-forming immunoassays in Vero cells.

This assay was also performed using THP-1 cells, as described previously [23]. The 10-fold serial dilutions of plasma were

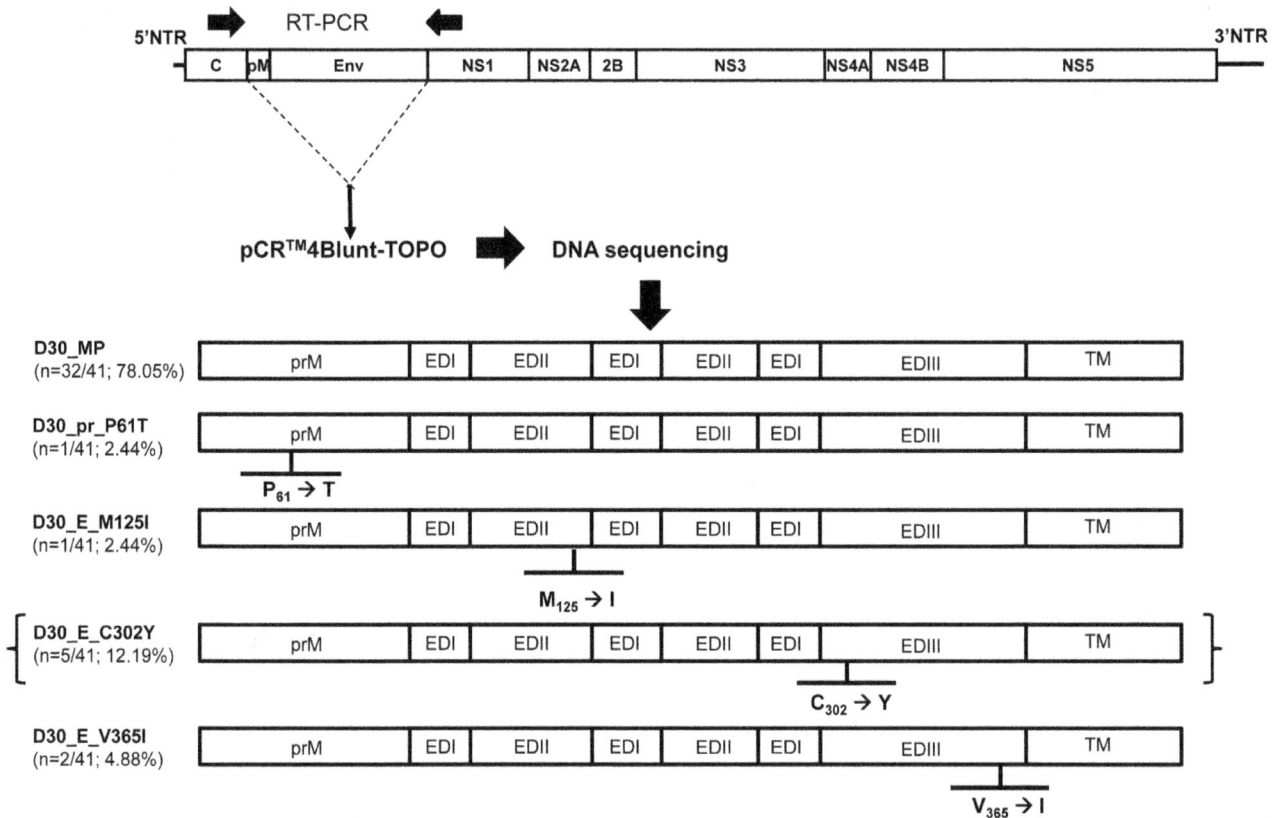

Figure 1. Construction of recombinant DENVs based on virus samples from patient plasma. RNA was extracted from the plasma of patient D30 and the prM-E encoding region of DENV was amplified by RT-PCR and cloned into the pCR4Blunt-TOPO vector for DNA sequence analysis. Representative prM-E region variants were selected and used to construct full-length DENV cDNA clones based on plasmid pmMW/R05-624. The resultant full-length cDNAs containing D30-derived variants were used as templates for RNA synthesis, and in vitro-transcribed viral RNAs were transfected into C6/36 cells. Supernatants from transfected cells were passaged once in C6/36 to obtain adequate quantities of viruses. EDI, envelope domain I. EDII, envelope domain II. EDIII, envelope domain III. TM, transmembrane. The recombinant DENV clone in brackets was excluded from further study due to an inadequate titer.

incubated with virus solution at 37°C for 30 minutes. THP-1 cells in serum-free medium were inoculated with these plasma-virus mixtures and incubated at 37°C for 2 hours. After adding RPMI-1640 medium supplemented with 2% FBS, the cells were incubated for a further 3 days at 37°C. Finally, the fluid fractions obtained after low-speed centrifugation were subjected to virus titration in focus-forming immunoassays using Vero cells, while total RNA was extracted from the cellular fractions using TRIzol reagent (Life technologies). The RNA was subjected to one-step quantitative (real-time) RT-PCR using the QuantiTect SYBR green RT-PCR kit (QIAGEN, Germany), according to the manufacturer's instructions. The data derived from real-time RT-PCR were analyzed using the $\Delta\Delta$Ct analysis method [33]. GAPDH was used as an internal control. The assays were performed in triplicate and the results were expressed as the mean ± standard deviations (SD).

Accession number

The prM-E sequences obtained from patient D30 were deposited in Genbank (http://www.ncbi.nlm.nih.gov/GenBank/) under accession numbers KF729018 - KF729022.

Ethics statement

All human specimens were collected using research protocols approved by the Ethics Committee of the Faculty of Tropical Medicine, Mahidol University, and written informed consent was obtained from all participants.

Results

Patient serum samples showed low ADE and high levels of virus neutralization

Initially, we examined virus neutralization and ADE induction using K562 as a host cell line. Anti-DENV antibodies and infectious DENV virions derived from the acute-phase serum of ten HTD dengue patients (six DF and four DHF patients) secondarily infected with DENV-1, -2, or -3 were used in the assays (Table 2). As shown in Figure 2, the titers of the different viruses from infected K562 cells in the absence of anti-DENV antibodies varied greatly, from around 10^4 in sample HTD45 to around 10^2 in sample HTD25, even though the K562 cells were infected at the same MOI. These results suggest that the susceptibility of K562 cells to DENV infection varied depending on the patient the virus sample was isolated from. High levels of virus neutralization (> x100–1000) were observed using samples from DF patients HTD26, HTD42, HTD27, HTD40, and HTD16, as well as samples from DHF patients HTD6 and HTD25. For the remaining samples, zero (HTD45, a DHF patient) or low levels (> x100; HTD7, a DF patient; and HTD49, a DHF patient) of virus neutralization were observed. There was

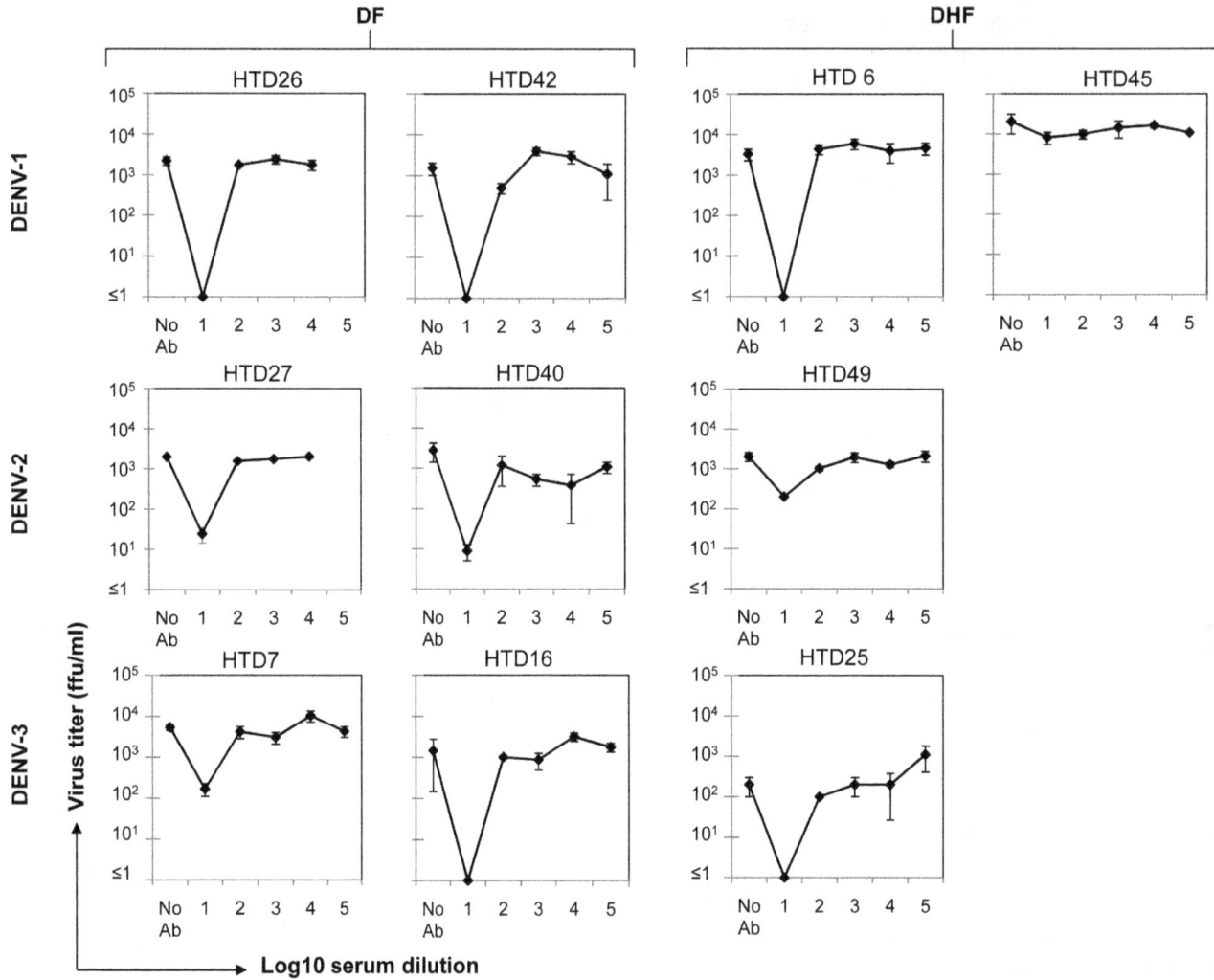

Figure 2. Low ADE when using serum and viruses from DENV-patients. Serum samples (DENV-1, DENV-2, and DENV-3) from HTD dengue patients with DF and DHF symptoms were ultracentrifuged to precipitate DENV virions which were used in assays without any subsequent passage in cells. The supernatant fractions were heat-inactivated at $56°C$ for 30 minutes and then serially diluted 10-fold. The dilutions were mixed for 30 minutes at $37°C$ with the precipitated virions from autologous plasma at an MOI of 0.02. The virus-antibody complexes were added to K562 cells and incubated for 2 hours at $37°C$ before the addition of maintenance medium supplemented with 2% FBS. The cells were then incubated for a further 3 days. Supernatants were harvested for virus titration by focus-forming immunoassay in Vero cells, and the results are expressed as FFU/ml. The mean $\pm$ SD of triplicate experiment is shown. 'No Ab' means virus infection in the absence of plasma. The 'No Ab' value was used as a baseline for calculating virus infection enhancement.

little or no evidence of ADE under these assay conditions when antibody and virus samples from any of the ten patients were used, regardless of virus serotype or disease severity.

We also assessed sera from four HTD patients for neutralization activity and ADE levels using antibodies from different patients infected with the same DENV serotype. Although we used heterologous sera from different patients, the antibodies neutralized heterologous virus infections at low serum dilutions (1Log_{10}) and no ADE induction has been observed (Figure S1).

These results clearly demonstrate that antibodies present in the ten serum samples from DF and DHF patients infected with DENV-1, -2, or -3, were not able to induce serum-derived DENV infection enhancement in K562 cells. In addition, eight out of ten sera neutralized the major virus population with which the patient had been infected. Despite the fact that the samples contained polyclonal antibodies, these results show that the majority of

antibodies induced by the infecting virus prevented the virus from infecting K562 cells.

Laboratory-adapted strains of DENV show high levels of ADE and low neutralization activity in the presence of patient sera

Previously, we reported that the majority of HuMAbs (prepared by fusing PBMC from dengue patients at the acute phase of a secondary DENV-2 infection with SPYMEG cells) showed ADE activity in assays employing THP-1 cells and the DENV-2 strain 16681 [23]. Here, we examined ADE activity using laboratory-adapted strains of DENV and patient sera as a source of anti-DENV antibodies (Figure 3). Serotypes of the laboratory-adapted strains used in the ADE assay were the same as those identified in the patients: DENV-1 strain 16007 for patients HTD26, HTD42, HTD6, and HTD45; DENV-2 strain 16681 for patients HTD27,

Table 2. DENV serotypes, viremia titer, and anti-DENV antibody isotypes in DENV-infected patients.

ID[a]	Symptom[b]	Serotype[c]	Viremia titers[d] (ffu/mL sera)	IgM[e] Index	Interpretation	IgG[f] Index	Interpretation	Virus infection[g] IgM/IgG	Interpretation
HTD6	DHF	DV1	$(7.72\pm1.84)\times10^5$	0.78	Neg	1.14	Pos	0.68	Secondary
HTD7	DF	DV3	$(4.80\pm1.05)\times10^5$	0.84	Neg	4.86	Pos	0.17	Secondary
HTD16	DF	DV3	$(3.88\pm0.78)\times10^4$	0.85	Neg	3.96	Pos	0.21	Secondary
HTD25	DHF	DV3	$(1.08\pm0.12)\times10^5$	2.27	Pos	4.17	Pos	0.54	Secondary
HTD26	DF	DV1	$(4.49\pm0.75)\times10^5$	0.59	Neg	2.97	Pos	0.20	Secondary
HTD27	DF	DV2	$(4.52\pm1.07)\times10^5$	0.50	Neg	1.67	Pos	0.30	Secondary
HTD40	DF	DV2	$(3.88\pm0.45)\times10^5$	0.46	Neg	1.82	Pos	0.25	Secondary
HTD42	DF	DV1	$(3.41\pm0.99)\times10^7$	0.77	Neg	2.49	Pos	0.31	Secondary
HTD45	DHF	DV1	$(6.57\pm3.76)\times10^5$	0.51	Neg	3.61	Pos	0.14	Secondary
HTD49	DHF	DV2	$(4.68\pm0.43)\times10^4$	1.25	Pos	1.49	Pos	0.84	Secondary
[h]D30	DHF	DV2	ND	4.54	Pos	6.59	Pos	0.69	Secondary

[a]ID, patient identification.
[b]Dengue disease was determined by examining the clinical symptoms of patients according to the WHO criteria.
[c]DENV serotype was determined by RT-PCR with universal and serotype-specific primers [31].
[d]Viremia titers were determined in a focus-forming immunoassay in semi-adherent K562 cells [30].
[e]IgM in patient serum was detected by Dengue Virus IgM Capture DxSelect. An index value of >1.00 was interpreted as positive (POS) and an index value of <1.00 was interpreted as negative (NEG).
[f]IgG in patient serum was detected by Dengue Virus IgG DxSelect. An index value of >1.00 was interpreted as positive (POS) and an index value of <1.00 was interpreted as negative (NEG).
[g]Cases with an IgM/IgG index ratio of ≤1.2 were diagnosed as secondary infections [32].
[h]Patient's blood specimen was used for huMAb preparation as described elsewhere [24]. ND, not detectable.

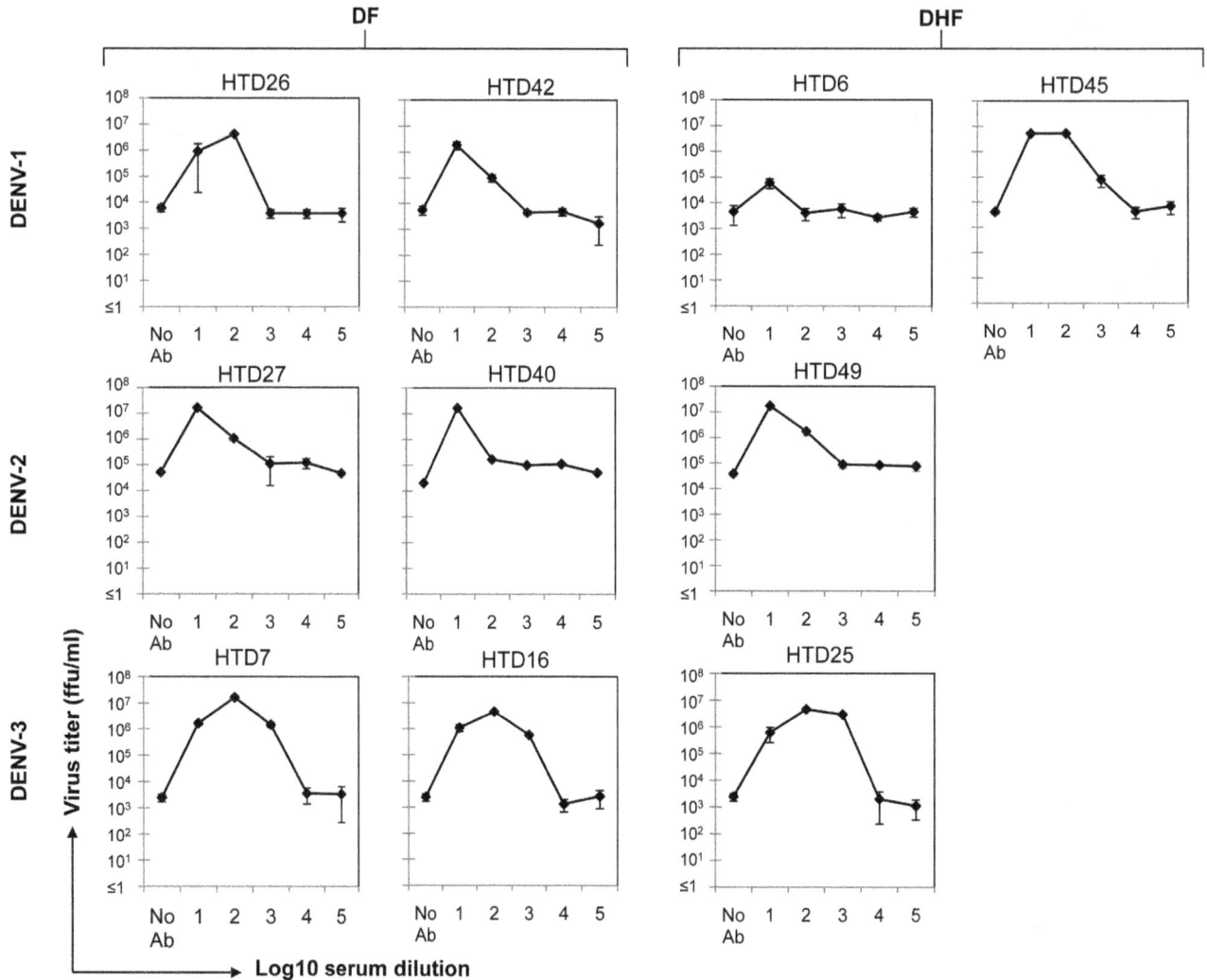

Figure 3. High levels of ADE when using patient plasma and laboratory-culture adapted DENV. Ultracentrifugation supernatants of patient sera were heat-inactivated at 56°C for 30 min, diluted 10-fold, and pre-mixed at an MOI of 0.02 with laboratory culture-adapted DENV-1, -2, and -3 for 30 minutes at 37°C. Virus-antibody complexes were added to K562 cells and incubated for 2 hours at 37°C. Maintenance medium supplemented with 2% FBS was then added before a further incubation for 3 days. Supernatants were harvested for virus titration in focus-forming immunoassays in Vero cells. Results are expressed as the mean ± SD of triplicate experiments. 'No Ab' means virus infection in the absence of plasma. The 'No Ab' value was used as a base line for calculating virus infection enhancement.

HTD40, and HTD49; and DENV-3 strain 16562 for patients HTD7, HTD16, and HTD25. The K562 cells used for these ADE assays were the same as those used in Figure 2.

ADE activity induced by sera from patients in the presence of laboratory-adapted virus strains was greatly increased (Figure 3). Furthermore, no virus neutralization was detected when using patient-derived sera and laboratory-adapted strains of DENV. ADE was highest (around ×10,000) in the serum sample obtained from HTD7 (a DF patient infected with DENV-3). ADE levels for DF patients HTD26, HTD40, HTD16 and for DHF patients HTD45 and HTD25 were around ×1,000. ADE in serum samples obtained from HTD27, HTD42 and HTD49 was ×100, and that for HTD6 (a DHF patient) was around ×10. Taken together, these results revealed that there was no correlation between the results of neutralization/ADE assays and the type of disease manifestation (DF or DHF), or the DENV serotype that caused the disease.

Replication kinetics of recombinant DENVs containing prM-E sequences obtained from virus samples of patients

Sequence variations in their prM-E encoding regions could be a reason for the observed differences in ADE and neutralization levels between serum-derived DENV and laboratory-adapted virus strains. Furthermore, serum-derived viruses might be present within immune complexes, which may render the viruses more sensitive to neutralization than laboratory-adapted strains. To test these hypotheses, we compared ADE levels induced by recombinant DENVs containing patient-derived prM-E gene sequences.

Using viral RNA extracted from the plasma of DHF patient D30 (D30-plasma), we constructed four infectious DENV cDNA clones harboring different amino acid substitutions within their prM-E region: R05/D30_MP, R05/D30_pr_P61T, R05/D30_E_M125I, and R05/D30_E_V365I. R05/D30_MP contained the prM-E gene sequence derived from a major DENV-2 population in D30-plasma (as was detected among 78.05% (32/41) of the clones). Other recombinant viruses with amino acid substitutions in the prM-E region were detected among 2.44% (1/41) of R05/D30_pr_P61T and R05/D30_E_M125I clones, among 4.88% (2/41) of the R05/D30_E_V365I clone, and among 12.19% (5/41) of the R05/D30_E_C302Y clone. Since we could not obtain a sufficient titer of R05/D30_E_C302Y, the remaining four recombinant viruses were assayed for levels of virus neutralization and ADE induction, and the levels were compared with those of parental R05-624 virus and DENV-2 strain 16681. A phylogenetic analysis of the D30 plasma-derived recombinant DENVs including the parental R05-624 clone, is shown in Figure S2. The five sequences of the prM-E region are closely related to each other and to those of Thai clinical isolates previously registered in the NCBI database.

Prior to investigating the recombinant viruses in neutralization and ADE assays, we validated the infectivity of the molecular clones in several different host cells, including C6/36, Vero, and K562. As shown in Figure 4A, DENV-2 16681 produced a significantly higher level of progeny viruses than the recombinant viruses or the parental R05-624 strain at all time points ($p < 0.05$ at Days 2, 3 and 5, $p < 0.01$ at Days 1 and 4). The rate of replication and virus production among the recombinant viruses was statistically significantly different at each time point. For instance, the replication rates of R05/D30_MP and R05/D30_E_V365I were significantly higher than those of R05/D30_pr_P61T, R05/D30_ E_M125I and parental R05-624 strain during the first 2 days of infection ($p < 0.01$). By contrast, the replication kinetics of DENV-2 strain 16681 in Vero cells were similar to those of all four recombinant viruses including the parental R05-624 strain during the first 3 days of virus infection, except on Days 4 and 5 post-infection ($p < 0.01$). Although R05/D30_E_M125I showed similar replication kinetics, the overall level of virus production was significantly lower than that of the other strains ($p < 0.01$; Figure 4B).

Virus production in the culture fluids of K562 cells differed between recombinant viruses and control viruses. The R05/D30_pr_P61T strain did not produce progeny viruses in K562 cells (Figure 4C). R05/D30_MP, R05/D30_E_V365I and DENV-2 16681 showed replication kinetics similar to those of R05/D30_E_M125I and the parental R05-624 strain; however, overall virus production of the latter two was significantly lower, especially at Days 2 ($p < 0.05$) and 3 ($p < 0.01$) post-infection. In addition, the recombinant viruses, as well as the parental R05-624 virus and DENV-2 16681 showed declining virus production levels in K562 cells at 4 days post-infection, a time point at which virus production was still increasing in C6/36 and Vero cells.

Virus neutralization and ADE levels of recombinant DENVs are affected by HuMAb

Virus neutralization and ADE assays were performed in K562 cells using recombinant viruses and DENV-2 strain 16681. Similar to the results shown in Figure 3, replication of the DENV-2 strain 16681 was strongly enhanced, as shown by 10^5-fold increases in the peak enhancement titer (PENT); however, the virus was resistant to neutralization (Figure 5A, Supplemental Figure S3A). Also, the virus titer of DENV-2 16681 was significantly higher than that of other viruses when serum was added at $2\mathrm{Log}_{10}$ to $5\mathrm{Log}_{10}$ dilutions ($p < 0.01$; Figure 5A). Conversely, the parental R05-624 virus and all D30-derived recombinant viruses (except R05/D30_pr_P61T) were positive for both virus neutralization and ADE activity. Interestingly, the titers of the recombinant viruses in the absence of antibodies were only 10-30 fold higher than that of R05/D30_E_M125I ($p < 0.05$), whereas the virus titers at the PENT were 260-560 fold higher than that of R05/D30_E_M125I ($p < 0.01$).

Antibody preparations from individual patient plasma would be expected to contain polyclonal antibodies that recognize different virion surface epitopes; thus they would be expected to react

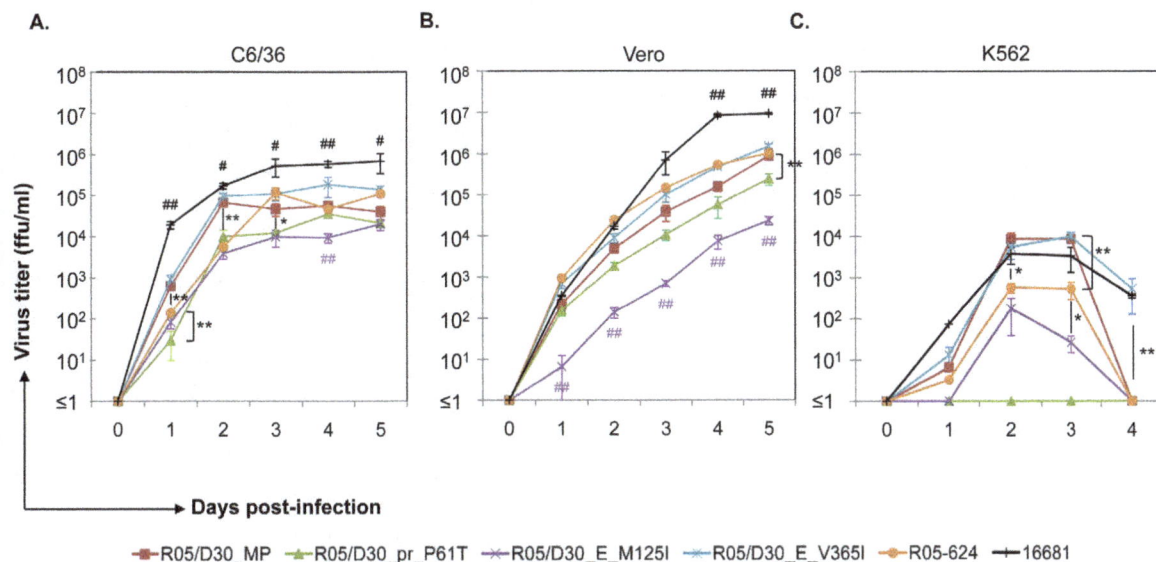

Figure 4. Replication kinetics of recombinant DENVs. DENV-2 16681 or individual recombinant DENVs were used to infect C6/36 (A) and Vero cells (B) at an MOI of 0.001, or K562 cells (C) at an MOI of 0.1. After 2 hours of incubation, the supernatants were removed and cells were washed twice with plain medium before the addition of maintenance medium supplemented with 2% FBS. For infected C6/36 and Vero cells, the supernatants were harvested daily. For infected K562 cells, both the culture medium and infected cells were harvested and centrifuged. Virus titers in the supernatants were determined in focus-forming assays in Vero cells. Results are expressed as mean ± SD of triplicate experiment (*$p < 0.05$ and **$p < 0.01$, unpaired two-tailed Student's t-test, n = 3 per point). Statistically significant differences between data points are indicated by # (# $p < 0.05$, ## $p < 0.01$).

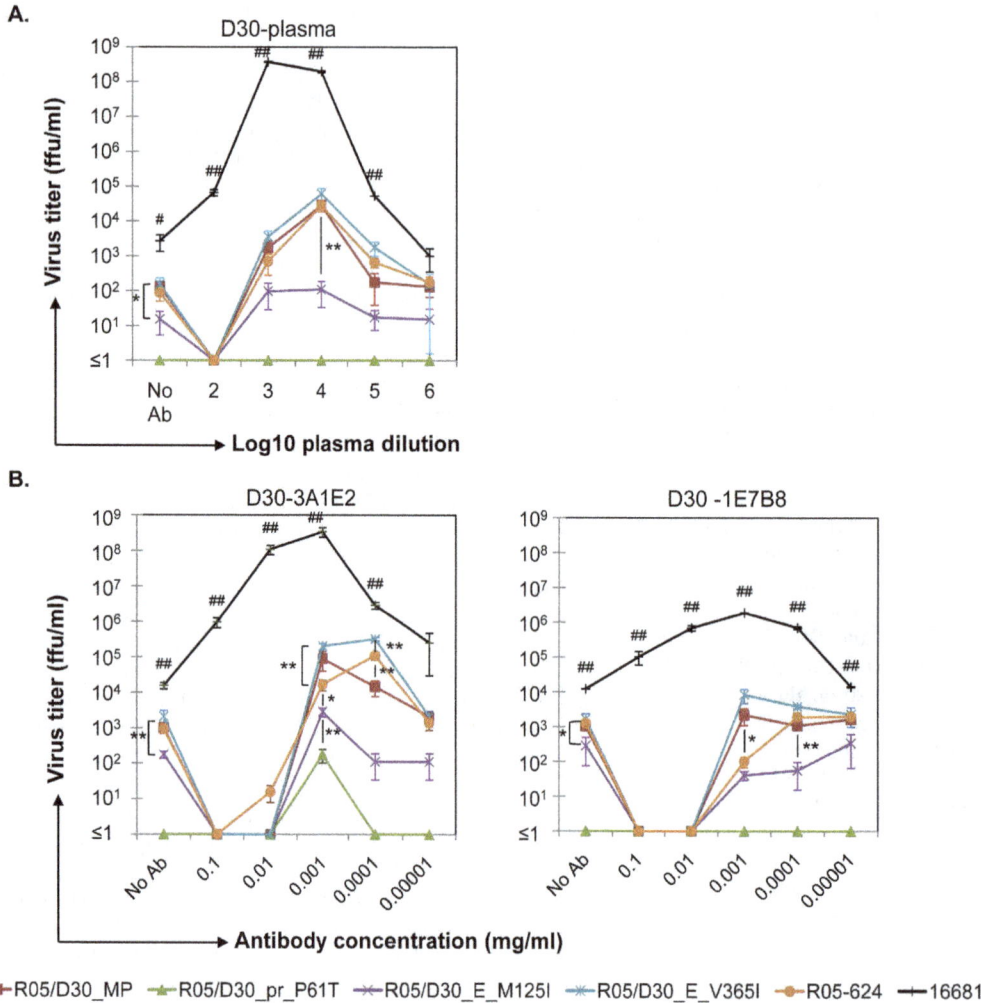

Figure 5. ADE levels of recombinant DENVs or DENV-2 strain 16681 exposed to D30-plasma or HuMAbs. A heat-inactivated D30-plasma sample (A) or purified human MAbs derived from patient D30 (B) were serially diluted 10-fold in RPMI-1640 medium and incubated with either DENV-2 16681 or individual recombinant DENVs for 30 min at an MOI of 0.1. Virus-antibody complexes were added to K562 cells and incubated for a further 2 h; maintenance medium was then added (without washing the cells) to yield a FBS final concentration of 2%. Cells and supernatants were collected on Day 3 post-infection. Virus titers in the supernatants were determined in focus-forming immunoassays in Vero cells. Results are expressed as the mean ± SD from two independent experiments performed in triplicate (*$p<0.05$ and **$p<0.01$, unpaired two-tailed Student t-test, n = 3 per point). Statistically significant differences between data points are indicated by # (# $p<0.05$, ## $p<0.01$).

differently with the viral population(s) used in the assays. To analyze whether the polyclonal nature of antibodies in patient plasma was responsible for our observations, we used two HuMAbs previously prepared from PBMC isolated from the same DHF patient, D30 [23].

As shown in Figure 5 and S3, the viruses that showed the highest and lowest ADE (R05/D30_E_V365I and R05/D30_E_M125I, respectively) yielded similar results when either D30-derived plasma (Figure 5A) or a D30-derived HuMAb (D30-3A1E2) were used in the assay (Figure 5B). Interestingly, HuMAb D30-3A1E2, but not D30-plasma, increased the production of R05/D30_pr_P61T ~ 7-fold. On the other hand, another D30-derived HuMAb, D30-1E7B8, showed strong neutralization activity against all of the cloned viruses and against the parental R05-624 strain. However, it showed weak ADE against the D30-derived recombinant viruses and the parental R05-624 strain, and weaker ADE activity than HuMAb D30-3A1E2 in presence of DENV-2 16681.

Although R05/D30_MP, R05/D30_E_V365I, and the control DENV-2 strain 16681 showed similar virus production levels in K562 cells (Figure 4C), PENT for DENV-2 16681 was significant higher (1.38×10^5 fold) than that of the other two strains (2.17×10^2 fold for R05/D30_MP and 4×10^2 fold for R05/D30_E_V365I; $p<0.01$; Supplemental Figure S3A). The level of ADE (3.25×10^2 fold) in the presence of the parental R05-624 virus was not different from that in the presence of the other two virus variants, R05/D30_MP and R05/D30_E_V365I (Figure 5), although overall virus production was significantly lower ($p<0.01$; Figure 4C). The PENT for all infectious clones, including parental R05-624, occurred at a plasma dilution of 4Log$_{10}$, while the plasma dilution peak for DENV-2 16681 was 3Log$_{10}$ (Figure 5A). When the DENV-2 strain 16681 was assayed, virus production increased by more than 10^4-fold over that of the control (no anti-DENV antibodies) in the presence of 0.001 mg/ml HuMAb D30-3A1E2. (Figure 5B and Figure S3B, left panel). Also, the PENT for R05/D30_E_V365I and the parental R05-624 strain occurred in the presence of 0.0001 mg/ml HuMAb D30-3A1E2 (Figure 5B and Figure S3B, right panel). Nevertheless, the PENT for D30 E_M125I was significantly lower than that of other viruses when either plasma or HuMAb were used ($p<0.01$; Figure S3).

Data from our previous paper showed that HuMAb D30-1E7B8 reacts with the full-length E protein, but not with truncated forms of E, indicating that this HuMAb recognizes a conformational epitope [23]. This HuMAb neutralized or blocked all virus replication at a concentration of 0.01–0.1 mg/ml (Figure 5B, right panel); however, it enhanced DENV-2 strain 16681 infection by approximately 100-fold at a lower concentration (0.001 mg/ml).

While other studies [21,23,30] used virus titers assessed in focus-forming immunoassays in Vero cells to estimate the MOI, our data demonstrated that virus titers assessed in K562 cells were more favorable to estimate optimal MOI for replication kinetics in K562 cells and ADE assays than Vero cells. When using virus titers assessed in K562 cells to estimate MOI for virus infection, we found that replication rates and virus production levels in K562 cells of recombinant DENVs, parental R05-624 strain and DENV-2 16681 were significantly higher than those when assessed in Vero cells ($p<0.05$ at Days 2 and $p<0.01$ at Days 3 post-infection; Supplemental Figure S4A). Furthermore, optimal MOI estimated from virus titers assessed in K562 cells resulted in statistically significantly higher virus titers at PENT of all viruses ($p<0.05$), except R05/D30_pr_P61T (Figure S4B).

Comparison of K562 and THP-1 cells for ADE activity measurement

Previous studies assayed ADE in K562 [10,26,34], THP-1 [23,35–37] or BHK [38,39] cells. Therefore, we used both THP-1 and K562 cells to assay ADE (Supplemental Figure S5). D30-plasma was serially diluted 10-fold and mixed with the D30-derived recombinant viruses, the parental R05-624 virus, and the DENV-2 strain 16681 at an MOI of 0.1 for each virus. After incubation for 30 min, THP-1 cells were infected with the mixture. On day 3 post-infection, total RNA extracted from the cell fraction was subjected to quantitative RT-PCR (Supplemental Figure S5A). The fluid fraction was titrated in a focus-forming immunoassay in Vero cells (Supplemental Figure S5B). High levels of ADE activity were observed for DENV-2 16681 ($p<0.05$ for fold enhancement and $p<0.01$ for virus titer), but not for the other recombinant DENVs (Supplemental Figure S5A and S5B). The same virus and antibody samples were then subjected to ADE assays in K562 cells under the conditions shown in Figure S4B (Supplemental Figure S5C). Again, DENV-2 16681 showed high level of ADE, whereas the D30-derived recombinant viruses showed only low ADE levels.

Discussion

This study examines virus neutralization and ADE activity *in vitro* using the K562 cell line along with polyclonal antibodies and DENV derived from the serum of dengue patient during the acute phase of a secondary DENV infection. The data demonstrate that serum from patients showed high levels of virus neutralization and low levels of ADE activity in the presence of viruses isolated from the same patients, whereas there was no neutralization and high levels of ADE activity in the presence of serotype-matched laboratory strains. Thus, the source of the virus had a profound effect on virus neutralization and ADE. We showed that DENV derived from patient sera were susceptible to neutralization but exhibited no ADE activity when pre-incubated with autologous serum. In most of these cases, the serum had opposing effects when assayed using laboratory strains of DENV matched to the serotype

isolated from the patient. This difference could be due to unidentified viral factor(s), as well as to the properties of anti-DENV antibodies present in the patient serum.

The K562 cell line is often used to assay the ADE activity of DENV because it expresses activating FcγRIIa receptors but not inhibitory FcγRIIb receptors [34,40–42]. Complement was excluded from our system by heating plasma at 56°C for 30 min before the assay. Hence the observed virus neutralization could only be due to the blocking of DENV replication by the specific antibodies. As DENV-containing immune complexes have been detected in patient plasma [43–45], the virus fractions used in our experiments may have contained virus-antibody complexes that augment virus replication in K562 in the absence of serum antibodies. However, the results reported herein show that addition of the antibody fraction of autologous serum at a 1Log$_{10}$ dilution diminished or blocked the infection in K562 cells by virus-antibody complexes by 10-fold to 1000-fold.

Most studies on ADE indicate that human sera obtained from patients with a secondary DENV infection possess the ability to enhance infection of cell lines by laboratory-adapted DENV *in vitro* [23,46,47]. Some studies used clinical isolates prepared from dengue patient plasma, which had been passaged in cell lines [38,48]. Therefore, we used laboratory-grown DENV with a serotype identical to that of the serotype detected in patient plasma. The results were in agreement with other findings: all ten sera from dengue patients with secondary infections enhanced antibody-dependent DENV infection of K562 cells. As seen in other studies [23,38,47], we also found that there was no correlation between *in vitro* ADE activity and disease severity. In the present study, only one out of ten serum samples (HTD45) was incapable of virus neutralization. Further investigations using more serum samples are necessary to confirm and extend these findings.

When using antibodies derived from patient serum, we found that the neutralization and ADE activities when assayed with autologous viruses were contrary to those when using serotype-matched laboratory strains. This may be due to considerable prM-E amino acid sequence diversity between serum-derived viruses and laboratory strains. Due to the nature of viral quasi-species, viruses derived from an individual patient's serum or plasma comprise a mixture of variants. Each of these variants would be expected to respond differently to an anti-DENV antibody obtained from autologous serum or plasma. Laboratory-adapted viruses are usually selected for their ability to grow *in vitro* and may have adapted to serial passage in tissue culture. To test this hypothesis, we utilized recombinant DENV containing the prM-E region derived from virus populations in plasma of DHF patient D30 to investigate whether amino acid substitutions in this region can affect ADE. ADE was higher in the presence of the DENV-2 16681 control virus than in the presence of any of the viral clones; this was true irrespectively of whether autologous plasma or HuMAb were used in the assay. The nucleotide sequence homology between the prM-E region of the DENV-2 16681 and that of the major DENV-2 population in D30-plasma, and between DENV-2 16681 and the parental R05-624 virus were 97.2 and 96.9%, respectively. The possibility that one or more nucleotide changes in the viral genome, particularly in the prM-E encoding region of the laboratory-adapted virus produced an "enhancing epitope" requires further investigation.

Another explanation for the differences in ADE activity between patient-derived and laboratory-adapted strains of DENV could be that serum-derived antibodies bind to virions as a complex; thus they are found in the precipitate fraction of plasma. Such bound antibodies may play a role in virus neutralization and would be absent from assays using laboratory strains. Therefore, we examined the neutralization and ADE activity of recombinant DENVs containing the prM-E region of DENV2 from patient D30 to ensure the absence of any immune complexes. Interestingly, the parental R05-624 virus and all the D30-derived cloned viruses were positive for both virus neutralization and ADE activity. We observed high levels of virus neutralization at high antibody concentrations when using plasmid-derived virus variants and the parental R05-625. When we used D30-plasma and HuMAb-D30-3A1E2, virus infection increased by 10-fold to 100-fold at low antibody concentrations. These results concur with other findings, i.e., that ADE can occur in the presence of neutralizing antibodies, but only at very low or sub-neutralizing antibody concentrations [7,23,49]. These plasmid-derived viruses, although identical in sequence to viruses detected in patient plasma, had been passaged once in C6/36 cells, which could have introduced mutations in their genomes outside prM-E affecting ADE.

Although the levels of ADE induced by D30-plasma or HuMAb D30-3A1E2 were comparable, HuMAb D30-1E7B8 exhibited strong neutralizing activity but did not induce ADE activity when assayed in the presence of recombinant DENVs. However, this antibody increased DENV-2 16681 replication by 100-fold. These results suggest that ADE and neutralization of DENV are the overall outcome of a combination of diverse DENV variants and their specific antibodies. As shown in Figure 5, HuMAb D30-3A1E2 was likely the main antibody in D30-plasma since it elicited a similar pattern of ADE induction to the D30-plasma. This ADE effect could overcome the strong neutralizing ability of HuMAb D30-1E7B8.

In conclusion, this study demonstrates that DENVs derived from patient serum elicit patterns of ADE that are different from those of laboratory-grown DENVs. Therefore, it is important to be careful when interpreting the enhancing or neutralizing effects of antibodies when using different sources of DENV. Furthermore, we also demonstrate that a single amino acid substitution in E, V365I, can affect ADE. However, the mechanism by which this amino acid position influences ADE requires further investigation.

Supporting Information

Figure S1 Comparison of ADE among heterologous DENV isolates of the same serotype. Serum samples (DENV-1, DENV-2, and DENV-3) from HTD dengue patients (three with DF and one with DHF clinical manifestations) were ultracentrifuged to precipitate the DENV virions. The supernatant fractions were heat-inactivated at 56°C for 30 minutes, and then serially diluted 10-fold. The dilutions were mixed with serum-derived viruses from the precipitate fraction of autologous plasma for 30 minutes at 37°C at an MOI of 0.02. The virus-antibody complexes were added to K562 cells and incubated for 2 hours at 37°C before the addition of maintenance medium supplemented with 2% FBS. The cells were then incubated for a further 3 days. Supernatants were harvested for virus titration in a focus-forming immunoassay in Vero cells. The results are expressed as FFU/ml. The mean ± SD of triplicate experiments is shown. 'No Ab' means virus infection in the absence of plasma. 'No Ab" values were used as a baseline for calculating virus infection enhancement. **Ab** in bold type indicates antibody from a DHF patient. (*$p<0.05$ and **$p<0.01$, unpaired two-tailed Student's t-test, n = 3 per point). # indicates a statistically significant difference between one specific point and the others (# $p<0.05$, ## $p<0.01$).

Figure S2 Phylogenetic tree of the prM-E encoding region of the infectious molecular clones. The phylogenetic tree was based on the nucleotide sequences of the prM-E region of the molecular clones derived from patient D30, the parental clone R05-624 and sequences from the NCBI database that were registered as the DENV-2 "Asian I" genotype from Thailand. The phylogenetic tree was generated using the Maximum Likelihood algorithm based on the Tamura-Nei model with bootstrapping (500 iterations). Evolutionary analyses were conducted in MEGA5.

Figure S3 Peak enhancing titers (PENT) of recombinant DENVs. Fold-enhancement was calculated from the virus titer data in Figure 5 by dividing the average number of foci at the highest virus titer in the presence of antibody by the average number of foci in the absence of antibody. Results are expressed as mean ± SD from two independent experiments performed in triplicate. (*$p<0.05$ and **$p<0.01$, unpaired two-tailed Student's t-test, n = 3 per point). Statistically significant differences between specific points and the others are indicated by # (# $p<0.05$, ## $p<0.01$). n.s., not significant.

Figure S4 Replication kinetics and ADE of recombinant DENVs in K562 cells. (A) Virus titers of the recombinant viruses, parental strain R05-624, and DENV-2 16681 were assessed in a focus-forming immunoassay in Vero cells and K562 cells to estimate optimal MOI. K562 cells were infected with DENV at an MOI of 0.1 after virus titration in Vero (dashed lines) or K562 cells (solid lines). After incubation at 37°C for 2 hours, viruses were removed and the infected cells were washed before the addition of maintenance medium supplement with 2% FBS. Supernatant were harvested consecutively within 4 days for virus titration in focus-forming immunoassay in Vero cells. Results are expressed as the mean ± SD of triplicate experiments. (B) For the ADE assay, 10-fold dilutions of heat-inactivated D30-plasma were pre-incubated with the recombinant virus variants, the parental R05-624 strain, or DENV-2 16681 at an MOI of 0.1 (which was estimated from virus titers assessed in Vero (solid bars) and K562 cells (open bars)). Then, the virus-antibody complexes were added to K562 cells and incubated for a further 2 h. Maintenance medium was added to yield a final FBS concentration of 2%. Cells and supernatants were collected on Day 3 post-infection. Virus titers in the supernatants were determined in a focus-forming immunoassay in Vero cells. Fold-enhancement was calculated by dividing the average number of foci at the highest virus titer in the presence of antibody by the average number of foci in the absence of antibody. Results are expressed as the mean ± SD from two independent experiments performed in triplicate. (*$p<0.05$ and **$p<0.01$, unpaired two-tailed Student's t-test, n = 3 per point).

Figure S5 ADE assays for recombinant DENVs in THP-1 and K562 cells (A) Heat-inactivated D30-plasma was serially diluted 10-fold in medium, and the dilutions were incubated at an MOI of 0.1 with recombinant DENVs derived from patient D30 plasma. Virus-antibody complexes were incubated with THP-1 cells for another 2 hours before adding maintenance medium. On day 3 post-infection, cells were harvested and DENV replication analyzed via one-step quantitative RT-PCR. The virus-antibody complexes were added to K562 cells and treated as described for THP-1 cells. On day 3 post-infection, the culture fluids from the samples in Figure A (B) and the infected K562 cells (C) were collected and their titers were determined in a focus-forming immunoassay in Vero cells. Results are expressed as the mean ± SD of triplicate experiments.

Acknowledgments

MOCID was established by the Research Institute for Microbial Diseases, Osaka University, Japan and Faculty of Tropical Medicine, Mahidol University, Thailand. We are grateful to Dr. Pratap Singhasivanon (Faculty of Tropical Medicine, Mahidol University), Dr. Yoshiharu Matsuura (Research Institute for Microbial Diseases, Osaka University), and Dr. Naokazu Takeda (RCC-ERI, Research Institute for Microbial Diseases, Osaka University) for their valuable help with this study.

Author Contributions

Conceived and designed the experiments: PC TK TO KI. Performed the experiments: PC. Analyzed the data: PC. Contributed reagents/materials/analysis tools: PC OP TS AY MS. Wrote the paper: PC KI. Bioinformatic: AY. Manuscript editing: TK TO TS PR. Provided oversight, support, and recruitment of study participants, as well as sample management: TO TK PR.

References

1. Kuhn RJ, Zhang W, Rossmann MG, Platnev SV, Corver J, et al. (2002) Structure of dengue virus: implications for flavivirus organization, maturation, and fusion. Cell 108: 717–725.
2. van der Schaar HM, Wilschut JC, Smit JM (2009) Role of antibodies in controlling dengue virus infection. Immunobiology 214: 613–629.
3. Midgley CM, Bajwa-Joseph M, Vasanawathana S, Limpitikul W, Wills B, et al. (2011) An in-depth analysis of original antigenic sin in dengue virus infection. J Virol 85: 410–421.
4. Sangkawibha N, Rojanasuphot S, Ahandrik S, Viriyapongse S, Jatanasen S, et al. (1984) Risk factors in dengue shock syndrome: a prospective epidemiologic study in Rayong, Thailand. I. The 1980 outbreak. Am J Epidemiol 120: 653–669.
5. Guzmán MG, Kouri GP, Bravo J, Soler M, Vazquez S, et al. (1990) Dengue hemorrhagic fever in Cuba, 1981: a retrospective seroepidemiologic study. Am J Trop Med Hyg 42: 179–184.
6. Rothman AL (2010) Cellular immunology of sequential dengue virus infection and its role in disease pathogenesis. Curr Top Microbiol Immunol 338: 83–98.
7. Halstead SB, O'Rourke EJ (1977) Dengue viruses and mononuclear phagocytes. I. Infection enhancement by non-neutralizing antibody. J Exp Med 146: 201–217.
8. Sabin AB (1952) Research on dengue during World War II. Am J Trop Med Hyg 1: 30–50.
9. García G, Sierra B, Pérez AB, Aguirre E, Rosado I, et al. (2010) Asymptomatic dengue infection in a Cuban population confirms the protective role of the RR variant of the FcγRIIa polymorphism. Am J Trop Med Hyg 82: 1153–1156.
10. Libraty DH, Acosta LP, Tallo V, Segubre-Mercado E, Bautista A, et al. (2009) A prospective nested case-control study of dengue in infects: Rethinking and refining the antibody-dependent enhancement dengue hemorrhagic fever model. PLoS Med 6: e1000171.
11. Balsitis SJ, Coloma J, Castro G, Alava A, Flores D, et al. (2009) Tropism of dengue virus in mice and human defined by viral nonstructural protein 3-specific immunostaining. Am J Trop Med Hyg 80: 416–424.
12. Jessie K, Fong MY, Devi S, Lam SK, Wong KT (2004) Localization of dengue virus in naturally infected human tissues, by immunohistochemistry and in situ hybridization. J Infect Dis 189: 1411–1418.
13. Baclig MO, Gervacio LT, Suarez LA, Buerano CC, Matias RR, et al. (2010) Flow cytometric analysis of dengue virus-infected cells in peripheral blood. Southeast Asian J Trop Med Public Health 41: 1352–1358.
14. Durbin AP, Vargas MJ, Wanionek K, Hammond SN, Gordon A, et al. (2008) Phenotyping of peripheral blood mononuclear cells during acute dengue illness demonstrates infection and increased activation of monocytes in severe cases compared to classic dengue fever. Virology 376: 429–435.
15. King AD, Nisalak A, Kalayanrooj S, Myint KS, Pattanapanyasat K, et al. (1999) B cells are the principal mononuclear cells infected by dengue virus. Southeast Asian J Trop Med Public Health 30: 718–728.
16. Srikiatkhachorn A, Wichit S, Gibbons RV, Green S, Libraty DH, et al. (2012) Dengue viral RNA levels in peripheral blood mononuclear cells are associated with disease severity and pre-existing dengue immune status. PLoS One 7: e51335.
17. Huang KJ, Yang YC, Lin YS, Huang JH, Liu HS, et al. (2006) The dual-specific binding of dengue virus and target cells for the antibody-dependent enhancement of dengue virus infection. J Immunol 176: 2825–2832.
18. Dejnirattisai W, Jumnainsong A, Onsirisakul N, Fitton P, Vasanawathana S, et al. (2010) Cross-reacting antibodies enhance dengue virus infection in humans. Science 328: 745–748.
19. Beltramello M, Williams KL, Simmons CP, Macagno A, Simonelli L, et al. (2010) The human immune response to dengue virus is dominated by highly cross-reactive antibodies endowed with neutralizing and enhancing activity. Cell Host Microbe 8: 271–183.
20. Rodenhuis-Zybert I, Moesker B, de Silva Voorham JM, der Ende-Metselaar H, Diamond MS, et al. (2011) A fusion-loop antibody enhances the infectious properties of immature flavivirus particles. J Virol 85: 11800–11808.
21. Hughes HR, Crill WD, Chang GJ (2012) Manipulation of immunodominant dengue virus E protein epitopes reduces potential antibody-dependent enhancement. Virol J 9: 115.
22. da Silva Voorham JM, Rodenhuis-Zybert IA, Ayala Nunez NV, Colpitts TM, van der Ende-Metselaar H, et al. (2012) Antibodies against the envelope glycoprotein promote infectivity of immature dengue virus serotype 2. PLoS One 7: e29957.
23. Sasaki T, Setthapramote C, Kurosu T, Nishimura M, Asai A, et al. (2013) Dengue virus neutralization and antibody-dependent enhancement activities of human monoclonal antibodies derived from dengue patients at acute phase of secondary infection. Antiviral Res 98: 423–431, 2013.
24. Guy B, Chanthavanich P, Gimenez S, Sirivichayakul C, Sabchareon A, et al. (2004) Evaluation by flow cytometry of antibody-dependent enhancement (ADE) of dengue infection by sera from Thai children immunized a live-attenuated tetravalent dengue vaccine. Vaccine 22: 3563–74.
25. Guy B, Barrere B, Malinowski C, Saville M, Teyssou R, et al. (2011) From research to phase III: preclinical, industrial and clinical development of the Sanofi Pasteur tetravalent dengue vaccine. Vaccine 29: 7229–7241.
26. Konishi E, Tabuchi Y, Yamanaka A (2010) A simple assay system for infection-enhancing and –neutralizing antibodies to dengue type 2 virus using layers of semi-adherent K562 cells. J Virol Methods 163: 360–367.
27. Halstead SB, Simasthien P (1970) Observations related to the pathogenesis of dengue hemorrhagic fever. II. Antigenic and biologic properties of dengue viruses and their association with disease response in the host. Yale J Biol Med 42(5): 276–92.
28. Kubota-Koketsu R, Mizuta H, Oshita M, Ideno S, Yunoki M, et al. (2009) Broad neutralizing human monoclonal antibodies against influenza virus from vaccinated healthy donors. Biochem Biophys Res Commun 387: 180–185.
29. Falconar AK (1999) Identification of an epitope on the dengue virus membrane (M) protein defined by cross-protective monoclonal antibodies: design of an improved epitope sequence based on common determinants present in both envelope (E and M) proteins. Arch Virol 144: 2313–2330.
30. Kurosu T, Khamlert C, Phanthanawiboon S, Ikuta K, Anantapreecha S (2010) Highly efficient rescue of dengue virus using a co-culture system with mosquito/mammalian cells. Biochem Biophys Res Commun 394: 398–404.
31. Yenchitsomanus P, Sricharoen P, Jaruthasana I, Pattanakitsakul S, Nitayaphan S, et al. (1996) Rapid detection and identification of dengue viruses by polymerase chain reaction (PCR). Southeast Asian J Trop Med Public Health 27: 228–236.
32. Shu PY, Chen LK, Chang SF, Yueh YY, Chow L, et al. (2003) Comparison of capture immunoglobulin M (IgM) and IgG Enzyme-linked immunosorbent assay (ELISA) and nonstructural protein NS1 serotype-specific IgG ELISA for differentiation of primary and secondary dengue virus infections. Clin Diagn Lab Immunol 10: 622–630.
33. Schmittgen TD, Livak KJ (2008) Analyzing real-time PCR data by the comparative C_T method. Nat Protoc 3: 1101–1108.
34. Boonnak K, Slike BM, Donofrio GC, Marovich MA (2013) Human FcγRII cytoplasmic differentially influence antibody-mediated dengue virus infection. J Immunol 190: 5659–5665.
35. Chareonsirisuthigul T, Kalayanarooj S, Ubol S (2007) Dengue virus (DENV) antibody-dependent enhancement of infection upregulates the production of anti-inflammatory cytokines, but suppresses anti-DENV free radical and pro-inflammatory cytokine production, in THP-1 cells. J Gen Virol 88: 365–375.
36. Paradkar PN, Ooi EE, Hanson BJ, Gubler DJ, Vasudevan SG (2011) Unfolded protein response (UPR) gene expression during antibody-dependent enhanced infection of cultured monocytes correlates with dengue disease severity. Biosci Rep 31: 221–230.
37. Modhiran N, Kalayanarooj S, Ubol S (2010) Subversion of innate defenses by the interplay between DENV and pre-existing enhancing antibodies: TLRs signaling collapse. PLoS Negl Trop Dis 4: e924.
38. Moi ML, Lim Ck, Tajima S, Kotaki A, Saijo M, et al. (2011) Dengue virus isolation relying on antibody-dependent enhancement mechanism using FcγR-expressing BHK cells and a monoclonal antibody with infection-enhancing capacity. J Clin Virol 52: 225–230.
39. Moi ML, Takasaki T, Saijo M, Kurane I (2013) Dengue virus infection-enhancing activity of undiluted sera obtained from patients with secondary dengue virus infection. Trans R Soc Trop Med Hyg 107: 51–58.
40. Littaua R, Kurane I, Ennis FA (1990) Human IgG Fc receptor II mediates antibody-dependent enhancement of dengue virus infection. J. Immunol. 144: 3183–3186.
41. Rodrigo WW, Jin X, Blackley SD, Rose RC, Schlesinger J (2006) Differential enhancement of dengue virus immune complex infectivity mediated by

signaling-competent and signaling-incompetent human FcγRIA (CD64) or FcγRIIA (CD32). J Virol 80: 10128–10138.

42. Rodrigo WW, Block OK, Lane C, Sukupolvi-Petty S, Goncalvez AP, et al. (2009) Dengue virus neutralization is modulated by IgG antibody subclass and Fcgamma receptor subtype. Virology 394: 175–182.

43. Ruangjirachuporn W, Boonpucknavig S, Nimmanitya S (1979) Circulating immune complexes in serum from patients with dengue haemorrhagic fever. Clin Exp Immunol 36: 46–53.

44. Wang WK, Chen HL, Yang CF, Hsieh SC, Juan CC, et al. (2006) Slower rates of viral load and virus-containing immune complexes in patients with dengue hemorrhagic fever. Clin Infect Dis 43: 1023–30.

45. Moi ML, Lim CK, Kotaki A, Takasaki T, Kurane I (2011) Detection of higher levels of dengue viremia using FcγR-expressing BHK-21 cells than FcγR-negative cells in secondary infection but not in primary infection. J Infect Dis 203: 1405–1414.

46. Kou Z, Lim JY, Beltramello M, Quinn M, Chen H, et al (2011) Human antibodies against dengue enhance dengue viral infectivity without suppressing type I interferon secretion in primary human monocytes. Virology 410: 240–247.

47. Setthapramote C, Sasaki T, Puiprom O, Limkittikul K, Pitaksajjakul P, et al. (2012) Human monoclonal antibodies to neutralize all dengue virus serotypes using lymphocytes from patients at acute phase of the secondary infection. Biochem Biophy Res Commun 423: 867–872.

48. Laoprasopwattana K, Libraty DH, Endy TP, Nisalak A, Chunsuttiwat S, et al. (2005) Dengue virus enhancing antibody activity in preillness plasma does not predict subsequent disease severity of viremia in secondary DV infection. J Infect Dis 192: 510–519.

49. Rodenhuis-Zybert IA, Wilschut J, Smit JM (2010) Dengue virus life cycle: viral and host factors modulating infectivity. Cell Mol Life Sci 67: 2773–2786.

14

Spatiotemporal Characterizations of Dengue Virus in Mainland China: Insights into the Whole Genome from 1978 to 2011

Hao Zhang[1,2], Yanru Zhang[1], Rifat Hamoudi[3,4], Guiyun Yan[5], Xiaoguang Chen[2]*, Yuanping Zhou[1]*

1 Department of Infectious Diseases, Nanfang Hospital, Southern Medical University, Guangzhou, Guangdong Province, China, **2** Key Laboratory of Prevention and Control for Emerging Infectious Diseases of Guangdong Province, School of Public Health and Tropical Medicine, Southern Medical Guangzhou, Guangdong Province, China, **3** Department of Pathology, Rockefeller Building, University College London, London, United Kingdom, **4** UCL Cancer Institute, Paul O Gorman Building, University College London, London, United Kingdom, **5** Program in Public Health, University of California Irvine, Irvine, California, United States of America

Abstract

Temporal-Spatial of dengue virus (DENV) analyses have been performed in previous epidemiological studies in mainland China, but few studies have examined the whole genome of the DENV. Herein, 40 whole genome sequences of DENVs isolated from mainland China were downloaded from GenBank. Phylogenetic analyses and evolutionary distances of the dengue serotypes 1 and 2 were calculated using 14 maximum likelihood trees created from individual genes and whole genome. Amino acid variations were also analyzed in the 40 sequences that included dengue serotypes 1, 2, 3 and 4, and they were grouped according to temporal and spatial differences. The results showed that none of the phylogenetic trees created from each individual gene were similar to the trees created using the complete genome and the evolutionary distances were variable with each individual gene. The number of amino acid variations was significantly different ($p = 0.015$) between DENV-1 and DENV-2 after 2001; seven mutations, the N290D, L402F and A473T mutations in the E gene region and the R101K, G105R, D340E and L349M mutations in the NS1 region of DENV-1, had significant substitutions, compared to the amino acids of DENV-2. Based on the spatial distribution using Guangzhou, including Foshan, as the indigenous area and the other regions as expanding areas, significant differences in the number of amino acid variations in the NS3 ($p = 0.03$) and NS1 ($p = 0.024$) regions and the NS2B ($p = 0.016$) and NS3 ($p = 0.042$) regions were found in DENV-1 and DENV-2. Recombination analysis showed no inter-serotype recombination events between the DENV-1 and DENV-2, while six and seven breakpoints were found in DENV-1 and DENV-2. Conclusively, the individual genes might not be suitable to analyze the evolution and selection pressure isolated in mainland China; the mutations in the amino acid residues in the E, NS1 and NS3 regions may play important roles in DENV-1 and DENV-2 epidemics.

Editor: Xia Jin, University of Rochester, United States of America

Funding: This work was supported by the National Science Foundation of China (30771899) to YP Zhou, and National Institutes of Health grant R01AI083202 to XG Chen. The funders had no role in study design, data collection and analysis, decision to publish, or preparation of the manuscript.

Competing Interests: The authors have declared that no competing interests exist.

* E-mail: xgchen2001@hotmail.com (XGC); yuanpingzhou@163.com (YPZ)

Introduction

Dengue is one of the most globally important vector-born infectious diseases in tropic and sub-tropic areas. It is caused by the single-stranded, positive-sense RNA, dengue virus (DENV) which is the member of the *Flavivirus* genus and the *Flaviviridae* family. DENV consists of four antigenically related serotypes (DENV-1, DENV-2, DENV-3 and DENV-4). The viral genome is approximately 11 kb in length and contains a single open reading frame (ORF) that encodes three structural proteins, including the capsid (C), premembrane/membrane (PrM/M), and envelope (E) proteins and seven non-structural (NS) proteins (NS1, NS2A, NS2B, NS3, NS4A, NS4B and NS5); this ORF is flanked by the 5′- and 3′-non-translated regions (5NTR/3NTR).

In mainland China, dengue fever cases have been reported every year since 1997, especially in the Guangdong province [1,2,3]. All four DENV serotypes have been epidemic. DENV-1 was responsible for dengue fever (DF) epidemics in Guangdong province in 1979 and 1985 [4]; several outbreaks caused by the

same virus were also reported in 1991, and from 1995 to 2010 [1,2,5,6]. DENV-2 caused DF epidemics in Hainan province in 1985, in Guangxi province in 1988, in Guangdong province in 1993, 1998 and 2001 and in Fujian province in 1999 [7]. DENV-3 has rarely caused epidemics in mainland China since 1982, and DENV-4 has always been sporadic and has consisted with other serotypes [7].

Co-circulation of multiple DENV serotypes, genotypes and clades in the same community has become common [8,9,10,11]. At present, the most widely accepted method for genotyping DENV involves the phylogenetic analysis of gene sequences, in particular the E gene [12,13]. Recent research has shown that individual genes, except the 5NTR gene, are suitable for genotyping DENV using the phylogenetic method in Thailand [14], a country in which dengue is seriously epidemic. The E gene of DENV has also been widely used in molecular and evolution analyses in mainland China [15,16,17]. Since the first documented DENV infection in Foshan in 1978, DENV has spread into mainland China during the last 30 years. However, there is a lack of research evaluaing whether the individual genes, including E gene, are suitable for genotyping the dengue viruses, as well as few analyses of their evolution and selection pressures. Recently, complete genome analysis of the West Nile virus and Japanese encephalitis virus, which belongs to the same family as DENV, has been shown to be a powerful tool for evaluating the relatedness and for reconstructing the evolutionary history and phylogeography of these viruses [18,19,20,21,22,23,24,25,26]. Spatial and temporal analyses of dengue fever cases in Guangdong province showed that the geographic range of the dengue fever epidemic has expanded during recent years [27]; counties around the Pearl River Delta area and the Chaoshan Region are at an increased risk for dengue fever [28]. Therefore, the characteristics of DENV epidemics in mainland China need to be described according to spatial and temporal analyses.

In this study, a total of 40 complete genome sequences of DENV (19 DENV-1; 11 DENV-2; 6 DENV-3; 4 DENV-4) were downloaded from GenBank and analyzed using bioinformatics methods. The two aims of this study were to determine whether individual genes are suitable for genotyping DENV and to characterize the molecular epidemiology and virology of the DENVs using the complete genome sequence by spatial and temporal analyses.

Materials and Methods

Virus

The complete sequences of dengue viruses were downloaded from GenBank (http://www.ncbi.nlm.nih.gov/genbank/). There were 19 DENV-1, 11 DENV-2, 6 DENV-3 and 4 DENV-4 viruses. The details of these viruses are shown in Table 1.

Genotyping Method

Phylogenetic analysis was performed on a gene-by-gene basis using the sequences of the coding region and the non-coding region of 40 DENV strains isolated in mainland China. Sequence alignments were performed using the Clustal W program, which resulted in alignments of the complete sequence and for each individual gene sequence for each of the four DENV serotypes. Maximum likelihood (ML) phylogenetic trees were then estimated

using the MEGA (Molecular Evolutionary Genetics Analysis) 5.05 software. To determine the support for a particular grouping on the phylogenetic trees, bootstrap re-sampling analyses was performed using 1000 replicate neighbor-joining trees estimated by using the ML substitution model.

The Evolutionary Distance of DENV using Individual Genes

The overall evolutionary distance of DENV using individual genes was determined using the Mega 5.05 software after the sequences were aligned. To determine the support for the distance calculating, bootstrap re-sampling analyses was performed using 1000 replicate neighbor-joining trees estimated using the ML substitution model.

Variations of Amino Acids (AAs) in DENV-1, DENV-2, DENV-3 and DENV-4

The ORF gene was obtained by manually removing the 5NTR and 3NTR region. The number of amino acid changes was observed in the four dengue serotypes compared to each standard dengue strain (DENV-1: Hawaii, EU848545; DENV-2: New guinea-C, AF038403; DENV-3: H87, M93130; DENV-4: H241, AY947539). When a significant difference was observed in the equality of variances ($p<0.1$), the Kruskal-Wallis statistic was used to compare the number of AA variations among the four DENV-1, DENV-2, DENV-3 and DENV-4 groups, and Student's t-test was used to compare DENV-1 and DENV-2 isolates in 2001–2010 group, when the data were not significant according to the normality and equality of variances ($p>0.1$). A one-way ANOVA test was used to compare the AA changes between the 17 DENV-1 and 8 DENV-2 viruses isolated during the past recent 20 years (1990–2010) because the data were not significant according to normality and equality of variances ($p>0.1$) analyses. According to the geography of these DENV-1 and DENV-2 isolates, the changes in AAs were also compared using the Kruskal-Wallis (significant differences in normality) or Student't- t-test (non-significant differences in normality). All tests were two-sided, and a $p<0.05$ value was considered statistically significant. The differences in normality and equality of variances were considered

Table 1. The overall distance of DENV-1 and DENV-2 from individual genes.

Gene Area	DENV-1 Mean ± Standard Deviation (M±SD)	DENV-2 Mean ± Standard Deviation (M±SD)
Whole genome	0.081±0.004	0.089±0.003
5'UTR	0.011±0.005	0.039±0.011
C	0.041±0.007	0.076±0.017
prM	0.055±0.009	0.098±0.022
E	0.084±0.009	0.079±0.008
NS1	0.091±0.015	0.089±0.011
NS2A	0.073±0.007	0.111±0.014
NS2B	0.094±0.02	0.099±0.021
NS3	0.082±0.009	0.092±0.009
NS4A	0.126±0.026	0.052±0.007
NS4B	0.073±0.011	0.092±0.012
NS5	0.080±0.007	0.072±0.006
3'UTR	0.035±0.007	0.017±0.006

significant when the p<0.1. This statistical analysis was performed using the SPSS software package (version 13.0).

Recombination Analysis

All the DENV-1 and DENV-2 isolates were analyzed using "DataMonkey" (available online: http://www.datamonkey.org/). The recombination events of the dengue viruses were analyzed using the genetic algorithm (GARD). The GARD method for detecting recombination was demonstrated in a previous study [29]. The neighbor-joining trees between the breakpoints were also demonstrated.

Results

To determine which gene is suitable for intra-serotype identification, phylogenetic analysis was performed separately using the sequences of the complete genome, the ORF region and each gene. Fourteen phylogenetic trees were generated using the ML method for the DENV-1 and DENV-2 serotypes (1 tree/1 gene). The bootstrap value was added to each major node. A bootstrap value is close to 100% at the nodes indicated, a more accurate genotype identification. A clade supported by a bootstrap value of at least 90% was considered highly significant. As a result of the small number of DENV-3 and DENV-4, these phylogenetic trees were not analyzed.

According to the different serotypes, location (Guangzhou and other regions) and isolation year, the AA variations were also determined to explain the DENV epidemic in mainland China using the ORF and individual genes.

Genotyping DENV-1

Phylogenetic analysis of DENV-1 included the creation of 14 ML trees derived from the complete genome sequence, the ORF and each gene (Figure 1). The ML trees generated from the ORF and the E region (1485 bp) were similar to the tree generated from the complete genome sequence; however, the trees generated from the ORF and the E gene were each supported by bootstrap values of less than 90% at some of the major nodes (Figure 1). The trees from other genes, including the 5′NTR (95 bp), C (342 bp), PrM (498 bp), NS1 (1056 bp), NS2A (654 bp), NS2B (390 bp), NS3 (1857 bp), NS4A (450 bp), NS4B (747 bp), NS5 (2706 bp) and 3′NTR (418 bp), were different from the tree generated using the complete sequence (Figure. 1). Therefore, all ML trees generated from the DENV-1 isolates showed different topology, suggesting that none of gene regions can be representatively used to describe the molecular characteristics of DENV-1 viruses in mainland China.

Genotyping DENV-2

Phylogenetic analysis of DENV-2 included the creation of 14 ML trees derived from the complete, the ORF and each gene (Figure 2). The ML tree generated from the ORF was the same as the tree generated using the complete sequence, and the topological structure of the tree generated using the NS3 gene region was similar to the one generated using the complete sequence; however, the trees generated from the NS3 region were each supported by bootstrap values of less than 90% at the major nodes (Figure 2). The trees from each of the genes, including the 5′NTR, C, PrM, E, NS1, NS2A, NS2B, NS4A, NS4B, NS5 and 3′NTR genes, were different from the tree generated for the complete sequence (Figure 2), Therefore, all of the ML trees generated for DENV-2 showed different topology, which suggests none of these gene regions, except for the ORF, can be

representatively used to describe the molecular characteristics of DENV-2 in mainland China.

The Overall Evolutionary Distance of DENV

This analysis was performed for DENV-1 and DENV-2. The evolutionary distances were similar for the NS5 (0.080 ± 0.007, 0.072 ± 0.006), NS3 (0.082 ± 0.009, 0.092 ± 0.009) and NS1 (0.089 ± 0.011, 0.089 ± 0.011) regions for DENV-1 and DENV-2, compared to the distance of the whole genome (DENV-1:0.081 ± 0.004 and DENV-2:0.089 ± 0.003); the distance of the E gene was relatively far (DENV-1:0.084 ± 0.009 and DENV-2:0.079 ± 0.011), which demonstrates that the variability of the E gene. The evolutionary distances of other individual genes are detailed in Table 1.

Amino Acid Sequence Variations in the DENV-1, DENV-2, DENV-3 and DENV-4 Viruses

The AA changes were significantly different in the ORF region of the four DENV groups ($\chi^2 = 14.8$, p = 0.002, Table 2). There were more changes in the AAs in the DENV-1 group (mean rank: 27), followed by DENV-4 group (mean rank: 22). As for the four groups based on the serotypes (DENV-1 and DENV-2) and the isolation year, a significant difference was shown in these four groups (F = 3.9, p = 0.024), while there was a significant difference in the AA changes between the two groups of the DENV-1 and DENV-2 strains isolated from 2001–2010 (p = 0.022, 89.2 ± 14.2 vs. 64 ± 6.7, Table 3). The AA changes in the E (Z = 2.96, p = 0.003) and NS1 (F = 0.4, p = 0.006) genes were significantly different between the DENV-1 and DENV-2 isolates from 2001–2010, as shown by the AA variations between these two genes (M±SD: 16.8 ± 2.4 vs. 11 ± 0.8; 15.3 ± 3.0 vs. 7.5 ± 1.7, respectively). According to the alignment of these DENV-1 and DENV-2 isolates, the N290D, L402F and A473T mutations in the E gene and the R101K, G105R, D340E and L349M mutations in the NS1 gene region of the DENV-1 isolates may be significant, while these AAs in the DENV-2 isolates have not been changed (Figure 3). The AA changes were more numerous in the viruses from Guangzhou, including the first reported dengue case in Foshan, than in the viruses from dengue epidemics outside of Guangzhou (NS1 of DENV-3: t = 2.3, p = 0.034; NS1, NS2B and NS3 of DENV-2: t = 2.7, 2.9, Z = 2.2; p = 0.024, 0.016, 0.042, Table 4).

Recombination Analysis

No recombination events were shown in the inter-serotype between DENV-1 and DENV-2, while significant recombination events were shown in the intra-serotype of DENV-1 and DENV-2. In DENV-1, seven breakpoints (location: 991, 1687, 5557, 6199, 6496, 7657 and 10321) were found, but only the first six breakpoints showed significant differences (P<0.01). Four breakpoints (location: 991, 1687, 5557 and 7657) occurred in the two isolates FJ196847 and FJ196848, while the remaining two breakpoints (location: 6199, 6496) were observed in the five isolates DQ193572, JQ048541, EU359008, FJ176780 and FJ196843 (Figure 4). In DENV-2, except for one non-significant breakpoint (location 1687), eight breakpoints (location: 760, 1459, 3823, 4996, 5260, 8290, 9452 and 10189) were observed. All of these breakpoints were found in the isolates FJ196851, FJ196852, FJ196853 and FJ196854 (Figure 4).

Discussion

Phylogenetic analysis of the gene sequences obtained directly from patient sera provides a rapid approach for discriminating

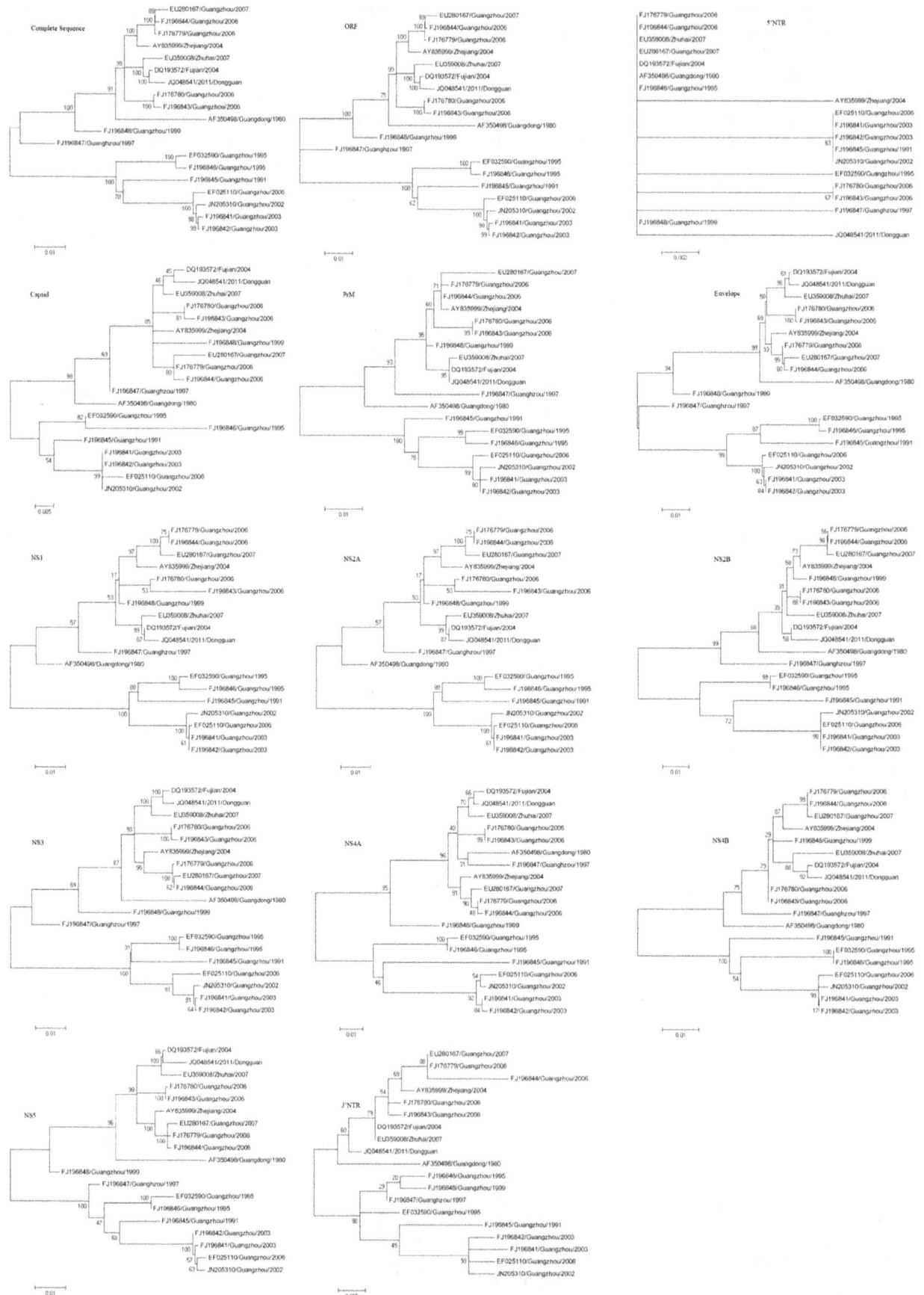

Figure 1. Phylogenetic analysis of DENV-1 as determined from 14 ML trees derived from the complete genome, ORF and individual gene sequence.

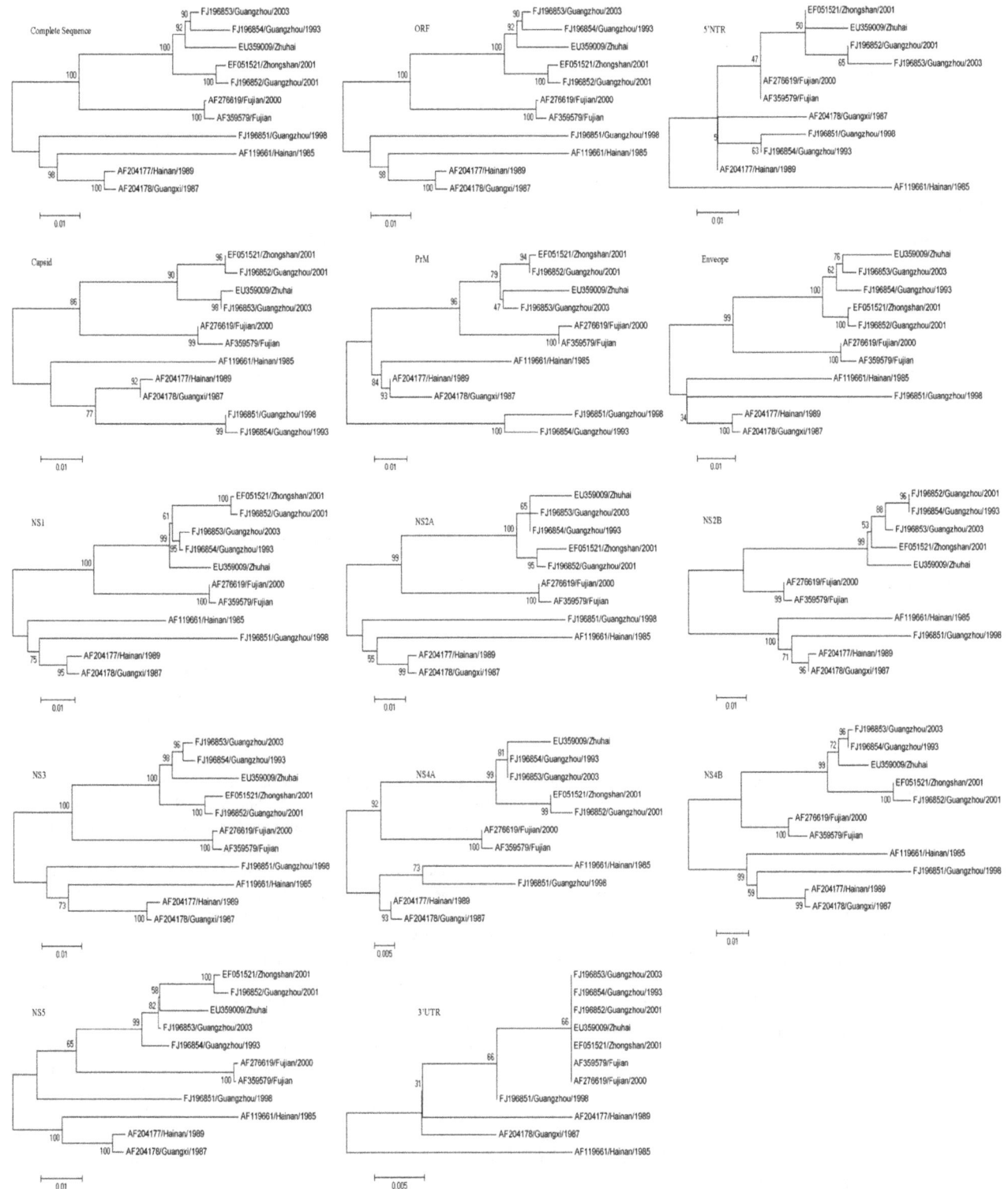

Figure 2. Phylogenetic analysis of DENV-2 as determined from 14 ML trees derived from the complete genome, ORF and individual gene sequence.

	290	402	473	101 105	340 349
EU848545/DENV-1/Hawaii/1944	NKLTLKGMSY	MLEATARGAR	RSASLSMTCI	RKMIGPQPME	DKEENLVKSL
DQ193572/Fujian/2004	DKLTLKGMSY	MFEATARGAR	RSTSLSMTCI	KKMIRPQPME	EKEENLVKSM
FJ196843/Guangzhou/2006	DKLTLKGMSY	MFEATARGAR	RSTSLSMTCI	KKMIRPQPME	EKEENLVKSM
FJ176780/Guangzhou/2006	DKLTLKGMSY	MFEATARGAR	RSTSLSMTCI	KKMIRPQPME	EKEENLVKSM
FJ176779/Guangzhou/2006	DKLTLKGMSY	MFEATARGAR	RSTSLSMTCI	KKMIRPQPME	EKEENLVKSM
EU280167/Guangzhou/2007	DKLTLKGMSY	MFEATARGAR	RSTSLSMTCI	KKMIRPQPME	EKEENLVKSM
FJ196844/Guangzhou/2006	DKLTLKGMSY	MFEATARGAR	RSTSLSMTCI	KKMIRPQPME	EKEENLVKSM
AY835999/Zhejiang/2004	DKLTLKGMSY	MFEATARGAR	RSTSLSMTCI	KKMIRPQPME	EKEENLVKSM
EU359008/Zhuhai/2007	DKLTLKGMSY	MFEATARGAR	RSTSLSMTCI	KKMIRPQPME	EKEENLVKSM
FJ196841/Guangzhou/2003	DKLTLKGVSY	MFEATARGAR	RSTSLSMTCI	KKMIRPQPME	EKEENLVKSM
FJ196842/Guangzhou/2003	DKLTLKGVSY	MFEATARGAR	RSTSLSMTCI	KKMIRPQPME	EKEENLVKSM
EF025110/Guangzhou/2006	DKLTLKGVSY	MFEATARGAR	RSTSLSMTCI	KKMIRPQPME	EKEENLVKSM
JN205310/Guangzhou/2002	DKLTLKGVSY	MFEATARGAR	RSTSLSMTCI	KKMIRPQPME	EKEENLVKSM
FJ390389/DENV-2/New Guinea-C	DKLQLKGMSY	MFETTMRGAK	RSTSLSVSLV	KRSLRPQPTE	EKEENLVNSL
FJ196852/Guangzhou/2001	DKLQLKGMSY	MFETTMRGAK	RSTSLSVSLV	KRSLRPQPTE	EKEENLVNSL
EF051521/Zhongshan/2001	DKLQLKGMSY	MFETTMRGAK	RSTSLSVSLV	KRSLRPQPTE	EKEENLVNSL
FJ196853/Guangzhou/2003	DKLQLKGMSY	MFETTMRGAK	RSASLSVSLV	KRSLRPQPTE	EKEENLVNSL
EU359009/Zhuhai/2007	DKLQLKGMSY	MFETTMRGAK	RSTSLSVSLV	KRSLRPQPTE	EKEENLVNSL
	E (290-299aa)	E (401-410aa)	E (471-480aa)	NS1 (101-110aa)	NS1 (340-349aa)

Figure 3. Special mutations in the E and NS1 gene regions of the DENV-1 isolates collected after 2000, compared with DENV-2.

dengue viruses according to serotype, genotype and clade. This molecular epidemiological typing technique is widely used and accepted for the genotyping of dengue viruses. Thus far, nearly all phylogenetic analyses on DENV in mainland China have used the nucleotide sequence of the E gene to identify the genotypes for the DENV-1, DENV-2, DENV-3 and DENV-4 viruses [15,16], and the E gene has not been evaluated to determine whether it is suitable for use in genotyping the virus. Additionally, spatial and temporal analyses were performed in previous epidemiological studies [27,28], but few have been analyzed using the whole genome of the dengue virus.

In the present study, phylogenetic analyses were performed using the nucleotide sequences of the complete genome, the ORF and individual coding and non-coding genes from 19 DENV-1 and 11 DENV-2 isolates from mainland China. The results showed that the E gene would not improve the stratification of the different genotypes. Although the E gene has been thought to be effective in genotyping the dengue viruses, the topology and its overall evolutionary distance did not support its use in analyzing the evolution and selection pressure of dengue virus in mainland China (Figure 1 and Table 1). These results suggest that the viral evolution in the different genetic groups reflects differences in both the individual coding and non-coding genes. The topologies from these genes were not similar to the topology from the complete sequence. Additionally, this study showed that the ORF gene might be useful for genotyping and clade identification for the majority of the DENV-2 isolates analyzed. In the DENV-1 isolates, according to the topology from the complete sequence, the viruses could be classified into three genotypes and five clades,

while one of the nodes was less than 90% certain according to the ORF gene (Figure 1: A, B). Thus, the ORF gene cannot be used to analyze the evolutionary distance and the selection pressure of the DENV-1 isolates from mainland China. These results greatly differ from a previously published study [14]. The reasons for these different results may be due to the different epidemic locations, the modes of evolution of the dengue viruses and different epidemic years. Additionally, this study had several limitations, including a small sample size. Therefore, if the aim of a study is to classify the dengue virus for the study of viral evolution and selection pressure, then there are no other target sequence(s) that can be selected apart from the complete sequences for the DENV-1 and DENV-2 isolates and the ORF gene for DENV-2 in mainland China.

Recently, the E gene region has been widely used for molecular characterization. However, the evolution of DENV involves not only in the E gene, but also other regions, particularly in the non-structural region, such as the NS1, NS2A, NS4B and NS5 regions [30,31,32]. In our study, there were significant differences not only in the AA variations of E gene region, but also in non-structural region. Therefore, phylogenetic analysis with the E gene region cannot replace the molecular characteristics of DENV in the study of viral evolution and selection pressure. Dengue has been epidemic in mainland China for 30 years. Mutations in regions other than the E gene may also influence the biological characteristics of DENV. Additionally, recombination events were observed in the E gene region of DENV-1 and DENV-2. Thus, the E gene might not be suitable for use in analyzing the molecular characteristics of the dengue virus in mainland China.

Table 2. Comparison of the AA variations in the complete sequences of isolates from the four serotypes in mainland China.

Dengue serotype	Strains (accession number/geography/year)	AA variations, Mean±Standard Deviation (M±SD)	Kruskal-Wallis Test
DENV-1	EF032590/Guangzhou/1995	85±3	$\chi^2 = 14.8$
	FJ196846/Guangzhou/1995		p = 0.002
	FJ196848/Guangzhou/1999		
	JN205310/Guangzhou/2002		
	EF025110/Guangzhou/2006		
	FJ176779/Guangzhou/2006		
	FJ176780/Guangzhou/2006		
	FJ196843/Guangzhou/2006		
	FJ196844/Guangzhou8/2006		
	AY834999/Zhejiang/2004		
	DQ193572/Fujian/2004		
	EU280167/Guangzhou/2007		
	EU359008/Zhuhai/2007		
	FJ196841/Guangzhou/2003		
	FJ196842/Guangzhou/2003		
	FJ196845/Guangzhou/1991		
	FJ196847/Guangzhou/1997		
	JQ048541/Dongguan/2011		
DENV-2	AF350498/Guangdong/1980	63±6	
	AF119661/Hainan/1985		
	AF204177/Hainan/1989		
	AF204178/Guangxi/1987		
	AF276619/Fujian/2000		
	AF359579/Fujian/1999		
	EF051521/Zhongshan/2001		
	EU359009/Zhuhai/2007		
	FJ196851/Guangzhou/1998		
	FJ196852/Guangzhou/2001		
	FJ196853/Guangzhou/2003		
	FJ196854/Guangzhou/1993		
DENV-3	AF317645/Guangxi,	59±9	
	EU367962/China		
	GU189648/Zhejiang/2009		
	GU363549/Guangzhou/2009		
	JF504679/Zhejiang/2009		
	JN662391/Guangzhou/2009		
DENV-4	FJ196849/Guangzhou/1978,	82±9	
	FJ196850/Guangzhou/1990		
	JF741967/Guangzhou/2010		
	JQ822247/Zhejiang/2009		

According to the number of AA variations in the four serotypes of DENV, the most variable AA sequence belonged to the DENV-1 serotype. This finding is consistent with the fact that the frequency of epidemics caused by the DENV-1 serotype is the highest [7,33]. Interestingly more AA changes were observed in DENV-4 than in DENV-2 and DENV-3; however, the frequencies of DENV-2 (10 epidemics) and DENV-3 (8 epidemics) epidemics were more than that of DENV-4 (4 epidemics) [7,33]. In other Southeast Asian countries, such as Thailand and Malaysia, the frequency of DENV-4 epidemic was also reported to be very low [34,35,36]. Thus, we conclude that a silent epidemic of DENV-4 may exist in Southeast Asian countries. However, few studies show the serotypes of the population with dengue in Southeast Asian countries. Therefore, a large epidemic survey is needed to prove this conclusion.

The AA changes of the DENV-1 isolates from 2001 to 2010 were more numoerous than those of the DENV-2 isolates from 2001 to 2010, and no significant difference was found between the

Table 3. Comparison of the AA variations between the two serotypes in mainland China.

Dengue serotype	Group	Strains (accession number/ geography/year)	AA variations in full-length (M±SD)	One-way ANOVA	AA variations of E (M±SD)§	AA variations of NS1(M±SD)⁎
DENV-1	1	FJ196845/Guangzhou/1991	82.0±6.7	F = 3.9	–	–
		FJ196846/Guangzhou/1995		p = 0.024		
		EF032590/Guangzhou/1995				
		FJ196848/Guangzhou/1999				
		FJ196847/Guangzhou/1997				
	2	JN205310/Guangzhou/2002				
		FJ196841/Guangzhou/2003,	89.2±14.2		16.8±2.4	15.3±3.0
		FJ196842/Guangzhou/2003				
		AY835999/Zhejiang/2004				
		DQ193572/Fujian/2004				
		EF025110/Guangzhou/2006				
		FJ176779/Guangzhou/2006				
		FJ176780/Guangzhou/2006				
		FJ196843/Guangzhou/2006				
		FJ196844/Guangzhou/2006				
		EU280167/Guangzhou/2007				
		EU359008/Zhuhai/2007				
DENV-2	3	FJ196854/Guangzhou/1993	74.8±7.8		–	–
		FJ196851/Guangzhou/1998				
		AF359579/Fujian/1999				
		AF276619/Fujian/2000				
	4	EF051521/Zhongshan/2001	64±6.7		11±0.8	7.5±1.7
		FJ196852/Guangzhou/2001				
		FJ196853/Guangzhou/2003				
		EU359009/Zhuhai/2007				

Note: "§": Mann-Whitney U test, Z = 2.96, p = 0.003; "⁎": Student's t-test: t = 4.89, p<0.001; "−": No statistics.

DENV-1 and DENV-2 isolates from 1991 to 2000. Seven mutations were observed in the DENV-1 isolates, including the N290D, L402F and A473T mutations in the E gene region and the R101K, G105R, D340E and L349M mutations in the NS1 region, while no mutation was found in the DENV-2 in these locations (Figure 3). The E protein consists of three domains, designated as domains I (amino acids 1–51, 132–192 and 280–295), II (amino acids 52–131 and 193–279) and III (amino acid 296–393). In this study, one mutation occurred in domain I, which is an elongated domain, and the other two mutations were not found in these three domains. However, a recent research showed

that the penultimate interaction, which involves the 402F residue, has hydrophobic contact with a conserved surface on domain II [37]. That study showed that it is important for DENV that the mutations occur in the E gene region. The NS1 protein plays a significant role in immune evasion during infection [38,39]; thus, adaptive AA mutations may have occurred after 2001 to enhance the virus' susceptibility to the human immune system. This may be one explanation for the high frequency of DENV-1 epidemics compared to that of DENV-2 after 2001.

The NS3 protein is a multifunctional enzyme with separate active sites involved in viral RNA replication and capping,

Table 4. AA variations in DENV-1 and DENV-2 between the Guangzhou city and other regions.

	DENV-1		Statistic	P value	DENV-2		Statistics	P value
	Guangzhou (14 strains)	Other regions (5 strains)			Guangzhou (4 strains)	Other regions (7 strains)		
NS1	–	–	–	–	10±3.7	5.7±1.6	t = 2.7	0.024
NS2B	–	–	–	–	3.3±1.0	1.7±0.8	t = 2.9	0.016
NS3	12.1±2.0	9.8±1.8	t = 2.3	0.034	12.8±1.5	8.4±4.5	Z = 2.2	0.042

Note: "−": No statistics; "t": using student-t test; "Z": using Mann-Whitney test.

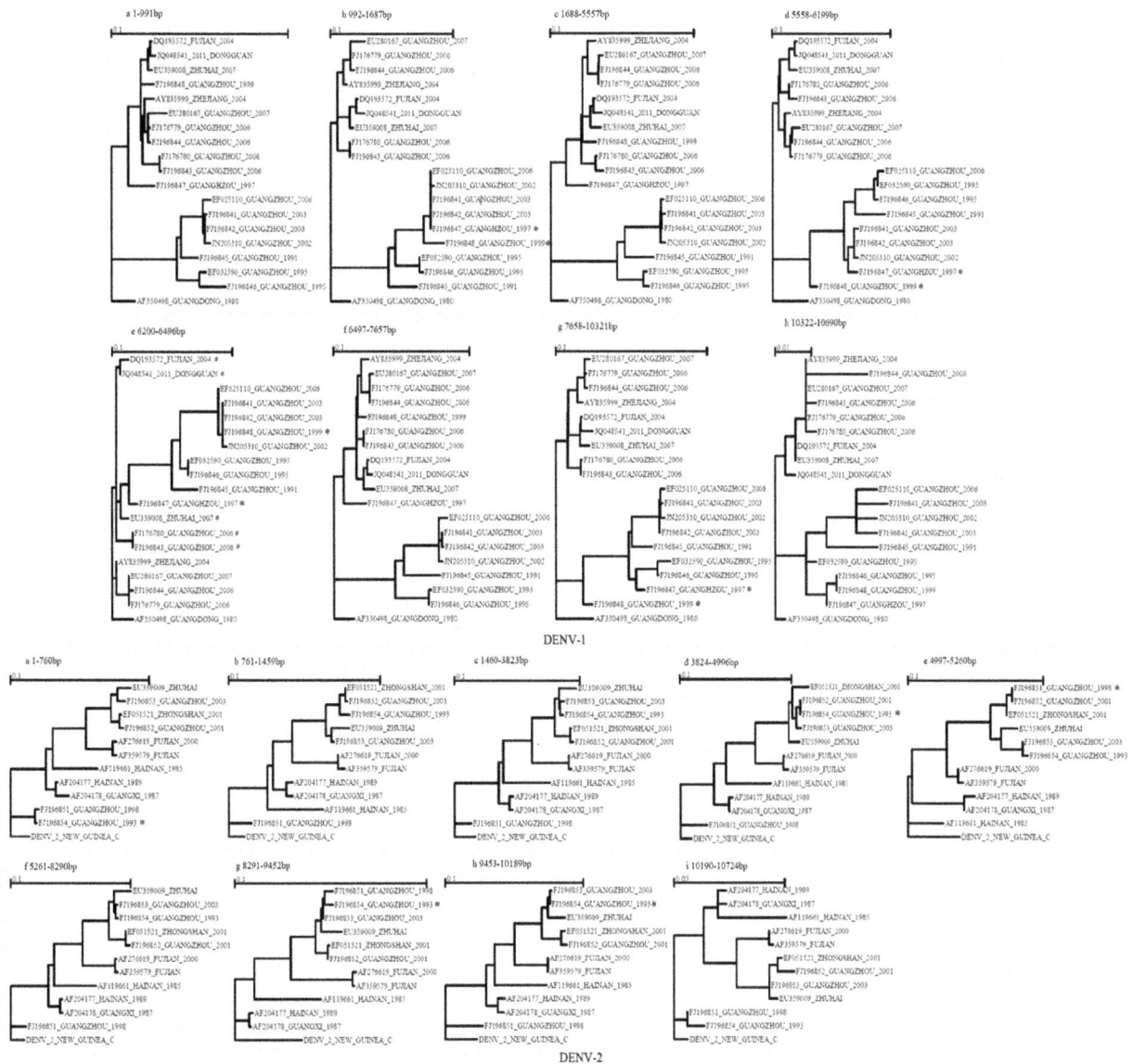

Figure 4. Phylogenetic analysis based on the breakpoints of DENV-1 and DENV-2 according to Datamonkey.

including helicase, nucleoside 5′-triphosphatase (NTPase) and RNA 5′-triphosphatase (RNPase) activities [40]. Therefore, mutations in this gene could have significant effects on viral replication. In mainland China, there are significant differences in the mutations within the NS3 region between the Guangzhou isolates and the other regional isolates of DENV-1 and DENV-2. An increase in the AA mutation frequency of the Guangzhou isolates increased the survival opportunity of the virus, which may explain why dengue is mainly epidemic in Guangzhou compare to other sub-tropic areas of mainland China.

Conclusion

According to this study, the complete sequence of DENV-1, as well as the complete genome or ORF sequence of DENV-2, is suitable or use in analyzing viral evolution and selection pressure, whereas the E genes are not. Additionally, the mutations in the E and NS1 regions may have had effects on the DENV-1 epidemics since 2001, and mutations in the NS3 region might affect the DENV-1 and DENV-2 epidemics in different regions.

Author Contributions

Conceived and designed the experiments: XGC YPZ GY. Performed the experiments: HZ. Analyzed the data: HZ YZ GY. Contributed reagents/materials/analysis tools: XGC YPZ YZ. Wrote the paper: HZ. Revised the paper: RH. Responsible for the supervision of the project and final approval of the version: XGC YPZ.

References

1. Luo H, He J, Zheng K, Li L, Jiang L (2002) Analysis on the epidemiologic features of Dengue fever in Guangdong province, 1990–2000. Zhonghua Liu Xing Bing Xue Za Zhi 23: 427–430.

2. Liang WJ, He JF, Luo HM, Zhou HQ, Yang F, et al. (2007) [Epidemiological analysis of dengue fever in Guangdong province, 2001–2006]. South China Journal of Preventive Medicine 5: 4–5.

3. Fan J, Lin H, Wang C, Bai L, Yang S, et al. (2013) Identifying the high-risk areas and associated meteorological factors of dengue transmission in Guangdong Province, China from 2005 to 2011. Epidemiol Infect: 1–10.

4. Qiu FX, Gubler DJ, Liu JC, Chen QQ (1993) Dengue in China: a clinical review. Bull World Health Organ 71: 349–359.

5. Peng HJ, Lai HB, Zhang QL, Xu BY, Zhang H, et al. (2012) A local outbreak of dengue caused by an imported case in Dongguan China. BMC Public Health 12: 83.

6. Jiang L, Wu X, Wu Y, Bai Z, Jing Q, et al. (2013) Molecular epidemiological and virological study of dengue virus infections in Guangzhou, China, during 2001–2010. Virol J 10: 4.

7. Wu JY, Lun ZR, James AA, Chen XG (2010) Dengue Fever in mainland China. Am J Trop Med Hyg 83: 664–671.

8. Klungthong C, Zhang C, Mammen MJ, Ubol S, Holmes EC (2004) The molecular epidemiology of dengue virus serotype 4 in Bangkok, Thailand. Virology 329: 168–179.

9. Rico-Hesse R (2003) Microevolution and virulence of dengue viruses. Adv Virus Res 59: 315–341.

10. Zhang C, Mammen MJ, Chinnawirotpisan P, Klungthong C, Rodpradit P, et al. (2005) Clade replacements in dengue virus serotypes 1 and 3 are associated with changing serotype prevalence. J Virol 79: 15123–15130.

11. Zhang C, Mammen MJ, Chinnawirotpisan P, Klungthong C, Rodpradit P, et al. (2006) Structure and age of genetic diversity of dengue virus type 2 in Thailand. J Gen Virol 87: 873–883.

12. Hillis DM (1998) Taxonomic sampling, phylogenetic accuracy, and investigator bias. Syst Biol 47: 3–8.

13. Lemmon AR, Milinkovitch MC (2002) The metapopulation genetic algorithm: An efficient solution for the problem of large phylogeny estimation. Proc Natl Acad Sci U S A 99: 10516–10521.

14. Klungthong C, Putnak R, Mammen MP, Li T, Zhang C (2008) Molecular genotyping of dengue viruses by phylogenetic analysis of the sequences of individual genes. J Virol Methods 154: 175–181.

15. Wu W, Bai Z, Zhou H, Tu Z, Fang M, et al. (2011) Molecular epidemiology of dengue viruses in southern China from 1978 to 2006. Virol J 8: 322.

16. Jiang L, Wu X, Wu Y, Bai Z, Jing Q, et al. (2013) Molecular epidemiological and virological study of dengue virus infections in Guangzhou, China, during 2001–2010. Virol J 10: 4.

17. Jiang LY, Cao YM, Xu Y, Jing QL, Cao Q, et al. (2012) Epidemiological situation and the E gene evolution of dengue virus in Guangzhou, 2011. Zhonghua Liu Xing Bing Xue Za Zhi 33: 1273–1275.

18. Mohammed MA, Galbraith SE, Radford AD, Dove W, Takasaki T, et al. (2011) Molecular phylogenetic and evolutionary analyses of Muar strain of Japanese encephalitis virus reveal it is the missing fifth genotype. Infect Genet Evol 11: 855–862.

19. Tang WF, Ogawa M, Eshita Y, Aono H, Makino Y (2010) Molecular evolution of Japanese encephalitis virus isolates from swine in Oita, Japan during 1980–2009. Infect Genet Evol 10: 329–336.

20. Carney J, Daly JM, Nisalak A, Solomon T (2012) Recombination and positive selection identified in complete genome sequences of Japanese encephalitis virus. Arch Virol 157: 75–83.

21. Davis CT, Ebel GD, Lanciotti RS, Brault AC, Guzman H, et al. (2005) Phylogenetic analysis of North American West Nile virus isolates, 2001–2004: evidence for the emergence of a dominant genotype. Virology 342: 252–265.

22. Grinev A, Daniel S, Stramer S, Rossmann S, Caglioti S, et al. (2008) Genetic variability of West Nile virus in US blood donors, 2002–2005. Emerg Infect Dis 14: 436–444.

23. Herring BL, Bernardin F, Caglioti S, Stramer S, Tobler L, et al. (2007) Phylogenetic analysis of WNV in North American blood donors during the 2003–2004 epidemic seasons. Virology 363: 220–228.

24. May FJ, Davis CT, Tesh RB, Barrett AD (2011) Phylogeography of West Nile virus: from the cradle of evolution in Africa to Eurasia, Australia, and the Americas. J Virol 85: 2964–2974.

25. Sotelo E, Fernandez-Pinero J, Llorente F, Aguero M, Hoefle U, et al. (2009) Characterization of West Nile virus isolates from Spain: new insights into the distinct West Nile virus eco-epidemiology in the Western Mediterranean. Virology 395: 289–297.

26. Zehender G, Ebranati E, Bernini F, Lo PA, Rezza G, et al. (2011) Phylogeography and epidemiological history of West Nile virus genotype 1a in Europe and the Mediterranean basin. Infect Genet Evol 11: 646–653.

27. Wang C, Yang W, Fan J, Wang F, Jiang B, et al. (2013) Spatial and Temporal Patterns of Dengue in Guangdong Province of China. Asia Pac J Public Health.

28. Li Z, Yin W, Clements A, Williams G, Lai S, et al. (2012) Spatiotemporal analysis of indigenous and imported dengue fever cases in Guangdong province, China. BMC Infect Dis 12: 132.

29. Kosakovsky PS, Posada D, Gravenor MB, Woelk CH, Frost SD (2006) Automated phylogenetic detection of recombination using a genetic algorithm. Mol Biol Evol 23: 1891–1901.

30. Rodriguez-Roche R, Villegas E, Cook S, Poh KP, Hinojosa Y, et al. (2012) Population structure of the dengue viruses, Aragua, Venezuela, 2006–2007. Insights into dengue evolution under hyperendemic transmission. Infect Genet Evol 12: 332–344.

31. Anoop M, Mathew AJ, Jayakumar B, Issac A, Nair S, et al. (2012) Complete genome sequencing and evolutionary analysis of dengue virus serotype 1 isolates from an outbreak in Kerala, South India. Virus Genes 45: 1–13.

32. Anez G, Morales-Betoulle ME, Rios M (2011) Circulation of different lineages of dengue virus type 2 in Central America, their evolutionary time-scale and selection pressure analysis. PLoS One 6: e27459.

33. Jiang L, Wu X, Wu Y, Bai Z, Jing Q, et al. (2013) Molecular epidemiological and virological study of dengue virus infections in Guangzhou, China, during 2001–2010. Virol J 10: 4.

34. Klungthong C, Zhang C, Mammen MJ, Ubol S, Holmes EC (2004) The molecular epidemiology of dengue virus serotype 4 in Bangkok, Thailand. Virology 329: 168–179.

35. Sabchareon A, Sirivichayakul C, Limkittikul K, Chanthavanich P, Suvanna-dabba S, et al. (2012) Dengue infection in children in Ratchaburi, Thailand: a cohort study. I. Epidemiology of symptomatic acute dengue infection in children, 2006–2009. PLoS Negl Trop Dis 6: e1732.

36. AbuBakar S, Wong PF, Chan YF (2002) Emergence of dengue virus type 4 genotype IIA in Malaysia. J Gen Virol 83: 2437–2442.

37. Klein DE, Choi JL, Harrison SC (2013) Structure of a dengue virus envelope protein late-stage fusion intermediate. J Virol 87: 2287–2293.

38. Avirutnan P, Punyadee N, Noisakran S, Komoltri C, Thiemmeca S, et al. (2006) Vascular leakage in severe dengue virus infections: a potential role for the nonstructural viral protein NS1 and complement. J Infect Dis 193: 1078–1088.

39. Sun DS, King CC, Huang HS, Shih YL, Lee CC, et al. (2007) Antiplatelet autoantibodies elicited by dengue virus non-structural protein 1 cause thrombocytopenia and mortality in mice. J Thromb Haemost 5: 2291–2299.

40. Benarroch D, Selisko B, Locatelli GA, Maga G, Romette JL, et al. (2004) The RNA helicase, nucleotide 5′-triphosphatase, and RNA 5′-triphosphatase activities of Dengue virus protein NS3 are Mg^{2+}-dependent and require a functional Walker B motif in the helicase catalytic core. Virology 328: 208–218.

15

A Meta-Analysis of the Diagnostic Accuracy of Two Commercial NS1 Antigen ELISA Tests for Early Dengue Virus Detection

Vivaldo G. da Costa*, Ariany C. Marques-Silva, Marcos L. Moreli*

Virology Laboratory, Federal University of Goiás, Jataí, Brazil

Abstract

Background: Dengue virus (DENV) NS1 antigen detection is regarded as an early diagnostic marker. Accordingly, several studies have evaluated the performance of tests that utilize NS1 capture, but the results of individual studies may be limited due to the restricted sample size of the patients recruited. Therefore, our objective was to perform a meta-analysis of the diagnostic accuracy of two commercial NS1 ELISAs (Panbio and Platelia).

Methods and Results: Studies of interest were found in PubMed, Embase and Google Scholar databases using defined inclusion/exclusion criteria. A total of 30 studies containing 12,105 total enrolled patients were included. The results were as follows: 1) Panbio assays showed low overall performance, sensitivity 66% (95% confidence interval (CI) 61–71), specificity 99% (95% CI 96–100), positive likelihood ratio (LR+) 98 (95% CI 20–464), negative likelihood ratio (LR-) 0.3 (95% CI 0.2–0.4), diagnostic odds ratio (DOR) 289 (95% CI 59–1412); 2) Platelia assays showed high overall performance, sensitivity 74% (95% CI 63–82), specificity 99% (95% CI 97–100), LR+ 175 (95% CI 28–1099), LR- 0.3 (95% CI 0.2–0.4), DOR 663 (95% CI 98–4478). The lowest sensitivity values were for secondary infections (57% [95% CI 47–67] and 66% [95% CI 53–77] for Panbio and Platelia, respectively) and for the detection of DENV4. Regarding clinical manifestations, the sensitivity of Platelia was 69% (95% CI 43–86) and 60% (95% CI 48–70) for fever and dengue hemorrhagic fever, respectively. In addition, the sensitivity of both tests was slightly lower for samples from Southeast Asia and Oceania.

Conclusion: DENV1 samples gave higher sensitivity results for both tests. We observed that factors negatively influencing the tests, such as the type of infection, geographical origins of samples and viral serotypes, require further investigation to optimize the diagnostic accuracy.

Editor: Ana Fernandez-Sesma, Icahn School of Medicine at Mount Sinai, United States of America

Funding: This study was supported by grant no. 201310267000308 from the Fundação de Amparo à Pesquisa do Estado de Goiás (FAPEG). VGC received fellowship from FAPEG. The funders had no role in study design, data collection and analysis, decision to publish, or preparation of the manuscript.

Competing Interests: The authors have declared that no competing interests exist.

* E-mail: vivbiom@gmail.com (VGC); mlmoreli@jatai.ufg.br (MLM)

Introduction

Dengue is a pandemic disease that has been neglected but is reemerging, putting approximately three billion people in tropical and subtropical regions at risk of this viral infection [1,2]. Therefore, dengue poses a major threat to the public health systems of many countries, considering the occurrence of millions of cases and thousands of deaths annually [3].

Dengue virus (DENV), genus *Flavivirus*, is antigenically classified into four serotypes (DENV1-4). DENV is an arbovirus (Arthropod-borne virus) and is increasingly infecting humans, with the incidence of dengue showing a 30-fold increase within the last 50 years [3–6]. Dengue disease results in a wide clinical spectrum with undifferentiated febrile symptoms, hindering early diagnosis and clinical management. Thus, DENV infections can be asymptomatic or present as the classical clinical picture of dengue fever (DF). In revised WHO classification system (2009), DF was divided into dengue with or without warning signs and severe dengue. We will use the classification into DF/dengue hemor-

rhagic fever (DHF)/or dengue shock syndrome (DSS), since it continues to be widely used [2,7].

Laboratory techniques involved in the diagnosis of DENV are based on the detection of viral genetic material, the specific detection of IgG/IgM antibodies and the detection of viral antigens, such as nonstructural protein 1 (NS1) [8–10]. NS1 is a glycoprotein that is abundantly produced by viruses in the early stages of infection, and it is found within the infected cells, in the cell membranes and secreted into the extracellular spaces [11,12]. Therefore, one advantage of laboratory methods that perform NS1 antigen capture is the precocity of this marker, present at the onset of symptoms, in contrast to IgM, which is detected later, beginning at the fifth day of disease.

Currently, several laboratory methods that use the capture of DENV NS1 antigen are available [13–17]. The successful implementation of these methods reflects on the good performance of these tests. Despite the existence of several studies evaluating tests for an NS1 capture ELISA assay, no meta-analysis evaluating the diagnostic accuracy of these commercial kits has been performed. Due to the limited sample size of patients recruited in individual studies, meta-analysis may increase the accuracy of estimates of individual studies. Therefore, we conducted a meta-analysis of the accuracy of diagnosis for Panbio NS1 and Platelia NS1 ELISA assay kits to obtain the overall estimated and summarized performance of the tests in the detection of DENV.

Materials and Methods

Search strategy

This meta-analysis was guided by the standard PRISMA protocol (Preferred Reporting Items for Systematic reviews and Meta-analysis (Table S1)) and methods proposed by the Cochrane Collaboration [18,19]. PubMed; Embase and Google Scholar databases were searched for articles using a combination of descriptors to select the studies of interest.

Study selection

After finding previously published studies in the databases with the descriptors "dengue" OR "dengue virus" AND "diagnosis" OR "ELISA NS1" OR "early diagnostic" OR "diagnostic accuracy" OR "performance test", we performed an analysis on the inclusion/exclusion criteria.

As inclusion criteria, we used studies that evaluated the sensitivity and specificity parameters of ELISA kits involving the capture of dengue NS1 antigen and the Panbio (Alere, Brisbane, Australia) or Platelia (Marnes-la-Coquette, France; Hercules, CA, USA (Bio-Rad)) kits.

As exclusion criteria, we did not review studies that were not published in English, Spanish or Portuguese or studies with limited information for calculating sensitivity and specificity. We excluded specific articles types, for instance review articles, comments, the editorial, letters and conference abstract. Additionally, two authors reviewed the studies independently, in case of disagreement a third author was consulted.

Data extraction

The following data from each study included in the meta-analysis were extracted: author, year of publication, place of study, gender, age and number of participants, method of diagnosis, study design, sensitivity and specificity data, positive predictive value (PPV) and negative predictive value (NPV). The data to be extracted were analyzed in the following subgroups: classification of infection, viral serotype, period of the collection of samples, geographic origin of patients and clinical picture presented. Subsequently, the data related to the accuracy of the diagnosis were plotted on a 2×2 contingency table.

Quality assessment

The analysis of the quality of the studies was performed based on a tool known as the quality assessment of diagnostic accuracy studies (QUADAS), which allows for the identification of important design elements in diagnostic accuracy studies [20]. The QUADAS tool consists of 14 key items (sufficient test description and reference, representative spectrum, reported withdrawals and indeterminate results, relevant clinical information, index test results blinded, definition positive test result, cutoff values, complete verification of diagnosis, avoided clinical review bias, appropriate selection and reference standard, and acceptable detail between tests). Items are evaluated using a score of "low", "high", or "obscure", which are formulated for an answer as "no", "yes" and "unclear", respectively, that may indicate low or high risk of publication bias. Each of 14 items was scored from 1 to 0, with a total quality score between 11 and 14 was considered

"good", between 7 and 10, "moderate", and 6 or less was considered "poor".

Statistical analysis

STATA IC/64 software (version 13.1, College Station, TX) with MIDAS and METANDI commands was used for the meta-analysis. For correction in the cells containing zero values, correction factors from METANDI commands were used.

The sensitivity (true positive rate), specificity (true negative rate), positive likelihood ratio and negative (LR+, or LR-, is estimated by the ratio of the proportion of positive, or negative, tests in the diseased versus no-diseased subjects) and diagnostic odds ratio (DOR is calculated as the LR+ divided by the LR-), with a confidence interval (CI) of 95%, were obtained for each study and subsequently combined. Cochran Q chi-square test and the I^2 statistic were explored to assess the heterogeneity of the included studies. Random-effects model was used if the result of the Q test was significant ($p < 0.05$) and $I^2 > 50\%$. The meta-regression was planned to be used if there was high heterogeneity ($I^2 > 50\%$) [21]. Additionally, an hierarchical summary receiver operating characteristic (HSROC) type curve of the selected studies was then plotted with the software. The HSROC curve is a bivariate model that provides information on the overall performance of a test through different thresholds. We also constructed the summary receiver operating characteristics (SROC) curve and the respective area under the curve that serves a global measure of the test performance [22].

To assess potential publication bias, we used the Deeks funnel plot, with $p < 0.05$ indicating the presence of publication bias [23]. Fagan nomograms, a two-dimensional graphical tool for estimating how much the result of a diagnostic test changes the probability that a patient has a disease, was also used to estimate the clinical value of the index test, which is based on the LR+ and LR- obtained from the meta-analysis [24].

Results

Our search found 672 citations related to dengue through the combined application of descriptors in the three databases described above. During the final stage of selection, we excluded five studies that only assessed the sensitivity of laboratory methods or did the overlap the results of the two tests in their analysis [13-17]. After the exclusion criteria were applied, 30 baseline studies remained [25-54], which were included in our meta-analysis because they involved experimental research evaluating the diagnostic accuracy of the Panbio or Platelia kits, which used NS1 antigen capture in an indirect ELISA format. The results of our literature search are shown in Figure 1.

Among the studies included in the meta-analysis, there were a total of 12,105 patients recruited. These patient samples were collected from 17 countries in Latin America, Asia and Oceania, and the most studies were conducted in Brazil (27%) [29,34,37,41,45,47,52,54], Vietnam (13%) [32,33,36,49], Malaysia (13%) [26,36,42,46] and Thailand (13%) [31,36,43,48]. Regarding the design of the studies, they were classified into two types: prospective and retrospective cohorts, of which only twelve reported that their samples were collected during dengue outbreaks [25,26,30,37,39,40,44,45,51-54]. Typically, most samples were collected until the sixth day of the onset of symptoms [25,27,28,30-37,40-42,47,49,50,52-54]. The data extracted from the final selection are shown in Table 1.

The QUADAS tool consists of 14 items, and the results of the analysis can be seen in Figure 2. The quality of all studies was generally moderate, with median QUADAS score of 9 (Table S2).

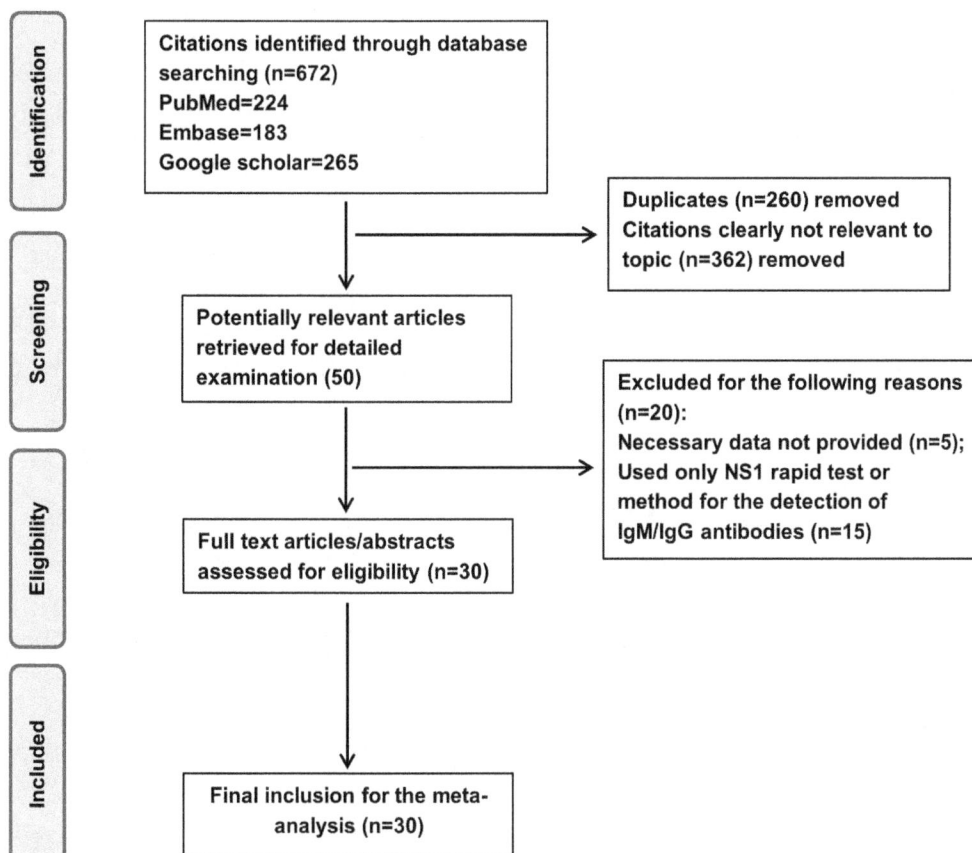

Figure 1. Flowchart of the steps performed in the meta-analysis.

However, the items related to the determination of the indeterminate results, including relevant clinical information (classification DF or DHF) and disclosure of the cut-off and blinding of samples before processing by laboratory tests, were evaluated items that presented more risk of bias. Additionally, the Deeks funnel plot did not show potential publication bias for the two subgroups of studies (p = 0.56 and p = 0.09) (Figure S1), yet a significant amount of heterogeneity were detected for the two tests (I^2 ranged from 85% to 97%). Meta-regression showed that the covariates, origin of the samples, period of sample collection and retrospective *versus* prospective samples were items that contributed to diversity among studies (Table S3).

Overall accuracy of the Panbio and Platelia commercial kits

Among the selected studies, 16 assessed the trials of Panbio [27,28,30,35–41,45,47,48,50–52] and 23 assessed the trials of Platelia [25–27,29–39,42–44,46,47,49,50,53,54]. In relation to Panbio, the sensitivity, specificity, LR+, LR- and DOR overall were 66% (95% CI 61–71), 99% (95% CI 96–100), 98 (95% CI 19–367), 0.3 (95% CI 0.2–0.4) and 289 (95% CI 59–1412), respectively. Similarly, the values for Platelia were 74% (95% CI 63–82), 99% (95% CI 97–100), 175 (95% CI 28–1099), 0.3 (95% CI 0.2–0.4) and 663 (95% CI 98–4478), respectively. The area under summary ROC curve were 0.84 (95% CI 0.80–0.87 (Panbio)) and 0.96 (95% CI 0.94–0.97 (Platelia)) (Figure S2) and the graphs of the HSROC curves of the individual studies for the

diagnostic accuracy of two tests analyzed are shown in Figure 3A–B.

Accuracy of the tests on the viral serotype and classification of infection

When evaluating the accuracy of tests for sensitivity, DOR, LR+ and LR- for serotype DENV1, we obtained the following values: 81% (95% CI 73–87), 702 (95% CI 101–4842), 136 (95% CI 23–806) and 0.2 (95% CI 0.1–0.3), respectively, for Panbio. Similarly, the values for Platelia were 90% (95% CI 81–95), 5460 (95% CI 131-225878), 526 (95% CI 12-21602) and 0.09 (95% CI 0.04–0.19).

For DENV2, pooled sensitivity was 74% (95% CI 67–80), DOR was 507 (95% CI 55–4663), LR+ and LR- were 133 (95% CI 17-1023) and 0.3 (95% CI 0.2–0.4), respectively, for Panbio. In Platelia, pooled sensitivity was 73.3% (95% CI 61–83), DOR was 714 (95% CI 37-13466), LR+ and LR- were 191 (95% CI 12-3090) and 0.26 (95% CI 0.17–0.4), respectively.

For DENV3, pooled sensitivity was 70.7% (95% CI 63–78), DOR was 481 (95% CI 33-6869), LR+ and LR- were 141 (95% CI 11-1780) and 0.3 (95% CI 0.2–0.4), respectively, for Panbio. In Platelia, pooled sensitivity was 83% (95% CI 75–89), DOR was 2353 (95% CI 72-7e+4), LR+ and LR- were 397 (95% CI 12-13119) and 0.16 (95% CI 0.11–0.25), respectively.

For DENV4, pooled sensitivity was 37% (95% CI 26–50), DOR was 18 (95% CI 6–63), LR+ and LR- were 12 (95% CI 4–38) and 0.6 (95% CI 0.5–0.8), respectively, for Panbio. In Platelia, pooled sensitivity was 58% (95% CI 30–81), DOR was 96848 (95% CI

Table 1. Summary of the included studies.

Ref.	Study Design	Location	Sample (n)	Sex	Median Age, y	Results PANBIO Sen.% (95% CI)	Spec.% (95% CI)	PPV% (95% CI)	NPV% (95% CI)	Results PLATELIA Sen.% (95% CI)	Spec.% (95% CI)	PPV% (95% CI)	NPV% (95% CI)	Dengue prevalence (%)	Diagnostic method
25	Cohort, prospective	French Guiana	349	Female 75%	33					88.7 (84–92.4)	100 (84.9–100)	89.8	100	72	ELISA; RT-PCR; VI
26	Cohort, retrospective	Malaysia	354	NR	NR					93.4	100	100	98.9	37.5	ELISA; RT-PCR; VI
27	NR	Puerto Rico	253	NR	NR	64.9 (58.2–71.1)	97.8 (88.4–99.6)	100 (97.2–100)	39.3 (30.7–48.5)	83.2 (77.5–87.7)	100 (92.1–100)	100 (97.2–100)	62.5 (51–72.8)	82	ELISA; Real time RT-PCR; VI
28	Cohort, prospective	Laos	92	NR	NR	63.2 (53.4–73)	100	100	79.4 (71.2–87.7)					41	ELISA; RT-PCR
29	Cohort, prospective	Brazil	250	Male 58%	35					85.4	94	81	95.6	32	ELISA; Real time RT-PCR; VI
30	Cohort, retrospective	French Guiana	320	NR	NR	55.1 (49–61.2)	97.9 (88.9–99.9)	75.2	98	82.4 (77.3–86.7)	100 (92.6–100)	100	100	69	ELISA; ICG; RT-PCR; VI
31	Cohort, prospective	Thailand	235	Male 56.2%	17.8					63.2 (55.7–70)	98.4 (91.7–99.7)	99	52.5	72.8	ELISA; RT-PCR; VI
32	Cohort, prospective	Vietnam	138	Male 44.9%	16					83.2 (75.5–89.3)	100 (86.7–100)	100 (97.2–100)	38.2 (22.2–56.4)	90	ELISA; RT-PCR
33	NR	Vietnam	459	Male 55%	18.3					37	99.5	90.9	92.2	12	ELISA; RT-PCR
34	Cohort, prospective	Brazil	92	NR	NR					70 (59–79.2)	100 (54.1–100)	100 (94–100)	18.7 (7.2–36.4)	93	ELISA; Real time RT-PCR
35	NR	Venezuela	147	NR	NR	60.9 (50.4–70.5)	94.4 (80.9–99.4)	100	41.4	71.3 (61–80)	86.1 (70.9–94.4)	100	49	59	ELISA; ICG; RT-PCR; VI
36	Cohort, prospective	M	2259	NR	NR	52	90	76.2	90	66	100	82.3	100	76	ELISA; RT-PCR; VI
37	Cohort, retrospective	Brazil	450	NR	NR	72	100	100	78	84	99	98	86	49	ELISA; RT-PCR; VI
38	Cohort, retrospective	Colombia	310	NR	NR	71.1 (64.6–77)	89.1 (80.9–94.7)	94 (89.1–97.1)	56.6 (48.1–64.8)	70.8 (64.1–76.8)	92.3 (84.8–96.9)	95.5 (91–98.2)	57.5 (49.1–65.7)	70	ELISA; RT-PCR; VI
39	Cohort, prospective	Singapore	433	NR	NR	67 (57.3–75.7)	100 (96.4–100)	100 (96.4–100)	73.5 (64.3–81.4)	81.7 (73.1–88.4)	100 (96.4–100)	100 (96.4–100)	83.3 (75.3–88.2)	37	ELISA; ICG; RT-PCR
40	Cohort, prospective	India	2070	NR	NR	61.4	100	100	100					41	ELISA; RT-PCR;
41	Cohort, prospective	Brazil	86	Female 62.5%	27	50 (29.9–70.1)	100 (94–100)	66	84.8					30	ELISA; RT-PCR; VI
42	Cohort, prospective	Malaysia; China; India	558	Male 62%	26					91.6	100	92.3	95.8	34	ELISA; Real time RT-PCR; VI
43	Cohort, prospective	Thailand	85	NR	NR					76.4	100 (82.8–100)	100	62	65	ELISA; ICG; VI

Table 1. Cont.

Ref.	Study Design	Location	Sample (n)	Sex	Median Age, y	Results[PANBIO] Sen.% (95% CI)	Spec.% (95% CI)	PPV% (95% CI)	NPV% (95% CI)	Results[PLATELIA] Sen.% (95% CI)	Spec.% (95% CI)	PPV% (95% CI)	NPV% (95% CI)	Dengue prevalence (%)	Diagnostic method
44	Cohort, prospective	Cambodia	339	Female 52.3%	4					57.7 (51.4–63.8)	100	100	41.8 (34.7–49.2)	72	ELISA; RT-PCR; VI
45	Cohort, retrospective	Brazil	450	NR	NR	80	100	100	100					51	ELISA; RT-PCR; VI
46	NR	Malaysia	208	NR	NR					83.7	90.4	86	95	38	ELISA; RT-PCR
47	Cohort, prospective	Brazil	147	NR	NR	87.5	71	68	85	95	47	58	92	47	ELISA; ICG; HI
48	NR	Thailand-Myanmar	162	Male 60.5%	23	54.6 (42–66)	100 (96–100)	100 (91–100)	73.2 (64.4–80.8)					44	ELISA; Real time RT-PCR
49	Cohort, prospective	Vietnam	116	NR	NR					64.7 (54.5–74.9)	95.8 (87.8–100)	73.9	96	82	ELISA; RT-PCR
50	Cohort, retrospective	Thailand	626	NR	NR	44.8 (38–51)	93.2 (88–97)	87.5	92.5	56.5 (50–63)	100 (98–100)	84	100	71	ELISA; RT-PCR; HI
51	Cohort, prospective	Indonesia	503	NR	NR	56.4	100	100	43					42	ELISA; RT-PCR; VI
52	Cohort, prospective	Brazil	220	NR	NR	82	91	85	89					31	ELISA; RT-PCR
53	Cohort, retrospective	Indonesia	275	Male 68%	30.7					46.8 (40.2–53.3)	100	100	32	80	ELISA; RT-PCR;
54	Cohort, prospective	Brazil	119	NR	NR					0	100	0	51	49	ELISA; RT-PCR; VI

Abbreviations: Ref, Reference studies; y, year; Sen., Sensitivity; Spec., Specificity; NR, Not reported; M, Multicenter; HI, Hemagglutination inhibition; ICG, Immunochromatographic; VI, Virus isolation.

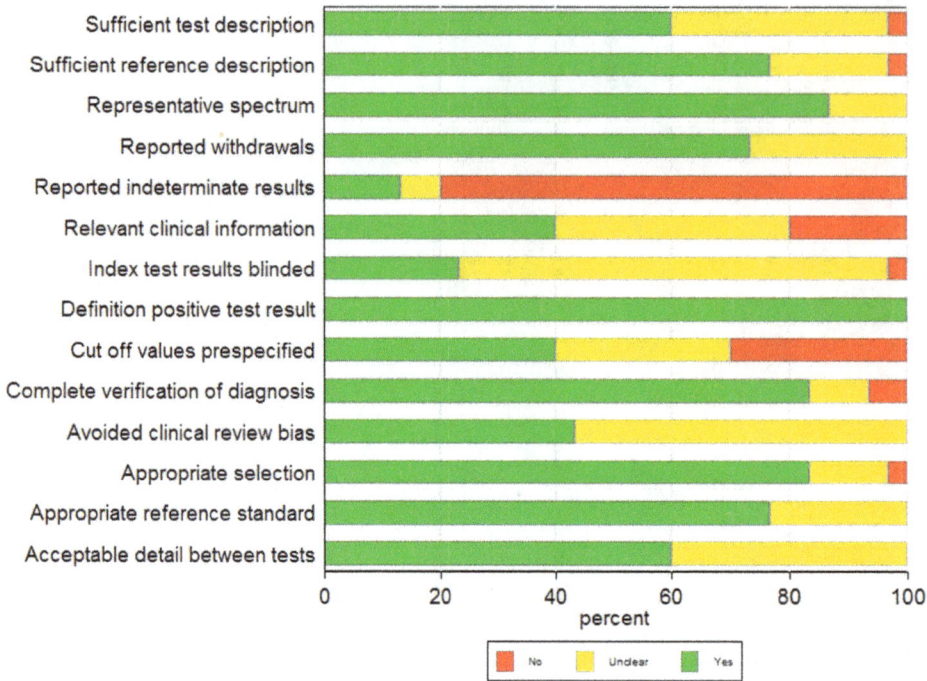

Figure 2. The assessment of methodological quality items shown for all included studies. Proportions of studies rated as "yes", "no", or "unclear" for each QUADAS item.

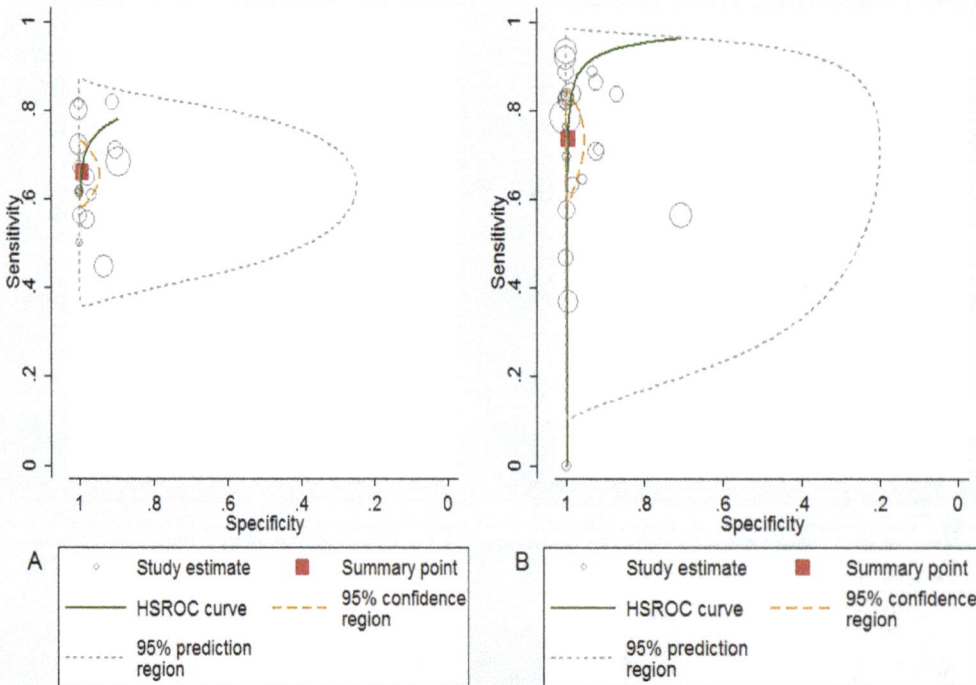

Figure 3. HSROC plot displaying diagnostic accuracy results of included studies. Panbio (A) and Platelia (B) kits. The circle diameter (study estimate) is proportional to the weight given to each study. Summary sensitivity and specificity is marked by a red square.

14–6e+8), LR+ and LR- were 41006 (95% CI 6–3e+8) and 0.4 (95% CI 0.2–0.8), respectively.

Regarding the classification of dengue primary or secondary infection types, the following global estimates for primary infection were obtained for the parameters of sensitivity, DOR, LR+ and LR-: 75% (95% CI 66–82.5), 7114 (95% CI 18–2e+6), 1761 (95% CI 5-601666) and 0.24 (95% CI 0.17–0.34), respectively, for Panbio, and 94.6% (95% CI 91–97), 2036 (95% CI 341–12130), 110 (95% CI 23–518) and 0.05 (95% CI 0.03–0.09), respectively, for Platelia. For secondary infection, these laboratory indices were 57% (95% CI 47–67), 3443 (95% CI 12–9e+5), 1484 (95% CI 6–4e+5) and 0.4 (95% CI 0.3–0.5), respectively, for Panbio, and 66% (95% CI 53–77), 632 (95% CI 47–8374), 216 (95% CI 13–3453) and 0.3 (95% CI 0.2–0.5), respectively, for Platelia.

Accuracy of the tests regarding clinical manifestations of dengue

To verify whether patients with moderate clinical forms (DF) or severe dengue (DHF/DSS) showed significant variations in the performance of the tests, we performed a global estimate of the accuracy of the tests. In this case, only Platelia was used for laboratory evaluation of the different clinical forms of the patients. Only five studies performed this calculation, with forest plot of sensitivity showing values that ranged from 25% to 95%

(Figure 4A–B). The pooled sensitivity was 69% (95% CI 43–86) and 60% (95% CI 48–70) for DF (A) and DHF (B), respectively.

DOR and post-test probability

The DOR is commonly considered a global measure of test performance that summarizes the diagnostic accuracy of the index test as a single number that describes how many times greater the chance is of getting a positive result in a person with the disease than in someone without the disease. As described above, the values of DOR were considerably high due to the high values of sensitivity and principally of the specificity observed in this study. In this case, a function of DOR plotted on the graph would present an exponential behavior, rising abruptly and presenting a clear positive correlation with the sensitivity and specificity [55,56].

To obtain the post-test probability, we used Fagan's nomogram for which we performed a simulation of an environment that had a prevalence of 37% for dengue disease, with base on the studies selected. Thus, the probability in this model of someone having the disease and not being detected by the NS1 Panbio ELISA test was 17%. In the same situation for the NS1 Platelia ELISA test, a negative result was associated with 13% of individuals with the disease (Figure 5A–B). In contrast, the post-test probability of sick patients with a positive test was 98% and 99%, respectively, for

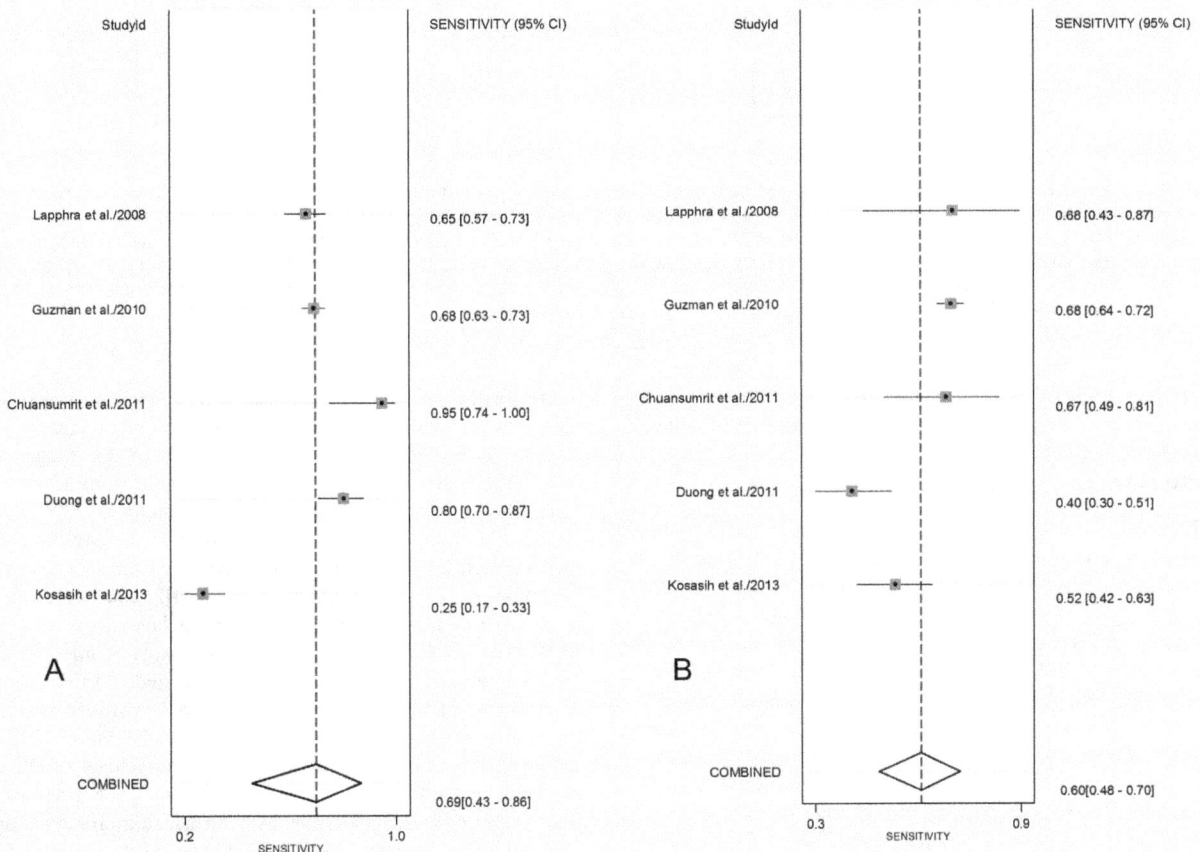

Figure 4. Forest plot of the sensitivity of Platelia kit. Forest plot of the sensitivity of each study and pooled sensitivity for studies that distinguished clinical features of patients infected with DENV into DF (A) and DHF (B). The sensitivity is represented by the circles in squares and the horizontal lines represent the point estimate (95% CI for each included study). Diamonds represent the pooled estimate (95% CI).

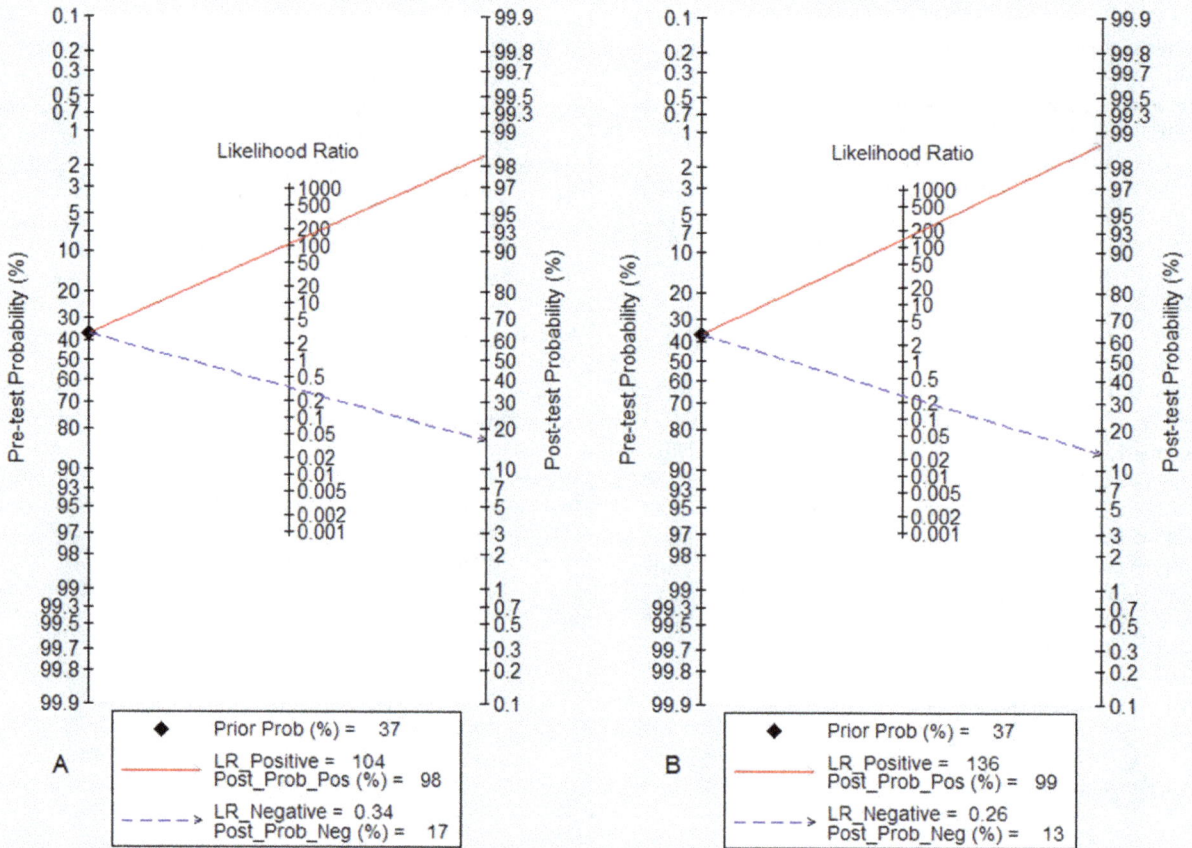

Figure 5. Fagan's nomogram for the calculation of post-test probabilities. A pre-test probability of 37% for dengue disease was fixed, which was estimated by the number of symptomatic cases in selected studies. (A) Panbio had a post-test probability of 98%. For Platelia kits (B) post-test probability was 99%, ie, with an estimated prevalence of 37%, if this patient tests positive, the post-test probability that she truly has dengue would be 99% (solid line in red). On the other hand, if patient tests negative, the post-test probability that she truly has dengue would be 17% (A) or 13% (B) (blue dotted line). The results were obtained by the following calculations: pretest odds = prevalence/1-prevalence; post-test odds = pretest odds x LR- (LR+); post-test probability = post-test odds/1+post-test odds. LR, likelihood ratio.

Panbio and Platelia. Thus, showing that these tests specifically capture the NS1 antigen is important in the diagnosis of dengue.

Discussion

The studies included in this meta-analysis had a global sensitivity and specificity ranging from 45% to 100% and 71% to 100%, respectively, for Panbio and ranging from 0% to 95% and from 47% to 100%, respectively, for Platelia. When we performed an overall estimate of sensitivity, a superiority of Platelia (74% [95% CI 63–82]) over Panbio (66% [95% CI 61–71]) was detected. With respect to this increased sensitivity of the former test, there are no hypotheses explaining this outcome, but it has been observed that viral serotype can influence the accuracy of the test, thereby changing the sensitivity and resulting in both the Panbio and Platelia tests having higher sensitivity for DENV1. However, there were more participants with DENV1 included for analysis using the Platelia test [25,27,28,30,35–37,39,44,47,53], a fact that may have influenced the overall estimate, although our results are similar to the scientific literature, which demonstrates a higher sensitivity for Platelia.

Our findings in relation to the sensitivity of the tests against viral serotypes are partially consistent with the scientific literature, with a lower sensitivity observed for both tests (37% for Panbio and 58% for Platelia) for DENV4. However, some studies have also reported a lower sensitivity for Platelia for DENV2 [30,35,36,47,50]. The low accuracy of the Panbio during an epidemic of DENV4 and Platelia were recently analyzed by Colombo et al. [52] and Sea et al. [54], who observed the occurrence of false negatives. It is not yet known why the NS1 ELISA has a lower sensitivity in the patients infected with DENV4, but some hypotheses can be postulated: (i) there could be quantitative differences in the secreted NS1 form, depending on the viral serotype, which may lead to less availability of NS1 and reduced chances of detection, (ii) the higher incidence of DENV4 in secondary infections, and (iii) there could be presence of polymorphism in the NS1 gene associated with immune epitopes. However, these speculations require additional studies to confirm them.

In silico analysis using the Virus Pathogen Resource software (ViPR: www.viprbrc.org) to assess the degree of variability of the NS1 protein of DENV1-4 serotypes of the complete sequences from Asia (1466 strains) *versus* South America (476 strains) revealed the existence of significant variability between NS1 sequences. At least 83 amino acid positions were identified (Table S4). However, in the known consensus NS1 region "[111]LRYSWKTWGKA[121]" [57], there was only one polymorphism (replacing R with K at position 112) in DENV4; this polymorphism was found in 23 strains from South America and Asia. Thus, it appears that this polymorphism is not the main factor influencing the test but will be important for understanding whether external variant amino acids can have some influence on the immune epitope.

The detection and semi-quantitation of NS1 is proportional to the optical density (OD) measured at 450/620 nm [10]. The kits that were analysed determine the cut off by the average and standard deviations of the OD values from calibrators and the values are expressed in scales that can be interpreted as negative, indeterminate or positive. The calibration curve for the detection of NS1 is obtained by comparing different dilutions of the antigen, and the resulting values are expressed in OD units, as measured using an ELISA reader. Accordingly, Young et al. [12] calculated the linear portion of the standard curve to determine the serum NS1 concentration, obtaining a minimum threshold of 4 ng/ml. If there are quantitative differences in the secretion of NS1, depending on the different DENV serotypes, this could reduce the sensitivity of the test when certain dilutions are made. Indeed, if NS1 DENV4 is present in smaller amounts, it would be interesting to increase the detection test by obtaining a new calibration curve with lower dilutions of the test samples.

The determination of dengue diagnosis only with clinical and epidemiological data may result in errors [58,59]. To circumvent this problem, a laboratory diagnosis is crucial for correct identification. One of the main benefits of laboratory methods is to allow the screening of patients suspected of such diseases to implement the most appropriate clinical management and to provide greater efficiency of the epidemiological surveillance system. The epidemiological surveillance systems are important in the control of outbreaks, as in cases of dengue, where movement of a new serotype of DENV often proceeds to epidemic proportions. The constant occurrence of dengue outbreaks can result in a higher incidence of secondary infections, which are positively correlated with a higher risk of DSS [60]. In this context, a lower sensitivity in patients with secondary infections was found for both analyzed tests, a fact that is worrisome because it would be useful to have a better test accuracy at this stage, due to the possibility of these patients progressing to more severe forms of the disease.

The "original antigenic sin" proposed by Sabin (1952) notes that, in successive infections by DENV, antibody memory may confer only transient protection against heterologous serotype infections, so that antibodies generated in secondary infections would be more effective in the neutralizing the viral serotype that caused the primary infection instead of the secondary one. The overall assessment of the sensitivity of both kits indicated that it was considered elevated in patients with primary infection (77% Panbio; 95.5% Platelia). In contrast, in secondary infections, there was a loss of sensitivity for both kits (24% for Panbio and 31% for Platelia). It is likely that this is due to the increased supply of antibodies, although weakly neutralizing [61], binding to the NS1 antigen. Accordingly, to increase the sensitivity of the tests, complex NS1 antibodies are separated by treatment of the test samples with acid [62]. Although this method has improved the sensitivity of the tests, only one study [31] among the ten that distinguished the types of infections [26,28,29,32,37,39,45,51,53] performed this step to dissociate antigen and antibody.

We conducted an overall estimate of the sensitivity of the kits correlated with the geographic origin of patients. The tests had a slight better accuracy for samples from Latin America, with values of 70% (95% CI 63–76 [Panbio]) and 80% (95% CI 75–85 [Platelia]), while these rates for patients who were from Southeast Asia and Oceania were 59% (95% CI 51–66 [Panbio]) and 73% (95% CI 61–82 [Platelia]). From these findings, it cannot be inferred that there were significant differences between geographical origins because even these results differ from the multicenter study conducted by Guzman et al. [36]. We believe that the differences in the sensitivity of the tests are most likely attributed to the process of the epidemiological evolution of DENV serotypes, in which a greater restriction of species from the same geographical region may be the result of the viral ancestral lineage [63]. This theory is supported by a phylogenetic analysis that elucidated the origins and molecular evolution of DENV in different geographic regions of world and showed the high genetic diversity of dengue, in which there are several clusters of different sublineages even within a single genotype [64]. In this context, Watanabe et al. [65], through studies in mice, have found that the secretion of NS1 is dependent on the viral strain. This reinforces the idea that co-circulating viral strains can affect the accuracy of tests that detect the NS1 antigen.

Although we mention above that the observed differences in laboratory parameters, in association with different geographical origins of patients, are mainly due to a process of molecular evolution of DENV, we cannot rule out the influence of the host in these molecular dynamics. In this sense, Mairiang et al. [66] found that there are several interactions between the protein of DENV and human and mosquito hosts. Therefore, there may be an interaction between the genotype of the host and the pathogen (DENV), although this has been demonstrated only in the main dengue vector, *Aedes aegypti* [67]. While the host may influence the molecular dynamics of the evolution of the pathogen, to what extent this influences the pathogen infecting humans in certain geographical regions and how this may affect the laboratory methods used should be defined to improve the performance of assays.

The DOR obtained in this meta-analysis was on average usually greater than 500. In fact, the high variations of values for sensitivity and specificity were also reflected in the DOR, which may vary from zero to infinity with higher values denote a better discriminatory diagnostic test [56]. Additionally, the post-test (Fagan's nomogram) probability was also high (Figure 5A–B), indicating a good clinical utility of the tests, although caution is needed in their interpretation because the samples included in the studies were mostly from symptomatic patients suspected of dengue, which increased the overall rates of prevalence.

In addition to the NS1 ELISA, there are immunochromatographic methods, which are known as rapid tests because results are obtained on average within 30 minutes. Several studies have evaluated the NS1 rapid tests, with sensitivities ranging from 51% to 90% [13–17,38]. So although very good methods for identification of DENV infections exist and are in use, it is prudent to include additional methods whenever possible. We believe that one of the best choices is the combination of NS1 ELISA methods and an NS1 rapid test, along with a method for detection of IgG to increase sensitivity in secondary type infections.

Our meta-analysis had several limitations. First, there are two generations of the Panbio NS1 ELISA, and the latest second-generation kit had a higher sensitivity. Among the analyzed studies, few authors identified the generation of the kits used in their experiments, so our overall estimate of the sensitivity of Panbio could be influenced by this aspect. Second, although the specificity was almost 100%, it should be noted that only a few authors used a different pathological group of dengue, while most used samples from healthy individuals and blood donors. We understand that this happens because of the abundance and ease of obtaining these samples, but it is critical to avoid biases and to test the assays more in relation to other *flavivirus* and similar diseases. Third, only a third of the studies made a distinction between or disclosed the serotypes of DENV. Perhaps this factor, along with precocity of the samples, had a greater influence on the accuracy of tests. Fourth, there was statistically significant heterogeneity across the included studies. In an effort to explore source of heterogeneity, meta-regression revealed that origin, period and retrospective samples might is causing diversity on sensitivity and specificity. Fifth, only a few studies reported that the samples were from primary or secondary infections. Sixth, we used available data to calculate the sensitivity up to the sixth day of blood collection; however, some studies had a period of sample collection lasting until the ninth day of the febrile phase and this factor can also significantly compromise the accuracy of tests. Finally, data were not divided into additional groups based on other variables, such as gender or age, due to the limitations of original information for each patient included in the studies.

In conclusion, despite the above limitations mentioned, this meta-analysis showed a good overall estimate of sensitivity ranging from 66% (95% CI 61–71 [Panbio]) to 74% (95% CI 63–82 [Platelia]). Specificity was near 100% for both kits. The main factors influencing the diagnostic accuracy were the type of infection (primary *versus* secondary), viral serotype, geographical origins of samples and how early the samples were collected. However, to what extent and how these factors affect the diagnostic accuracy require more studies in order to optimize these tests.

Supporting Information

Figure S1 Deek's funnel plot asymmetry test for publication bias. Deek's funnel plot asymmetry test not suggested potential publication bias (p = 0.56 in the Panbio kit (a)), (p = 0.09 in the Platelia kit (b)).

Figure S2 Summary ROC curve plot with sensitivity and specificity for Panbio (A) and Platelia (B). Each large X represents individual study in meta-analysis. Summary operating point is a single sensitivity/specificity point estimated by the results of studies. AUC = area under the curve.
(TIF)

Table S1 PRISMA Checklist.

Table S2 Methodological quality of the 30 included studies.

Table S3 Univariate meta-regression analyses of the sensitivity and specificity.

Table S4 Amino acid positions of NS1 identified with significant variations. The positions and variability were obtained by the crossing of the NS1 strains DENV1-4 from Asia and South America.

Author Contributions

Conceived and designed the experiments: VGC MLM. Performed the experiments: VGC ACMS MLM. Analyzed the data: VGC ACMS. Contributed reagents/materials/analysis tools: VGC. Wrote the paper: VGC.

References

1. Hotez PJ, Bottazzi ME, Franco-Paredes C, Ault SK, Periago MR (2008) The neglected tropical diseases of Latin America and the Caribbean: a review of disease burden and distribution and a roadmap for control and elimination. PLoS Negl Trop Dis 2: e300. doi:10.1371/journal.pntd.0000300. PubMed: 18820747.
2. WHO (2009) Dengue guidelines for diagnosis, treatment, prevention and control. Available: http://whqlibdoc.who.int/publications/2009/9789241547871_eng.pdf. Accessed 2013 December 16.
3. Guzman MG, Halstead SB, Artsob H, Buchy P, Farrar J, et al. (2010) Dengue: a continuing global threat. Nat Rev Microbiol 8: S7–S16. doi: 10.1038/nrmicro2460. PubMed: 21079655.
4. Chambers TJ, Hahn CS, Galler R, Rice CM (1990) Flavivirus genome organization, expression, and replication. Annu Rev Microbiol 10: 649–688. doi: 10.1146/annurev.mi.44.100190.003245. PubMed: 2174669.
5. Phillips ML (2008) Dengue reborn: widespread resurgence of a resilient vector. Environ Health Perspect 116: A382–8. PubMed: 18795135.
6. Tabachnick WJ (2010) Challenges in predicting climate and environmental effects on vector-borne disease episystems in a changing world. J Exp Biol 213: 946–954. doi: 10.1242/jeb.037564. PubMed: 20190119.
7. Martina BE, Koraka P, Osterhaus AD (2009) Dengue virus pathogenesis: an integrated view. Clin Microbiol Rev 22: 564-8. doi: 10.1128/CMR.00035-09. PubMed: 19822889.
8. Lai YL, Chung YK, Tan HC, Yap HF, Yap G, et al. (2007) Cost-effective real-time reverse transcriptase PCR (RT-PCR) to screen for Dengue virus followed by rapid single-tube multiplex RT-PCR for serotyping of the virus. J Clin Microbiol 45: 935–941. doi: 10.1128/JCM.01258-06. PubMed: 17215345.
9. Alexander DQF, Aralí MVR, Elvira OR, Angel VCL (2006) Evaluation of IgM determination in acute serum for the diagnosis of dengue in an endemic area. Enferm Infecc Microbiol Clin 24: 90–92. PubMed: 16545316.
10. Alcon S, Talarmin A, Debruyne M, Falconar A, Deubel V, et al. (2002) Enzyme-linked immunosorbent assay specific to dengue virus type 1 nonstructural protein NS1 reveals circulation of the antigen in the blood during the acute phase of disease in patients experiencing primary or secondary infections. J Clin Microbiol 40: 376–381. doi: 10.1128/JCM.40.2.376-381.2002. PubMed: 11825945.
11. Shu PY, Huang JH (2004) Current advances in dengue diagnosis. Clin Diagn Lab Immunol 11: 642–650. doi: 10.1128/CDLI.11.4.642–650.2004. PubMed: 15242935.
12. Young PR, Hilditch PA, Bletchly C, Halloran W (2000) An antigen capture enzyme-linked immunosorbent assay reveals high levels of the dengue virus protein NS1 in the sera of infected patients. J Clin Microbiol 38: 1053–1057. PubMed: 10698995.
13. Kumarasamy V, Chua SK, Hassan Z, Wahab AHA, Chem YK, et al. (2007) Evaluating the sensitivity of a commercial dengue NS1 antigen-capture ELISA for early diagnosis of acute dengue virus infection. Singapore Med J 48: 669–73. PubMed: 17609831.
14. Chuansumrit A, Chaiyaratana W, Pongthanapisith V, Tangnararatchakit K, Lertwongrath S, Yoksan S (2008) The use of dengue nonstructural protein 1 antigen for the early diagnosis during the febrile stage in patients with dengue infection. Pediatr Infect Dis J 27: 43–48. PubMed: 18162937.
15. McBride WJH (2009) Evaluation of dengue NS1 test kits for the diagnosis of dengue fever. Diagn Microbiol Infect Dis 64: 31–36. doi: 10.1016/j.diagmicrobio.2009.01.002. PubMed: 19232865.
16. Bisordi I, Rocco IM, Suzuki A, Katz G, Silveira VR, et al. (2011) Evaluation of dengue NS1 antigen detection for diagnosis in public health laboratories, São Paulo state, 2009. Rev Inst Med Trop Sao Paulo 53: 315–20. PubMed: 22183454.
17. Felix AC, Romano CM, Centrone CC, Rodrigues CL, Villas-Boas L, et al. (2012) Low sensitivity of NS1 protein tests evidenced during a dengue type 2 virus outbreak in Santos, Brazil, in 2010. Clin Vaccine Immunol 19: 1972–76. doi: 10.1128/CVI.00535-12. PubMed: 23100478.
18. Moher D, Liberati A, Tetzlaff J, Altman DG, et al. (2009) Preferred reporting items for systematic reviews and meta-analyses: the PRISMA statement. PLoS Med 6: e1000097. doi: 10.1371/journal.pmed.1000097. PubMed: 19621072.
19. Higgins JPT, Green S, editors (2011) Cochrane handbook for systematic reviews of interventions. Version 5.1.0:6.4.1. The Cochrane Collaboration; Available: http://www.cochrane-handbook.org. Accessed 2013 October 10.
20. Whiting P, Rutjes AWS, Reitsma JB, Bossuyt PMM, Kleijnen J (2003) The development of QUADAS: a tool for the quality assessment of studies of

diagnostic accuracy included in systematic reviews. BMC Med Res Methodol 3: 25. doi: 10.1186/1471-2288-3-25. PubMed: 14606960.

21. Higgins JP, Thompson SG, Deeks JJ, Altman DG (2003) Measuring inconsistency in meta-analyses. BMJ 327: 557–560. doi: 10.1136/bmj.327.7414.557. PubMed: 12958120.

22. Jones CM, Athanasiou T (2005) Summary receiver operating characteristic curve analysis techniques in the evaluation of diagnostic tests. Ann Thorac Surg 79: 16–20. doi: 10.1016/j.athoracsur.2004.09.040. PubMed: 15620907.

23. Deeks JJ, Macaskill P, Irwig L (2005) The performance of tests of publication bias and other sample size effects in systematic reviews of diagnostic test accuracy was assessed. J Clin Epidemiol 58: 882–893. doi: 10.1016/j.jclinepi.2005.01.016. PubMed: 16085191.

24. Fagan TJ (1975) Letter: Nomogram for Bayes theorem. N Engl J Med 293: 257. doi: 10.1056/NEJM197507312930513. PubMed: 1143310.

25. Dussart P, Labeau B, Lagathu G, Louis P, Nunes MRT, et al. (2006) Evaluation of an enzyme immunoassay for detection of dengue virus NS1 antigen in human serum. Clin Vaccine Immunol 13: 1185–89. doi: 10.1128/CVI.00229-06. PubMed: 16988003.

26. Kumarasamy V, Wahab A, Chua SK, Hassan Z, Chem YK, et al. (2007) Evaluation of a commercial dengue NS1 antigen-capture ELISA for laboratory diagnosis of acute dengue virus infection. J Virol Methods 140: 75–79. Available: http://dx.doi.org/10.1016/j.jviromet.2006.11.001. Accessed 2013 December 14.

27. Bessoff K, Delorey M, Sun W, Hunsperger E (2008) Comparison of two commercially available dengue virus (DENV) NS1 capture enzyme-linked immunosorbent assays using a single clinical sample for diagnosis of acute DENV infection. Clin Vaccine Immunol 15: 1513–18. doi: 10.1128/CVI.00140-08. PubMed: 18685015.

28. Blacksell SD, Mammen Jr MP, Thongpaseuth S, Gibbons RV, Jarman RG, et al. (2008) Evaluation of the Panbio dengue virus nonstructural 1 antigen detection and immunoglobulin M antibody enzyme-linked immunosorbent assays for the diagnosis of acute dengue infections in Laos. Diagn Microbiol Infect Dis 60: 43–49. doi:10.1016/j.diagmicrobio.2007.07.011. PubMed: 17889487.

29. Castro LA (2008) Avaliação da detecção da proteína NS1 no diagnóstico da infecção pelo vírus dengue-3 em comparação a outros métodos laboratoriais utilizados no diagnóstico da dengue. Dissertação de Mestrado em Imunologia Básica e Aplicada. Universidade de São Paulo, Ribeirão Preto, SP. 100p.

30. Dussart P, Petit L, Labeau B, Bremand L, Leduc A, et al. (2008) Evaluation of two new commercial tests for the diagnosis of acute dengue virus infection using NS1 antigen detection in human serum. PLoS Negl Trop Dis 2: e280. doi:10.1371/journal.pntd.0000280. PubMed: 18714359.

31. Lapphra K, Sangcharaswichai A, Chokephaibulkit K, Tiengrim S, Piriyakarnsakul W, et al. (2008) Evaluation of an NS1 antigen detection for diagnosis of acute dengue infection in patients with acute febrile illness. Diagn Microbiol Infect Dis 60: 387–91. doi:10.1016/j.diagmicrobio.2007.11.010. PubMed: 18191361.

32. Hang VT, Nguyet NM, Trung D, Tricou V, Yoksan S, et al. (2009) Diagnostic accuracy of NS1 ELISA and lateral flow rapid tests for dengue sensitivity, specificity and relationship to viraemia and antibody responses. PLoS Negl Trop Dis 3: e360. doi:10.1371/journal.pntd.0000360. PubMed: 19156192.

33. Phuong HL, Thai KTD, Nga TTT, Giao PT, Hung LQ, et al. (2009) Detection of dengue nonstructural 1 (NS1) protein in Vietnamese patients with fever. Diagn Microbiol Infect Dis 63: 372–78. doi: 10.1016/j.diagmicrobio.2008.12.009. PubMed: 19232866.

34. Poloni TRRS (2009) Detecção e tipificação do vírus da dengue por RT-PCR em tempo real. Dissertação de mestrado em Biociências Aplicadas à Farmácia. Universidade de São Paulo. Ribeirão Preto, SP. 56p.

35. Ramirez AH, Moros Z, Comach G, Zambrano J, Bravo L, et al. (2009) Evaluation of dengue NS1 antigen detection tests with acute sera from patients infected with dengue virus in Venezuela. Diagn Microbiol Infect Dis 65: 247–53. doi: 10.1016/j.diagmicrobio.2009.07.022. PubMed: 19733994.

36. Guzman MG, Jaenisch T, Gaczkowski R, Hang VTT, Sekaran SD, et al. (2010) Multi-country evaluation of the sensitivity and specificity of two commercially-available NS1 ELISA assays for dengue diagnosis. PLoS Neglected Trop Dis 4: e811. doi:10.1371/journal.pntd.0000811. PubMed: 20824173.

37. Lima MRQ, Nogueira RMR, Schatzmayr HG, Santos FB (2010) Comparison of three commercially available dengue NS1 antigen capture assays for acute diagnosis of dengue in Brazil. PLoS Negl Trop Dis 4: e738. doi:10.1371/journal.pntd.0000738. PubMed: 20625558.

38. Osorio L, Ramirez M, Bonelo A, Villar LA, Parra B (2010) Comparison of the diagnostic accuracy of commercial NS1-based diagnostic tests for early dengue infection. Virol J 7: 361. doi: 10.1186/1743-422X-7-361. PubMed: 21134275.

39. Pok KY, Lai YL, Sng J, Ng LC (2010) Evaluation of nonstructural 1 antigen assays for the diagnosis and surveillance of dengue in Singapore. Vector-Borne Zoonotic Dis 10: 1009–16. doi: 10.1089/vbz.2008.0176. PubMed: 20426686.

40. Singh MP, Majumdar M, Singh G, Goyal K, Preet K, et al. (2010) NS1 antigen as an early diagnostic marker in dengue: report from India. Diagn Microbiol Infect Dis 68: 50–54. doi: 10.1016/j.diagmicrobio.2010.04.004. PubMed: 20727470.

41. Araújo FMC, Brilhante RSN, Cavalcanti LPG, Rocha MFG, Cordeiro RA, et al. (2011) Detection of the dengue non-structural 1 antigen in cerebral spinal fluid samples using a commercially available enzyme-linked immunosorbent

assay. J Virol Methods 177: 128–31. doi: 10.1016/j.jviromet.2011.07.003. PubMed: 21798288.

42. Chua KB, Mustafa B, Abdul Wahab AH, Chem YK, Khairul AH, et al. (2011) A comparative evaluation of dengue diagnostic tests based on single-acute serum samples for laboratory confirmation of acute dengue. Malays J Pathol 33: 13–20. PubMed: 21874746.

43. Chuansumrit A, Chaiyaratana W, Tangnararatchakit K, Yoksan S, Flamand M, Sakuntabhai A (2011) Dengue nonstructural protein 1 antigen in the urine as a rapid and convenient diagnostic test during the febrile stage in patients with dengue infection. Diagn Microbiol Infect Dis 71: 467–69. doi: 10.1016/j.diagmicrobio.2011.08.020. PubMed: 21996098.

44. Duong V, Ly S, Try PL, Tuiskunen A, Ong S, et al. (2011) Clinical and virological factors influencing the performance of a NS1 antigen-capture assay and potential use as a marker of dengue disease severity. PLoS Negl Trop Dis 5: e1244. doi:10.1371/journal.pntd.0001244. PubMed: 21811645.

45. Lima MRQ, Nogueira RMR, Filippis AMB, Santos FB (2011) Comparison of two generations of the Panbio dengue NS1 capture enzyme-linked immunosorbent assay. Clin Vaccine Immunol 18: 1031–33. doi: 10.1128/CVI.00024-11. PubMed: 21525305.

46. Kassim FM, Izati MN, TgRogayah TAR, Apandi YM, Saat Z (2011) Use of dengue NS1 antigen for early diagnosis of dengue virus infection. Southeast Asian J Trop Med Public Health 42: 562–9. PubMed: 21706934.

47. Silva FG, Silva SJS, Rocco IM, Silveira VR, Suzuki A, et al. (2011) Evaluation of commercial kits for detecting the antigen NS1-dengue-São Paulo. Bepa 8: 14–26.

48. Watthanaworawit W, Turner P, Turner CL, Tanganuchitcharnchai A, Jarman RG, et al. (2011) A prospective evaluation of diagnostic methodologies for the acute diagnosis of dengue virus infection on the Thailand-Myanmar border. Trans R Soc Trop Med Hyg 105: 32–37. doi: 10.1016/j.trstmh.2010.09.007. PubMed: 21035827.

49. Anders KL, Nguyet NM, Quyen NTH, Ngoc TV, Tram TV, et al. (2012) An evaluation of dried blood spots and oral swabs as alternative specimens for the diagnosis of dengue and screening for past dengue virus exposure. Am J Trop Med Hyg 87: 165–70. doi: 10.4269/ajtmh.2012.11-0713. PubMed: 22764309.

50. Blacksell SD, Jarman RG, Gibbons RV, Tanganuchitcharnchai A, Mammen Jr MP, et al. (2012) Comparison of seven commercial antigen and antibody enzyme-linked assays for detection of acute dengue infection. Clin Vaccine Immunol 19: 804–10. doi: 10.1128/CVI.05717-11. PubMed: 22441389.

51. Aryati A, Trimarsanto H, Yohan B, Wardhani P, Fahri S, Sasmono RT (2013) Performance of commercial dengue NS1 ELISA and molecular analysis of NS1 gene of dengue viruses obtained during surveillance in Indonesia. BMC Infect Dis 13: 611. doi:10.1186/1471-2334-13-611. PubMed: 24571329.

52. Colombo TE, Vedovello D, Araki CS, Cogo-Moreira H, Dos Santos INP, et al. (2013) Dengue 4 false negative results by Panbio dengue early ELISA assay in Brazil. J Clin Virol 58: 710–13. doi: 10.1016/j.jcv.2013.10.021. PubMed: 24238889.

53. Kosasih H, Alisjahbana B, Widjaja S, Nurhayati, Mast Q, et al. (2013) The diagnostic and prognostic value of dengue nonstructural 1 antigen detection in a hyper-endemic region in Indonesia. PLoS One 8: e80891. doi:10.1371/journal.pone.0080891. PubMed: 24260501.

54. Sea VRF, Cruz ACR, Gurgel RQ, Nunes BTD, Silva EVP, et al. (2013) Underreporting of dengue-4 in Brazil due to low sensitivity of the NS1 Ag test in routine control programs. PLoS One 8: e64056. doi: 10.1371/journal.pone.0064056. PubMed: 23715529.

55. Buehler AM, Figueró M, Moreira FR, Cavalcanti AB, Sasse A, Berwanger O. Diretrizes metodológicas: elaboração de revisão sistemática e meta-análise de estudos diagnósticos de acurácia. Available: http://200.214.130.94/rebrats/publicacoes/dbrs_Diagn_v_final.pdf. Accessed 2013 December 17.

56. Glas AS, Lijmer JG, Prins MH, Bonsel GJ, Bossuyt PMM (2003) The diagnostic odds ratio: a single indicator of test performance. J Clin Epidemiol 56: 1129–35. doi:10.1016/S0895-4356(03)00177-X. PubMed: 14615004.

57. Falconar AK, Young PR, Miles MA (1994) Precise location of sequential dengue virus subcomplex and complex B cell epitopes on the nonstructural-1 glycoprotein. Arch Virol 137: 315–26. PubMed: 7944953.

58. Daumas RP, Passos SR, Oliveira RV, Nogueira RM, Georg I, et al. (2013) Clinical and laboratory features that discriminate dengue from other febrile illnesses: a diagnostic accuracy study in Rio de Janeiro, Brazil. BMC Infect Dis 8: 13–77. doi: 10.1186/1471-2334-13-77. PubMed: 23394216.

59. Terzian AC, Mondini A, Bronzoni RV, Drumond BP, Ferro BP, et al. (2011) Detection of Saint Louis encephalitis virus in Dengue-suspected cases during a dengue 3 outbreak. Vector Borne Zoonotic Dis 11: 291–300. doi: 10.1089/vbz.2009.0200. PubMed: 20645866.

60. Huy NT, Van Giang T, Thuy DH, Kikuchi M, Hien TT, et al. (2013) Factors associated with dengue shock syndrome: a systematic review and meta-analysis. PLoS Negl Trop Dis 7: e2412. doi:10.1371/journal.pntd.0002412. PubMed: 24086778.

61. Wahala WMPB, Silva AM (2011) The human antibody response to dengue virus infection. Viruses 3: 2374–95. doi: 10.3390/v3122374. PubMed: 22355444.

62. Koraka P, Burghoorn-Maas CP, Falconar A, Setiati T, Djamiatun K, et al. (2003) Detection of immune-complex-dissociated nonstructural-1 antigen in patients with acute dengue virus infections. J Clin Microbiol 41: 4154–59. doi: 10.1128/JCM.41.9.4154-4159.2003. PubMed: 12958240.

63. Costa RL, Voloch CM, Schrago CG (2012) Comparative evolutionary epidemiology of dengue virus serotypes. Infect Genet Evol 12: 309–314. doi: 10.1016/j.meegid.2011.12.011. PubMed: 22226705.

64. Weaver SC, Vasilakis N (2009) Molecular evolution of dengue viruses: contributions of phylogenetics to understand the history and epidemiology of the preeminent arboviral disease. Infect Genet Evol 9: 523–540. doi: 10.1016/j.meegid.2009.02.003. PubMed: 19460319.

65. Watanabe S, Tan KH, Rathore APS, Rozen-Gagnon K, Shuai W, et al. (2012) The magnitude of dengue virus NS1 protein secretion is strain dependent and does not correlate with severe pathologies in the mouse infection model. J Virol 86: 5508–14. doi: 10.1128/JVI.07081-11. PubMed: 22419801.

66. Mairiang D, Zhang H, Sodja A, Murali T, Suriyaphol P, et al. (2013) Identification of new protein interactions between dengue fever virus and its hosts, human and mosquito. PLoS One 8: e53535. doi:10.1371/journal.pone.0053535. PubMed: 23326450.

67. Fansiri T, Fontaine A, Diancourt L, Caro V, Thaisomboonsuk B, et al. (2013) Genetic mapping of specific interactions between *Aedes aegypti* mosquitoes and dengue viruses. PLoS Genet 9: e1003621. doi: 10.1371/journal.pgen.1003621. PubMed: 23935524.

16

Vectorial Capacity of *Aedes aegypti*: Effects of Temperature and Implications for Global Dengue Epidemic Potential

Jing Liu-Helmersson[1]*, Hans Stenlund[1], Annelies Wilder-Smith[1,2], Joacim Rocklöv[1]

1 Department of Public Health and Clinical Medicine, Epidemiology and Global Health, Umeå University, Umeå, Sweden, 2 Lee Kong Chian School of Medicine, Nanyang Technological University, Singapore, Singapore

Abstract

Dengue is a mosquito-borne viral disease that occurs mainly in the tropics and subtropics but has a high potential to spread to new areas. Dengue infections are climate sensitive, so it is important to better understand how changing climate factors affect the potential for geographic spread and future dengue epidemics. Vectorial capacity (VC) describes a vector's propensity to transmit dengue taking into account human, virus, and vector interactions. VC is highly temperature dependent, but most dengue models only take mean temperature values into account. Recent evidence shows that diurnal temperature range (DTR) plays an important role in influencing the behavior of the primary dengue vector *Aedes aegypti*. In this study, we used relative VC to estimate dengue epidemic potential (DEP) based on the temperature and DTR dependence of the parameters of *A. aegypti*. We found a strong temperature dependence of DEP; it peaked at a mean temperature of 29.3°C when DTR was 0°C and at 20°C when DTR was 20°C. Increasing average temperatures up to 29°C led to an increased DEP, but temperatures above 29°C reduced DEP. In tropical areas where the mean temperatures are close to 29°C, a small DTR increased DEP while a large DTR reduced it. In cold to temperate or extremely hot climates where the mean temperatures are far from 29°C, increasing DTR was associated with increasing DEP. Incorporating these findings using historical and predicted temperature and DTR over a two hundred year period (1901–2099), we found an increasing trend of global DEP in temperate regions. Small increases in DEP were observed over the last 100 years and large increases are expected by the end of this century in temperate Northern Hemisphere regions using climate change projections. These findings illustrate the importance of including DTR when mapping DEP based on VC.

Editor: Luciano A. Moreira, Centro de Pesquisas René Rachou, Brazil

Funding: This study is part of the DengueTools project [33] funded by the European Union Seventh Framework Programme FP7/2007-2013 under grant agreement no. 282589. The funders had no role in study design, data collection and analysis, decision to publish, or preparation of the manuscript.

Competing Interests: The authors have declared that no competing interests exist.

* E-mail: Jing.Helmersson@umu.se

Introduction

Dengue is a mosquito-borne viral infection and is a major public health concern [1]. Over 2.5 billion people – or 40% of the world population [1] – are at risk, and about 390 million people are infected annually [2]. Increased global connectivity and population movements affect the global distribution of both the dengue virus and its vectors [3–7] and this has facilitated the spread of dengue to new geographic areas. Therefore, it is important to understand the vector's potential capability to transmit dengue globally.

Weather and climate are important factors in determining mosquito behavior and the effectiveness of dengue virus transmission [8]. Compared to studies on malaria [9], however, research on the relationship between weather variables and dengue is mostly limited to average temperature values and these miss the important role of short-term variability [8,10]. Lambrechts et al. [11] demonstrated through combined experimental and simulation studies that the diurnal temperature range (DTR) has important effects on two parameters of *A. aegypti*: the infection and transmission probability. Carrington et al. [12] demonstrated the influence of DTR on the life cycle stages of *A. aegypti*. Using the

same daily average temperature but with small and large DTR to mimic the temperatures corresponding to the high and low seasons of dengue infection in Thailand, they demonstrated the negative influence of a large DTR on these vector parameters of dengue transmission by *A. aegypti*.

No study has considered the combined effect of temperature and DTR on all dengue vector parameters, especially vectorial capacity [8,10,13] (see Equation (1) below), although there are an increasing number of studies focusing on the relationship between temperature variation and health [14–16]. There are also no studies on dengue vectorial capacity that take DTR into consideration when using historic data and estimated projections of future climate scenarios. The few global mapping studies that estimate the impact of climate change scenarios on dengue are limited to long-term average climate [17,18] or temperature [10] estimates. Studying the impact of climate change on vector-borne diseases is hampered by the long time periods necessary for such studies and by the confounding socio-economic and behavioral factors that are associated with such long time periods [7,19,20]. However, it is important to understand the degree to which

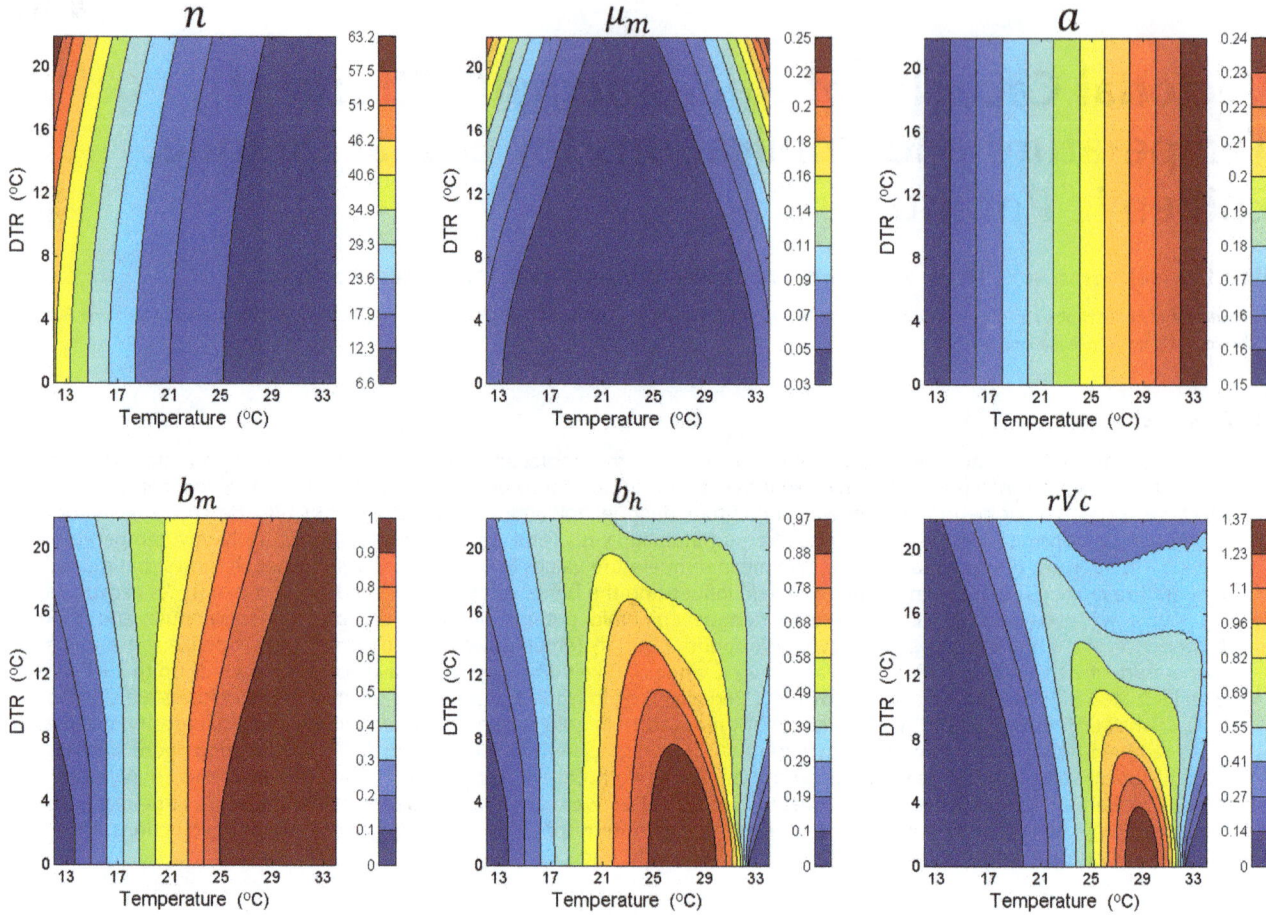

Figure 1. The effect of temperature and DTR on the vector parameters and relative vectorial capacity (rVc). Top row: n, μ_m, and a; bottom row: b_m, b_h, and rVc. Average daily temperature (the horizontal axis) and DTR (the vertical axis) both have units of °C. The color bar on the right side of each graph describes the value of the parameter. A higher rVc corresponds to a greater dengue epidemic potential.

climate change influences the potential for dengue epidemics, especially for populations currently living in non-endemic areas.

Vectorial capacity describes a vector's ability to spread disease among humans and takes into account host, virus, and vector interactions [21,22] assuming that all three of these parameters are present. It represents the average daily number of secondary cases generated by one primary case introduced into a fully susceptible population [21]. From the classical definition of Ross-McDonald [23], the relative vectorial capacity (rVc, the vectorial capacity relative to the vector-to-human population ratio) can be expressed as:

$$rVc = a^2 b_h b_m e^{-\mu_m n} / \mu_m \quad (1)$$

where the vector parameters used are 1) the average daily vector biting rate (a), 2) the probability of vector to human transmission per bite (b_h), 3) the probability of human to vector infection per bite (b_m), 4) the duration of the extrinsic incubation period (n), and 5) the vector mortality rate (μ_m). It is preferable to use the rVc when comparing dengue epidemic potential over space and time. A higher rVc indicates a higher potential for a dengue epidemic, and all of the rVc parameters depend on temperature [11,24–26] and DTR. Therefore, temperature can be either an effective barrier or a facilitator of vector-borne diseases [13].

To date, including both temperature and DTR has only been taken into account for two of the parameters – infection and transmission probability – that contribute to vectorial capacity for Dengue. Here we show the effect of temperature and its daily fluctuation on the five parameters of the primary dengue vector's capability to transmit the disease. Using temperature - driven models of rVc, we have estimated the global potential for dengue epidemic for the period of 1901–2099 using historical global temperature and future climate scenarios estimated from the highest levels of greenhouse emissions.

Results

Dependence of rVc (A. aegypti) parameters and rVc on temperature and DTR

To determine how the mean temperature (T) and its daily variation, DTR, affect dengue epidemic potential, contour plots (Figure 1) were created for each of the five *A. aegypti* parameters of the rVc equation. In the figure, mean temperatures range from 12°C to 34°C (x-axis) and the DTR ranges from 0°C to 22°C (y-axis). All parameters except biting rate show a nonlinear dependence on both T and DTR, which means that the parameters and rVc have different values at different values of T and DTR. The temperature dependence of these parameters and rVc at a DTR of 0°C is shown in Figure S1. The extrinsic incubation period, n, decreases as T increases and increases as DTR increases, and the variation is greater when T is near the lower extreme. The mortality rate, μ_m, increases when DTR increases at T near the two extremes but stays constant when T is in the middle (about 23°C). The biting rate, a, increases linearly with T and is independent of DTR. This is due to the cancellation of the positive change during the day by the negative change at night around the mean value of a. The probability of human to vector infection per bite, b_m, increases linearly with T when DTR is 0°C until a high T (26.1°C) and then becomes constant (see Figure S1). As DTR increases, b_m increases at low temperatures (<18°C), is constant around 19°C, and decreases at high temperatures (>20°C). The probability of vector to human transmission per bite, b_h, changes with T. When DTR is 0°C, b_m increases almost linearly at low T, reaches a peak value at middle T, and then decreases at high T (Figure S1A). As DTR increases, b_h increases at the low (<18°C) and very high (>32°C) extremes of temperature, is constant around 18°C, and decreases as temperature increases from 18°C to 32°C.

The dependence of rVc on T and DTR (Figure 1, bottom right) shows a similar pattern as that of b_h. As shown in Figure S1B, when DTR = 0°C, rVc has a bell-shaped temperature dependence that peaks at $T = 29.3$°C and decreases below and above this temperature. rVc shows a complex pattern as DTR increases from 0°C to 22°C. rVc increases monotonically when $T < 20$°C and $T > 32$°C and it increases slowly over a peak and then decreases when T is in the range of 20°C $< T \leq 32$°C. The peak height becomes smaller as the temperature approaches 29.3°C. Thus the effect of a high DTR, compared to zero or a low value, is to increase rVc if T is low ($T < 20$°C) or very high ($T > 32$°C) and to decrease the rVc in between the two ends (20°C $< T \leq 32$°C). The reason for this behavior is elaborated more in the Supplementary Information S1. Figures S1C and S1D show rVc for two mean temperatures: $T = 14$°C (temperate climate regions such as summer in Northern Europe) and 26°C (tropical climate regions such as Thailand throughout the year). A small DTR (<10°C) increases rVc for tropical areas but a large DTR reduces it. In cold regions, DTR raises rVc continuously and the higher the DTR the greater the increase in rVc. The increase of rVc in cold regions is much larger than the reduction of rVc in tropical regions when DTR is 20°C. In other words, the effect of DTR is to reduce the differences in rVc or the dengue epidemic potential between cold/mild (including extremely hot) and warm/hot (subtropical and tropical) areas. At any one location, the larger the DTR, the more effect it exerts on the rVc value of that location.

Mapping of global dengue epidemic potential

Global dengue epidemic potential is estimated through rVc, as shown in Figure 2, where rVc was averaged for the highest three consecutive months of the year (will be called "high rVc period") over the period of 1980 to 2009. The effect of DTR is illustrated by comparing the rVc calculated based on monthly T alone (Fig. 2A) with that based on T and DTR (Fig. 2B). The blue color indicates that potential for dengue transmission is unlikely when rVc is below the value of 0.05 per day. With T alone (Fig. 2a), the majority of the Northern Hemisphere does not appear to be a climatically conducive area for dengue transmission.

Assuming that the human to mosquito ratio, m, equals 1 and using a typical infectious period of 5 days, the threshold value for a dengue epidemic outbreak using rVc is estimated to be 0.2 per day (see Supplementary Information S1). In the maps, any area colored orange or red would exceed the threshold for a dengue outbreak when other necessary conditions were also met (sufficient presence of humans, viruses, and vectors). Under these conditions

and criteria, the dengue epidemic potential is limited to the tropical and subtropical regions and covers most of the Southern Hemisphere (Fig. 2A), the southern tip of Europe, the Middle East, and the southern parts of the US and China. Most of the land masses in the Northern Hemisphere are below the critical value.

When the influence of T and DTR are considered (Fig. 2B), the temperate regions show increased rVc values and warmer/hot regions show reduced rVc values that are still much higher than the values in the temperate regions and are above the threshold. The maximum value of rVc is reduced from 1.37 to 1.18 per day. The areas where rVc is above the threshold value of 0.2 per day include Central Europe (the majority of Spain, part of France, Ukraine, etc.), southern Russian, the Middle East, the majority of the non-mountainous areas of China, the majority of the US, and all of Africa. Tropical and subtropical regions show a reduction in rVc, e.g. Southeast Asia, large parts of Central and South America, Africa, and Australia. Nevertheless, rVc is still sufficiently high to result in sustained transmission in these tropical and subtropical regions. Thus, the main effect of DTR is to increase (by a relatively large percentage) the overall dengue epidemic potential in temperate climates and reduce (by a relatively small percentage) the dengue epidemic potential in the tropical regions.

Figure 3 shows the dengue epidemic potential for the highest three consecutive months of the year where DTR was included in the present (1980–2009) rVc estimates (Figure 3A) and the projected rVc estimates for the future (2070–2099) time period (Figure 3B) under a high greenhouse emission scenario (RCP8.5, see Methods section for definition) [27–29]. It is apparent from Figure 3B that the majority of the Northern Hemisphere is projected to have a higher epidemic potential in this period. This effect of temperature on the dengue epidemic potential is projected to occur in most parts of Europe, Asia, and North America including parts of Sweden, Finland, Russia, Alaska, and Canada. Only Greenland and the very northern parts of Canada and Russia are projected to have sufficiently low temperatures to limit the dengue epidemic potential. On the other hand, the magnitude of the dengue epidemic potential is reduced in tropical and subtropical areas, including South Asia, Central and South America, Australia, and Africa, but the reduction would not eliminate the potential risk of sustained dengue epidemics.

Similar to the comparison of the high rVc period (Fig. 3), Figure 4 shows the dengue epidemic potential based on annual average of rVc for the present (1980–2009) (Figure 4A) and future (2070–2099) (Figure 4B) time periods. Using the annually averaged rVc, we show the same trend as for the highest three consecutive month average although with less magnitude and smaller geographic areas affected. There is an obvious increase in dengue epidemic potential in areas in the Northern Hemisphere but a reduction in magnitude in the near-equator belt over the 200-year time span.

The changes in dengue epidemic potential over time are shown in Figure 5 (averaged for the highest three consecutive months) and Figure 6 (averaged annually) using the rVc difference between the present and the past (Figures 5A and 6A) and between the projected future scenario and the present (Figures 5B and 6B). Cold colors indicate decreases in dengue epidemic potential and warm colors indicate increases. Figure 5A (high rVc period) and 6A (annual) show the differences in rVc between the present (1980–2009) and the past (1901–1930) when DTR is included. During the high rVc period (Fig. 5A), rVc did not change in most world regions (white), some reductions (blue) were found around the equator and tropical deserts and some increases (yellow, orange, and red) were seen in some temperate regions in Southern

A

B

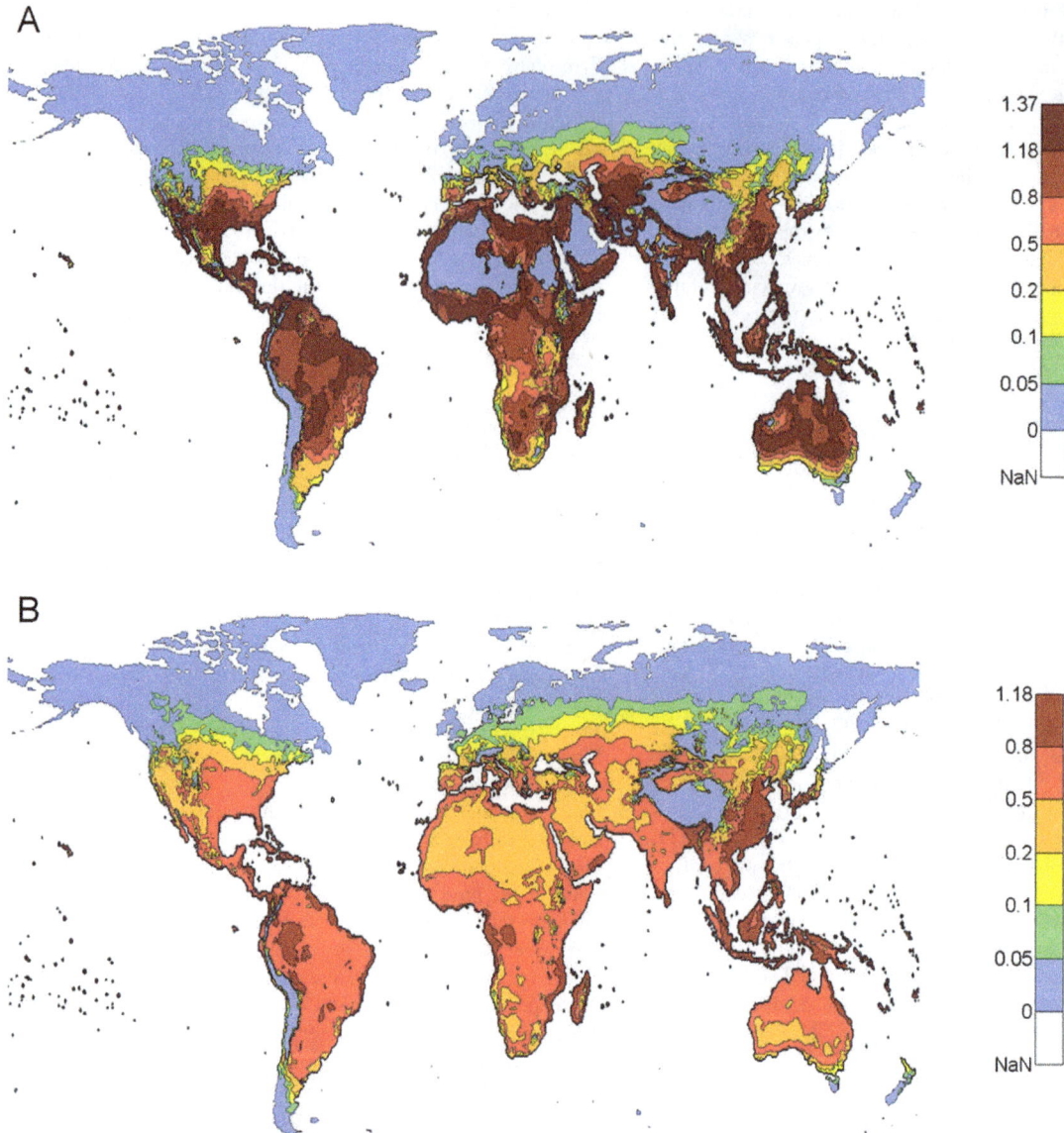

Figure 2. The effect of DTR on global dengue epidemic potential (*rVc*). **A)** Using only monthly *T*. **B)** Using monthly *T* and DTR. For each location (0.5×0.5 degree), the *rVc* is averaged over the highest three consecutive months of the year from 1980 to 2009. The color bar describes the values of the *rVc*.

Europe, the Mediterranian, East Asia, Australia, southeastern parts of South America, large parts of the US, and southern parts of Africa. Using annually averaged *rVc*, very few changes were found between the present and the past (Fig. 6A). The changes were mainly limited to increases and were mainly located in the Southern Hemisphere including the southeastern part of South America and the southern part of Africa.

Figures 5B and 6B show predicted differences in *rVc* between the future (2070–2099) and the present (1980–2009) when DTR was included. Under a projected climate change scenario, during the high *rVc* period (Figure 5B) the increase in dengue epidemic potential is dramatic (warm colors) and covers large portions of the Northern Hemisphere and the very southern parts of Southern Hemisphere. The reduction in *rVc* is also large in terms of both magnitude and spatial area and covers the tropical and subtropical belt (blue) along the equator and a large part of the Southern Hemisphere. For annually averaged *rVc* (Figure 6B), the increase

in *rVc* covers a large portion of the Northern Hemisphere as well as the southern part of the Southern Hemisphere. The area where the *rVc* is reduced is mainly around the equator and extends to the southern part of the Southern Hemisphere. In both Figure 5 and Figure 6, the change in *rVc* is much larger in the projected future than in the past (Figures 5B and 6B relative to Figures 5A and 6A). Therefore, compared to the intensity and spatial area over the past century, projected climate change suggests rather large increases in the epidemic potential of dengue at the end of the 21st century in temperate regions of the world, particularly in the Northern Hemisphere.

Discussion

We show that *T* and DTR are intrinsically related to the dengue epidemic potential. We find that diurnal temperature variations

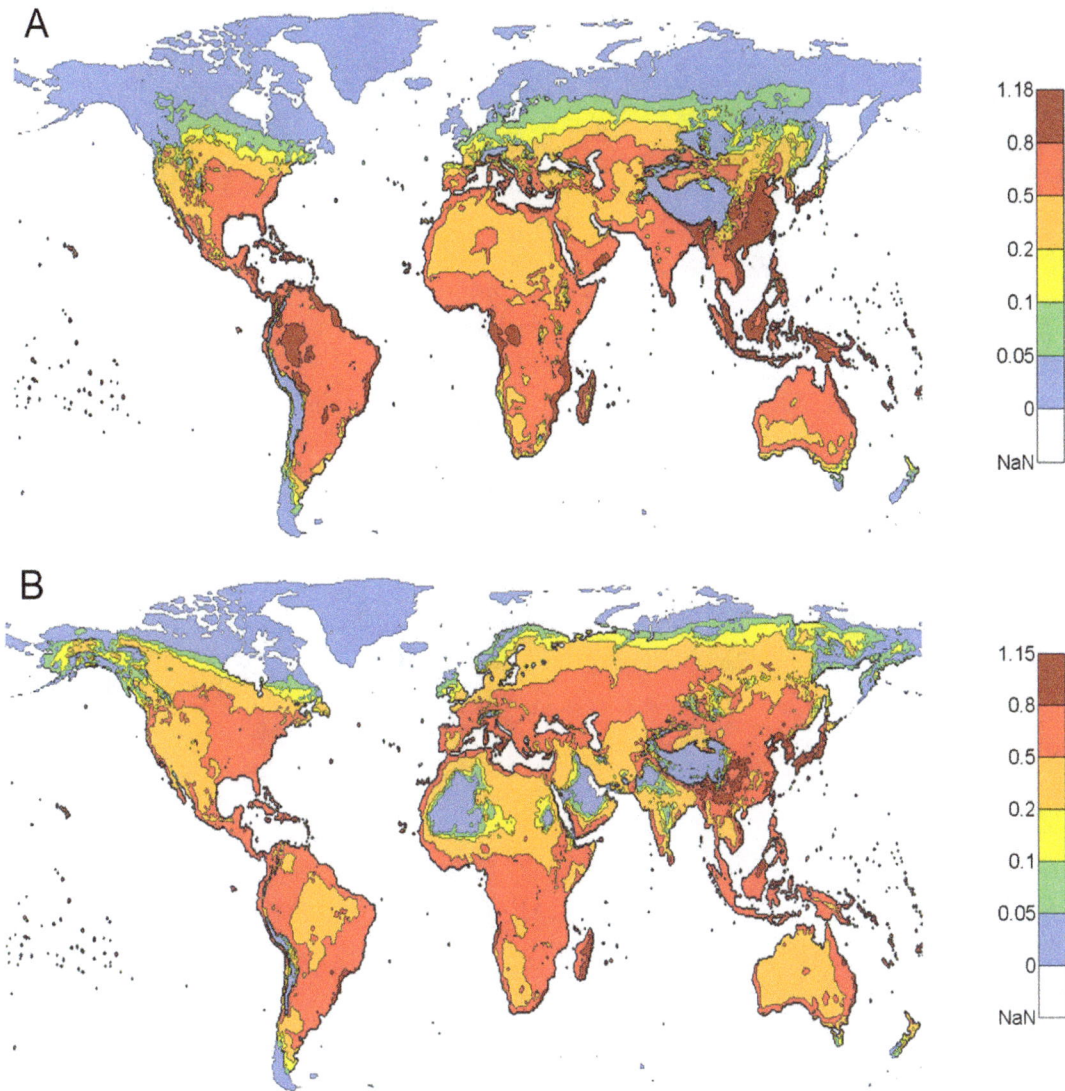

Figure 3. Global maps of dengue epidemic potential (rVc) for the highest three consecutive months of the year. A) Present (1980–2009) (same as Fig. 2B). **B)** Future (2070–2099) under RCP8.5 from five global climate models. In A) and B), DTR was included. The color bar describes the values of the rVc.

are particularly important for the understanding of dengue in temperate regions of the Northern Hemisphere.

We found that the optimal T for *A. aegypti* to transmit dengue is around 29.3°C when DTR = 0°C and that this is reduced to 20°C when the DTR increases to 20°C. The dependence of dengue epidemic potential (the rVc) on T and DTR is two-fold: for cold to temperate areas ($T<20$°C) and extremely hot areas ($T>32$°C), increasing DTR (from 0°C to 22°C) raises the dengue epidemic potential by a relatively large percentage from its low or zero value, and in subtropical and tropical regions (20°C≤T≤32°C) increasing DTR causes the dengue epidemic potential to increasing to a peak value and then to decrease. The peak height is reduced as the average temperature approaches 29.3°C, which is the optimal temperature for rVc when DTR is 0°C. In other words, extreme temperature ranges (either too cold or too hot) are not optimal for *A. aegypti*. When T is far from the optimal temperature for dengue transmission, the effect of DTR is to increase rVc both above and below 29.3°C. On the other hand, when T is near the optimal temperature, the effect of a small DTR

is to increase rVc but a large DTR decreases rVc (see Supplementary Information S1 for detailed discussion). Therefore, large daily temperature fluctuations facilitate or inhibit the dengue epidemic potential depending on the daily T.

The similarity in contour maps for vector to human transmission probability, b_h, and rVc indicates the importance of b_h in affecting the dengue epidemic potential. The dependence of b_h on temperature is consistent with the findings of Lambrechts et al. [11], but the non-linear increase in the relation between n and DTR differs from Lambrechts et al.'s simulation results. They found an independent relation between n and DTR when using a sinusoidal function for DTR (Fig. S2A) but a decrease of n with DTR when using the Parton-Logan function (a sinusoidal increase during the daytime and an exponential decrease during the night) (Fig. S2B).

When examining dengue epidemic potential globally, the obvious difference between Figures 2A and 2B shows an overall increase in areas with high rVc (larger than threshold value) when DTR is included (more areas with orange and red colors). DTR

A

B

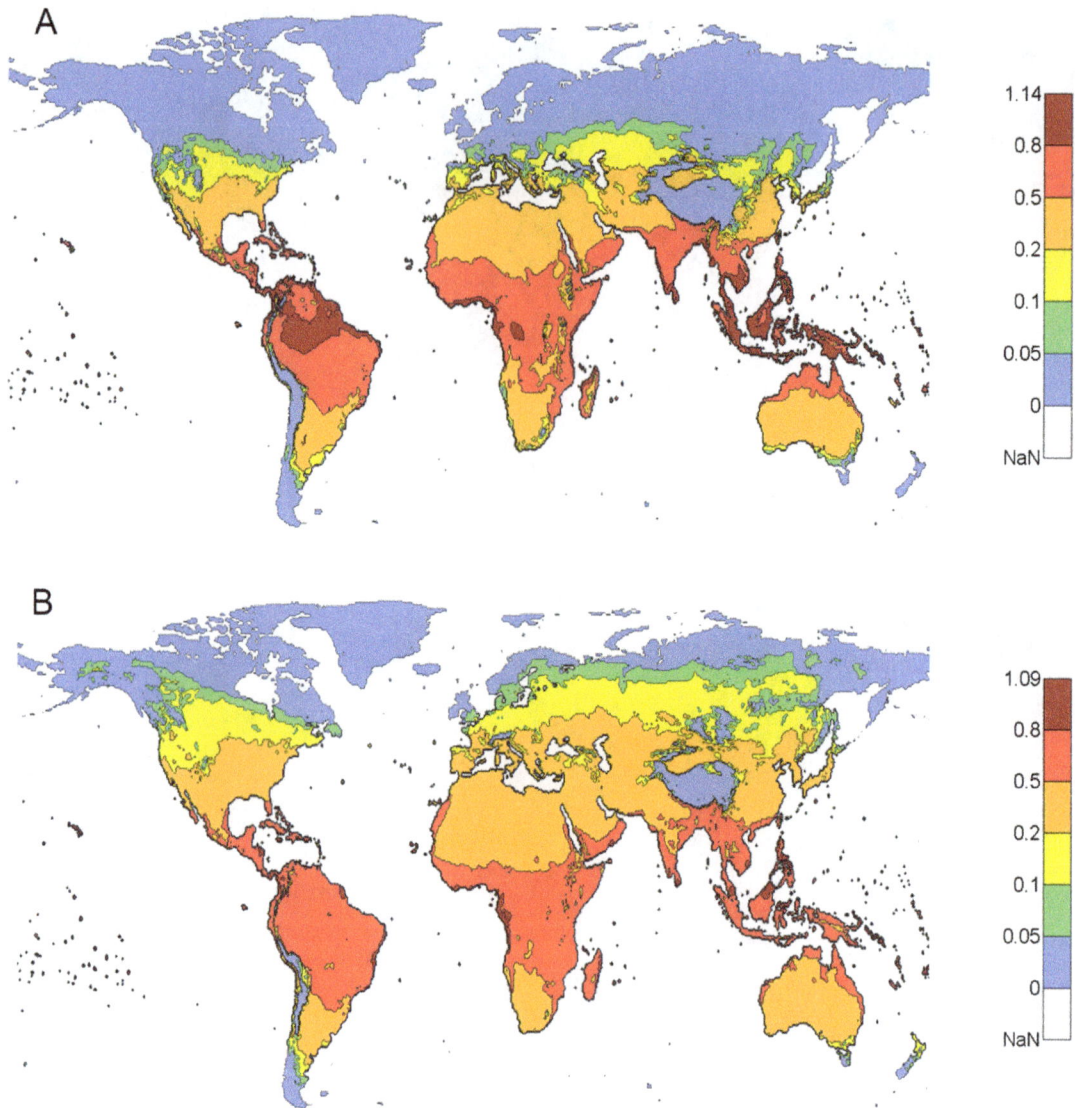

Figure 4. Global maps of dengue epidemic potential using annually averaged rVc**. A**) Present scenario (1980–2009). **B**) Future scenario (2070–2099) under RCP8.5 from five global climate models. In A) and B), DTR was included. The color bar describes the values of rVc.

also increases the magnitude of the rVc value, especially in the areas where T is normally cold to mild or extremely hot. In the tropical regions, however, the magnitude of dengue epidemic potential is mostly reduced when DTR is included but still well above the threshold value. The magnitude of the change on a relative scale is large for regions with cold to mild as well as extremely hot climates and small for areas with a tropical or subtropical climate. In absolute values of rVc, the dengue epidemic potential is still much higher in tropical and subtropical areas than other areas. With DTR included and using projected (30 year average) temperature under a high greenhouse emission scenario (RCP8.5) at the end of this century, a large increase of dengue epidemic potential in both intensity and areas is observed as shown in Figure 3 and Figure 4 – especially in the Northern Hemisphere – compared to the estimate based on the present temperature. The change in dengue epidemic potential has been more dramatic in this century than the last century as shown in Figure 5 and Figure 6. The dengue epidemic potential based on

annually averaged rVc shows the same trend with less magnitude than that based on the average of the high rVc period.

Dengue transmission in temperate regions will, in reality, increase only when the other necessary conditions are met: the presence of susceptible humans, the establishment and proliferation of the dengue vector, the introduction of the dengue virus, and conducive human behavior and ecological and socioeconomic conditions [5,18,20,29].

The dengue vectors *A. aegypti* and *A. albopictus* have already become established in new areas and are spreading further north, for example, into Europe [30,31]. Global travel and trade provide many opportunities to introduce the dengue virus into uninfected areas [3–7] as demonstrated by the recent dengue outbreak in Madeira and a vector survey in Europe [30,32,33]. Thus it is important to develop a new generation of dengue mathematical models that give insights into the possible interactions of climate, global travel, human and vector density distribution, and other

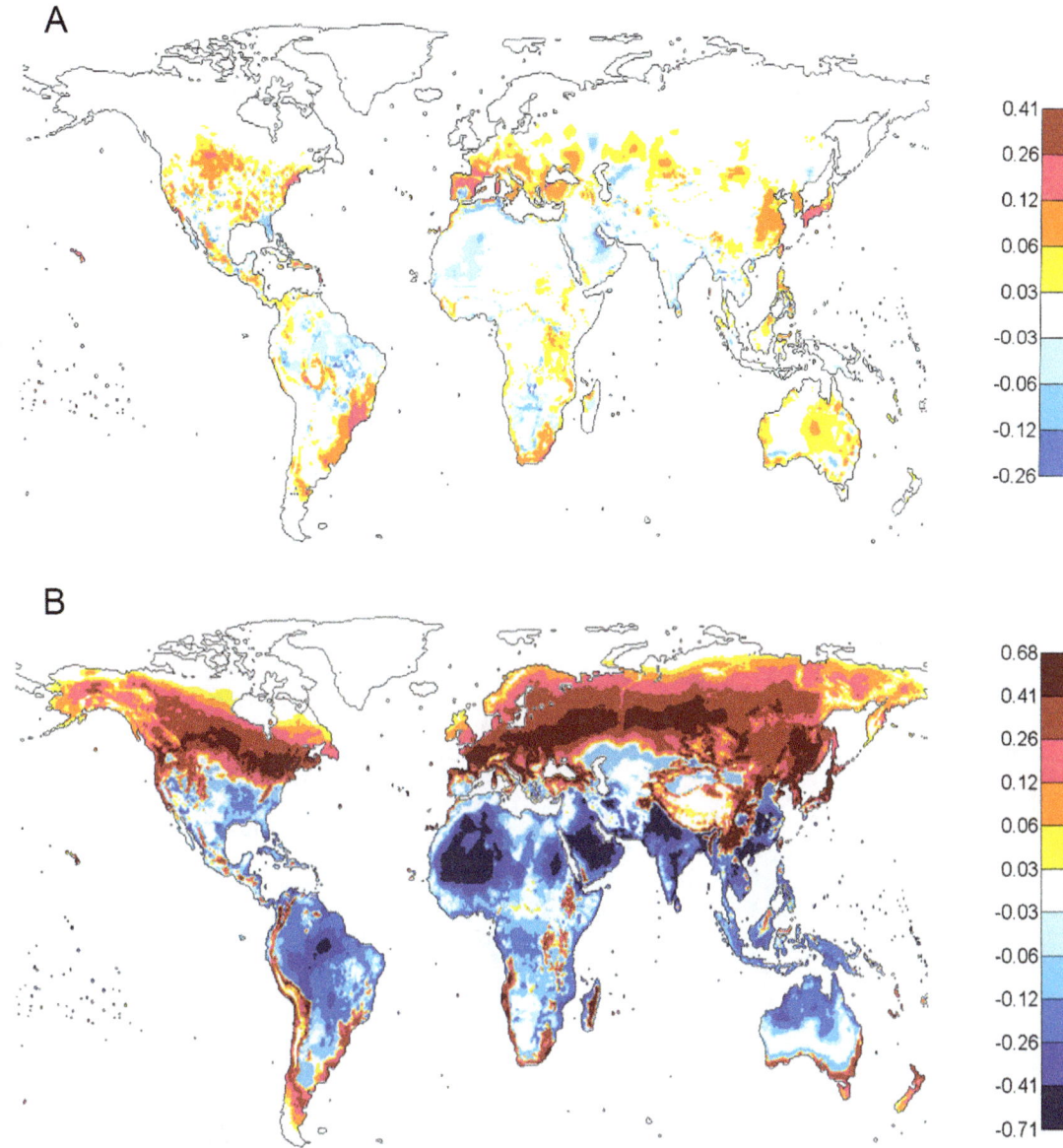

Figure 5. Trend of global dengue epidemic potential (rVc) for the highest three consecutive months of the year. Differences in averaged rVc based on 30 year averages of temperature and DTR. **A)** Differences between 1980–2009 and 1901–1930. **B)** Differences between 2070–2099 and 1980–2009. The mean value of rVc was averaged from five global climate models under RCP8.5. The color bar describes the values of the rVc.

environmental factors on global dengue epidemic potential. This work is a first step toward the realization of this goal.

Conclusions

Based on our temperature and DTR-driven relative vectorial capacity estimates, we found a strong temperature dependence of the dengue epidemic potential. It peaks at a mean temperature of 29.3°C when DTR is 0°C and at 20°C when DTR is 20°C. Increasing average temperatures up to 29°C leads to an increased potential for a dengue epidemic, but temperatures above 29°C reduces the potential. In tropical areas where the mean temperatures are close to 29°C, a small DTR increases the dengue epidemic potential while a large DTR reduces it. In cold to temperate or extremely hot climates where the mean temperatures

are far from 29°C, increasing DTR increases the dengue epidemic potential and the larger the DTR, the greater the dengue epidemic potential. Incorporating these findings using historical and predicted temperature and DTR over a two hundred year period (1901–2099), we found an increasing trend for global dengue epidemic potential in temperate regions over time. Small increases in epidemic potential were observed over the last 100 years and large increases are expected by the end of this century in temperate Northern Hemisphere regions using climate change projections. These findings illustrate the importance of including DTR when mapping the dengue epidemic potential using vectorial capacity.

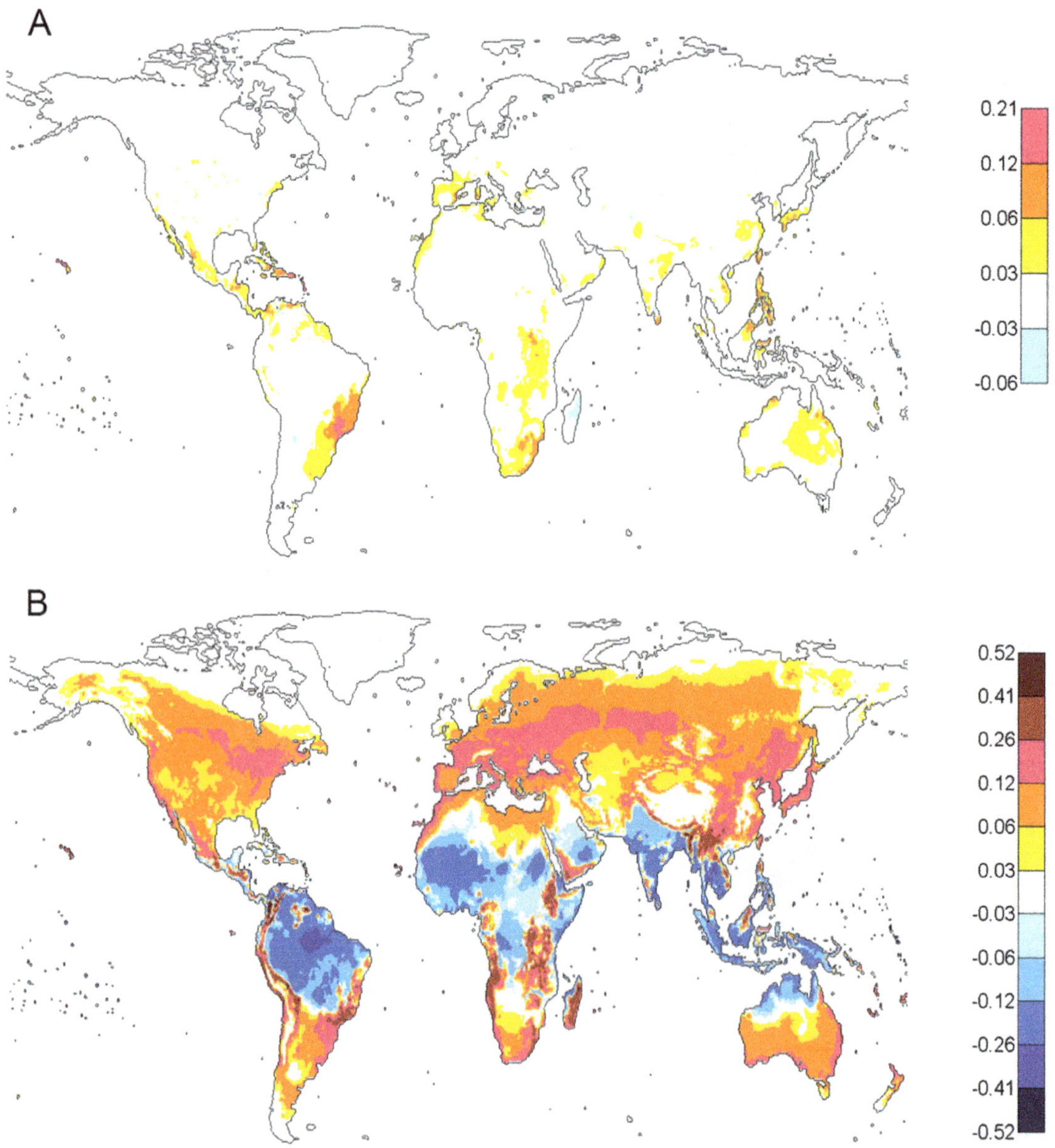

A

B

Figure 6. Trend of annually averaged global dengue epidemic potential (rVc). Differences in rVc based on 30-year averages of temperature and DTR. **A)** Differences between 1980–2009 and 1901–1930. **B)** Differences between 2070–2099 and 1980–2009. The mean value of rVc was averaged from five global climate models under RCP8.5. The color bar describes the values of the rVc.

Methods

Effect of temperature on dengue relative vectorial capacity – rVc

The associations of all five vector parameters a, b_h, b_m, n, and μ_m with temperature were determined for the primary dengue vector A. aegypti from the peer-reviewed literature. These are listed in relation to T from which the relation to DTR is derived.

1) **Biting rate** (a). The average blood meal frequency (a) of female A. aegypti collected weekly increased linearly with weekly T in Thailand after converting weeks to days [24]:

$$a(T) = 0.0043T + 0.0943 \quad (day^{-1}) \quad (21°C \leq T \leq 32°C) \quad (2)$$

The relationship is statistically significant ($p = 0.05$ and $R^2 = 0.08$).

2) **The probability of infection from humans to vector per bite** (b_m). Based on empirical data for various flaviviruses (West Nile virus, Murray Valley encephalitis virus, and St. Louis encephalitis virus), Lambrechts et al. derived the relationships between temperature and the probability of infection (see Supplementary Information S1) [11]:

$$b_m(T) = \begin{cases} 0.0729T - 0.9037 & (12.4°C \leq T \leq 26.1°C) \\ 1 & (26.1°C < T < 32.5°C) \end{cases} \quad (3)$$

This relationship is piecewise linear, with increasing probability starting at 12.4°C and a constant probability of one above 26.1°C.

3) The probability of transmission from vector to human per bite (b_h). Lambrechts et al. also described the equations for the probability of human infection using thermodynamic functions [11,34]:

$$b_h(T) = 0.001044T(T-12.286)\sqrt{32.461-T}\text{(for }12.286°\text{C}\leq T < 32.461°\text{C)}$$ (4)

b_h increases almost linearly with T for $12.3°\text{C}\leq T<26°\text{C}$, decreases sharply when $T>28°\text{C}$, and decreases to zero when $T\geq32.5°\text{C}$.

4) Extrinsic incubation period (n). Based on experimental data for the range of 12°C to 36°C [35,36], an exponential function was used to fit the data, although other functions could also be used [26].

$$n(T) = 4 + e^{5.15-0.123T}$$ (5)

5) Mortality rate (μ_m). Experiments by Yang et al. [25] on female *A. aegypti* mosquitos over the temperature range of $10.54°\text{C}\leq T\leq33.41°\text{C}$ found the mortality rate ranged from 0.027 (0.27%) per day to 0.092 (0.92%) per day with the highest survival at $T=27.6°\text{C}$ and the lowest survival at $T<14°\text{C}$ and $T>32°\text{C}$. They used a 4th order polynomial function to fit the data:

$$\mu_m(T) = 0.8692 - 0.1590T + 0.01116T^2 - 3.408\times10^{-4}T^3 + 3.809\times10^{-6}T^4$$ (6)

The relationships of vector parameters in equations (2) through (6) provide the basis for incorporating the influence of DTR in rVc (equation (1)) by assuming a sinusoidal hourly temperature variation between the two extremes ($T\pm\text{DTR}/2$) within a period of 24 hours. The corresponding contour plots for the parameters and rVc (Figure 1) were calculated and averaged over a day with variable T and DTR.

Global mapping of the dengue epidemic potential

From the CRU online database, time series of monthly T and DTR were obtained all over the world for the period of January 1901 to December 2009 [37]. CRU-TS v3.1 data was used for grid boxes of 0.5 by 0.5 degrees (about 50×50 km at the equator) latitude and longitude.

For each month, a running 30-year average of T and DTR was calculated. rVc was then calculated for each month including and excluding the average DTR. When DTR was included, the daily temperature was assumed to take a sinusoidal form around its mean. Maps were generated based on either annual average rVc or the highest calculated monthly average rVc occurring in a consecutive three-month period in each grid box (location).

For the future projection of rVc for the period of 2070–2099, temperature projections were based on the RCP8.5 emission scenario [27,28,38] and the mean rVc values based on CMIP5 [39,40] general circulation models were calculated and mapped. The modeling used the average outcome of five different global circulation models (GCMs) as described in [21,23,24]. RCP stands for *representative concentration pathways* and describes the forcing of greenhouse gases used to project future climate changes. The most extreme one, RCP8.5, displays a continuous rise in radiative forcing during the 21st century leading to a value of about 8.5 Wm^{-2} in 2100 [38].

Limitations of the methods used

Vector parameters and their dependence on temperature were based on studies on *A. aegypti* for various virus serotypes in different regions of the world. Inconsistencies in methods and different errors in data processing and data fitting are to be expected. In addition, due to limited information this study did not distinguish between different virus serotypes and virus titers (dosages) that can affect the parameters [26]. Furthermore, we extended the daily biting rate $a(T)$ from the low temperature limit of 21°C down to 12.4°C. This extension was based on the fact that the measured a varies slowly with T as shown in equation (2) in the observed range ($21°\text{C}\leq T\leq32°\text{C}$, $p=0.05$) in Thailand and shows an even flatter linear increase in Puerto Rico ($a(T)=0.01T+1.05$ ($week^{-1}$), $p=0.37$). We expect that our extension would not substantially affect rVc. The exponential fitting of n in equation (5) with three constants based on experimental data is not unique because the temperature range is less than one order of magnitude. Other relationships, such as polynomials, might work as well. We chose the exponential function because it has been used in other modeling of n in malaria-carrying mosquitoes [8]. Within the range of temperature used in this estimation of n, the rVc is not likely to be affected by the fitting equations used.

When including DTR, we chose the simple sinusoidal function instead of the Parton-Logan function or other more sophisticated temperature variations [11] so as to match the monthly data on T and DTR. DTR from the present CRU data were used for projected climate change. This might be reasonable because the uncertainty of the future projected temperature is large and the error introduced by DTR is less important.

Finally, our results provide insights into the potential role of temperature and DTR on dengue but do not provide projections of numbers of actual cases because transmission requires the following four conditions: 1) susceptible humans, 2) abundant vector, 3) virus introduction, and 4) conducive weather/climate. Here we consider only one, the role of temperature, and assume that the other conditions are already met. This method can overestimate the dengue epidemic potential for areas where there are no humans, vectors, or viruses. Thus, it is called epidemic *potential* and not *risk*. Reported case mapping might be closer to reality, but this provides limited insights into how changing conditions could affect future disease burdens.

Mosquitoes are not inert, and they actively avoid extremes of temperatures by seeking out microenvironments that buffer extreme ambient temperature. *A. aegypti* in particular is tightly tied to, and highly buffered by, humans and the land use associated with the urbanization and transport of people and goods that have increased with globalization. The natural history of dengue is complex and involves the interplay of many factors such as climate, ecology, vector biology, and human drivers that are influenced by demographic and societal changes, socioeconomic conditions, human behavior, etc. Therefore, the true dengue risk in a specific area might be quite different from our estimation based on the vectorial capacity and the influence of climate. However, as a first approximation, this study improves our current understanding of dengue epidemic potential. Our approach is based on evidence from the scientific literature on transmission dependencies on weather and climate and synthesizes many research studies on vector parameters. It provides a basis for the improvement of dengue modeling based on weather and climate data, and it provides one possibility for how the dengue transmission potential could change as the global climate continues to change.

Supporting Information

Figure S1 The dependence of vector parameters and relative vectorial capacity (rVc) **on temperature and DTR.** A) Vector parameters from the literature. Different scales are used for each parameter to be able to put them on the same graph. B) rVc dependence on temperature when DTR is 0°C. C) and D) DTR dependence of rVc at average temperatures of 26°C and 14°C, respectively.

References

1. World Health Organization (WHO) (2012) Dengue and severe dengue – Fact sheet N°117. Available: http://www.who.int/mediacentre/factsheets/fs117/en/#. Accessed 03 December 2012.
2. Bhatt S, Gething PW, Brady OJ, Messina JP, Farlow AW, et al. (2013) The global distribution and burden of dengue. Nature 12060.
3. Huang Z, Das A, Qiu Y, Tatem AJ (2012) Web-based GIS: the vector-borne disease airline importation risk (VBD-AIR) tool. Int J Health Geogr 11: 33.
4. Randolph SE, Rogers DJ (2010) The arrival, establishment and spread of exotic diseases: patterns and predictions. Nat Rev Microbiol 8: 361–371.
5. Reiter P (2010) Yellow fever and dengue: a threat to Europe? Euro Surveill 15: 19509.
6. Tatem AJ, Rogers DJ, Hay SI (2006) Global transport networks and infectious disease spread. Adv Parasitol 62: 293–343.
7. Wilder-Smith A, Gubler DJ (2008) Geographic expansion of dengue: the impact of international travel. Med Clin North Am 92: 1377–1390.
8. Massad E, Coutinho F, Lopez L, Silva d (2011) Modeling the impact of global warming on vector-borne infections. Physics of Life Reviews 8: 169–199.
9. Gething PW, Boeckel TPV, Smith DL, Guerra CA, Patil AP, et al. (2011) Modelling the global constraints of temperature on transmission of Plasmodium falciparum and P. vivax Parasites & Vectors 4.
10. Patz JA, Martens WJ, Focks DA, Jetten TH (1998) Dengue fever epidemic potential as projected by general circulation models of global climate change. Environ Health Perspect 106: 147–153.
11. Lambrechts L, Paaijmans KP, Fansiri T, Carrington LB, Kramer LD, et al. (2011) Impact of daily temperature fluctuations on dengue virus transmission by Aedes aegypti. Proc Natl Acad Sci U S A 108: 7460–7465.
12. Carrington LB, Seifert SN, Willits NH, Lambrechts L, Scott TW (2013) Large diurnal temperature fluctuations negatively influence Aedes aegypti (Diptera: Culicidae) life-history traits. Journal of medical entomology. Proc Natl Acad Sci USA 50: 43–51.
13. Descloux E, Mangeas M, Menkes C, Lengaigne M, Leroy Aea (2012) Climate-Based Models for Understanding and Forecasting Dengue Epidemics. PLoS Negl Trop Dis 6: 1470.
14. Paaijmans K, Blanford S, Bell A, Blanford J, Read A, et al. (2010) Influence of climate on malaria transmission depends on daily temperature variation PNAS
15. Raffel T, Romansic J, Halstead N, McMahon T, Venesky M, et al. (2012) Disease and thermal acclimation in a more variable and unpredictable climate. Nature Climate Change 3: 146–151.
16. Gosling S, Mcgrego rG, Lowe J (2009) Climate change and heat-related mortality in six cities Part 2: climate model evaluation and projected impacts from changes in the mean and variability of temperature with climate change. Int J Biometeorol 53: 31–51.
17. Hales S, de Wet N, Maindonald J, Woodward A (2002) Potential effect of population and climate changes on global distribution of dengue fever: an empirical model. Lancet 360: 830–834.
18. Astrom C, Rocklov J, Hales S, Beguin A, Louis V, et al. (2013) Potential Distribution of Dengue Fever Under Scenarios of Climate Change and Economic Development. Ecohealth.
19. Reiter P, Lathrop S, Bunning M, Biggerstaff B, Singer D, et al. (2003) Texas lifestyle limits transmission of dengue virus. Emerg Infect Dis 9: 86–89.
20. Beebe N, Cooper R, Mottram P, Sweeney A (2009) Australia's dengue risk driven by human adaptation to climate change. PLoS Negl Trop Dis 3: 429.
21. Garrett-Jones C (1964) Prognosis for Interruption of Malaria Transmission through Assessment of the Mosquito's Vectorial Capacity. Nature 204: 1173–1175.

22. Liu-Helmersson J (2012) Mathematical Modeling of Dengue -Temperature Effect on Vectorial Capacity. Master of Science Thesis. Available: http://www.phmed.umu.se/digitalAssets/104/104555_jing-helmersson.pdf: Umeå University; 2012. Accessed 11 December 2012.
23. Anderson R, May R (1991) Infectious Diseases of Humans: Dynamics and Control. Oxford Oxford University Press.
24. Scott TW, Amerasinghe PH, Morrison AC, Lorenz LH, Clark GG, et al. (2000) Longitudinal studies of Aedes aegypti (Diptera: Culicidae) in Thailand and Puerto Rico: blood feeding frequency. J Med Entomol 37: 89–101.
25. Yang HM, Macoris ML, Galvani KC, Andrighetti MT, Wanderley DM (2009) Assessing the effects of temperature on the population of Aedes aegypti, the vector of dengue. Epidemiol Infect 137: 1188–1202.
26. Focks DA, Daniels E, Haile DG, Keesling JE (1995) A simulation model of the epidemiology of urban dengue fever: literature analysis, model development, preliminary validation, and samples of simulation results. Am J Trop Med Hyg 53: 489–506.
27. ISI-MIP (2013) Inter-Sectoral Impact Model Intercomparison Project. Available: www.isi-mip.org. Accessed 07 April 2013.
28. Warszawski L, Frieler K, Huber V, Piontek F, Serdeczny O, et al. (2013) The Inter-Sectoral Impact Model Intercomparison Project (ISI–MIP): Project framework. Proceedings of the National Academy of Sciences.
29. Hempel S, Frieler K, Warszawski L, Schewe J, Piontek F (2013) A trend-preserving bias correction – the ISI-MIP approach. Earth Syst Dynam Discuss 4: 49–92.
30. Marí R, Peydró RJ (2012) Re-Emergence of Malaria and Dengue in Europe, Current Topics in Tropical Medicine; Rodriguez-Morales A, editor: InTech.
31. European Centre for Disease Prevention and Control (ECDC) (2009) Technical Report - Development of Aedes albopictus risk maps Stockholm: ECDC.
32. Sousa C, Clairouin M, Seixas G, Viveiros B, Novo M, et al. (2012) Ongoing outbreak of dengue type 1 in the Autonomous Region of Madeira, Portugal: preliminary report. Euro Surveill 17: 20333.
33. European Centre for Disease Prevention and Control (2012) Epidemiological update: Outbreak of dengue in Madeira, Portugal 14 Feb 2013. Stockholm: ECDC.
34. Brière J, Pracros P, Roux AL, Pierre J (1999) A novel rate model of temperature dependent development for arthropods. Environ Entomol 28: 22–29.
35. Watts D, Burke D, Harrison B, Whitmire R, Nisalak A (1987) Effect of temperature on the vector efficiency of Aedes aegypti for dengue 2 virus. Am J Trop Med Hyg 36: 143–152.
36. McLean D, Clarke A, Coleman J, Montalbetti C, Skidmore A, et al. (1974 Feb) Vector capability of Aedes aegypti mosquitoes for California encephalitis and dengue viruses at various temperatures. Can J Microbiol 20: 255–262.
37. Jones P, Harris I (2008) CRU Time Series (TS) high resolution gridded datasets. University of East Anglia Climatic Research Unit (CRU). NCAS British Atmospheric Data Centre.
38. Goosse H, Barriat P, Lefebvre W, Loutre M, Zunz V (2013) Chapter 6.1.2 Representative concentration pathways (RCPs). Introduction to climate dynamics and climate modeling. Available: http://www.elic.ucl.ac.be/textbook.
39. Taylor KE, Stouffer RJ, Meehl GA (2011) An Overview of CMIP5 and the Experiment Design. Bulletin of the American Meteorological Society 93: 485–498.
40. CMIP5 (2013) Coupled Model Intercomparison Project Phase 5. WCRP - World Climate Research Programme. Available: http://cmip-pcmdi.llnl.gov/cmip5/. Accessed 15 April 2013.

Acknowledgments

We thank Dr. Kristie Ebi, Peter Byass and Mikkel Quam for editing the manuscript. We acknowledge the ISI-MIP project for providing the climate change scenario data used in the projections [21] [28].

Author Contributions

Conceived and designed the experiments: JR. Performed the experiments: JLH. Analyzed the data: JLH HS JR. Contributed reagents/materials/analysis tools: HS. Wrote the paper: JLH JR AWS.

17

Distribution of Fitness in Populations of Dengue Viruses

Md Abu Choudhury[1]*, William B. Lott[1,2], John Aaskov[1]

1 Institute of Health and Biomedical Innovation, Queensland University of Technology, Brisbane, Queensland, Australia, 2 School of Chemistry, Physics, and Mechanical Engineering, Science and Engineering Faculty, Queensland University of Technology, Brisbane, Queensland, Australia

Abstract

Genetically diverse RNA viruses like dengue viruses (DENVs) segregate into multiple, genetically distinct, lineages that temporally arise and disappear on a regular basis. Lineage turnover may occur through multiple processes such as, stochastic or due to variations in fitness. To determine the variation of fitness, we measured the distribution of fitness within DENV populations and correlated it with lineage extinction and replacement. The fitness of most members within a population proved lower than the aggregate fitness of populations from which they were drawn, but lineage replacement events were not associated with changes in the distribution of fitness. These data provide insights into variations in fitness of DENV populations, extending our understanding of the complexity between members of individual populations.

Editor: Lark L. Coffey, University of California Davis, United States of America

Funding: The work was supported by National Health and Medical Research Council of Australia, under grant 497203, Cook Estate and QUT Postgraduate Research Scholarships, Queensland University of Technology. The funders had no role in study design, data collection and analysis, decision to publish, or preparation of the manuscript.

Competing Interests: The authors have declared that no competing interests exist.

* Email: nahidqut13@gmail.com

Introduction

Dengue viruses (DENVs) are the world's most important mosquito-borne viral pathogens for humans in terms of morbidity, mortality and economic impact. DENVs consist of four antigenically distinct serotypes (DENV 1–4), which cause a wide spectrum of clinical manifestations. An estimated 3.6 billion people in the global population and approximately 120 million travellers are at risk of DENV infection. The number of dengue cases reported annually is 50–100 million, with approximately 24,000 deaths in children [1–4]. There is no commercially available DENV vaccine or DENV specific antiviral therapies, despite more than fifty years of research in this field [5].

DENV is a single stranded, positive sense RNA virus belonging to the genus *Flavivirus* (family *Flaviviridae*). Due to the error prone nature of the RNA-dependent RNA polymerase (RdRP) and genome recombination [6–8], DENVs raise significant genetic diversity during their replication [9]. Phylogenetic studies of DENV serotypes showed that they form diverse phylogenetic clusters, that consist of multiple distinct lineages [10,11]. The lineage extinction and replacement on a regular basis is the most surprising feature of DENVs evolutionary dynamics [10]. A lineage that persists for a number of years at a given geographical location sometimes becomes extinct, as an entirely new lineage takes over [12]. Lineage replacement events on a regional scale are well documented. For example, DENV-1 lineage replacements were observed in Myanmar, Cambodia, Thailand in the late 1990s [13], in the mid-1990s [12,14] and in the early 2000s [15] respectively. Similarly, DENV-2 lineage replacements were observed in Vietnam in the early 2000s [16]. DENV-3 lineage replacements were observed in Sri Lanka in the late 1980s [17], and in Thailand in the early 1990s [18]. And DENV-4 lineage replacements were observed in Puerto Rico during the 1980s and 1990s [19]. A more global lineage replacement event has also been reported [20], in which DENV-2 lineages from Southeast Asia displaced the American DENV-2 lineage in the Americas during the early 1990s.

Exploring the causes of DENV lineage replacement has important implications for dengue epidemiology and control [14,17,20–23]. As DENV antigenic properties often differ between lineages, understanding the mechanisms that underlie lineage turnover will influence vaccine design [14,24], and the putative mechanisms of lineage replacement are used to develop prediction models for future dengue epidemics [14,16]. Despite this potential significance, there are multiple explanations exists on whether lineage replacement events result from the random sampling of viral variants during genetic bottlenecks due to the stochastic nature of DENV transmission, or from variations in fitness within discrete viral populations. For the purposes of this work, fitness is defined as the ability of DENV-1 virions to replicate in cultured cells.

Some phylogenetic studies have suggested that observed DENV lineage replacement events were due to either a higher viraemia in the human host [16] or enhanced infectivity in mosquito vectors [14,25–27], while others suggested that the data were more consistent with stochastic events [13,18]. With respect to viral fitness in other systems, fewer than 5% of members of Vesicular stomatitis virus (VSV) populations were reported to be more fit than the population from which they were drawn [28], and mixtures of Ross river virus (RRV) populations containing less than 1% of a virulent strain nonetheless displayed a virulent phenotype [29]. Despite these observations, the distribution of fitness in DENV populations has been not yet been quantified and correlated with epidemiological patterns, like lineage extinction and replacement during transmission. Here, we measured distribution of fitness within DENV populations with differing epidemiological histories and correlated them with observed lineage extinction and replacement events.

Materials and Methods

Ethics statement

This study was approved by the Queensland University of Technology Research Ethics Unit (Ethics No. 0700000910). As no patient tissue was employed in this study, the University Ethics Unit did not require informed patient consent. All patient identifiers were removed from dengue virus samples before they were used for research purposes.

Study population

Viruses were recovered from acute phase sera from dengue patients admitted to the Yangon Children's Hospital [30]. Strains of DENV used in the study, which are described in Table 1, were passaged once in C6/36 before sequencing.

Cell lines and virus isolation

Cell lines were maintained in RPMI-1640 medium (Invitrogen) supplemented with 10% (v/v) heat-inactivated fetal bovine serum (FBS) (Invitrogen) and 1% (v/v) L-Glutamine (200 mM) Penicillin (10,000 units) Streptomycin (10 mg/ml) (Sigma). C6/36 cells were incubated at 30°C and all others were at 37°C in an atmosphere of 5% CO_2/air. Viruses were isolated in C6/36 cells from serum samples collected from Myanmar by using a previously published protocol [31].

Cell culture ELISA

Monolayers of cells in 96-well plates (Nunc) were infected with 200 μl tenfold dilution of DENV and incubated for 8 days. Culture supernatant from each culture was removed and cell monolayers were fixed with 5% (v/v) formaldehyde in PBS for 30 minutes at room temperature. After four washes with PBS-T, 100 μl 0.5% (v/v) triton X-100 in PBS was added to the

monolayers for 5 minutes at room temperature. After a further three washes with PBS-T, the cells were blocked with 2% (w/v) skim milk in PBS for 30 minutes at room temperature. HRP labelled 6B6C-1 antibody [32] was diluted 1:3000 with 2% (w/v) skim milk in PBS and 100 μl were added to each well and incubated for 1 hour at room temperature. Cells then were washed six times with PBS-T and 50 μl TMB solution was added. Virus infected cells were stained blue.

Immunofluorescence assays

Confluent adherent (C6/36, BHK-21 clone 15, HuH-7 and HS1) and non-adherent (K562 and U937) cells in 12 well plates were infected with 200 μl DENV (DENV-1, -2, -3, -4) in serum-free RPMI-1640. After 1 hour of infection, 1 ml RPMI-1640 containing 2% v/v FBS was added to each well and incubated for 12 days. Supernatant from each culture was removed after 12 days. 5 μl of cell suspensions from each dilution were added to each well of a 12 well, teflon coated, immunofluorescence slides (ICN Biomedicals). Excess liquid was aspirated from the spots and cells were air dried for 15 minutes at room temperature before being fixed in ice cold acetone for 4 minutes. 50 μl of a anti-DENV monoclonal antibody solution (M10 for anti- DENV-1, 3H5 for anti-DENV-2, 5D4 for anti-DENV-3 and 1H10 for anti-DENV-4) [33] were added to each spot and incubated for one hour at room temperature. The slides then were washed three times with PBS, each for 10 minutes. 50 μl of a secondary antibody solution composed of a 1:30 dilution of fluorescein isothiocyanate (FITC) labeled anti-mouse IgG (Dako) and a 1:80 dilution of FITC labeled rabbit anti-human IgM (Dako) in PBS was added to each spot and incubated for 45 minutes at room temperature. The slides were washed with PBS three times again each for 10 minutes. Cover slips were mounted on the slides and the cells examined under a fluorescent microscope (Eclipse, Nikon) using ploem illumination. The images were recorded using photometric CoolSnap (Nikon). Cells were considered infected if a clear green fluorescence was observed in the cytoplasm of the

Table 1. Strains of DENV-1 used.

Serotype	Strain	Country	Date of Isolation	Accession number	Source	Passage number
DENV-1	31459	Myanmar	1998	AY588272	[67]	P1 in C6/36
	31987	Myanmar	1998	AY588273	[67]	P1 in C6/36
	32514	Myanmar	1998	AY600860	[67]	P1 in C6/36
	36957	Myanmar	2000	AY620951	[67]	P1 in C6/36
	43826	Myanmar	2001	DQ264966	[34]	P1 in C6/36
	44988	Myanmar	2002	AY726552	Unpublished	P1 in C6/36
	47317	Myanmar	2002	KF559253	This study	P1 in C6/36
	47662	Myanmar	2002	DQ265041	[34]	P1 in C6/36
	49440	Myanmar	2002	DQ265137	[34]	P1 in C6/36
	62690	Myanmar	2005	KF559255	This study	P1 in C6/36
	68417	Myanmar	2007	KF559256	This study	P1 in C6/36
	80579	Myanmar	2009	KF559257	This study	P1 in C6/36
	Infectious clone	Myanmar	2002	KF559254	This study	1 X BHK, 1 X C6/36
DENV-2	New Guinea C	New Guinea	1944	AF038403	[68]	Multiple, unknown
DENV-3	H87	Philippines	1956	M93130	[69]	Multiple, unknown
DENV-4	H241	Philippines	1956	AY947539	Novartis Institute for Tropical Diseases	Multiple, unknown

infected cells. Fluorescent and transmitted light images were recorded for each field.

Indirect ELISA

50 µl of supernatant from DENV infected, or uninfected cell cultures were diluted with an equal volume of chilled borate saline (B.S) pH 9.0 (B.S) and added to 96 well ELISA plates (Maxisorb, Nunc) at 4°C for 24 hours. The plates then were washed five times with PBS-T and 100 µl of HRP-labeled 6B6C-1 diluted in 1:6000 in PBS-T was added to each well and incubated for 45 minutes at room temperature. The plates then were washed six times with PBS-T and 100 µl soluble TMB (ELISA Systems) was added to each well and incubated for 20 minutes for colour to develop. 50 µl of 1 M sulphuric acid (H_2SO_4) was added to each well to stop the reaction. The absorbance in each well was determined with an ELISA plate reader (Beckman Instruments) at a wavelength of 450 nm against a blank of 620 nm.

Assay for distribution of fitness

DENVs were diluted two-fold (1 in 2 to 1 in 128) to provide a theoretical "one infectious unit" of virus as an input to individual cell cultures in 96-well plates i.e. ~66 of the 96 well C6/36 cells monolayer's were infected. Two wells in each 96-well plate (A1 and B1) were infected with undiluted DENV as control (Fig. S1). Yield of prototypes strains of DENV, in cultures of *A. albopictus* (C6/36) cells, infected with ten-fold dilutions was peak at about 8 days irrespective of MOI (Figure S2). Eight days after infection, the culture supernatant from each of the 96-wells was transferred into corresponding wells in a second 96-well plate. The amount of virus released from cells in each culture was determined by indirect ELISA in the second plate described previously (Fig. S1). We calculated mean and +/−2 standard deviations of the control values to determined 95 confidence interval of the range for statistically valid comparison with the fitness of individual populations. Cell monolayers in the original plate were stained for DENV E protein by cell ELISA as described previously.

RNA extraction and RT-PCR and sequencing

RNA was extracted from 140 µl samples of virus using the QIAamp Viral RNA mini kit (Qiagen), according to the manufacturer's instructions. RNA was quantified by spectrophotometry. Equal amounts of RNA were used for RT. Complementary DNA (cDNA) was produced from the RNA of DENV using random hexanucleotide primers (Boehringer Mannheim) and expand reverse transcriptase (Expand RT; Roche). Briefly, 1 µl random hexamer primers (200 ng/µl) was added to 11 µl RNA in a 0.5 ml tube (LabAdvantage) and the mixture was incubated at 65°C for 5 minutes in a heating block before being placed on ice for 2 minutes. Four microliters of 5x RT buffer (Roche), 1 µl 100 mM DTT (Roche), 1 µl 10 mM dNTPs (Roche), 1 µl RNAse inhibitor (40 unit/µl; Roche) and 1 µl expand RT (50 unit/µl) were added to the tube and the volume made up to 20 µl with nuclease free water. RT reactions were incubated at 55°C for 1.5 hours. The primers used for PCR amplification corresponded to a region of the E of DENV-1, which were: D1 843F, 5′-ATGCCATAGGAACATCC 3′ and D1 2465R, 5′-TTGGTGA-CAAAAATGCC 3′. Five microliters of 10x Expand high fidelity PCR buffer with 15 mM MgCl2 (Roche), 1 µl 10 mM dNTP, 2 µl forward primer (100 ng/µl), 2 µl reverse primer (100 ng/µl), 0.75 µl Expand high fidelity PCR system (3.5 unit/µl; Roche), 5 µl cDNA and 34.25 µl nuclease free water were mixed to make the total volume of 50 µl. PCR was performed using cycling conditions of 94°C for 2 minutes for one cycle and then 92°C for 30 seconds, 58°C for 40 seconds and 68°C for 2.30 minutes for 10 cycles, 92°C for 30 seconds, 58°C for 30 seconds and 68°C for 3 minutes for 10 cycles, 92°C for 30 seconds, 58°C for 30 seconds and 68°C for 3.30 minutes for 18 cycles run for 39 cycles followed by 68°C for 10 minutes for final extension. PCR products were electrophoresed on 1.0% agarose in 1x TBE buffer and products of the correct size were gel purified with the MinElute PCR purification kit (Qiagen), according to the manufacturer's instructions. The purified DNA (100 ng per 300 bp of product) was added to 3.2 pmol of oligonucleotide primers (forward and reverse) in a final volume of 12 µL. The remaining sequencing reaction was performed by Australian Genome Research Facility Ltd (AGRF), Brisbane. Sequencing was performed on automated ABI 3730 DNA Analyzer (Applied Biosystems) using dye-terminator chemistry.

Sequence Alignments and Phylogenetic Analysis

Alignment of the consensus sequences were performed using the ClustalW program in the Geneious Pro 6.1. The aligned nucleic acid sequences were used to construct bootstrapping phylogenetic tree using the Neighbor-joing tree building method and Tamura-Nei genetic distance model in the Geneious Pro 6.1.

Results

Phylogenetic relationship between DENV-1 isolates

Analyses of Myanmar DENV-1 E gene sequences from Genbank and unpublished sequences (Table 1) produced a phylogenetic tree with five distinct branches (Fig. 1). Lineage A contained the first DENV-1 isolate recovered in Myanmar (Burma, Bur76 and Mya76). This lineage became extinct in 1998, about the same time lineages B and C appeared. No examples of lineage B have been recovered since 2002, but lineage C was still circulating in 2008. Lineage D was first detected in 2006, and was still circulating in 2008. The single example of lineage E, which was most closely related to DENV-1 from Vietnam, did not appear to have established cycles of transmission and was excluded from analysis. For the purposes of analysis, lineages A and B are considered to have become extinct in 1998 and 2002, respectively. Lineages C and D were deemed to be still circulating in 2008. The strains in bold type in Figure 1 were regarded as representative of their lineage and were used in subsequent studies.

Susceptibility of vertebrate and invertebrate cell lines to infection with DENV

Because subsequent fitness studies required that DENV be cultured in both mosquito and relevant human cell lines, the susceptibility of C6/36 (mosquito) cells and a range of human cell lines (HuH7, HepG2, HC04, K562, U937, HS1 and SW987) to DENV infection was determined. Baby Hamster kidney (BHK-21) cells were included as a control substrate. With the exception of HuH7 cells, the human cell lines were uniformly refractory to infection with prototype strains of DENV (Table S1). Subsequent experiments with low passage DENV isolates and other DENV populations of interest were performed only in C6/36 and HuH7 cells (Table 2). As subsequent experiments required serum-free cell culture, the yield of DENV isolated from C6/36 cells cultured with and without a FBS supplement was assayed (Table 2) and showed no significant difference ($p > 0.05$, student t-test). As previously observed (Table S1), the yield of DENV from HuH7 cells was consistently lower than that from C6/36 cells. C6/36 mosquito cells were as much as one million times more sensitive to infection with low passage strains of DENV-1. No DENV production was

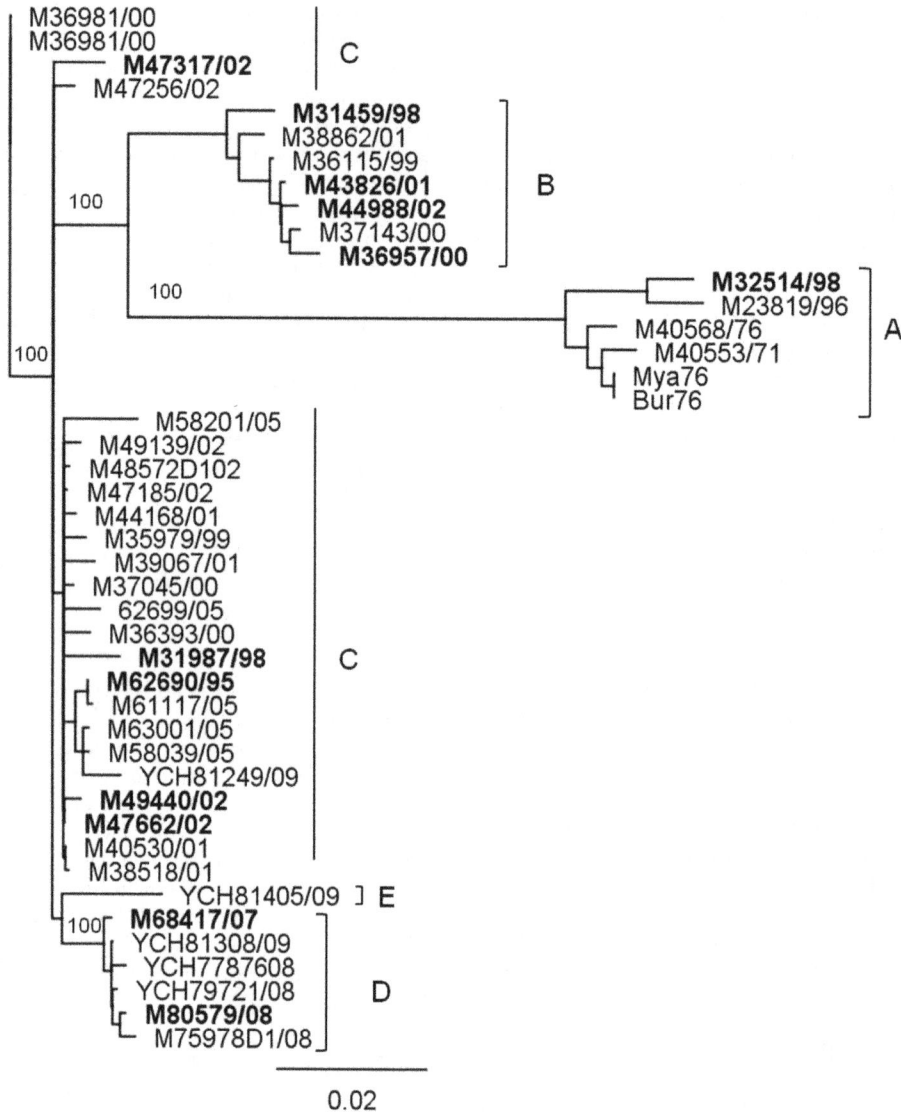

Figure 1. Phylogenetic analysis of the E gene of DENV-1 showing lineage extinction and replacement of DENV-1 in Myanmar.
Bootstrap values (100 replications) for key nodes are shown. A distance bar is shown below the tree. Lineage A, B and E are extinct and lineage C and D are still circulating. Strains selected for study have been highlighted.

detectable in HuH7 cells infected with 8 of the 20 DENV strains studied.

Distribution of fitness within population of DENV-1

Stocks of viruses from the three lineages in Fig. 1 (A, B, C) were limit diluted to provide a theoretical "one infectious unit"/200 µl inoculum (i.e. 65 of the 96 wells contained infectious virus) and used to infect monolayers of C6/36 cells in 96 well plates. Eight days after infection, at the time of peak virus production (Fig. S2), the amount of virus released from C6/36 cells in each well was determined by indirect ELISA (Fig. S1). The amount of virus from cultures infected with one infectious dose of virus was compared with that of the population from which it was derived i.e. cell monolayers in the 96 well plate infected with corresponding undiluted stock virus. The mean absorbance (±2 s.d.) was calculated for the duplicate control wells containing undiluted stock of the DENV-1 population being analysed (A1, B1; Fig. S1). Supernatants from cultures giving rise to an ELISA absorbance

similar to the mean (±2 s.d.) for cultures A1, B1 (undiluted stocks of virus) were regarded as having the same fitness is the population from which they were derived. Supernatants from cultures giving rise to an ELISA absorbance of more than 2 s.d. less than the mean for cultures A1 and B1 were regarded as less fit. Supernatants from cultures giving rise to an ELISA absorbance of more than 2 s.d. greater than the mean for A1 and B1 were regarded as more fit. The numerical fitness distribution within each of these classifications (more, average, less fit) is presented in Table S3. The distribution of fitness within populations of DENV-1 (lineages A, B and C) is shown in Fig. 2.

Less than 2 per cent (fewer than 1 in 94) of the members of DENV-1 populations collected in 1998 (lineages A, B, C) were more fit than the population from which they were drawn ($p<$ 0.05, Chi-Square-test) (Fig. 2).

Members of all populations recovered after 1998 contained some members (14.1% to 45.71%) that were more fit than the population from which they were derived except for the sample

Table 2. Infectivity of dengue viruses (DENVs) for mosquito (C6/36) and human (HuH7) cell lines.

Dengue virus		Titre of virus (log$_{10}$TCID/ml)			
Serotype	Strain	C6/36 without FBS	C6/36 with FBS	HuH7 without FBS	HuH7 with FBS
DENV-1	Hawaii	6.5	5.5	<1.0	<1.0
	31459	7.0	6.5	<1.0	2.0
	31987	5.5	5.0	<1.0	3.0
	32514	7.0	6.5	3.0	3.0
	62699	6.0	4.5	<1.0	<1.0
	63001	5.5	5.0	<1.0	2.0
	75971	5.5	5.5	<1.0	2.0
	84077	8.0	7.5	3.0	3.0
	84558	7.5	7.0	<1.0	2.0
	I. C	7.5	7.0	<1.0	4.0
DENV-2	New Guinea C	8.0	8.0	4.0	4.0
	I. C	8.0	8.0	4.0	4.0
DENV-3	H87	7.5	7.5	<1.0	2.0
	82899	7.0	5.5	<1.0	<1.0
	83468	5.0	4.5	<1.0	<1.0
	84014	7.0	6.5	<1.0	<1.0
	84700	4.5	3.5	<1.0	<1.0
DENV-4	H241	7.0	7.0	<1.0	2.0
	84711	6.5	5.5	<1.0	<1.0
	84087	7.0	6.5	<1.0	<1.0

DENVs isolated from clinical patients in C6/36 were infected in C6/36 and Huh7 with ten-fold dilutions to determine the relative titres in both cell types. Both cells (C6/36 and Huh7) were infected at the same time with the same dilution of DENVs to determine the relative titres.
I.C. Infectious clone derived DENV-2.

recovered in 2000 (36957/00, lineage B) which showed an increase in the prevalence of more fit members. Most of the post-1998 samples were recovered after the explosive outbreak of DENV-1 infection in Myanmar in 2001 and showed an increase in the prevalence of more fit members. While DENV populations of both lineages B and C appeared to be gaining (14.1% to 45.71%) more fit members, only lineage C has survived.

Fitness distribution in lineage B and C represents a polarization of fitness which increased in both numbers (more and less fit). We observed that 75% of the viral strains were polarized in extinct lineage B, whereas only 20% of the viral strains were polarized in circulating lineage C, ($P = 0.09$, Pearson Chi-square statistics = 2) (Table 3). We considered the fitness was being polarized when more than 33% (one third) populations were more and less fit than average fitness. We excluded linage A from this analysis because of limited number of samples for statistically valid comparison.

Discussion

DENV lineage turnover is commonly observed in DENV evolution, but it is unclear whether lineage replacement events are caused by selective pressure or by random sampling during transmission. While DENV populations are highly diverse [18,34–39], the overall fitness of a DENV population in an individual host is unlikely to be simply the sum of individual fitness. Other similarly diverse arboviruses exhibit characteristics consistent with synergy within their viral populations. For example, less than 5 per cent of VSV virions within a population were more fit than the population from which they were drawn [28], and RRV

populations containing less than 1% of a virulent strain nevertheless displayed a virulent phenotype [29]. Recent observations that defective DENV genomes can be complemented by fully competent genomes to overcome the defect [31] supports the concept of cooperativity within DENV populations. To date, there has been no attempt to quantify the distribution of fitness within DENV populations, and to correlate these data with epidemiological patterns. Here we report the distribution of fitness within populations of DENVs collected from Myanmar between 1998 and 2005.

Our observation that all members of DENV-1 populations collected in 1998 were less fit than the overall fitness of the populations from which they were drawn regardless of lineage (Fig. 2) is consistent with extensive complementation among the 90–99% of DENV genomes that are incapable of self-replication [16,40,41]. The distribution of fitness appeared to polarise in subsequent years, in which the fraction of the population that was more fit than the overall population fitness increased. This was especially apparent for lineage B from 1998 to 2002 (Fig. 2). The proportion of individuals in DENV-1 populations that were more fit than the population as a whole increased after the explosive outbreak of DENV-1 infection in 1998, suggesting that more fit viruses may have been selected during the rapid transmission accompanying the outbreak. However, an increase in the proportion of "more fit" members of a DENV population did not guarantee survival of a lineage, as lineage B became extinct between 2002 and 2005.

We observed a trend (although statistically not significant, $P = 0.09$, Pearson Chi-square statistics = 2) that fitness of extinct

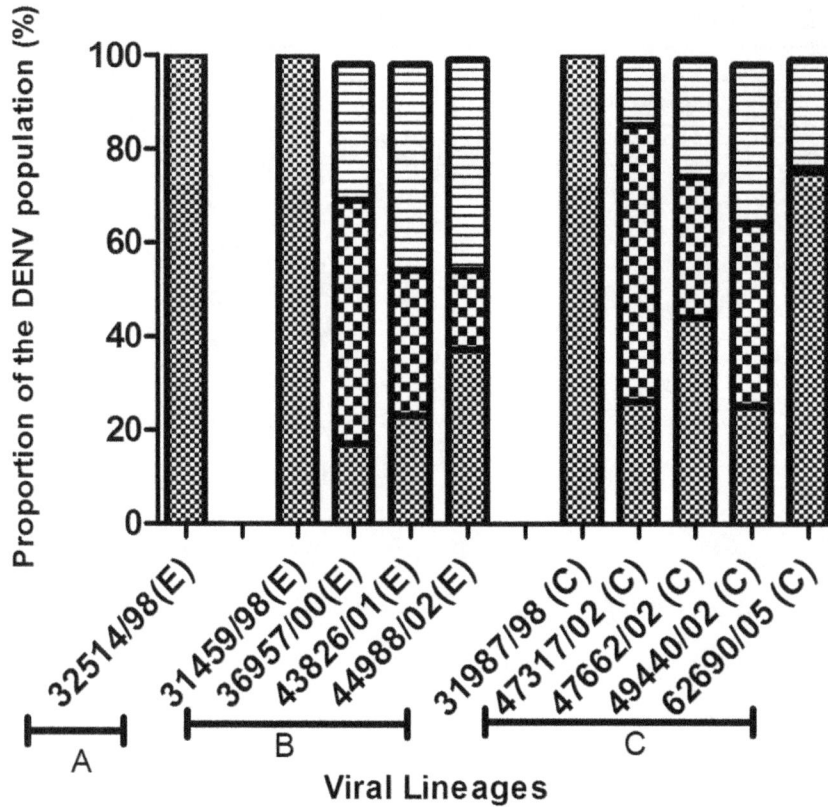

Figure 2. Distribution of fitness within populations of DENV-1 from four lineages. Populations are identified as strain/year/E (extinct) or C (circulating); proportion more fit than the population average indicated horizontal hatch, same fit as the original population indicated as bold squares and less fit than the original population indicated as small squares.

lineage was more polarised (>50%) than circulating lineage. It is possible that polarisation of fitness within a lineage population in which the "more fit" viruses specialising in high virus titre support the "less fit" viruses within the same population. If true, the less fit viruses presumably specialise in some other characteristics which are important for lineage survival (i.e. increased replication rate or increased ability to evade the host immune system), and similarly support more fit viruses within their lineage population. Such specialisation represents a loss of fitness homogeneity that could result in populations that are more vulnerable to stochastic sampling (bottleneck) effects. For example, the distribution of fitness of a small-sized random sample from a homogeneous 1998 lineage population would likely represent of the overall population with respect to fitness distribution, and thus would likely maintain the cooperative characteristics of the population from which it was drawn. However, the fitness distribution of a similarly small-sized random sample from the polarised 2002 lineage population would be less likely to accurately represent the fitness distribution of the source population. If the random sample were to contain insufficient numbers of more fit viruses to effectively support the less fit viruses, the lineage would become vulnerable to extinction. However, more data would be required to verify this interpretation as this is not statistically significant ($P = 0.09$, Pearson Chi-square statistics = 2) (Table 3). The results could be statistically significant if we had sufficient number of samples. Unfortunately, in this study our sample numbers are not high. Further studies required with large number of samples to determine whether

Table 3. Relationship between DENV lineage extinction and polarization in fitness in populations.

DENV fitness polarization	Lineage		Total
	Extinct	**Circulating**	
Polarized	3	1	4
Non-polarized	1	4	5
Total	4	5	9

75% of the extinct viral strains were polarized and 80% of the circulating strains were non-polarized. We have conducted a Chi-square test of independence to test the null hypothesis that there is no association between polarization and virus extinction. The test results show that there is no statistically significant association between polarization and virus extinction (Pearson Chi- square statistic = 2.7, $p = 0.09$).

fitness polarisation in DENV population has any impact on lineage extinction.

We observed no association between the distribution of fitness of members with DENV-1 populations in mosquito cells and the survival or extinction of a lineage of viruses (Fig. 2). However, there was an increase in the proportion of more fit members during and after the 2001–2002 outbreaks, suggesting that there may have been some selection for DENV that grew to high titre in mosquitoes. This observation has two caveats. The first is that there was an increase in the proportion of more fit members in population 36957/00, compared to 31459/98 (clade B) *before* the outbreak began (36957/00 was recovered in the dengue season of 2000 in which the number of reported cases was low). The second is that the half life of an *Aedes aegypti* mosquito in Thailand (and presumably in neighbouring Myanmar) is only 7–8 days [42] and so selection might be for a virus that replicated faster rather than one that grew to high titre. However, DENV, which grows to high titre, may also reach significant titres earlier.

Fitness can be defined as a measure of the ability to replicate (and produce infectious progeny) in a host [43,44] but a more appropriate definition could be a measure of the ability to be transmitted, i.e. to infect the next host in a transmission cycle. While transmissibility is probably the most relevant measure for a virus like DENV, with infection cycles involving alternate human and mosquito hosts, technical constraints prevented this measure being used. In this study, fitness was defined as the yield of DENV-1 virions from infected cells.

An indirect ELISA procedure was employed to estimate the quantity of DENV virions released into a culture supernatant (see Materials and Methods). It was accepted that a proportion of these would contain genomes that were not infectious. However, given the complexity of the interactions between RNA genomes e.g. complementation, interference by sub-genomic RNA etc., the yield of virions was a more relevant measure of productive infection than estimates of either the number of infectious virus particles (able to infect cell substrate) or of genome copy number.

A comparison of titres of DENV in patients measured as infectious virus or as genome copy number suggested that copy number values are 10–100 times higher than infectious titres [16,40,41]. That the individual members of DENV populations might vary in their fitness is not surprising given that there are reports of virions with genomes with mutations and indels giving rise to intragenic stop codons as well as genomes with deletions of thousands of nucleotides [31,34,37,45–49] There also is an extensive literature describing non-lethal changes that effect DENV replication [50–53]. Taken together with the comments above, it is unlikely that an individual cell is infected by a single DENV genome. For these reasons, a unit, "one infectious dose" has been used in this study and has been derived statistically, i.e. if 96 infectious units of virus in 9.6 ml are aliquoted uniformly into 96 wells of a microtitre plate, only 65 wells will contain virus (some wells will contain more than one infectious dose). While this is a weakness of this approach, there was no alternative, and the same methodology was used for all populations, so enabling comparisons to be made.

It was important to select appropriate human and mosquito cell lines for a suitable surrogate to measure fitness *in vitro*. The primary and/or major sites of DENV replication in humans are not known yet. Therefore, it was unclear what cells or cell lines might be appropriate substrates for experiments relevant to the human condition. A survey of the literature (Table S2) suggested DENV could be identified most commonly in the liver, as it was associated with liver dysfunction [54–56] and pathology [55,57–59] but it was not clear whether this was due to the extensive

phogocytic activity of the liver [60–65] or that cells in the liver are more susceptible to infection than those in other tissues. However, in this study, all human cell lines including a number of liver cell lines, were extremely refractory to infection by the low passage DENV-1 (Table 2). The use of HuH7 cells in this study reflected that these cells appeared to be the best available rather than that they were a productive cell substrate. Other investigators [66] have struggled to find human cell lines that are uniformly susceptible to infection by DENV from patient serum or by low passage DENV isolates.

These investigations focussed on DENV infections in C6/36 mosquito cells. Mosquito cell is not a perfect representation to measure fitness; however, it is representation of mosquito vectors. Additional information may have been revealed if similar studies were undertaken in human cells, and more informative changes may have been revealed if similar studies were undertaken in human cells. However, it was not possible to identify a human cell line that was sufficiently susceptible to infection with all low passage strains of DENV (Table 2). Furthermore, the most susceptible human cell line, HuH7, required a FBS supplement for growth and the FBS reduced the sensitivity of the ELISA method employed to quantitate DENV in culture supernatants.

This study has provided clear evidence that the lineage turnover in DENV transmission is not due to any selective pressures because of the variation in fitness within populations. While we observed a trend that fitness of extinct lineage DENV populations was more polarised than circulating lineage, impact of polarisation of fitness in population in DENV lineage extinction need to be further explored. As Myanmar is a hyperendemic country, the presence of multiple DENV serotypes may result in complex patterns of cross-immunity, which might determine which clades survive and which become extinct [13,30]. The explanation for clade replacement may lie with the phenotype of the host with the more susceptible hosts (host proteins able to support the replication of DENV most efficiently; the innate immune system least able to resist infection) being infected more readily after appearance of a new clade such that, after several years, the virus struggles to survive. A new clade, with a different phenotype, may be able to exploit hosts which the resident clade is struggling to infect.

Supporting Information

Figure S1 Distribution of fitness within populations of DENV-1. Serial dilutions of DENV were added to 94 wells of 96 well plates containing monolayers of C6/36 cells. Undiluted virus was added to the two remaining wells shown within bracket. Eight days later the supernatants from the cultures were transferred to 96 well ELISA plates and the cell monolayers stained for DENV antigen by indirect ELISA. The amount of DENV in each supernatant was quantified by indirect ELISA.

Acknowledgments

The authors thank Dr. Francesca Frentiu for important comments on previous version of this manuscript and Dr. Shahera Banu for helping in statistical analysis.

Author Contributions

Conceived and designed the experiments: MAC JA. Performed the experiments: MAC. Analyzed the data: MAC WBL JA. Contributed reagents/materials/analysis tools: JA. Wrote the paper: MAC JA.

References

1. Halstead SB (2007) Dengue. Lancet 370: 1644–1652.
2. WHO (2012) Dengue and severe dengue [Online]. World Health Organization: Available: http://www.who.int/mediacentre/factsheets/fs117/en/index.html Accessed 2012 Jan 1.
3. Ooi E-E, Gubler DJ (2009) Global spread of epidemic dengue: the influence of environmental change. Future Virology 4: 571–580.
4. Wilder-Smith A, Gubler DJ (2008) Geographic expansion of dengue: the impact of international travel. Medical Clinics of North America 92: 1377–1390.
5. Wilder-Smith A, Ooi EE, Vasudevan SG, Gubler DJ (2010) Update on dengue: epidemiology, virus evolution, antiviral drugs, and vaccine development. Current Infectious Disease Reports 12: 157–164.
6. Craig S, Thu HM, Lowry K, Wang X-F, Holmes EC, et al. (2003) Diverse dengue type 2 virus populations contain recombinant and both parental viruses in a single mosquito host. Journal of Virology 77: 4463–4467.
7. Aaskov J, Buzacott K, Field E, Lowry K, Berlioz-Arthaud A, et al. (2007) Multiple recombinant dengue type 1 viruses in an isolate from a dengue patient. Journal of General Virology 88: 3334–3340.
8. Worobey M, Rambaut A, Holmes EC (1999) Widespread intra-serotype recombination in natural populations of dengue virus. Proceedings of the National Academy of Sciences of the United States of America 96: 7352–7357.
9. Holmes EC, Burch SS (2000) The causes and consequences of genetic variation in dengue virus. Trends in Microbiology 8: 74–77.
10. Holmes EC, Twiddy SS (2003) The origin, emergence and evolutionary genetics of dengue virus. Infection, Genetics and Evolution 3: 19–28.
11. Weaver SC, Vasilakis N (2009) Molecular evolution of dengue viruses: Contributions of phylogenetics to understanding the history and epidemiology of the preeminent arboviral disease. Infection, Genetics and Evolution 9: 523–540.
12. Zhang C, Mammen MP, Chinnawirotpisan P, Klungthong C, Rodpradit P, et al. (2005) Clade replacements in dengue virus serotypes 1 and 3 are associated with changing serotype prevalence. Journal of Virology 79: 15123–15130.
13. Thu HM, Kym L, Jiang L, Hlaing T, Holmes EC, et al. (2005) Lineage extinction and replacement in dengue type 1 virus populations are due to stochastic events rather than to natural selection. Virology 336: 163–172.
14. Lambrechts L, Fansiri T, Pongsiri A, Thaisomboonsuk B, Klungthong C, et al. (2012) Dengue-1 virus clade replacement in Thailand associated with enhanced mosquito transmission. Journal of Virology 86: 1853–1861.
15. Duong V, Simmons C, Gavotte L, Viari A, Ong S, et al. (2011) Genetic diversity and lineage dynamic of dengue virus serotype 1 (DENV-1) in Cambodia. Infection, Genetics and Evolution: 1–10.
16. Ty Hang VT, Holmes EC, Veasna D, Quy NT, Tinh Hien T, et al. (2010) Emergence of the Asian 1 genotype of dengue virus serotype 2 in Viet Nam: In vivo fitness advantage and lineage replacement in South-East Asia. PLoS Neglected Tropical Diseases 4: e757.
17. Messer WB, Gubler DJ, Harris E, Sivananthan K, de Silva AM (2003) Emergence and global spread of a dengue serotype 3, subtype III virus. Emerging Infectious Diseases 9: 800–809.
18. Wittke V, Robb TE, Thu HM, Nisalak A, Nimmannitya S, et al. (2002) Extinction and rapid emergence of strains of dengue 3 virus during an Interepidemic period. Virology 301: 148–156.
19. Bennett SN, Holmes EC, Chirivella M, Rodriguez DM, Beltran M, et al. (2003) Selection-driven evolution of emergent dengue virus. Molecular Biology and Evolution 20: 1650–1658.
20. Rico-Hesse R, Harrison LM, Salas RA, Tovar D, Nisalak A, et al. (1997) Origins of dengue type 2 viruses associated with increased pathogenicity in the Americas. Virology 230: 244–251.
21. Gubler DJ, Suharyono W, Lubis I, Eram S, Gunarso S (1981) Epidemic dengue 3 in central Java, associated with low viremia in man. American Journal of Tropical Medicine and Hygiene 30: 1094–1099.
22. Gubler DJ, Reed D, Rosen L, Hitchcock JR (1978) Epidemiologic, clinical, and virologic observations on dengue in the Kingdom of Tonga. American Journal of Tropical Medicine and Hygiene 27: 581–589.
23. Steel A, Gubler DJ, Bennett SN (2010) Natural attenuation of dengue virus type-2 after a series of island outbreaks: a retrospective phylogenetic study of events in the South Pacific three decades ago. Virology 405: 505–512.
24. Wahala WM, Donaldson EF, de Alwis R, Accavitti-Loper MA, Baric RS, et al. (2010) Natural strain variation and antibody neutralization of dengue serotype 3 viruses. PLoS Pathogens 6: e1000821.
25. Anderson JR, Rico-Hesse R (2006) Aedes aegypti vectorial capacity is determined by the infecting genotype of dengue virus. American Journal of Tropical Medicine and Hygiene 75: 886–892.
26. Armstrong PM, Rico-Hesse R (2003) Efficiency of dengue serotype 2 virus strains to infect and disseminate in Aedes Aegypti. American Journal of Tropical Medicine and Hygiene 68: 539–544.
27. Hanley K, Nelson J, Schirtzinger E, Whitehead S, Hanson C (2008) Superior infectivity for mosquito vectors contributes to competitive displacement among strains of dengue virus. BMC Ecology 8: 1.
28. Duarte EA, Novella IS, Ledesma S, Clarke DK, Moya A, et al. (1994) Subclonal components of consensus fitness in an RNA virus clone. Journal of Virology 68: 4295–4301.
29. Taylor WP, Marshall ID (1975) Adaptation studies with Ross River virus: laboratory mice and cell cultures. Journal of General Virology 28: 59–72.
30. Thu HM, Lowry K, Myint TT, Shwe TN, Han AM, et al. (2004) Myanmar dengue outbreak associated with displacement of serotypes 2, 3, and 4 by dengue 1. Emerging Infectious Diseases 10: 593–597.
31. Li D, Lott WB, Lowry K, Jones A, Thu HM, et al. (2011) Defective interfering viral particles in acute dengue infections. PLoS One 6: e19447.
32. Roehrig JT, Day JW, Kinney RM (1982) Antigenic analysis of the surface glycoproteins of a Venezuelan equine encephalomyelitis virus (TC-83) using monoclonal antibodies. Virology 118: 269–278.
33. Henchal EA, Gentry MK, McCown JM, Brandt WE (1982) Dengue virus-specific and flavivirus group determinants identified with monoclonal antibodies by indirect immunofluorescence. American Journal of Tropical Medicine and Hygiene 31: 830–836.
34. Aaskov J, Buzacott K, Thu HM, Lowry K, Holmes EC (2006) Long-term transmission of defective RNA viruses in humans and Aedes mosquitoes. Science 311: 236–238.
35. Chao DY, King CC, Wang WK, Chen WJ, Wu HL, et al. (2005) Strategically examining the full-genome of dengue virus type 3 in clinical isolates reveals its mutation spectra. Virology Journal 2: 72.
36. Thai KTD, Henn MR, Zody MC, Tricou V, Nguyet NM, et al. (2012) High-resolution analysis of intrahost genetic diversity in dengue virus serotype 1 infection identifies mixed infections. Journal of Virology 86: 835–843.
37. Wang WK, Lin SR, Lee CM, King CC, Chang SC (2002) Dengue type 3 virus in plasma is a population of closely related genomes: quasispecies. Journal of Virology 76: 4662–4665.
38. Zhang C, Mammen MP Jr, Chinnawirotpisan P, Klungthong C, Rodpradit P, et al. (2006) Structure and age of genetic diversity of dengue virus type 2 in Thailand. Journal of General Virology 87: 873–883.
39. Parameswaran P, Charlebois P, Tellez Y, Nunez A, Ryan EM, et al. (2012) Genome-wide patterns of intrahuman dengue virus diversity reveal associations with viral phylogenetic clade and interhost diversity. Journal of Virology 86: 8546–8558.
40. Vaughn DW, Green S, Kalayanarooj S, Innis BL, Nimmannitya S, et al. (2000) Dengue viremia titer, antibody response pattern, and virus serotype correlate with disease severity. Journal of Infectious Diseases 181: 2–9.
41. Houng HS, Chung-Ming Chen R, Vaughn DW, Kanesa-thasan N (2001) Development of a fluorogenic RT-PCR system for quantitative identification of dengue virus serotypes 1–4 using conserved and serotype-specific 3' noncoding sequences. Journal of Virological Methods 95: 19–32.
42. Harrington LC, Buonaccorsi JP, Edman JD, Costero A, Kittayapong P, et al. (2001) Analysis of survival of young and old Aedes aegypti (Diptera: Culicidae) from Puerto Rico and Thailand. Journal of Medical Entomology 38: 537–547.
43. Domingo E, Holland JJ (1997) RNA virus mutations and fitness for survival. Annual Review of Microbiology 51: 151–178.
44. Domingo E, Escarmis C, Menendez-Arias L, Holland J (1999) Viral quasispecies and fitness variations. In: Domingo E, Webster, R and Holland, J., editor. Origin and Evolution of Viruses. London: Academic Press. 141–161.
45. Noppornpanth S, Smits SL, Lien TX, Poovorawan Y, Osterhaus AD, et al. (2007) Characterization of hepatitis C virus deletion mutants circulating in chronically infected patients. Journal of Virology 81: 12496–12503.
46. Pacini L, Graziani R, Bartholomew L, De Francesco R, Paonessa G (2009) Naturally occurring hepatitis C virus subgenomic deletion mutants replicate efficiently in Huh-7 cells and are trans-packaged in vitro to generate infectious defective particles. Journal of Virology 83: 9079–9093.

47. Cattaneo R, Schmid A, Eschle D, Baczko K, ter Meulen V, et al. (1988) Biased hypermutation and other genetic changes in defective measles viruses in human brain infections. Cell 55: 255–265.

48. Brinton MA (1982) Characterization of West Nile virus persistent infections in genetically resistant and susceptible mouse cells. I. Generation of defective nonplaquing virus particles. Virology 116: 84–98.

49. Wang W-K, Sung T-L, Lee C-N, Lin T-Y, King C-C (2002) Sequence diversity of the capsid gene and the nonstructural gene NS2B of dengue-3 virus in vivo. Virology 303: 181–191.

50. García-Arriaza J, Domingo E, Briones C (2007) Characterization of minority subpopulations in the mutant spectrum of HIV-1 quasispecies by successive specific amplifications. Virus Research 129: 123–134.

51. Clyde K, Kyle JL, Harris E (2006) Recent advances in deciphering viral and host determinants of dengue virus replication and pathogenesis. Journal of Virology 80: 11418–11431.

52. Hsieh SC, Zou G, Tsai WY, Qing M, Chang GJ, et al. (2011) The C-terminal helical domain of dengue virus precursor membrane protein is involved in virus assembly and entry. Virology 410: 170–180.

53. Lin SR, Zou G, Hsieh SC, Qing M, Tsai WY, et al. (2011) The helical domains of the stem region of dengue virus envelope protein are involved in both virus assembly and entry. Journal of Virology 85: 5159–5171.

54. Nguyen TL, Nguyen TH, Tieu NT (1997) The impact of dengue hemorrhagic fever on liver function. Research in Virology 148: 273–277.

55. Wahid SF, Sanusi S, Zawawi MM, Ali RA (2000) A comparison of the pattern of liver involvement in dengue hemorrhagic fever with classic dengue fever. Southeast Asian Journal of Tropical Medicine and Public Health 31: 259–263.

56. Mohan B, Patwari AK, Anand VK (2000) Hepatic dysfunction in childhood dengue infection. Journal of Tropical Pediatrics 46: 40–43.

57. Bhamarapravati N, Tuchinda P, Boonyapaknavik V (1967) Pathology of Thailand hemorrhagic fever: a study of 100 autopsy cases. Annals of Tropical Medicine and Parasitology 61: 500–510.

58. Burke T (1968) Dengue hemorrhagic fever: a pathological study. Transactions of the Royal Society of Tropical Medicine and Hygiene 62: 682–692.

59. Bhamarapravati N (1989) Hemostatic defects in dengue hemorrhagic fever. Reviews of Infectious Diseases 11 Suppl 4: S826–829.

60. Huerre MR, Lan NT, Marianneau P, Hue NB, Khun H, et al. (2001) Liver histopathology and biological correlates in five cases of fatal dengue fever in Vietnamese children. Virchows Archiv 438: 107–115.

61. Rosen L, Drouet MT, Deubel V (1999) Detection of dengue virus RNA by reverse transcription-polymerase chain reaction in the liver and lymphoid organs but not in the brain in fatal human infection. American Journal of Tropical Medicine and Hygiene 61: 720–724.

62. Jessie K, Fong MY, Devi S, Lam SK, Wong KT (2004) Localization of dengue virus in naturally infected human tissues, by immunohistochemistry and in situ hybridization. Journal of Infectious Diseases 189: 1411–1418.

63. Couvelard A, Marianneau P, Bedel C, Drouet MT, Vachon F, et al. (1999) Report of a fatal case of dengue infection with hepatitis: demonstration of dengue antigens in hepatocytes and liver apoptosis. Human Pathology 30: 1106–1110.

64. Ramos C, Sanchez G, Pando RH, Baquera J, Hernandez D, et al. (1998) Dengue virus in the brain of a fatal case of hemorrhagic dengue fever. Journal of Neurovirology 4: 465–468.

65. Rosen L, Khin MM, Tin U (1989) Recovery of virus from the liver of children with fatal dengue: reflections on the pathogenesis of the disease and its possible analogy with that of yellow fever. Research in Virology 140: 351–360.

66. Diamond MS, Edgil D, Roberts TG, Lu B, Harris E (2000) Infection of human cells by dengue virus is modulated by different cell types and viral strains. Journal of Virology 74: 7814–7823.

67. Myat Thu H, Lowry K, Myint TT, Shwe TN, Han AM, et al. (2004) Myanmar dengue outbreak associated with displacement of serotypes 2,3, and 4 by dengue 1. Emerging Infectious Diseases 10: 593–597.

68. Gruenberg A, Woo W, Biedrzycka A, Wright PJ (1988) Partial nucleotide sequence and deduced amino acid sequence of the structural proteins of dengue virus type 2, New Guinea C and PUO-218 strains. The Journal of general virology 69: 1391–1398.

69. Osatomi K, Sumiyoshi H (1990) Complete nucleotide sequence of dengue type 3 virus genome RNA. Virology 176: 643–647.

18

Galectin-1 Exerts Inhibitory Effects during DENV-1 Infection

Karina Alves Toledo[1,9]**, Marise Lopes Fermino**[2,9]**, Camillo del Cistia Andrade**[2]**, Thalita Bachelli Riul**[2]**,
Renata Tomé Alves[2]**, Vanessa Danielle Menjon Muller**[2]**, Raquel Rinaldi Russo**[2]**, Sean R. Stowell**[3]**,
Richard D. Cummings[3]**, Victor Hugo Aquino**[2]**, Marcelo Dias-Baruffi**[2]*****

1 Department of Biological Sciences, Universidade Estadual Paulista – UNESP (FCL-Assis), Assis, Brazil, 2 Departmento de Análises Clínicas, Toxicológicas e Bromatológicas, Faculdade de Ciências Farmacêuticas de Ribeirão Preto, Universidade de São Paulo, Ribeirão Preto, Brazil, 3 Emory University School of Medicine, Atlanta, Georgia, United States of America

Abstract

Dengue virus (DENV) is an enveloped RNA virus that is mosquito-transmitted and can infect a variety of immune and non-immune cells. Response to infection ranges from asymptomatic disease to a severe disorder known as dengue hemorrhagic fever. Despite efforts to control the disease, there are no effective treatments or vaccines. In our search for new antiviral compounds to combat infection by dengue virus type 1 (DENV-1), we investigated the role of galectin-1, a widely-expressed mammalian lectin with functions in cell-pathogen interactions and immunoregulatory properties. We found that DENV-1 infection of cells in vitro exhibited caused decreased expression of Gal-1 in several different human cell lines, suggesting that loss of Gal-1 is associated with virus production. In test of this hypothesis we found that exogenous addition of human recombinant Gal-1 (hrGal-1) inhibits the virus production in the three different cell types. This inhibitory effect was dependent on hrGal-1 dimerization and required its carbohydrate recognition domain. Importantly, the inhibition was specific for hrGal-1, since no effect was observed using recombinant human galectin-3. Interestingly, we found that hrGal-1 directly binds to dengue virus and acts, at least in part, during the early stages of DENV-1 infection, by inhibiting viral adsorption and its internalization to target cells. To test the in vivo role of Gal-1 in DENV infection, Gal-1-deficient-mice were used to demonstrate that the expression of endogenous Galectin-1 contributes to resistance of macrophages to in vitro-infection with DENV-1 and it is also important to physiological susceptibility of mice to in vivo infection with DENV-1. These results provide novel insights into the functions of Gal-1 in resistance to DENV infection and suggest that Gal-1 should be explored as a potential antiviral compound.

Editor: Tian Wang, University of Texas Medical Branch, United States of America

Funding: This work was supported by Fundação de Coordenação de Aperfeiçoamento de Pessoal de Nível Superior (CAPES - Grant 23038.039425–42/2008), Conselho Nacional de Pesquisa e Desenvolvimento Científico e Tecnológico (CNPq – Grants: 576322/2008–3 and 487351/2012–6) and Fundação de Amparo à Pesquisa do Estado de São Paulo (FAPESP – Grant 2013/07340–1) to MDB. The funders had no role in study design, data collection and analysis, decision to publish, or preparation of the manuscript.

Competing Interests: The authors have declared that no competing interests exist.

* Email: mdbaruff@fcfrp.usp.br

9 These authors equally contributed to this work.

Introduction

Dengue is a mosquito-borne viral disease of expanding geographical range and incidence, it is estimated that up to 3.6 billion people live in endemic regions [reviewed in reference 1]. Recent estimates indicated that the number of infections worldwide is 400 million with ~500,000 episodes of severe dengue, and <20,000 dengue related deaths per year [1].

Dengue is predominantly transmitted by the mosquito *Aedes agypti* and is caused by dengue viruses (DENV), a group of four serologically distinct positive strand RNA viruses: DENV-1, DENV-2, DENV-3, and DENV-4. They belong to the Flaviviridae family and genus Flavivirus (reviewed in [2]). Infection with any serotype can induce a range of disease from sub-clinical to a severe disorder. The severe disorder is associated with hemorrhage and plasma leakage which are recognized as dengue hemorrhagic fever (DHS) or dengue shock syndrome (DSS) [3,4]. There are currently no specific treatments for dengue disease [5], and

therefore, only supportive care is given [6]. Thus, antiviral compounds need to be identified in view of the spread of dengue disease throughout the world [5].

To identify control mechanisms for Dengue disease, we investigated the physiological functions of an endogenous innate immune protein named galectin-1 (Gal-1), a β-galactoside-binding lectin, in controlling infection caused by dengue virus (DENV-1). Galectin-1 is a ubiquitously expressed lectin, and can occur in both intracellular (cytoplasm and nucleus) as well as extracellular (cell surface and serum) compartments, despite the lack of a signal peptide for classical secretion [7]. Galectin-1 is differentially expressed by various normal and pathological tissues, including muscle, heart, liver, kidney, prostate, lymph nodes, spleen, thymus, placenta, testis, retina and also in immune and non-immune cells [8]. For instance, during infection or inflammation, Gal-1 may be released by infected epithelium, activated macrophages, and endothelial cells [8]. In fact, concerning endothelial cells, it has been extensively demonstrated that Gal-1 contributes to multiple steps of the angiogenesis cascade and then it has pro-angiogenic activity (reviewed in [9]).

Gal-1 exists in a monomer-dimer equilibrium, and in its dimeric form, the lectin can mediate cell-cell or host-pathogen interactions [10,11,12], similar to other members of the galectin family [13,14] and other mammalian lectin families [15]. It has been extensively shown that it presents an immunomodulatory effect on microbial infections [16]. This lectin has a role in viral infections but its mechanisms and physiological functions are not clear. While some groups have reported an antiviral activity of Gal-1 during infections caused by Nipah virus [17,18], Nodavirus [19], Influenza virus [20] and human simplex virus 1 (HSV-1) [21], other groups have reported that Gal-1 promotes infections caused by human immunodeficiency virus 1 (HIV-1) [22-27], HSV-1 [28] and human T-lymphotropic virus 1 HTLV-1 [29].

To our knowledge, the role of Gal-1 in DENV infection is yet to be evaluated. Here we show that both endogenous and exogenous Gal-1 inhibits DENV-1 infectivity, both in *in vitro* and *in vivo* infection in mice. Our results suggest that recombinant Gal-1 might have potential use as a novel approach to control DENV-1-induced pathology.

Materials and Methods

Cell lineages

The mosquito cell lineage from *Aedes albopictus* (C6/36) was cultivated at 28°C in L-15 medium (Leibovitz) (Cultilab, Campinas, Brazil) supplemented with 0.3% tryptose phosphate broth, 0.02% glutamine, 1% minimum essential medium (MEM) non-essential amino acids solution and 5% fetal bovine serum (Hyclone, Logan, USA). Vero-E6 (African green monkey kidney, ATCC CCL-81) cells were grown at 37°C in DMEM (Gibco, Life Technologies, Gaithersburg, MD, USA) supplemented with 10% fetal bovine serum. The human urinary bladder carcinoma cells (ECV-304, ATCC CRL-1998) were maintained at 37°C in RPMI-1640 medium (Gibco). Human lung microvascular endothelial cell lineage (HMVEC-L; ATCC CC2527) was cultivated in EC growth medium (EBM-2; Cambrex, Walkersville, MD, USA) containing 5% fetal bovine serum, human recombinant epidermal growth factor, human recombinant insulin-like growth factor-1, human basic fibroblast growth factor, vascular endothelial growth factor, hydrocortisone, ascorbic acid, gentamicin, and amphotericin B.

DENV-1

The stock of the DENV-1 (strain Mochizuki, GenBank: AB074760.1) was prepared in C6/36 cells and titrated by plaque formation on Vero-E6 cells, as described previously [30]. Supernatants containing virus were collected and stored at −80°C for use in *in vitro* assays. *In vivo* assays were performed with the DENV-1 mouse brain-adapted strain, generated from Mochizuki strain in the same manner as described in reference [31]. Mouse-brain adapted DENV-1 was used on in vivo assays because non-adapted mouse strains do not readily replicate or cause pathology in immunocompetent mice, which is the case of mice used in the present study. Therefore, mouse-adapted DENV is lethal after intracranial challenge, and this severity parameter was used here to assess the physiological impact of Gal-1.

Mice and survival study

Gal-1-deficient (*Lgals1*−/−) mice and age-matched wild-type (WT) mice on a C57Bl-6 background were used in experimental DENV-1 infections. For mortality assays, groups ranging from six to eight 3-day-old mice from both WT and *Lgals1*−/− lineages were infected with mouse-brain adapted DENV-1 as previously described, with modifications [31,32]. Briefly, mice were intracerebrally injected with 10^6 virions diluted in a total volume of 10 μl of phosphate buffer after anesthetization with a mixture of 10 mg/Kg of xylasine (Dopalen Vetbrands) and 100 mg/Kg of ketamine (Dopaser Hertap Caller). The brain macerates from non-infected mice were used for mock infection. The brains from non-infected and infected mice were collected after animals were euthanized by inhalation of carbon dioxide. Subsequent to the intracranial inoculation mice were examined daily, and mortality rates, as a direct result of the infection, were recorded up to 10 days post-infection. After this period, the surviving animals were euthanized by inhalation of carbon dioxide.

Macrophage cultures

Resident macrophages were obtained from peritoneal washouts of 4–6 weeks-old WT and *Lgals1*−/− mice, after euthanasia by inhalation of carbon dioxide. Cells were suspended in RPMI-1640 medium supplemented with 10% of fetal bovine serum and allowed to attach onto 24-well plates. After an overnight incubation period, unattached cells were removed and adherent cells (macrophages) were used for *in vitro* infection with DENV-1 or submitted to Gal-1 expression analysis using Western Blot assay or conventional PCR methods.

Ethical aspects

The present study uses death endpoint as a direct result from infection with DENV-1 and without humane euthanasia. This choice was strongly justified based on the following reasons: 1) the alternative use of humane endpoints based on clinical criteria was not possible since the earlier and reliable indicators of disease severity biomarkers had not been established or validated at the times the experiments were performed; 2) Our study was designed so that the survival assay consisted of a total of 35 mice from each lineage. If we had proposed to establish and validate biomarkers for severity, in order to use a humane endpoint, we would have had to use a much larger number of mice, which in our view would be unnecessary and raise other ethical concerns; 3) The mouse strain C57BL-6 was used in our study because its genetic counterpart, the *Lgals1*−/− mice, is naturally resistant to infection with DENV-1, so it was necessary to use a high inoculum in newborn mice, which promotes death during the acute infection; 4) All mouse experiments were performed under approved conditions in accordance to Faculdade de Ciências Farmacêuticas de Ribeirão Preto – Universidade de São Paulo (USP) Institutional Animal Care and User Committee approved protocols. The Ethics Committee on Animal Research of the University of São Paulo approved all the procedures described (Protocol Number: 10.1.1300.53.0).

Human recombinant Galectin-1 (hrGal-1) and Galectin-3 (hrGal-3)

Recombinant forms (dimeric and monomeric) of human galectin-1 (hrGal-1) and human galectin-3 were prepared based on procedures previously described [33–36]. In addition, purified hrGal-1 was treated with 100 mM iodoacetamide (Sigma-Aldrich, MO, USA) in 100 mM lactose/PBS overnight at 4°C, as described [10,18,22,33]. To ensure that hrGal-1 and hrGal-3 samples were endotoxin free, Detoxi-Gel Endotoxin removing gel (Pierce Biotechnology, Rockford, IL) was used. The activity of all produced galectins was assessed by hemagglutination. Biotinylation of hrGal-1 was performed using sulfo-NHS-LC-biotin (sulfosuccinimidyl 6-[biotinamido] hexanoate) (Pierce), according to the manufacturer's recommendations.

In vitro viral infection

Indicated cell lineages were inoculated with DENV-1 (MOI 0.5) or vehicle solution (supernatant from non infected cells) and cultivated for 24, 48, 72, 96 or 120 hours, as indicated, at $37°C$ in a humidified, CO_2-controlled atmosphere in appropriate medium supplemented with 10% FBS. Following, supernatants of culture were recovered for determination of viral load. Gal-1 effects were assessed by incubating cells, virus or both with the indicated concentrations of this lectin for 1 hour at $37°C$ before viral inoculum, as indicated. To evaluate the involvement of Gal-1 CRD in its antiviral activity the treatments were done in the presence of 10 mM lactose or sucrose.

Adsorption and Internalization assays

Adsorption and internalization assays were performed as described previously [37] with modifications. For adsorption assays, ECV-304 cells were seeded in 24-well plates and infected with DENV-1 with a MOI of 10, in the presence or absence of 10 μM of hrGal-1, for 1 hour at $4°C$. Following, cells were washed twice with PBS and immediately submitted to total RNA extraction or stored at $-80°C$ until the time of use. For the internalization assays, cells were seeded in 24-well plates and inoculated with DENV-1 (MOI 10), for 1 hour at $4°C$. After the incubation period, the inoculum was removed by 2 washes with PBS. The cells were then incubated with medium containing or not 10 μM of hrGal-1, for additional 1 hour at $37°C$. The cells were then washed with PBS and treated with citrate buffer for 1 min to inactivate the adsorbed but not internalized virus. Finally, cells were washed with PBS to remove citrate buffer and stored at $-80°C$ for subsequent quantification of viral load.

Real-Time and conventional PCR

Viral loads were quantified in the culture supernatants using a one-step quantitative Real-Time PCR [38]. The total viral RNA purified from 1×10^7 PFU of DENV-1 were 10-fold serially diluted to generate a standard curve. The viral RNA was purified using the QIAamp Viral RNA minikit (QIAGEN; Hamburg, Germany). Quantitative PCR reaction was carried out with the SuperScript III Platinum SYBR Green One-Step qRT-PCR kit (Invitrogen, Life Technologies) in a One-Step Real-Time PCR RT-PCR (Applied Biosystems, Life Technologies). Triplicate reactions were performed for each sample, and a no template control was included as a negative control. The primer sequences used for DENV-1 detection were RNC5-S: 5'-3'AGTTGTTAGTC-TACGTGGACCGA and RNC5-C: 5'-3'CGCGTTTCAGCA-TATTGAAAG.

Qualitative analysis of Gal-1 mRNA expression on WT and $Lgals1^{-/-}$ cells was performed using conventional RT-PCR. Total RNA was purified using RNeasy Protect Mini Kit (QIAGEN) and cDNA obtained using M-MLV reverse transcriptase (1U) and oligo dT primers (both from Invitrogen, Life Technologies). PCR amplification was performed with primers for mouse Gal-1 (pFBNdgal-1: 5'-3'CGGATCCCATATGGCCTGTGGTCTG and pRHXgal-1: 5'-3'GCTCG AGAAGCTTTCACTCAA-AGGCC) and β-actin (Fb-actin: 5'-3'CCCTAGGC ACCA-GGGTGTGA and Rb-actin 5'-3':GCCATGTTCAATGGGG-TACTTC).

Virucidal assay

The virucidal activity of hrGal-1 was assessed as described in reference [37], with modifications. Briefly, DENV-1 (2×10^5 PFU) was incubated at $37°C$ for 1 hour in presence or absence of 10 μM of hrGal-1. The incubation was performed in presence of absence of RNAse A (150 mg/mL, Sigma-Aldrich). After one hour, the viral RNA was purified using QIAamp Viral RNA minikit and the samples were subjected to Real-Time PCR as described above. Purified viral RNA, treated or not with RNAse A, was used as positive control of reaction.

Enzyme-linked Immunosorbent Assay

Soluble Gal-1 present in the culture supernatants was quantified by ELISA. Briefly, 96-well microplates were coated with rabbit polyclonal anti-Gal-1 antibody (1 μg/ml, produced in our laboratory). Plates were washed (PBS-Tween 0.05%) and incubated for 2 h at $37°C$ with blocking buffer (PBS/FBS 3%). Next, supernatant samples were added to plates and incubated at room temperature for 2 hours. After extensive washing, a chicken polyclonal anti-Gal-1 antibody (2 μg/ml; produced in our laboratory), diluted in PBS/FBS 3%, was added to each well and incubated for 1 h, at $37°C$. After washing, wells were incubated with HRP-conjugated donkey anti-chicken IgY (Jackson ImmunoResearch, West Grove, PA, USA) for 1 h, at $37°C$. Subsequently; substrate solution (substrate buffer, 1% TMB and 1% H_2O_2) was added. After a 20 min incubation period at room temperature, the reaction was stopped by addition of stop solution (5.5% H_2SO_4). Absorbance was determined at 450 nm using an ELISA reader (Thermo Labsystems, Franklin, MA, USA). A standard curve ranging from 20 to 20,000 pg/ml of hrGal-1 was generated for each ELISA.

The ability of hrGal-1 to bind DENV-1 was also tested by ELISA. Each well in 96-well microtiter plates was coated with 1 μg of hrGal-1 or 1% BSA overnight at $4°C$. Plates were then rinsed once with PBS-Tween 0.05% and incubated with blocking buffer (PBS-Tween 0.05%, BSA 3%) for 2 hours at room temperature. After washing, serial two-fold dilutions of DENV-1 were added to each well and plates were incubated for 2 hours at room temperature. After three washes with PBS-Tween 0.05%, each well was incubated with mouse anti-E protein IgG (AbD Serotec, Raleigh, NC, USA) for 1 h, at $37°C$. Following this incubation step, plates were washed and incubated with HRP-conjugated donkey anti-mouse IgG (Jackson IR) for 1 h, at $37°C$. The development of peroxidase reaction was performed with TMB substrate, as describe above. To assess the participation of Gal-1 CRD on viral-lectin interactions, different concentrations of lactose or sucrose were added to wells before the addition of virus dilutions.

Flow cytometry

Measurement of free ligands for Gal-1 on ECV-304 cells surface was performed by incubating ECV-304 cells with 10 μM biotinylated-hrGal-1 for 1 hour at $4°C$, in presence or absence of 40 mM lactose or sucrose (Sigma-Aldrich). After washing, cells were incubated with streptavidin-FITC (Jackson IR) for 30 minutes at $4°C$, washed and fixed. Labeled cells were acquired on a FACS Canto (Becton Dickinson, Mountain View, CA, USA) and analyzed in the DIVA software (Becton Dickinson).

Cell death assay

Apoptosis and necrosis signals were investigated through propidium iodide (PI) and Annexin-V staining. Membrane permeability was evaluated in fresh ECV-304 cells, after immediate addition of propidium iodide (2 mg). DNA degradation was detected in ECV-304 cells gently resuspended in 0.3 ml hypotonic PI solution (PI, 50 µg/ml in 0.1% sodium citrate plus 0.1% Triton X-100; Sigma-Aldrich). Tubes were kept at 4°C for 16 hours in the dark. Cells treated with Camptothecin (CPT – 10 µM – Sigma-Aldrich) were used as positive inducer of cellular death.

Cell viability assay

Cell viability was measured by the colorimetric MTT (1-(4,5-Dimethylthiazol-2-yl)-3,5-diphenylformazan, Sigma-Aldrich) assay as previously described [39].

Western blot assay

Cells were lysed in sample buffer (62.5 M Tris, pH 6.8, 2% SDS (w/v), 5% glycerol (v/v), 30 µM phenol red and 0.9% β-mercaptoethanol) and incubated for 5 min at 100°C. Samples were resolved in 15% polyacrylamide gels and transferred onto nitrocellulose membranes (Amersham Biosciences, Uppsala, Sweden). After saturation with 5% non-fat dry milk, membranes were probed with mouse monoclonal anti-Gal-1 or mouse monoclonal anti-β-actin (Abcam, MA, EUA) for 2 hours at room temperature. After washing, membranes were incubated with HRP-conjugated donkey anti-mouse IgG (Jackson IR) for 45 minutes at room temperature. Bound antibodies were revealed by enhanced chemiluminescence using the ECL kit (Pierce).

Data Analysis

Statistically significant differences among groups were assayed using analysis of variance (ANOVA) (Bonferroni Dunn test). Values of $p < 0.05$ were considered significant results.

Results

Reduced expression of endogenous Gal-1 results in increased permissiveness to DENV-1 infection

To investigate the role of endogenous Gal-1 in the course of DENV infection, we infected three different cell lines with DENV. Vero-E6 cells are known to be permissive to all four dengue virus serotypes [40–42], while ECV-304 (a carcinoma cell lineage with endothelial characteristics) and lung microvascular endothelial cells (HMVEC-L) are known to be permissive to dengue virus serotype-2 [24,43–45]. Interestingly, ECV-304 and Vero-E6 cells express similar levels of Gal-1 protein, while HMVEC-L expressed somewhat higher levels of Gal-1 when compared to other cell lines tested (Figure 1A) and quantified by ImageJ program (Figure 1A). Next, cells were inoculated with DENV-1 (MOI 0.5) and cultivated for 72 hours, and the viral load was quantified from the culture supernatants by One Step Real-Time PCR. We found that Vero-E6 cells, which displayed the lowest Gal-1 expression level (Figure 1A), were highly permissive to DENV-1 infection (Figure 1B). In sharp contrast, we detected the lowest level of viral load in the supernatants of HMVEC-L cells (Figure 1B), which displayed the highest Gal-1 expression level (Figure 1A). To further investigate the relationship between Gal-1 levels and permissiveness to DENV infection, we infected the ECV-304 cells with DENV-1 for 72 h and evaluated Gal-1 expression by western blot. As shown in Figure 1C, the presence of DENV-1 decreased the expression of endogenous Gal-1 in comparison to that cells maintained in medium alone. In addition, ECV-304-infected cells secreted more Gal-1 to culture supernatants (Figure 1D), which could explain at least in part the reduction of cell-associated Gal-1 protein after infection (Figure 1C).

Treatment with recombinant hrGal-1 reduces viral production in DENV-1 virus-infected cells

Since Gal-1 expression levels seemed to be inversely correlated to DENV permissiveness, we therefore evaluate whether the addition of exogenous Gal-1 could interfere with DENV infection in vitro. First, we demonstrated that ECV-304 cells display Gal-1-specific binding sites because human recombinant Gal-1 (hrGal-1) was able to bind ECV-304 cell surfaces, and this binding is abrogated in the presence of lactose, a weak but effective inhibitor of Gal-1, but not by sucrose, an isomeric sugar that does not bind galectins (Figure 2A). Similar results were obtained using HMVEC-L and Vero-E6 cells (data not shown). Monolayers of ECV-304, Vero-E6 and HMVEC-L cells were treated with 10 µM of hrGal-1 for 1 hour at 37°C, followed by addition DENV-1 virus (MOI 0.5) for 72 hours, and the viral load was quantified from the culture supernatants. As demonstrated before (Figure 1B), EVC-304 and Vero-E6 cells are much more permissive to DENV-1 infection than HMVEC-L cells; however, all the three cell lines had a significant reduction in viral load (35% in Vero-E6 cells, 60% in ECV-304 cells and 65% HMVEC-L cells) when pre-treated with hrGal-1 (Figure 2B). The kinetics of DENV-1 infection was also monitored in EVC-304 cells, pretreated or not with hrGal-1, during a period of 120 hours after infection. As shown in (Figure 2C), at 48, 72, 96 and 120 hours postinfection, the viral loads detected in the supernatant of DENV-1-infected ECV-304 cells pre-treated with hrGal-1 were significantly lower compared with viral load recovered from the supernatants of Gal-1-untreated cells. We also found a dose-dependent inhibition of DENV-1 infection when ECV-304 cells were pretreated with increasing hrGal-1 concentrations for 1 hour before the infection (Figure 2D).

It has been shown that Gal-1 exists in a monomer-dimer equilibrium, and several important functions of this protein have been shown to be dependent on Gal-1 dimerization [8,36]. Therefore, we tested whether the inhibitory effect of Gal-1 on DENV-1 infection was dependent on its capacity to form dimers. Using a mutant Gal-1, which is unable to form dimers, we showed that the monomeric form of hrGal-1(m) had no capacity to reduce DENV-1 viral loads in the supernatant of EVC-304-infected cells compared with the hrGal-1 (d), indicating that dimerization is important for the inhibitor effects of Gal-1 on DENV-1 infection (Figure 2D). Importantly, we observed that this inhibitory effect was specific for hrGal-1 since galectin-3, another galectin binding protein from galectin family, and one which naturally occurs in multimeric forms, showed no inhibitory effect on vital load (Figure 2D).

To assess the involvement of the carbohydrate-recognition domain (CRD) of Gal-1 in this inhibitory effect, ECV-304 cells were pre-treated or not with hrGal-1 in presence or absence of a specific sugar inhibitor (lactose). Lactose blocked the inhibitory effect of hrGal-1 on DENV-1 infection, whereas sucrose did not block (Figure 2E), indicating a dependence of the Gal-1 CRD for these functions.

Inhibitory effect of Gal-1 on DENV-1 release is not associated with induction of cell death

We explored whether the antiviral effect of Gal-1 could be due to induction of cell death. Thus, we evaluated the apoptosis and necrosis of ECV-304 cells pre-treated or not with hrGal-1 and infected with DENV-1 virus. As can be seen in the Figure 3A, DENV-1-infected ECV-304 cells (pretreated or not with hrGal-1) did not show significant staining with either PI or Annexin-V-FITC, in contrast to cells treated with camptothecin, a positive

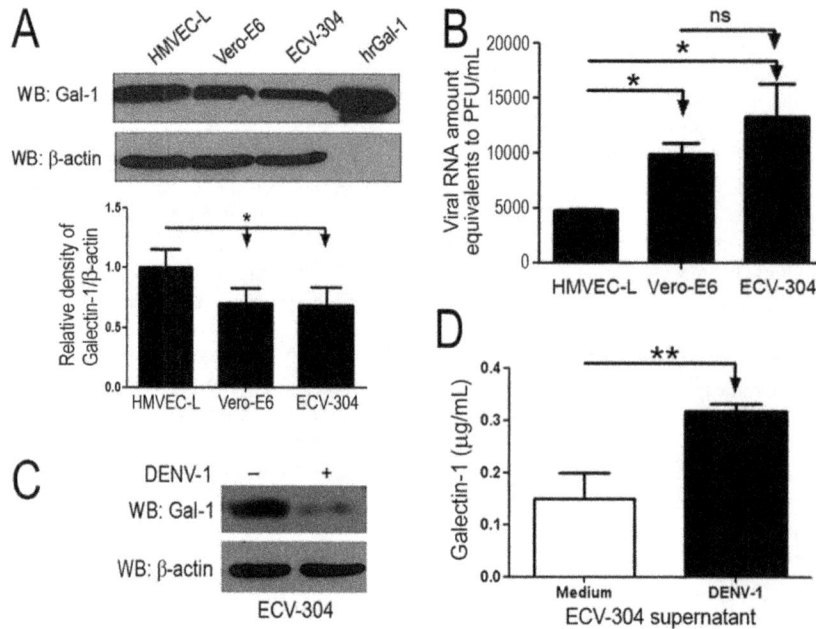

Figure 1. Lower expression of Gal-1 is correlated with higher viral loads produced by DENV-1-infected cells. (A) Gal-1 expression on HMVEC-L, Vero-E6 and ECV-304 cells was assessed by western blot method and normalized by β-actin endogenous control. The relative density of Gal-1 was determined by ImageJ software. **(B)** HMVEC-L, Vero-E6 and ECV-304 cells (2.5×10^4) were incubated with DENV-1 (MOI 0.5) for 72 hours at 37°C. At the end of incubation period, the total amounts of viral RNA in the cell-free supernatants were determined by Real-Time PCR, using a standard curve constructed from DENV-1 RNA purified from 1×10^7 PFU (PFU: plate formed units). Results are shown as Viral RNA amount equivalents to PFU/ml±SD from 3 independent assays performed in triplicates. **(C)** ECV-304 cells were inoculated with DENV-1 (MOI 0.5) or only with medium and cultivated for 72 hours at 37°C. Cells were analyzed for Gal-1 expression by western blot assay. **(D)** Soluble Gal-1 was detected in the supernatants from cell cultures using ELISA method (N = 3). *$p < 0.01$; **$p < 0.001$.

inducer of cell death. In order to confirm this result, we also checked the degradation of chromosomal DNA and cell viability by using the MTT assay. Corroborating our previous result using Annexin-V/PI staining, pretreatment of cells with hrGal-1 before DENV-1 infection did not cause any effect on DNA degradation and cell viability (Figure 3B and C, respectively). Cell viability and apoptosis assays performed in Vero-E6 and HMVEC-L cell lineages infected with DENV-1 in presence or absence of hrGal-1 provided similar results (data not shown). Altogether, these data indicate that Gal-1 inhibits DENV-1 infection without inducing cell death in infected cells.

hrGal-1 binds to DENV-1 and inhibits its adsorption and internalization processes in ECV-304 cells

To further investigate the inhibitory effect of exogenous Gal-1 on DENV-1 infection, we first checked whether Gal-1 was able to bind directly to the virus and exert any *direct virucidal* activity against DENV-1. As shown in Figure 4A, DENV-1 bound to immobilized hrGal-1 in a dose-dependent manner, whereas the virus failed to bind to BSA-coated wells. Unexpectedly, the binding of DENV-1 to hrGal-1 was not abolished by the addition of lactose, an inhibitor of carbohydrate binding (Figure 4A). This may mean that the affinity of binding between hrGal-1 and DENV-1 is extremely high toward immobilized hrGal-1, and thus not readily reversible by lactose, or binding occurs through a non-carbohydrate interaction to hrGal-1. We next evaluated whether hrGal-1 could affect virus adsorption and/or virus internalization. As shown in Figure 4B, hrGal-1 significantly inhibited virus adsorption at 4°C for 1 hour (Figure 4B) when hrGal-1 was present during the incubation. If adsorption took place in a hrGal-1-free medium, and the lectin was added at culture supernatants

when the temperature was raised at 37°C and maintained only additional 1 h of incubation, the virus yield also significantly decreased in comparison with untreated cultures (Figure 4B). A possible virucidal effect of hrGal-1 on DENV-1 was discarded by a virucidal assay (Figure 4C). Altogether, these results suggest that hrGal-1 may influence the early steps of DENV-1 infection. Finally, we investigated whether the inhibitory effects exerted by Gal-1 also depended on its interaction with the target cells. The pretreatment of DENV-1 with hrGal-1 [(DENV1+rhGal-1)+ ECV] led to a significant decrease in viral load in the culture supernatants (Figure 4D). However, when ECV-304 cells were treated with hrGal-1 before DENV infection [(ECV+rhGal-1)+ DENV1] or ECV-304 cells were treated concomitantly with hrGal-1 and DENV-1 (ECV+rhGal-1+DENV1), we observed an even greater reduction in the viral load in the culture supernatants (Figure 4D).

Absence of endogenous Gal-1 leads to early mortality of mice to DENV-1 infection

Based on the results presented so far and to better demonstrate the role of Gal-1 in controlling DENV-1 infection, we next infected newborn Gal-1-deficient ($Lgals1^{-/-}$) and wild-type mice with mouse-brain adapted DENV-1 virus and analyzed host survival for 10 days (Figure 5A). Although mice from both lineages displayed similar overall mortality rate, $Lgals1^{-/-}$ mice began to succumb earlier than WT mice: within the first 4 days post-infection, almost 60% of $Lgals1^{-/-}$ mice died, while 90% of WT mice survived up to 5 days past challenge (Figure 5A).

Since macrophages are important target for DENV virus in mouse models of dengue infection [46,47] and we demonstrated above that there is an inverse correlation between DENV

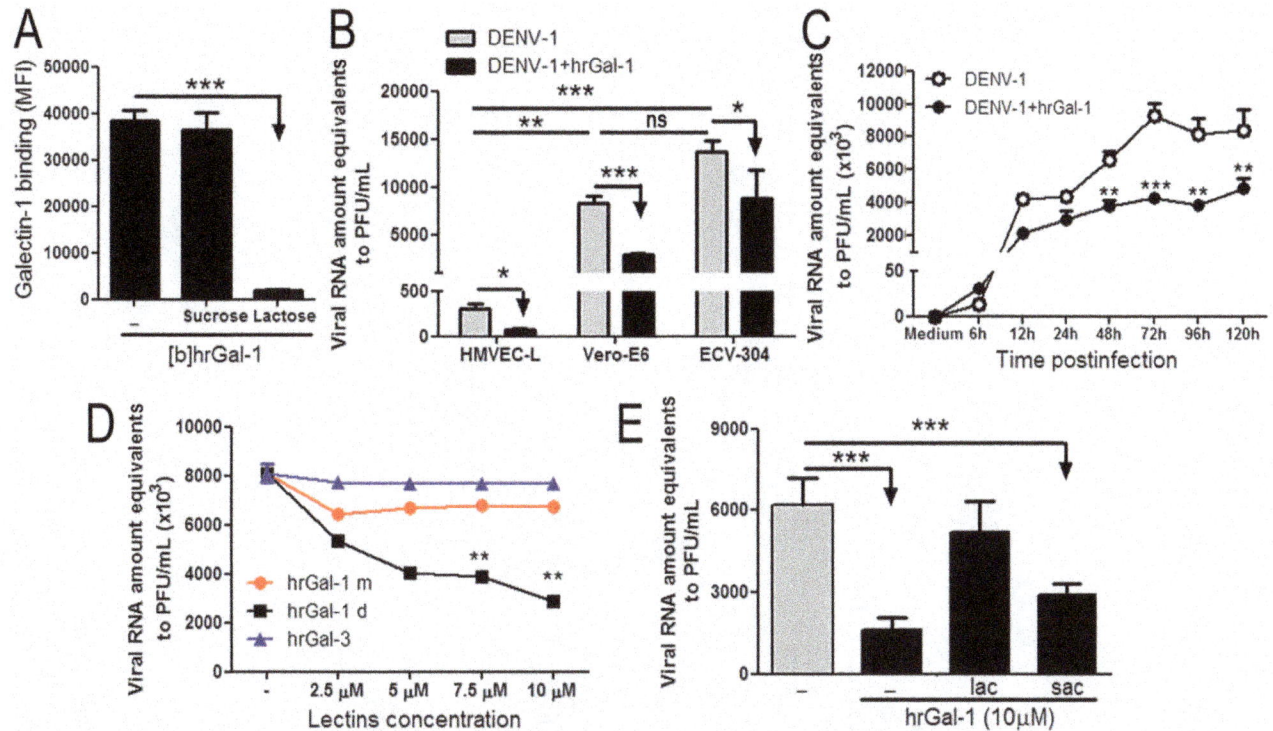

Figure 2. Treatment with human recombinant Gal-1 inhibits DENV-1 in vitro infection. (A) Biotinylated-hrGal-1 (20 µg/mL) was incubated with ECV-304 cells in presence or absence of 40 mM lactose or sucrose for 1 hour at 4°C. The binding of biotinylated-hrGal-1 to ECV-304 cells surfaces was detected by staining with streptavidin-FITC and measured by flow cytometry. The analysis was performed using a Diva software (Becton Dickson) and results are expressed as mean mean fluorescence intensity (MFI)±SD. Tests were performed in triplicates. **(B)** HMVEC-L, Vero-E6 and ECV-304 cells were incubated with 10 µM hrGal-1 or only medium for 1 hour at 37°C. Following, cells were inoculated with DENV-1 at a MOI of 0.5 and cultivated for 72 hours. At 72 hours postinfection the supernatants were collected and the viral RNA amounts were quantified by Real-Time PCR. Results are shown as Viral RNA amounts equivalent to PFU/ml±SD from 3 assays performed in triplicates. **(C)** ECV-304 cells were treated with hrGal-1 and infected with DENV-1 as described in (B) for 120 hours. The supernatants were collected at the indicated times postinfection and the viral loads were quantified by Real-Time PCR as described in (B). (N = 3) **(D)** ECV-304 cells were incubated with increased concentrations of monomeric-Gal-1 (hrGal-1 m), dimeric-Gal-1 (hrGal-1 d) or galectin-3 (hrGal-3) for 1 hour at 37°C before inoculation with DENV-1 (MOI 0.5). Cells were cultivated for 72 hours at 37°C and viral load was quantified as described in (A) (N = 3). **(E)** ECV-304 cells were treated with hrGal-1 (10 µM) in the presence of 40 mM lactose (LAC) or 40 mM sucrose (SUC) and then infected with DENV-1 as described in (B), for 72 hours. The viral load was quantified as described in (B). Data are representative from three independent experiments. *$p < 0.01$; **$p < 0.001$; ***$p < 0.0001$.

permissiveness and Gal-1 expression level, we evaluate the susceptibility of macrophages isolated from $Lgals1^{-/-}$ to DENV infection. As expected, macrophages from $Lgals1^{-/-}$ mice did not express Gal-1 mRNA or protein levels (Figure 5B). Corroborating the data obtained with endothelial cells (Figure 1A and 1B), we detected much higher viral load in the supernatant of $Lgals1^{-/-}$ macrophages than in the supernatants from WT macrophages (Figure 5C). This result suggests that endogenous Gal-1 contributes to mice resistance during infection with DENV-1.

Discussion

Here we demonstrated that both endogenous and exogenous Gal-1 reduces DENV-1 infection by inhibiting virus infection of mammalian cells. Our results show that, at least in part, the inhibition by Gal-1 involves the prevention of adsorption and internalization of dengue virus into target cells. Also, the inhibitory effect of Gal-1 on DENV-1 infection depends on carbohydrate recognition and Gal-1 dimerization.

Gal-1 is widely expressed in animal cells and tissues; it is expressed in the thymus and by lymphoid parenchymal epithelial cells, endothelial cells, trophoblasts, activated T and B cells, macrophages, follicular DCs, and CD4+CD25+ regulatory T cells

[12]. Gal-1 has an important immunomodulatory activity, playing essential roles during microbial infection by modulating both innate and adaptive immunity [16]. However, the role of Gal-1 in the context of viral infections is less clear. Gal-1 has an anti-viral effect on infections by Nipah virus [17,18], Nodavirus [19], Influenza virus [20] and HSV-1 [21]. In such cases, Gal-1 negatively controls the infection by both directly interacting with viral glycoproteins, and thus inhibiting their mobility, maturation and functions [18,40], and by affecting the immune response of the target cells after infection [17,19]. However, Gal-1 can also promote the infectivity of cells by HSV-1 [28], HIV-1 [22–27] and HTLV-1 [29]. In such cases Gal-1 acts as a soluble adhesion molecule that stabilizes virus attachment to host cells and facilitates their entry [20]. Concerning DENV, there are no data in the literature exploring the role of Gal-1 in the infection caused by any of the four DENV-serotypes.

The initial steps leading to DENV entry into the host cells for primary infection are very poorly understood. Here we demonstrated that ECV-304, Vero-E6 and HMVEC-L cell lineages and WT murine macrophages are permissive to DENV-1 infection, and all of them constitutively express Gal-1 (Figure 1A and 5B). However, Gal-1 expression on HMVEC-L cells is higher when compared with the other two cell lineages, and interestingly, the

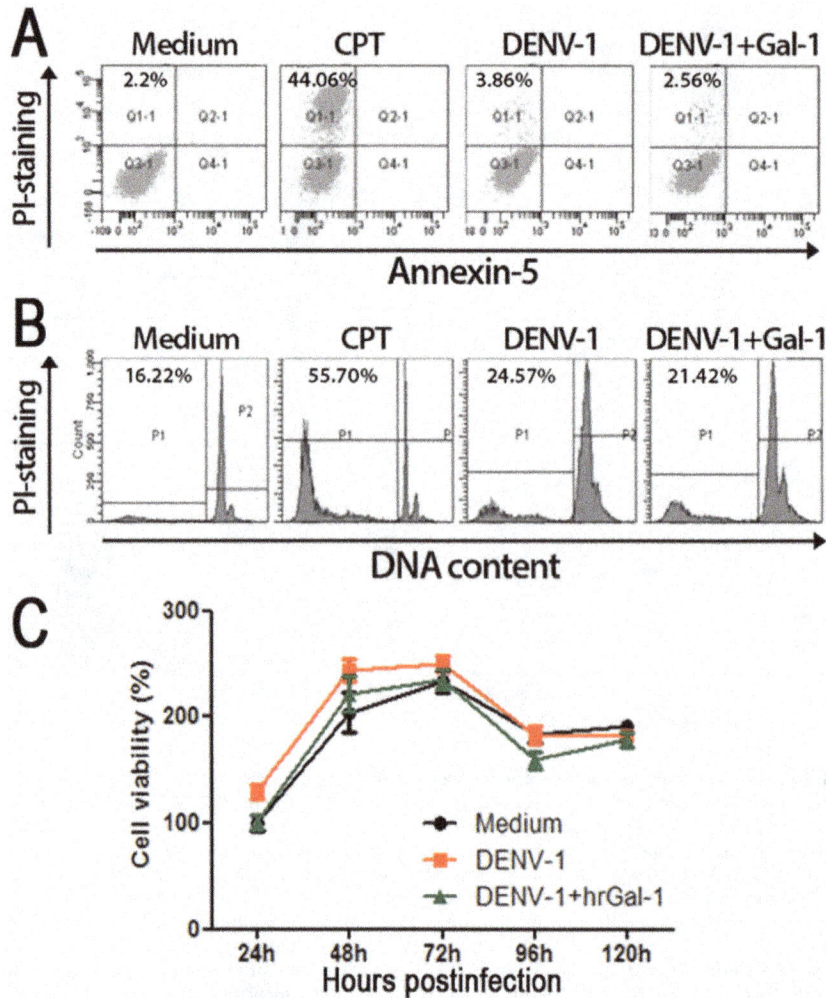

Figure 3. Gal-1 does not induce cell death during DENV-1 infection. (A and B) ECV-304 cells (2.5×10^4) were treated with hrGal-1 (10 µM) and infected with DENV-1 (MOI 0.5). At 72 hours postinfection, PI staining was used to evaluate the membrane permeability (A) and DNA degradation (B). For these purposes, PI was added to fresh cells or to permeabilized cells, respectively. Samples were acquired and analyzed by flow cytometry. Data is representative from three experiments with similar results. **(C)** ECV-304 cells were treated or not with 10 µM of hrGal-1 and infected with DENV-1 as described in (A). At the indicated times postinfection, cell viability was examined by MTT assay. Cells cultivated only with medium at 24 hours were designated as 100% of cell viability. Data is representative of 3 independent experiments performed in triplicates.

permissiveness of HMVEC-L cells to DENV-1 is lower than ECV-304 and Vero-E6 cells. On the other hand, macrophages with no expression of Gal-1 (*Lgals1*$^{-/-}$) are more permissive to DENV-1 infection. These data suggest an inverse correlation between Gal-1 expression and permissiveness to DENV-1 infection. It has been shown that dengue virus can interact with a large number of proteins [48], including the heat-shock protein 70 and DC-SIGN (a C-type mannose-binding lectin) [49]. It is also known that the galectins may form glycoprotein lattices on the cell surface [8,23], directly affecting their distribution, functions and endocytosis [18]. Since HMVEC-L cells present higher expression of Gal-1 compared with ECV-304 and Vero-E6, it is tempting to speculate that the membrane-associated Gal-1 may interact with DENV glycoprotein E to form lattices, and thus inhibit DENV-1 infectivity by reducing the entry of virus particles. It is also possible that Gal-1 could inhibit subsequent virus maturation, similar to the observed for Nipah virus [18].

Although we can not rule out that other factors could be also affecting HMVEC-L susceptibility, the possibility that Gal-1 might

restricts viral entry is corroborated by our findings, showing that addition of exogenous Gal-1 inhibits virus adsorption to ECV-304 cells and its internalization during *in vitro* infection (Figure 4B). This inhibitory effect is reflected on the decreased virus release at 72 hours postinfection, and it is observed not only in ECV-304 cells, but also in Vero-E6 and HMVEC-L cell lineages (Figure 2B). In this set of experiments we demonstrated that the inhibitory effect of Gal-1 on DENV-1 release depends on protein dimerization, previously demonstrated to be required for efficient cross-linking of functional receptors or for the formation of signaling lattices [50–52]. Also, hrGal-1 inhibitory effect was dependent on carbohydrate recognition as is specifically impaired by the presence of lactose (Figure 2E). Together, these findings support the idea that the inhibitory effect of Gal-1 partly involves extracellular activities of this protein, which may include the lattice-formation (which is CRD-dependent) and interferes with virus adsorption and internalization.

Gal-1 may also exert an inhibitory effect on DENV-1 release by affecting the host cell responses. It has been reported that Gal-1

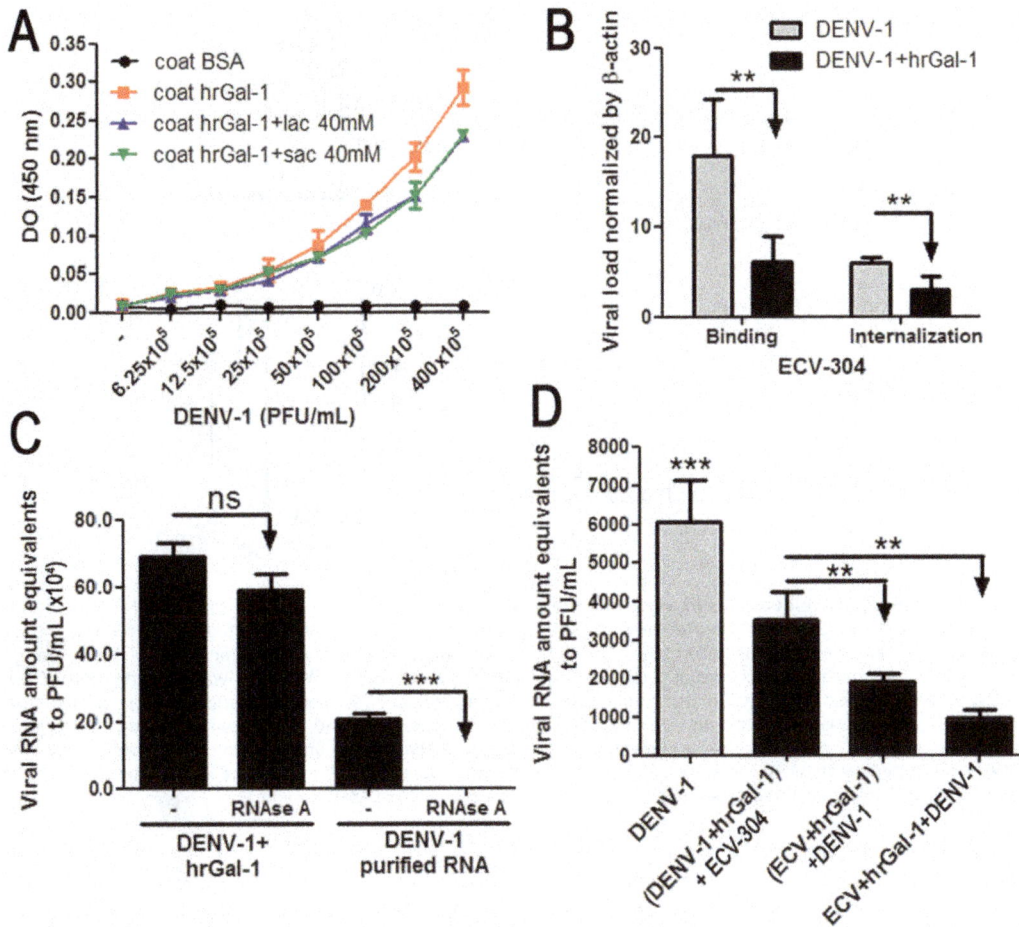

Figure 4. Gal-1 acts at early stages during DENV-1 infection. (A) Binding of DENV-1 to hrGal-1 in a dose-dependent manner. Serial two-fold dilutions of DENV-1 were applied to 96-well plates coated with 1 µg of hrGal-1 per well, and the bound virus particles were detected by ELISA with mouse anti-E protein antibody. BSA-coated wells served as the negative control. To assess the involvement of Gal-1 CRD, the assay was performed in presence of 40 mM lactose or sucrose. Each value represents the mean±the SD from 4 assays performed in duplicates. **(B)** Adsorption and internalization assays: for adsorption assay, ECV-304 cells were infected with DENV-1 at MOI of 10 in presence or absence of 10 µM hrGal-1 during 1 h at 4°C and then washed to remove viral inoculum. Cells were collected and the viral RNA was quantified by Real-Time PCR. Data was normalized by host β-actin expression. For internalization assay, ECV-304 cells were inoculated with DENV-1 (MOI of 10) at 4°C for 1 hour. Then, cells were washed and transferred to 37°C and hrGal-1 (10 µM) or only medium were added to culture. After 1 hour of incubation, non-internalized viruses were inactivated with citrate buffer and viral loads were quantified by Real-Time PCR. Data is presented as Viral RNA amount equivalents to PFU/mL±SD from 3 experiments assessed in triplicates. **(C)** For virucidal assay, DENV-1 was incubated with hrGal-1, in the presence or absence of RNAse. After 1 h incubation at 37°C, RNA was isolated and subjected to RT-Real-Time PCR. Purified viral RNA incubated or not with RNAse was used as control (N = 3). **(D)** ECV-304 cells were infected with DENV-1 at a MOI of 0.5 (DENV-1). For the treatments, hrGal-1 was incubated with ECV-304 and DENV-1 simultaneously (ECV+Gal-1+DENV), or hrGal-1 (10 µM) was pre-incubated with either ECV-304 cells or with DENV-1 (MOI 0.5) for 60 minutes before the inoculation (ECV+hrGal-1)+DENV versus (DENV+hrGal-1)+ECV, respectively. At 72 hours postinfection, supernatants were collected and the viral loads were quantified by Real-Time PCR (N = 3). **p<0.001; ***p<0.0001.

expression is altered after viral infections (*Helicobacter pylori* [53] e HTLV-1 [29]. We found decreased cellular Gal-1 expression accompanied of accentuated levels of Gal-1 in the supernatants from DENV1-infected ECV-304 cells at 72 hours postinfection (Figure 1C and 1D). It is possible that once released to the extracellular milieu, Gal-1 could act as an autocrine regulatory factor for endothelial cells to limit viral spread or act as potential damage-associated molecular pattern (DAMP) [54,55], thus interfering with the immune responses arising after DENV-1 infection.

It has been demonstrated that intracranial infection of mice on a C57Bl-6 background results in neurological abnormalities and death, but these mice does not show the most usual clinical signs observed in humans [30–33]. However, although we can not

extrapolate our data concerning the impact of Gal-1 in in vivo DENV-1 infection of mice to DENV-1 infection in humans, this approach allowed us to develop insights into the mechanisms behind Gal-1 effects.

The lethality of mice infected with DENV-1 is also associated with increased vascular permeability induced by an uncontrolled release of pro-inflammatory cytokines known as "Cytokine storm" [49,56]. Herein we demonstrated that newborn *Lgals1*[-/-] mice infected with DENV-1 start dying earlier than WT mice. This condition seems to be associated with the evidence that the *Lgals1*[-/-] macrophages (and probably other cell types as well) release higher amounts of virus particles at 72 hours post-infection, compared with the WT macrophages. Interestingly, there is uncertainty in the scientific community concerning DENV

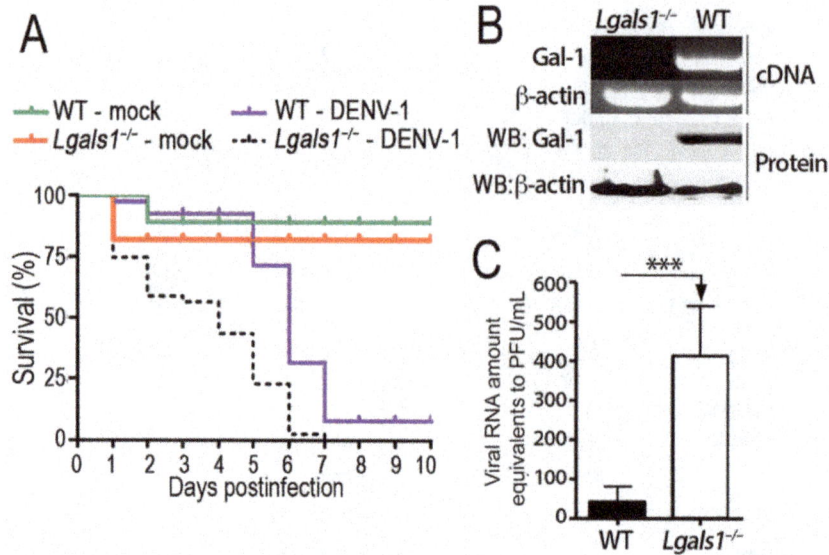

Figure 5. Gal-1 is physiologically relevant to in vivo infection with DENV-1. (A) Newborn WT and *Lgals1*$^{-/-}$ mice were intracerebraly infected with 10^6 PFU/ml of DENV-1 mouse-brain adapted or mock (supernatant from mouse brain not infected with DENV-1) and their mortality was monitored for 10 days. Results are shown as the percentage survival from five independent assays performed with 6–8 mice per group. **(B)** Total mRNA isolated from resident peritoneal macrophages of Gal-1-deficient (*Lgals1*$^{-/-}$) and wild-type (WT) mice was converted into cDNA and the Gal-1 expression was analyzed using conventional PCR. The β-actin gene was used as an endogenous control. Alternatively, total protein from *Lgals1*$^{-/-}$ and WT macrophages were isolated and Gal-1 expression was quantified by western blot assay and normalized to β-actin expression. **(C)** Peritoneal resident macrophages from *Lgals1*$^{-/-}$ or WT mice were cultivated (5x10^5/well) in 24-well plates and inoculated with DENV-1 at a MOI of 0.5. After 72 hours at 37°C, cell-free supernatants were recovered and the viral loads were determined by Real-Time PCR. Results are showed as Viral RNA amounts equivalent to PFU/ml±SD from three experiments assessed in triplicates. ***p<0.0001.

infectivity on macrophages. Some groups have noted that human and mouse macrophages are major cellular targets for DENV infection [46,49,57,58], but others suggests that the virus does not efficiently infect these cells in the absence of sub-neutralizing antibodies [59]. In our system, macrophages from WT mice were infected with DENV-1, however, the viral load from these cells was very low (viral RNA amount equivalent to 50 PFU/mL, Figure 5C), compared to viral load from other cell lineages (between 5,000 and 20,000 PFU/mL, Figure 1B). Nevertheless, the viral load in macrophages from *Lgals1*$^{-/-}$ animals was about eight times higher than that from WT macrophages, suggesting that endogenous Gal-1 contributes to resistance of mice to DENV-1 infection. The absence of Gal-1 in newborn *Lgals1*$^{-/-}$ mice may favor the establishment of a stronger cytokine storm in these mice later in the infection, since Gal-1 is classically known as an important anti-inflammatory factor [8,60]. Altogether, these conditions may contribute to the faster mortality observed in *Lgals1*$^{-/-}$ mice. Our results are in accordance to previous report showing that *Lgals1*$^{-/-}$ mice were also more susceptible to influenza virus infection compared with their WT counterparts [20].

Despite the increasing incidence of DENV as a human pathogen, there are no antiviral agents or vaccines for treatment or prevention [61]. Data presented here show that both endogenous and exogenous Gal-1 are inhibitory to DENV-1 infection. The differences between dengue pathogenesis in mouse and humans should be taken into account, but our results raise the possibility of using recombinant Gal-1 of as an additional/alternative method of treatment for dengue disease. This concept has also been advanced by others for the development of

therapeutic treatments for pathogenic and non-pathogenic diseases [8,62–64]. It has been shown that prophylactic or therapeutic administration of Gal-1 in animal experimental models of inflammatory diseases; cancer or neurodegeneration can ameliorate the disease symptoms or even the mice survival (reviewed in [8]). In the case of pathogenic diseases, the effects of recombinant Gal-1 administration are not well defined and have been shown to be context-dependent, since it can restrict or facilitate the infection [18,22,65]. Despite the difficulties in this field, the potential use of galectins as therapeutic targets has advanced. In the present work, we have shown that Gal-1 may interfere with the course of dengue virus infection probably through several mechanisms, including its participation in DENV-1 entry and cellular responses. Our future investigations aimed to elucidate the molecular mechanisms behind Gal-1 effects and also its roles during dengue human pathogenesis. Together, our study may promote the development of new drugs to combat the pathogenesis caused by this virus.

Acknowledgments

We thank Rubens Eduardo da Silva and Fabiana Rossetto de Morais for their excellent technical assistance with in vivo experiments and cytometry analysis, respectively.

Author Contributions

Conceived and designed the experiments: KAT MLF VHA MDB. Performed the experiments: KAT CDCA MLF RTA TBR VDMM RRR. Analyzed the data: KAT MLF CDCA TBR VDMM RRR VHA SRS RDC MDB. Contributed reagents/materials/analysis tools: VHA MDB. Wrote the paper: KAT MLF MDB.

References

1. Murray NE, Quam MB, Wilder-Smith A (2013) Epidemiology of dengue: past, present and future prospects. Clin Epidemiol 5: 299–309.

2. Beaumier CM, Gillespie PM, Hotez PJ, Bottazzi ME (2013) New vaccines for neglected parasitic diseases and dengue. Transl Res 162: 144–155.

3. Guzman MG, Kouri G (2002) Dengue: an update. Lancet Infect Dis 2: 33–42.

4. Halstead SB (2002) Dengue hemorrhagic fever: two infections and antibody dependent enhancement, a brief history and personal memoir. Rev Cubana Med Trop 54: 171–179.

5. Whitehorn J, Yacoub S, Anders KL, Macareo LR, Cassetti MC, et al. (2014) Dengue Therapeutics, Chemoprophylaxis, and Allied Tools: State of the Art and Future Directions. PLoS Negl Trop Dis 8: e3025.

6. NaTHNaC (2009) Dengue Fever. Health Protection Agency. Natural Travel Health Network and Centre.

7. Hughes RC (1997) The galectin family of mammalian carbohydrate-binding molecules. Biochem Soc Trans 25: 1194–1198.

8. Camby I, Le Mercier M, Lefranc F, Kiss R (2006) Galectin-1: a small protein with major functions. Glycobiology 16: 137R–157R.

9. Thijssen VL, Griffioen AW (2014) Galectin-1 and -9 in angiogenesis: A sweet couple. Glycobiology 24: 915–920.

10. Stowell SR, Cho M, Feasley CL, Arthur CM, Song X, et al. (2009) Ligand reduces galectin-1 sensitivity to oxidative inactivation by enhancing dimer formation. J Biol Chem 284: 4989–4999.

11. Barondes SH, Cooper DN, Gitt MA, Leffler H (1994) Galectins. Structure and function of a large family of animal lectins. J Biol Chem 269: 20807–20810.

12. Sato S, Ouellet M, St-Pierre C, Tremblay MJ (2012) Glycans, galectins, and HIV-1 infection. Ann N Y Acad Sci 1253: 133–148.

13. Stowell SR, Arthur CM, Dias-Baruffi M, Rodrigues LC, Gourdine JP, et al. (2010) Innate immune lectins kill bacteria expressing blood group antigen. Nat Med 16: 295–301.

14. Stowell SR, Arthur CM, McBride R, Berger O, Razi N, et al. (2014) Microbial glycan microarrays define key features of host-microbial interactions. Nat Chem Biol 10: 470–476.

15. Arthur CM, Cummings RD, Stowell SR (2014) Using glycan microarrays to understand immunity. Curr Opin Chem Biol 18: 55–61.

16. Cedeno-Laurent F, Dimitroff CJ (2012) Galectin-1 research in T cell immunity: past, present and future. Clin Immunol 142: 107–116.

17. Levroney EL, Aguilar HC, Fulcher JA, Kohatsu L, Pace KE, et al. (2005) Novel innate immune functions for galectin-1: galectin-1 inhibits cell fusion by Nipah virus envelope glycoproteins and augments dendritic cell secretion of proinflammatory cytokines. J Immunol 175: 413–420.

18. Garner OB, Aguilar HC, Fulcher JA, Levroney EL, Harrison R, et al. (2010) Endothelial galectin-1 binds to specific glycans on nipah virus fusion protein and inhibits maturation, mobility, and function to block syncytia formation. PLoS Pathog 6: e1000993.

19. Poisa-Beiro L, Dios S, Ahmed H, Vasta GR, Martínez-López A, et al. (2009) Nodavirus infection of sea bass (Dicentrarchus labrax) induces up-regulation of galectin-1 expression with potential anti-inflammatory activity. J Immunol 183: 6600–6611.

20. Yang ML, Chen YH, Wang SW, Huang YJ, Leu CH, et al. (2011) Galectin-1 binds to influenza virus and ameliorates influenza virus pathogenesis. J Virol 85: 10010–10020.

21. Rajasagi NK, Suryawanshi A, Sehrawat S, Reddy PB, Mulik S, et al. (2012) Galectin-1 reduces the severity of herpes simplex virus-induced ocular immunopathological lesions. J Immunol 188: 4631–4643.

22. Ouellet M, Mercier S, Pelletier I, Bounou S, Roy J, et al. (2005) Galectin-1 acts as a soluble host factor that promotes HIV-1 infectivity through stabilization of virus attachment to host cells. J Immunol 174: 4120–4126.

23. Mercier S (2008) Galectin-1 promotes HIV-1 infectivity in macrophages through stabilization of viral adsorption. Virology 371: 121–129.

24. St-Pierre C, Manya H, Ouellet M, Clark GF, Endo T, et al. (2011) Host Soluble Galectin-1 Promotes HIV-1 Replication through a Direct Interaction with Glycans of Viral gp120 and Host CD4. J Virol 85: 11742–11751.

25. St-Pierre C, Ouellet M, Giguère D, Ohtake R, Roy R, et al. (2012) Galectin-1-specific inhibitors as a new class of compounds to treat HIV-1 infection. Antimicrob Agents Chemother 56: 154–162.

26. Reynolds JL, Law WC, Mahajan SD, Aalinkeel R, Nair B, et al. (2012a) Morphine and galectin-1 modulate HIV-1 infection of human monocyte-derived macrophages. J Immunol 188: 3757–3765.

27. Reynolds JL, Law WC, Mahajan SD, Aalinkeel R, Nair B, et al. (2012b) Nanoparticle based galectin-1 gene silencing, implications in methamphetamine regulation of HIV-1 infection in monocyte derived macrophages. J Neuroimmune Pharmacol 7: 673–685.

28. Gonzalez MI, Rubinstein N, Ilarregui JM, Toscano MA, Sanjuan NA, et al. (2005) Regulated expression of galectin-1 after in vitro productive infection with herpes simplex virus type 1: implications for T cell apoptosis. Int J Immunopathol Pharmacol 18: 615–623.

29. Gauthier S, Pelletier I, Ouellet M, Vargas A, Tremblay MJ, et al. (2008) Induction of galectin-1 expression by HTLV-I Tax and its impact on HTLV-I infectivity. Retrovirology 5: 105.

30. Muller VD, Russo RR, Cintra AC, Sartim MA, Alves-Paiva Rde M, et al. (2012) Crotoxin and phospholipases A$_2$ from Crotalus durissus terrificus showed antiviral activity against dengue and yellow fever viruses. Toxicon 59: 507–515.

31. Gualano RC, Pryor MJ, Cauchi MR, Wright PJ, Davidson AD (1998) Identification of a major determinant of mouse neurovirulence of dengue virus type 2 using stably cloned genomic-length cDNA. J Gen Virol 79: 437–446.

32. Ip PP, Liao F (2010) Resistance to dengue virus infection in mice is potentiated by CXCL10 and is independent of CXCL10-mediated leukocyte recruitment. J Immunol 184.: 5705–5714.

33. Stowell SR, Qian Y, Karmakar S, Koyama NS, Dias-Baruffi M, et al. (2008) Differential roles of galectin-1 and galectin-3 in regulating leukocyte viability and cytokine secretion. J Immunol 180: 3091–3102.

34. Stowell SR, Karmakar S, Arthur CM, Ju T, Rodrigues LC, et al. (2009) Galectin-1 induces reversible phosphatidylserine exposure at the plasma membrane. Mol Biol Cell 20: 1408–1418.

35. Cho M, Cummings RD (1995) Galectin-1, a beta-galactoside-binding lectin in Chinese hamster ovary cells. I. Physical and chemical characterization. J Biol Chem 270: 5198–5206.

36. Cho M, Cummings RD (1996) Characterization of monomeric forms of galectin-1 generated by site-directed mutagenesis. Biochemistry 35: 13081–13088.

37. Koishi AC, Zanello PR, Bianco ÉM, Bordignon J, Nunes Duarte dos Santos C (2012) Screening of Dengue virus antiviral activity of marine seaweeds by an in situ enzyme-linked immunosorbent assay. PLoS One 7: e51089.

38. dos Santos HW, Poloni TR, Souza KP, Muller VD, Tremeschin F, et al. (2008) A simple one-step real-time RT-PCR for diagnosis of dengue virus infection. J Med Virol 80: 1426–1433.

39. Mosmann T (1983) Rapid colorimetric assay for cellular growth and survival: application to proliferation and cytotoxicity assays. J Immunol Methods 65: 55–63.

40. Lee JY, Kim JY, Lee YG, Byeon SE, Kim BH, et al. (2007) In vitro immunoregulatory effects of Korean mistletoe lectin on functional activation of monocytic and macrophage-like cells. Biol Pharm Bull 30: 2043–2051.

41. Agis-Juárez RA, Galván I, Medina F, Daikoku T, Padmanabhan R, et al. (2009) Polypyrimidine tract-binding protein is relocated to the cytoplasm and is required during dengue virus infection in Vero cells. J Gen Virol 90: 2893–2901.

42. Mosso C, Galván-Mendoza IJ, Ludert JE, del Angel RM (2008) Endocytic pathway followed by dengue virus to infect the mosquito cell line C6/36 HT. Virology 378: 193–199.

43. Warke RV, Xhaja K, Martin KJ, Fournier MF, Shaw SK, et al. (2003) Dengue virus induces novel changes in gene expression of human umbilical vein endothelial cells. J Virol 77: 11822–11832.

44. Warke RV, Becerra A, Zawadzka A, Schmidt DJ, Martin KJ, et al. (2008) Efficient dengue virus (DENV) infection of human muscle satellite cells upregulates type I interferon response genes and differentially modulates MHC I expression on bystander and DENV-infected cells. J Gen Virol 89: 1605–1615.

45. Vervaeke P, Alen M, Noppen S, Schols D, Oreste P, et al. (2013) Sulfated Escherichia coli K5 Polysaccharide Derivatives Inhibit Dengue Virus Infection of Human Microvascular Endothelial Cells by Interacting with the Viral Envelope Protein E Domain III. PLoS ONE 8(8): e74035.

46. Kyle JL, Beatty PR, Harris E (2007) Dengue virus infects macrophages and dendritic cells in a mouse model of infection. J Infect Dis 195: 1808–1817.

47. Prestwood TR, May MM, Plummer EM, Morar MM, Yauch LE, et al. (2012) Trafficking and replication patterns reveal splenic macrophages as major targets of dengue virus in mice. J Virol 86: 12138–12147.

48. Mairiang D, Zhang H, Sodja A, Murali T, Suriyaphol P, et al. (2013) Identification of new protein interactions between dengue fever virus and its hosts, human and mosquito. PLoS One 8: e53535.

49. Rodenhuis-Zybert IA, Wilschut J, Smit JM (2010) Dengue virus life cycle: viral and host factors modulating infectivity. Cell Mol Life Sci 67: 2773–2786.

50. Demetriou M, Granovsky M, Quaggin S, Dennis JW (2001) Negative regulation of T-cell activation and autoimmunity by Mgat5 N-glycosylation. Nature 409: 733–739.

51. Nieminen J, Kuno A, Hirabayashi J, Sato S (2007) Visualization of galectin-3 oligomerization on the surface of neutrophils and endothelial cells using fluorescence resonance energy transfer. J Biol Chem 282: 1374–1383.

52. Brewer CF, Miceli MC, Baum LG (2002) Clusters, bundles, arrays and lattices: novel mechanisms for lectin-saccharide-mediated cellular interactions. Curr Opin Struct Biol 12: 616–623.

53. Lim JW, Kim H, Kim KH (2003) Cell adhesion-related gene expression by Helicobacter pylori in gastric epithelial AGS cells. Int J Biochem Cell Biol 35: 1284–1296.

54. Sato S, St-Pierre C, Bhaumik P, Nieminen J (2009) Galectins in innate immunity: dual functions of host soluble beta-galactoside-binding lectins as damage-associated molecular patterns (DAMPs) and as receptors for pathogen-associated molecular patterns (PAMPs). Immunol Rev 230: 172–187.

55. Vasta GR (2009) Roles of galectins in infection. Nat Rev Microbiol 7: 424–438.

56. Munoz-Jordan JL, Sanchez-Burgos GG, Laurent-Rolle M, Garcia-Sastre A (2003) Inhibition of interferon signaling by dengue virus. Proc Natl Acad Sci USA 100: 14333–14338.

57. Kyle JL, Beatty PR, Harris E (2007) Dengue virus infects macrophages and dendritic cells in a mouse model of infection. J Infect Dis 195: 1808–1817.

58. Moreno-Altamirano MM, Sánchez-García FJ, Legorreta-Herrera M, Aguilar-Carmona I (2007) Susceptibility of mouse macrophage J774 to dengue virus infection. Intervirology 50: 237–239.

59. Wahala WM, Silva AM (2011) The human antibody response to dengue virus infection. Viruses 3: 2374–2395.

60. Salatino M, Croci DO, Bianco GA, Ilarregui JM, Toscano MA, et al. (2008) Galectin-1 as a potential therapeutic target in autoimmune disorders and cancer. Expert Opin Biol Ther 8: 45–57.

61. Acosta EG, Castilla V, Damonte EB (2009) Alternative infectious entry pathways for dengue virus serotypes into mammalian cells. Cell Microbiol 11: 1533–1549.

62. Horie H, Kadoya T, Sango K, Hasegawa M (2005) Oxidized galectin-1 is an essential factor for peripheral nerve regeneration. Curr Drug Targets 6: 385–394.

63. Kami K, Senba E (2005) Galectin-1 is a novel factor that regulates myotube growth in regenerating skeletal muscles. Curr Drug Targets 6: 395–405.

64. Kato T, Ren CH, Wada M, Kawanami T (2005) Galectin-1 as a potential therapeutic agent for amyotrophic lateral sclerosis. Curr Drug Targets 6: 407–418.

65. Zúñiga E, Gruppi A, Hirabayashi J, Kasai KI, Rabinovich GA, et al. (2001) Regulated expression and effect of galectin-1 on Trypanosoma cruzi-infected macrophages: modulation of microbicidal activity and survival. Infect Immun 69: 6804–6812

19

Association of HLA Class-I and Inhibitory KIR Genotypes in Gabonese Patients Infected by Chikungunya or Dengue Type-2 Viruses

Caroline Petitdemange[1,2,3], Nadia Wauquier[1,4], Jean-Michel Jacquet[5], Ioannis Theodorou[1,2,5], Eric Leroy[3,6], Vincent Vieillard[1,2,7]*

1 Sorbonne Universités, UPMC, Univ Paris 06, CR7, CIMI-Paris, Paris, France, 2 INSERM, U1135, CIMI-Paris, Paris, France, 3 Centre International de Recherches Médicales de Franceville, Unité des maladies Emergentes, Franceville, Gabon, 4 Metabiota Inc., San Francisco, California, United States of America, 5 AP-HP Hôpital Pitié-Salpêtrière, Département d'Immunologie, Paris, France, 6 IRD, Maladies Infectieuses et Vecteurs: Ecologie, Génétique, Evolution et Contrôle, Montpellier, France, 7 CNRS, ERL8255, CIMI-Paris, Paris, France

Abstract

Background: Natural killer (NK) cells provide defense in the early stages of the immune response against viral infections. Killer cell immunoglobulin-like receptors (KIR) expressed on the surface of NK cells play an important role in regulating NK cell response through recognition of human leukocyte antigen (HLA) class I molecules on target cells. Previous studies have shown that specific KIR/ligand combinations are associated with the outcome of several viral infectious diseases.

Methods: We investigated the impact of inhibitory and activating KIR and their HLA-class I ligand genotype on the susceptibility to Chikungunya virus (CHIKV) and Dengue virus (DENV2) infections. From April to July 2010 in Gabon, a large outbreak of CHIKV and DENV2 concomitantly occurred in two provinces of Gabon (Ogooué-Lolo and Haut-Ogooué). We performed the genotypic analysis of KIR in the combination with their cognate HLA-class I ligands in 73 CHIKV and 55 DENV2 adult cases, compared with 54 healthy individuals.

Results: We found in CHIV-infected patients that KIR2DL1 and KIR2DS5 are significantly increased and decreased respectively, as compared to DENV2[+] patients and healthy donors. The combination of KIR2DL1 and its cognate HLA-C2 ligand was significantly associated with the susceptibility to CHIKV infection. In contrast, no other inhibitory KIR-HLA pairs showed an association with the two mosquito-borne arboviruses.

Conclusion: These observations are strongly suggestive that the NK cell repertoire shaped by the KIR2DL1:HLA-C2 interaction facilitate specific infection by CHIKV.

Editor: Niklas K. Björkström, Karolinska Institutet, Sweden

Funding: This study was funded in part by the Institut National de la Recherche Médicale (INSERM), and the Université Pierre et Marie Curie, Paris, France. Vincent Vieillard is a researcher from the Centre National de la Recherche Scientifique (CNRS). The funders had no role in study design, data collection and analysis, decision to publish, or preparation of the manuscript.

Competing Interests: Nadia Wauquier is consultant at Metabiota Inc. The remaining authors declare no conflicts of interest. All authors have contributed to, seen, and approved the final, revised version of the manuscript.

* Email: vincent.vieillard@upmc.fr

Introduction

Chikungunya virus (CHIKV) and Dengue virus (DENV) are two mosquito-borne arboviruses transmitted by the *Aedes* genus. The diseases caused by these viruses have much in common in terms of symptoms, incubation period, clinical course, and symptomatic treatments. Both viruses have been recently proven responsible for major outbreaks leading to serious health and economical problems, and the rapid geographical expansion of their vector could potentially lead to a worldwide increased risk within non-immune populations [1,2]. However, unlike CHIKV, DENV strains are divided into four different serotypes (DENV1 to DENV4), which only confer short-term partial cross-protection against other strains, and contribute to the development of severe forms of Dengue fever (Dengue haemorrhagic fever/Dengue shock syndrome) [3]. Through active surveillance of acute febrile syndrome in Gabon, CHIKV and serotype 2 DENV (DENV2) were detected between 2007 and 2010, and have caused together a large simultaneous outbreak centered on Franceville in southeast Gabon in 2010 [4].

Although natural killer (NK) cells hold a central role early after number of viral infections, not only for viral containment but also for timely and efficient induction of adaptive responses, their role in the control of CHIKV and DENV2 infections is still poorly documented [5,6]. NK cells are controlled by a combination of activating and inhibitory receptors, and the integration of signals induced upon ligation of these receptors determines whether they become activated. These receptors include the killer cell immunoglobulin-like receptors (KIR) that encode for a family of highly polymorphic genes, and individual KIR haplotypes differ in number and identity of genes [7]. Expression of KIR receptors is very complex and controlled by a stochastic mechanism that shuts off expression of some receptors and not others in individual cells thereby allowing different NK cell clones to recognize different targets [8]. It is therefore unlikely for two unrelated individuals to share the same KIR genes or haplotypes and express the receptors. The KIR receptors are type I integral membrane glycoproteins that are usually expressed on the cell surface as monomers. The KIR receptors are named according to the number (i.e. 2 or 3) of Ig-like domains present in the extracellular region as well as the length (i.e. L: long or S: short) of their cytoplasmic tails. Functionally, KIR-L carry one or two tyrosine-based inhibition motifs (ITIMs), which contribute to inhibitory signaling whereas, KIR-S have a lysine residue in their trans-membrane domain that is required for pairing with the tyrosine-based activation motif (ITAM) - containing adaptor DAP12 [9]. The KIR family now includes seven inhibitory KIRs and six activating KIRs, in addition to KIR2DL4, which is an unusual activating member of the KIR family with inhibitory potential. KIRs bind polymorphic major histocompatibility complex (MHC) class-I molecules. For instance KIR2DL1/KIR2DS1 and KIR2DL2/KIR2DL3/KIR2DS2 bind group 2 (C2) and group 1 (C1) HLA-C alleles, respectively, whereas, KIR3DL1 recognizes HLA-Bw4 epitopes [8–10]. Besides their role in inhibiting NK cell function, combinations of KIR and HLA molecules also play an essential role during NK education, to establish self-tolerance and to shape the KIR repertoire of fully functional NK cells. Indeed functional maturation of NK cells requires specific interaction with MHC class I molecules [11]. However, MHC class I genes map to chromosome 6 whereas KIR genes map to chromosome 19 [7]. Therefore, the inheritance of each group of genes and the expression of the receptors and their ligands are physically independent of one another. It has become increasingly clear that the strength of KIR-HLA interactions has functional significance, and can influence the susceptibility to or the outcome of various infectious diseases, as previously shown for human immunodeficiency virus type 1 (HIV-1) and hepatitis C virus (HCV) [12,13], yet no such associations have been uncovered in the context of CHIKV and DENV infections. Therefore, this study was undertaken to determine the impact of inhibitory KIR and their HLA-class I ligand genotype on the susceptibility to CHIKV and DENV2 infections.

Materials and Methods

Ethics statement

The research we report here was conducted in accordance with the principals expressed in the Declaration of Helsinki and was approved by the relevant French and Gabonese institutional ethics panels. Following the 2010 Gabon outbreak, the public-health response was based on cooperation between the Gabonese Ministry of Health (MoH) and "Centre International de Recherches Médicales de Franceville" (CIRMF). All eligible participants were aged ≥18 years provided informed consent, but given the urgency of diagnosis and according to the MoH directives; only individual oral consent was required for sampling. All results were confidentially transmitted to the MoH. This procedure was approved by an Institutional Review Board ("Conseil Scientifique du CIRMF") and the Regional Health Director (Authorization N°139, May 27, 2010). The institutional review board of the Pitié-Salpêtrière Hospital (Comité de

Protection des personnes, Ile-de-France, Paris, France) also approved this study.

Study population

Peripheral blood samples from 73 CHIKV-infected (male: 44.7%; age mean: 37.5 yr), and 55 DENV-2-infected (male: 25.7%; age mean: 34.6 yr) patients were obtained between April and July 2010 during the simultaneous outbreak of CHIKV and DENV-2, which occurred in two provinces (Ogooue Lolo and Haut Ogooue) of southeast Gabon, occupied predominantly by the rural rainforest Kaningi population. Peripheral blood samples were collected on suspected adult cases during the first five days after the following symptoms: fever (>38.5°C), arthralgias, myalgias, headaches, rash, fatigue, nausea, vomiting, diarrhea or bleeding. Patients who met the case definition were sampled and tested for various arboviral RNA genomes, as described [4]. Each sample was negative for Yellow, West Nile and Rift Valley fevers, or malaria. As controls, 54 Gabonese healthy individuals were selected to match for origin, age (mean: 36.0 yr), and sex (male: 41%) [14]. This healthy control group was sampled between 2001 and 2007, before the first outbreak of CHIKV and DENV2, which occurred in Gabon from March 2007 [4,15].

Viral RNA extraction and quantification

Diagnosis for CHIKV or DENV fevers was confirmed and quantification performed using a standard quantitative real-time reverse-transcription polymerase chain reaction (qRT-PCR) method. Briefly, RNA was extracted from 140 µL of plasma using the QIAamp Viral RNA Mini kit (Qiagen). cDNA was synthesized using qRT-PCR with a 9500 thermocycler (Applied biosystems), and mixing 25 µL of extracted RNA with 25 µL of High Capacity cDNA kit (Applied Biosystems). Five µL of newly synthesized cDNA was used as template in 25 µL of Taqman universal PCR Master Mix with specific CHIKV or DENV primers for a partial envelope (E1) gene sequence of CHIKV (692 bp, position 10 138–10829 nt) and a partial envelope (E) gene sequence of DENV-2 (758 bp, position 1503–2260 nt). Amplifications were run in duplicate in a 7500 Real-time PCR system (Applied Biosystem), as described [4,5].

KIR and HLA genotyping

DNA was extracted from whole blood using QIAamp DNA blood mini kit (Qiagen). Inhibitory KIR genotyping was performed by PCR using the KIR typing kit (Miltenyi Biotec, Inc) following manufacturer's instructions, as previously performed [14], and then confirmed by PCR using standard primers, and internal controls, as previously described [16]. HLA-Class I alleles were hybridized using LABType SSO kit (One Lambda). HLA sequences were read with a LABScan 200 (Luminex Technology) and computer-assisted HLA Fusion software.

Statistical analysis

Fisher's exact test was used to compare results between healthy control and CHIKV$^+$ or DENV$^+$ patients. The P values of statistically significant differences were then corrected, by the formula $P^n = 1-(1-P)^n$, where n is the number of comparisons [17].

Results and Discussion

We studied variations in KIR polymporphic CMH class I genotypes and associations in CHIKV-, DENV2-infected patients and healthy individuals from Gabon.

Table 1. Diversity of the KIR genotypes in CHIKV and DENV2-infected patients compared with healthy controls from the same origin.

Genotype	KIR 2DL1	2DL2	2DL3	2DL4	2DL5	2DS1	2DS2	2DS3	2DS4	2DS5	3DL1	3DL2	3DL3	3DS1	3DP1	3DP2	CTRL (n=54) n	%	CHIKV+ (n=30) n	%	p	DENV-2+ (n=31) n	%	p
1 AA	+	−	+	+	−	−	−	−	+	−	+	+	+	−	+	+	13	24.0	2	6.7		5	16.1	
2 AB/BB	+	−	+	+	+	−	−	−	+	−	+	+	+	−	+	+	3	5.6					1	3.2	
3 AB/BB	+	−	+	+	+	−	−	−	+	+	+	+	+	−	+	+	2	3.7							
4 AB/BB	+	−	+	+	+	+	−	−	+	+	+	+	+	+	+	+	1	1.8							
5 AB/BB	+	+	−	+	+	−	+	−	+	+	+	+	+	−	+	+	3	5.6	2	6.7		1	3.2	
6 AB/BB	+	+	−	+	+	−	+	−	+	−	+	+	+	−	+	+	2	3.7					2	6.4	
7 AB/BB	+	+	−	+	+	+	−	−	+	−	+	+	+	−	+	+	1	1.8							
8 AB/BB	+	+	−	+	+	+	+	−	+	−	+	+	+	−	+	+	1	1.8	1	3.3		1	3.2	
9 AB/BB	+	+	+	+	+	+	+	+	+	−	+	+	+	−	+	+	1	1.8							
10 AB/BB	+	+	+	+	+	+	+	+	+	+	+	+	+	−	+	+	2	3.7					1	3.2	
11 AB/BB	+	+	+	+	+	+	+	+	+	+	+	+	+	+	+	+	1	1.8							
12 AB/BB	+	+	+	−	−	−	+	−	+	+	+	+	+	−	+	+	3	5.6	1	3.3				
13 AB/BB	+	+	+	+	+	−	+	−	+	−	+	+	+	−	+	+	3	5.6	1	3.3		2	6.4	
14 AB/BB	+	+	+	+	+	−	+	−	+	+	+	+	+	−	+	+	3	5.6	2	6.7		2	6.4	
15 AB/BB	+	+	+	+	+	−	+	−	+	−	+	+	+	+	+	+	11	20.3			0.006	1	3.2	
16 AB/BB	+	+	+	+	+	−	+	+	+	+	+	+	+	+	+	+	2	1.8						
17 AB/BB	+	+	+	+	+	−	+	−	+	+	+	+	+	+	+	+	2	3.7	2	6.7				
18 AB/BB	+	+	+	+	+	−	+	+	+	+	+	+	+	+	+	+	1	1.8						
19 AB/BB	+	+	+	+	+	−	−	−	+	−	+	+	+	−	+	+			1	3.3		1	3.2	
20 AB/BB	+	−	+	+	+	+	−	−	+	+	+	+	+	−	+	+			3	10.0	0.043	6	19.3	0.001
21 AB/BB	+	−	+	+	+	+	−	−	+	+	+	+	+	+	+	+			1	3.3		1	3.2	
22 AB/BB	−	+	−	+	+	−	+	−	+	+	+	+	+	−	+	+			1	3.3				
23 AB/BB	−	+	−	+	+	−	+	−	+	−	+	+	+	−	+	+			1	3.3				
24 AB/BB	+	+	+	+	−	−	−	−	+	−	+	+	+	+	+	+			2	6.7				
25 AB/BB	+	+	+	+	+	−	+	−	+	+	+	+	+	+	+	+			1	3.3				
26 AB/BB	+	+	−	+	+	−	+	−	+	−	+	+	+	−	+	+			1	3.3				
27 AB/BB	+	+	+	+	−	−	+	−	+	+	+	+	+	−	+	+			2	6.7				
28 AB/BB	+	+	+	+	+	−	+	−	+	+	+	+	+	+	+	+			2	6.7				
29 AB/BB	+	−	+	+	−	−	−	−	+	−	+	+	+	−	+	+			1	3.3				
30 AB/BB	+	+	+	+	−	−	+	+	+	+	+	+	+	+	+	+			1	3.3				
31 AB/BB	+	+	+	−	−	−	+	−	+	−	+	+	+	−	+	+			1	3.3		1	3.2	
32 AB/BB	+	+	+	−	−	−	+	−	+	+	+	+	+	−	+	+			1	3.3		1	3.2	
33 AB/BB	+	−	+	+	+	+	−	−	+	−	+	+	+	−	+	+						1	3.2	

Table 1. Cont.

Genotype	KIR																CTRL (n=54)		CHIKV+ (n=30)			DENV-2+ (n=31)		
	2DL1	2DL2	2DL3	2DL4	2DL5	2DS1	2DS2	2DS3	2DS4	2DS5	3DL1	3DL2	3DL3	3DS1	3DP1	3DP2	n	%	n	%	p	n	%	p
34 AB/BB	+	+	+	+	+	+	−	−	+	−	−	+	+	−	+	+						1	3.2	
35 AB/BB	+	−	+	+	−	−	+	−	+	−	+	+	+	−	+	+						1	3.2	
36 AB/BB	+	−	+	+	−	−	+	−	+	−	+	+	+	−	+	+						1	3.2	
37 AB/BB	+	−	+	+	−	−	−	−	+	−	−	+	+	−	+	+						1	3.2	

Initial analysis of the KIR locus among all participants identified 37 different genotypes [18,19]. Table 1 shows that the number of KIR genotypes in the different groups of patients varied from 18 to 21, with only KIR2DL4, KIR2DS4, KIR3DL3, KIR2DP1 and KIR3DP1 being detectable in all genotypes. All healthy and infected individuals possessed the framework genes (KIR2DL4, KIR3DL2 or KIR3DL3) [20]. This finding is biologically relevant to the studies showing that the NK cells lacking inhibitory receptors for self-MHC class I molecules could be hyporesponsive [21]. The frequency of individuals presenting an A/A genotype, containing only one activating gene (KIR2DS4), was higher in healthy individuals (24.0%) and DENV-2+ samples (16.7%), compared to CHIKV+ carriers (6.7%) (Table 1). The most represented AB/BB genotype in healthy donors (20.3%), genotype #15, was totally absent in CHIKV+ patients (p = 0.006), and only present in 1/31 (3.2%) DENV-2+ patient. Notably, in CHIKV+ patients, each genotype was only poorly represented, and a large proportion of them were not observed in healthy donors. In addition, the frequency of genotype #20 was significantly higher in CHIKV+ (p = 0.043) and DENV-2+ (p = 0.001) patients than in healthy donors (Table 1). Altogether these data suggest that CHIKV and DENV infections were characterized by KIR distributions that differed from healthy controls, suggesting that the KIR repertoire could contribute to an increased susceptibility to CHIKV and/or DENV infection.

We next compared individual inhibitory KIR genotypes in healthy volunteers to patients infected with CHIKV or DENV2. Percentages of KIR gene carriers in the Gabonese control samples (Table 2) were in accordance to other African cohorts [22,23]. In DENV2-infected patients, proportions of all activating and inhibitory KIRs were similar to the healthy control. However, Beltram et al. [24] have recently shown for DENV-3 in southern Brazil significant differences for the KIR2DS1, KIR2DS5 and KIR2DL5 genes. The differences with our data could be explained by the DENV serotype (DENV-2 vs DENV-3) and the origin of the populations under study. In contrast, the proportion of KIR2DL1 gene carriers significantly decreased amongst CHIKV+ (p^n = 0.0338), compared to Gabonese healthy controls. Notably, amongst the "KIR and Diseases Database" (htpp://www.allelefrequencies.net/diseases/) several other diseases were reported to be significantly associated with a modulation of KIR2DL1, including placental Malaria in pregnant Kenyan women [25]. However, for CHIKV-infection, it is important to note that decreased frequency of KIR2DL1 gene is very consistent with the significant cell-surface phenotypic down-modulation of KIR2DL1 inversely associated with the viral load, that we have previously observed in acute CHIKV-infection [5]. Of note, the proportion of KIR2DS5 is significantly increased in CHIKV-infected patients (p^n = 0.050) compared to healthy controls (Table 2), as previously observed in patients with HCV infection who cleared the virus in the association with a decreased of KIR2DL2/KIR2DS2 [26]. In addition, the presence of KIR2DS5 appears to be protective in ankylosing spondylitis, endometriosis and acute kidney graft rejection but a lack of KIR2DS5 and presence of C1 allotype was associated with rheumatoid arthritis [27]. KIR2DS5 code for surface receptor that trigger NK cell functions, although its ligand is unknown [28].

Since the interactions between KIR and their ligands are essential to control of NK cell function, we next evaluated the frequency of KIR genes in combination with the genes encoding their respective known ligands in the same patients. It is noteworthy that all Gabonese individuals, whatever their infectious status, had similar HLA-Bw4 genetic profiles (Figure 1A) which is consistent with what was observed in other African

Table 2. KIR genotypes and HLA ligand combinations in CHIV- and DENV2-infected patients, compared with healthy donors from the same Gabonese population.

	Control		CHIKV+				DENV-2+			
	n	%	n	%	p	p^n	n	%	p	p^n
Inhibitory KIR genotypes										
2DL1	54/54	100	63/73	86.1	0.0049	0.0338	52/52	100	ns	ns
2DL2	35/54	64.8	44/73	60.3	ns	ns	30/52	57.7	ns	ns
2DL3	43/54	79.6	48/73	65.7	ns	ns	41/52	78.8	ns	ns
2DL5	39/54	72.2	40/73	54.8	ns	ns	31/52	59.6	ns	ns
3DL1	54/54	100	73/75	97.3	ns	ns	47/50	94.0	ns	ns
3DL2	54/54	100	68/69	98.5	ns	ns	52/52	100	ns	ns
3DL3	54/54	100	69/69	100	ns	ns	52/52	100	ns	ns
Activating KIR genotypes										
2DL4	54/54	100	68/73	93.1	ns	ns	51/52	98.0	ns	ns
2DS1	10/54	18.5	11/55	20.0	ns	ns	15/52	28.8	ns	ns
2DS2	31/54	64.8	18/39	46.1	0.0237	ns	16/41	39.0	ns	ns
2DS3	19/54	35.2	7/36	19.4	ns	ns	6/36	16.7	ns	ns
2DS4	54/54	100	70/70	100	ns	ns	48/48	100	ns	ns
2DS5	18/54	33.3	33/56	58.9	0.0081	0.0489	23/52	44.2	ns	ns
3DS1	4/54	7.4	7/66	10.6	ns	ns	6/50	12.0	ns	ns
Inhibitory KIR-HLA associations										
C2+ in 2DL1+	32/47	68.1	44/48	91.6	0.0048	0.0238	26/40	65.0	ns	ns
C1+ in 2DL2+	20/31	64.5	21/33	63.4	ns	ns	14/22	63.6	ns	ns
C1+ in 2DL3+	27/38	71.0	18/40	45.0	ns	ns	21/31	67.7	ns	ns
C1+ in 2DL2/2DL3+	32/47	68.1	28/51	54.9	ns	ns	26/40	65.0	ns	ns
Bw4+ in 3DL1+	33/47	70.2	38/55	69.1	ns	ns	22/31	59.5	ns	ns
Inhibitory KIR3DL1+-HLA-Bw4 subtype associations										
Bw4-80Ile+	22/47	46.8	38/55	69.1	0.0274	ns	20/37	54.0	ns	ns
Bw4-80Trr+	12/47	25.5	1/55	1.8	0.0005	0.0011	3/37	8.1	0.0472	ns
Activating KIR-HLA associations										
C2+ in 2DS1+	7/8	87.5	8/8	100	ns	ns	9/12	75.0	ns	ns
C1+ in 2DS2+	18/22	64.3	12/17	70.6	ns	ns	10/12	83.3	ns	ns

P: Fisher exact test; P^n: The P values of statistically significant differences were then corrected by the formula $P^n = 1-(1-P)^n$, where n is the number of comparisons [17].

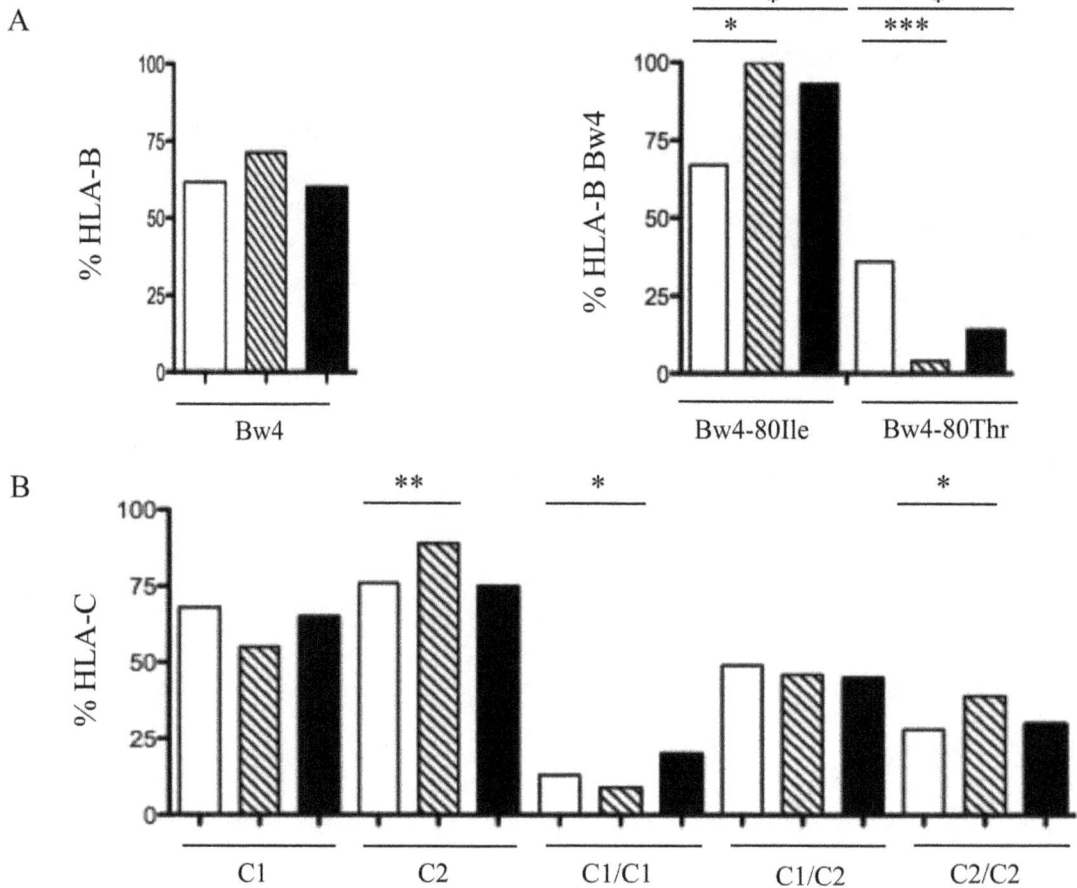

Figure 1. Allele frequency for HLA-B Bw4 (A) and HLA-C (B) subtypes in Gabonese individuals. The frequency of each variable is shown for non-infected controls (n = 54; open bars), CHIKV-infected patients (n = 60; hatched bars), and DENV2-infected patients (n = 45; closed bars). *P< 0.05; **P<0.001; ***P<0.0001.

cohorts [29]. However an increased frequency of HLA-B*44, an HLA-Bw4 allele, was recently associated with DENV3 severity in Brazilians [30]. This discrepancy suggests possible differences between the DENV serotypes and/or variations due to ethnicity. HLA-Bw4 (and not Bw6) allotypes serve as ligands for KIR3DL1 subtypes and subtypes are defined by amino-acid variations at positions 77–83 of the HLA-B molecules [7]. Table 2 shows similar proportions of HLA-Bw4 allele amongst KIR3DL1[+] samples, whatever the study group. HLA-Bw4 molecules are further divided into two groups on the basis of whether isoleucine (Ile) or threonine (Thr) residues are present at position 80, defining HLA-Bw4-80Ile and Bw4-80Thr, respectively [31]. According to Norman et al. [32] an unusual KIR3DL1/S1 evolution occurred in Africans. Thus, KIR3DL1/S1 locus encodes two lineages of polymorphic inhibitory KIR3DL1 allotypes and one lineage of conserved activating KIR3DS1. They also highlighted that random combination of polymorphic KIR3DL1 receptor and HLA-B ligands has vast potential for varying the NK cell response to infection [32]. Figure 1A shows that Bw4-80Thr alleles are significantly more common in CHIKV[+] patients than in both DENV2[+] and healthy individuals, individuals. We examined the combination of Bw4-80Ile/Thr and KIR3DL1 in the context of sensitivity to CHIKV or DENV2 infection, and only observed significant modulation for the combination KIR3DL1:Bw4-80Thr ($p^n = 0.001$), compared to healthy controls (Table 2). In agreement

with receptor-binding and lysis-inhibition data suggesting that HLA-Bw4-80Ile molecules are more effective ligands for KIR3DL1 than HLA-Bw4-80Thr [33], we have observed no significant phenotypic modulation of KIR3DL1 expression after acute CHIKV [5] and DENV2 (Petitdemange et al., Manuscript in preparation) infections. In contrast, for HIV-1 the KIR3DL1:HLA-Bw4-80Ile combination was described in association with disease severity [34].

HLA-C molecules are also dichotomized into two groups, based on their KIR specificity; HLA-C group 1 (C1) specifically binds to KIR2DL2/DL3 and HLA-C group 2 (C2) binds to KIR2DL1 [8]. The genetic combinations of KIR2DL2/DL3 or KIR2DS2 and HLA-C1 genes remained similar in infected and healthy Gabonese yet we have previously reported a clonal expansion of NK cells that co-express activating CD94/NKG2C and inhibitory KIR2DL2/DL3 receptors in direct association with the viral load during acute CHIKV-infection [5]. The combination of KIR2DL2/DL3 with HLA-C1 might therefore not be involved in susceptibility to CHIKV infection but the observed expansion of NK cells expressing these receptors suggests that this interaction is of importance during the development of the disease. For example, KIR2DL2/DL3:HLA-C1 interaction could be associated with the delayed progression to the development of persistent chronic inflammation in CHIKV-infected patients. Infiltrating activated NK cells were found in synovial tissue in close vicinity to chronically CHIKV-infected perivascular synovial macrophages [35]. Importantly, a significant increase in frequency of HLA-C2 was observed in CHIKV-infected patients (p = 0.0041), mainly of HLA-C2 homozygous subjects, compared to DENV$^+$ patients and controls (Figure 1B). More intriguingly, this HLA-C2 increased effect was also significantly observed in combination with KIR2DL1 (p = 0.0238) (Table 2). In this regard, however, it cannot be ruled out that these results were influenced by population demographic history; these results will need to be confirmed through the study of samples collected from other ethnic groups. Notably, this data highlights that CHIKV infection could be influenced by KIR2DL1/HLA-C2 interplay. Consistent with this notion we have previously shown a depletion of KIR2DL1$^+$ cells early after CHIKV infection, inversely associated with the viral load [5].

The finding that inhibitory interactions are protective against a viral infection initially seems counterintuitive. However, NK cells are held in check by their inhibitory receptors as originally proposed by the missing-self hypothesis' and loss of these interactions could be a key mechanism to allow NK cell activation [36]. *In vitro* studies with autologous influenza infected targets have shown that NK cells from individuals with KIR2DL3:HLA-C1 were activated more rapidly than those with KIR2DL1:HLA-C2 [37]. Consistently we previously showed that the KIR2DL1$^+$ NK cell depletion was associated with an expansion of KIR2DL2/

DL3$^+$ NKG2C$^+$ cells after acute CHIKV infection [5]. In summary, we can hypothesize that the expansion of highly functional NK cells and the development of a strong adaptive memory response, as previously described [5,38], are independent of a specific KIR/HLA pathway in DENV2 infection, but certainly associated to an interplay between KIR2DL1 and HLA-C2 in response to CHIKV infection. This study is an interesting first step towards understanding the different roles of KIR and their specific ligands in CHIKV and DENV2 infections. However, further studies will be necessary to conclude as to the role of these receptors and ligands in the context of susceptibility to these infections or in the development of the disease and chronic or hemorrhagic symptoms.

Acknowledgments

We thank Philippe Engandja from CIRMF (Franceville, Gabon) for technical assistance.

Author Contributions

Conceived and designed the experiments: CP EL VV. Performed the experiments: CP NW JMJ. Analyzed the data: CP NW IT EL VV. Contributed reagents/materials/analysis tools: NW EL. Wrote the paper: CP NW VV.

References

1. Pialoux G, Gauzere BA, Jaureguiberry S, Strobel M (2007) Chikungunya, an epidemic arbovirosis. Lancet Infect Dis 7: 319–327.
2. World Health Organization. Fact sheet no. 117: dengue and dengue haemorrhagic fever. Available: http://www.who.int/mediacentre/factsheets/fs117/en/. Accessed 2009.
3. Fried JR, Gibbons RV, Kalayanarooj S, Thomas SJ, Srikiatkhachorn A, et al. (2010) Serotype-specific differences in the risk of dengue hemorrhagic fever: an analysis of data collected in Bangkok, Thailand from 1994 to 2006. PLoS Negl Tro Dis 4: e617.
4. Caron M, Paupy C, Grard G, Becquart P, Mombo I, et al. (2012) Recent introduction and rapid dissemination of Chikungunya virus and Dengue virus serotype 2 associated with human and mosquito coinfections in Gabon, central Africa. Clin Infect Dis 55: e45–53.
5. Petitdemange C, Becquart P, Wauquier N, Béziat V, Debré P, et al. (2011) Unconventional repertoire profile is imprinted during acute chikungunya infection for natural killer cells polarization toward cytotoxicity. PLoS Pathog 7: e1002268.
6. Azeredo EL, De Oliveira-Pinto LM, Zagne SM, Cerqueira DI, Nogueira RM, et al. (2006) NK cells, displaying early activation, cytotoxicity and adhesion molecules, are associated with mild dengue disease. Clin Exp Immunol 143: 345–356.
7. Kulkarni S, Martin MP, Carrington M (2008) The Yin and Yang of HLA and KIR in human disease. Semin Immunol 20: 343–352.
8. Lanier LL (2005) NK cell recognition. Annu Rev Immunol 23: 225–274.
9. Falco M, Moretta L, Moretta A, Bottino C (2013) KIR and KIR ligand polymorphism: a new area for clinical applications? Tissue Antigens 82: 363–373.
10. Ivarsson MA, Michaëlsson J, Fauriat C (2014) Activating killer cell Ig-like receptors in health and disease. Front Immunol 5:184.
11. Anfossi N, André P, Guia S, Falk CS, Roetynck S, et al. (2006) Human NK cell education by inhibitory receptors for MHC class I. Immunity 25: 331–342.
12. Khakoo SI, Thio CL, Martin MP, Brooks CR, Gao X, et al. (2004) HLA and NK cell inhibitory receptor genes in resolving hepatitis C virus infection. Science 305: 872–874.
13. Martin MP, Qi Y, Gao X, Yamada E, Martin JN, et al. (2007) Innate partnership of HLA-B and KIR3DL1 subtypes against HIV-1. Nat Gen 39: 733–740.
14. Wauquier N, Padilla C, Becquart P, Leroy E, Vieillard V (2010) Association of KIR2DS1 and KIR2DS3 with fatal outcome in Ebola virus infection. Immunogenetics 62: 767–771.
15. Leroy EM, Nkoghe D, Ollomo B, Nze-Nkogue C, Becquart P, et al. (2009) Concurrent chikungunya and dengue virus infections during simultaneous outbreaks, Gabon, 2007. Emerg Infect Dis 15: 591–593.
16. Vilches C, Castaño J, Gómez-Lozano N, Estefanía E (2007) Facilitation of KIR genotyping by a PCR-SSP method that amplifies short DNA fragments. Tissue Antigens 70: 415–422.
17. Svejgaard A, Ryder LP (1994) HLA and disease associations: detecting the strongest association. Tissue Antigens 43: 18–27.
18. Martin MP, Single RM, Wilson MJ, Trowsdale J, Carrington M (2009) KIR haplotypes defined by segregation analysis in 59 Centre d'Etude Polymorphism Humain (CEPH) families. Immunogenetics 61: 79.
19. Hollenbach JA, Nocedal I, Ladner MB, Single RM, Trachtenberg EA (2012) Killer cell immunoglobulin-like receptor (KIR) gene content variation in the HGDP-CEPH populations. Immunogenetics 64: 719–737.
20. Vilches C, Parham P (2002) KIR: diverse, rapidly evolving receptors of innate and adaptive immunity. Annu Rev Immunol 20: 217–251.
21. Kim S, Poursine-Laurent J, Truscott SM, Lybarger L, Song YJ, et al. (2005) Licensing of natural killer cells by host major histocompatibility complex class I molecules. Nature 436: 709–713.
22. Norman PJ, Carrington CV, Byng M, Maxwell LD, Curran MD, et al. (2002) Natural killer cell immunoglobulin-like receptor (KIR) locus profiles in African and South Asian populations. Genes Immunol 3: 86–95.
23. Denis L, Sivula J, Gourraud PA, Kerdudou N, Chout R, et al. (2005) Genetic diversity of KIR natural killer cell markers in populations from France, Guadeloupe, Finland, Senegal and Réunion. Tissue Antigens 66: 267–276.
24. Beltrame LM, Sell AM, Moliterno RA, Clementino SL, Cardozo DM, et al. (2013) Influence of KIR genes and their HLA ligands in susceptibility to dengue in a population from southern Brazil. Tissue Antigens 82: 397–404.
25. Omosun YO, Blackstock AJ, Gatei W, Hightower A, van Eijk AM, et al. (2012) Differential association of gene content polymorphisms of killer cell immunoglobulin-like receptors with placental malaria in HIV− and HIV+ mothers. PLoS One 7: e38617.
26. Paladino N, Flores AC, Marcos CY, Fainboim H, Theiler G, et al. (2007) Increased frequencies of activating natural killer receptors are associated with liver injury in individuals who do not eliminate hepatitis C virus. Tissue Antigens 69:109–111.
27. Nowak I, Majorczyk E, Wiśniewski A, Pawlik A, Magott-Procelewska M, et al. (2010) Does the KIR2DS5 gene protect from some human diseases? PLoS One 5: e12381.
28. Della Chiesa M, Romeo E, Falco M, Balsamo M, Augugliaro R, et al. (2008) Evidence that the KIR2DS5 gene codes for a surface receptor triggering natural killer cell function. Eur J Immunol 38: 2284–2289.
29. Paximadis M, Mathebula TY, Gentle NL, Vardas E, Colvin M, et al. (2012) Human leukocyte antigen class I (A, B, C) and II (DRB1) diversity in the black and Caucasian South African population. Hum Immunol 73: 80–92.
30. Xavier Eurico de Alencar L, de Mendonça Braga-Neto U, José Moura do Nascimento E, Tenório Cordeiro M, Maria Silva A, et al. (2013) HLA-B*44 is associated with Dengue severity caused by DENV-3 in a Brazilian population. J Trop Med 2013: 648475.
31. Müller CA, Engler-Blum G, Gekeler V, Steiert I, Weiss E, et al. (1989) Genetic and serological heterogeneity of the supertypic HLA-B locus specificities Bw4 and Bw6. Immunogenetics 30: 200–207.
32. Norman PJ, Abi-Rached L, Gendzekhadze K, Korbel D, Gleimer M, et al. (2007) Unusual selection on the KIR3DL1/S1 natural killer cell receptor in Africans. Nat Genet 39: 1092–1099.

33. Carr WH, Pando MJ, Parham P (2005) KIR3DL1 polymorphisms that affect NK cell inhibition by HLA-Bw4 ligand. J Immunol 175: 5222–5229.

34. Parham P (2005) MHC class I molecules and KIRs in human history, health and survival. Nat Rev Immunol 5: 201–214.

35. Hoarau JJ, Jaffar Bandjee MC, Krejbich Trotot P, Das T, Li-Pat-Yuen G, et al. (2010) Persistent chronic inflammation and infection by Chikungunya arthritogenic alphavirus in spite of a robust host immune response. J Immunol 184: 5914–5927.

36. Ljunggren HG, Kärre K (1990) In search of the 'missing self': MHC molecules and NK cell recognition. Immunol Today 11: 237–244.

37. Ahlenstiel G, Martin MP, Gao X, Carrington M, Rehermann B (2008) Distinct KIR/HLA compound genotypes affect the kinetics of human antiviral natural killer cell responses. J Clin Invest 118: 1017–1026.

38. Wauquier N, Becquart P, Nkoghe D, Padilla C, Ndjoyi-Mbiguino A, et al. (2011) The acute phase of Chikungunya virus infection in humans is associated with strong innate immunity and T CD8 cell activation. J Infect Dis 204: 115–123.

20

Development, Characterization and Application of Monoclonal Antibodies against Brazilian Dengue Virus Isolates

Camila Zanluca[1,2♦], Giovanny Augusto Camacho Antevere Mazzarotto[1♦], Juliano Bordignon[1]*, Claudia Nunes Duarte dos Santos[1]*

1 Laboratório de Virologia Molecular, Instituto Carlos Chagas (ICC/Fiocruz/PR), Curitiba, Paraná, Brasil, **2** Programa de Pós-Graduação em Biologia Celular e Molecular, Universidade Federal do Paraná (UFPR), Curitiba, Paraná, Brasil

Abstract

Dengue is the most prevalent human arboviral disease. The morbidity related to dengue infection supports the need for an early, quick and effective diagnostic test. Brazil is a hotspot for dengue, but no serological diagnostic test has been produced using Brazilian dengue virus isolates. This study aims to improve the development of immunodiagnostic methods for dengue virus (DENV) detection through the production and characterization of 22 monoclonal antibodies (mAbs) against Brazilian isolates of DENV-1, -2 and -3. The mAbs include IgG2bκ, IgG2aκ and IgG1κ isotypes, and most were raised against the envelope or the pre-membrane proteins of DENV. When the antibodies were tested against the four DENV serotypes, different reactivity patterns were identified: group-specific, subcomplex specific (DENV-1, -3 and -4 and DENV-2 and -3) and dengue serotype-specific (DENV-2 or -3). Additionally, some mAbs cross-reacted with yellow fever virus (YFV), West Nile virus (WNV) and Saint Louis encephalitis virus (SLEV). None of the mAbs recognized the alphavirus Venezuelan equine encephalitis virus (VEEV). Furthermore, mAbs D3 424/8G, D1 606/A12/B9 and D1 695/12C/2H were used to develop a capture enzyme-linked immunosorbent assay (ELISA) for anti-dengue IgM detection in sera from patients with acute dengue. To our knowledge, these are the first monoclonal antibodies raised against Brazilian DENV isolates, and they may be of special interest in the development of diagnostic assays, as well as for basic research.

Editor: Nicholas J. Mantis, New York State Dept. Health, United States of America

Funding: The authors thank CNPq, CNPq/Prosul, Fiocruz, Fundação Araucária and Fundo Paraná and CNPq/CAPES PROCAD/Casadinho for financial support. CNDS is a CNPq fellowship recipient. The funders had no role in study design, data collection and analysis, decision to publish, or preparation of the manuscript.

Competing Interests: The authors have declared that no competing interests exist.

* Email: clsantos@tecpar.br (CNDS); julianobordignon@fiocruz.br (JB)

♦ These authors contributed equally to this work.

Introduction

Dengue is one of the most prevalent arboviral diseases in tropical and subtropical regions of the world. Over 40% of the world's population lives in areas at risk of transmission, and there are an estimated 390 million dengue infections each year, of which 96 million manifest disease symptoms [1]. Additionally, it is believed that ~500,000 cases result in severe disease and ~12,500 in death each year [2,3].

Dengue virus (DENV), the causative agent of dengue, is a positive-sense single-stranded RNA virus that belongs to the genus *Flavivirus*, family *Flaviviridae*. The virus is transmitted by *Aedes* (*Stegomyia*) mosquitoes and is classified into four antigenically distinct but closely related serotypes (DENV-1 to -4) [4]. All four DENV serotypes manifest in a wide spectrum of clinical presentations, including severe (hemorrhagic fever, DHF; or shock syndrome, DSS) and non-severe diseases (dengue fever, DF) [5]. DENV infection symptoms are not sufficiently specific to allow clinical differentiation from other acute febrile illnesses, especially in areas where multiple tropical diseases such as malaria, yellow fever, West Nile disease and Saint Louis encephalitis are endemic [6]. There are several dengue vaccine candidates under development, but none is licensed and available [7]. Additionally, there is no specific treatment for dengue, and the most effective protective measures are those that lower the risk of mosquito bites. Thus, early diagnosis is crucial to reducing morbidity and mortality from DHF and DSS.

Laboratory diagnosis of dengue is based on viral isolation in cell culture, reverse-transcriptase/polymerase-chain reaction (RT-PCR) and serological assays [8,9,10,11]. Several immunoassays for DENV, such as enzyme immunoassays, immunochromatographic and dot-blot assays, are commercially available [10,12,13,14,15]. The IgM antibody capture enzyme-linked immunosorbent assay (MAC-ELISA) is the assay of choice for the serological diagnosis of primary dengue-virus infection [11]. Combined with IgG titers, this assay allows the diagnosis of secondary dengue infection. Furthermore, both IgM and IgG dengue ELISAs are useful tools for seroepidemiological dengue surveillance and can be applied in studies of DENV pathogenesis and host-pathogen relationships [16,17].

Antibodies have been used in recent decades to diagnose several viral diseases and in investigations of viral structure [18,19,20,21,22]; however, the heterogeneity of the polyclonal antibodies used in tests can lead to problems in the interpretation, reproducibility and standardization of the assays. To overcome these limitations, several monoclonal antibodies (mAbs) able to bind to specific antigens have been developed [20,23,24,25]. The first serotype-specific mAbs against DENV were developed by Dittmar et al. (1980) [26]. Monoclonal antibodies against DENV have been successfully used for the identification of viral serotypes, flavivirus differentiation and epidemiological studies, as well as for dengue diagnosis and immunotherapy studies [10,27,28,29,30,31,32,33,34,35].

This study reports the development and characterization of twenty-two mAbs against Brazilian DENV isolates. From this panel, three mAbs were tested in an IgM capture assay for the detection of acute dengue patients in Brazil. The monoclonal antibodies generated were group-specific, subcomplex-specific and serotype-specific, representing essential tools for dengue- and serotype-specific diagnosis. Thus, these antibodies have the potential to increase the specificity and sensitivity of dengue diagnosis in Brazil and throughout South America.

Animals and Methods

Cell lines and viruses

The mouse myeloma cell line P3x63Ag8.653 (kindly supplied by Dr. Carlos R. Zanetti, from Laboratório de Imunologia Aplicada, at Universidade Federal de Santa Catarina, Florianópolis, Brazil; ATCC CRL-1580) and hybridomas were maintained in RPMI-1640 medium (Cultilab, Campinas, Brazil) supplemented with 20% fetal bovine serum (FBS–Gibco, Grand Island, USA), 23.8 mM sodium bicarbonate, 2.0 mM L-glutamine, 1.0 mM sodium pyruvate, 9.6 mM HEPES and antibiotics (100 IU/ml penicillin, 100 μg/ml streptomycin and 0.25 μg/ml amphotericin B – Sigma-Aldrich, Steinheim, Germany) at 37°C in a 5% CO_2 atmosphere. C6/36 Aedes albopictus cells (ATCC CRL-1660) were cultured in Leibovitz's L15 medium (Gibco) with 5% FBS, 25 μg/ml gentamicin (Gibco) and 0.27% tryptose at 28°C. Human-derived hepatoma cells (Huh7.5) (ATCC PTA-8561) and Vero E6 cells (Sigma, 85020206) were maintained in Dulbecco's Modified Eagle Medium/Nutrient Ham F12 (DMEM F12 – Gibco) with 10% FBS, 14.0 mM sodium bicarbonate and antibiotics (100 IU/ml penicillin, 100 μg/ml streptomycin) at 37°C in a 5% CO_2 atmosphere.

The serotypes DENV-1 (BR/01-MR and BR/90), -2 (BR/01-01 and ICC 266), -3 (290-02) and -4 (TVP 360) were used in this study. DENV-4 TVP 360 is a World Health Organization reference strain, kindly supplied by Dr. Ricardo Galler from Fundação Oswaldo Cruz, Rio de Janeiro, Brazil. DENV-1 BR/01-MR (GenBank AF513110.1) and BR/90 (GenBank AF226685.2); DENV-2 BR/01-01 (GenBank JX073928) and ICC 266 (not sequenced); and DENV3 290-02 (GenBank EF629369.1) are clinical isolates from dengue fever obtained in Brazil between 1990 and 2004. All viruses were amplified and titrated by the foci-forming assay in C6/36 cells [36]. The yellow fever virus (YFV) 17DD vaccine strain (BioManguinhos, Fiocruz, Brazil) was obtained after three passages and titration in Vero cells [37]. The Saint Louis encephalitis virus (SLEV) 78V6507 strain, isolated from Culex pipiens quinquefasciatus mosquitoes from Santa Fé Province, Argentina [38]; West Nile virus (WNV) E/7229/06, isolated from a dead horse from Buenos Aires Province, Argentina [39]; and Venezuelan equine encephalitis virus (VEEV) TC38 vaccine strain [40] were kindly supplied by Dr. Marta S.

Contiginani from Instituto de Virología Dr. J.M. Vanella, Facultad de Ciencias Médicas, Universidad Nacional de Córdoba.

Animals and immunization protocol

Ethics statements for all animal procedures were approved by the Ethical Committee on Animal Research of the Universidade Federal do Paraná under the protocol no. 23075.031314/2008-41. Four young adult (30- to 45-day-old) BALB/c mice were used in the immunization protocols for each DENV serotype. All animals were maintained at the Animal Facility of the Instituto Carlos Chagas – FIOCRUZ/PR with water and food ad libitum and a light-dark cycle of 12 h/12 h.

Animals were bled by caudal puncture for extraction of pre-immune serum and then immunized with five doses of 1×10^6 ffu$_{C6/36}$/dose/animal of DENV-1 (BR-01/MR), -2 (BR/01-01) or -3 (BR 290-02). Doses were administered via the intraperitoneal (doses 1 and 3), intradermal (doses 2 and 4) or intravenous route (dose 5), with 1-week intervals between doses. Complete Freund's adjuvant was used in dose 1 (Sigma-Aldrich), and Alu-Gel-S was used in doses 2 to 4 (Serva, Heidelberg, Germany). No adjuvant was used in the fifth dose.

Production of monoclonal antibodies

Three days after the final immunization, the mice were anesthetized with ketamine/xylazine (100 and 10 mg/kg, respectively) via the intraperitoneal route and bled by cardiac puncture to obtain post-immune sera. After post-immune sera were obtained, the animals were euthanized by cervical dislocation. Their spleens were removed aseptically, and splenocytes were fused with P3x63Ag8.653 cells using polyethylene glycol (MW 3000–3700; Sigma-Aldrich), as previously described [20]. Hybrid cells were selected by growth in RPMI-1640 (as described above) plus 100 μM hypoxanthine, 0.4 μM aminopterine and 16 μM thymidine (HAT medium–Sigma-Aldrich) for 14 days. The hybridoma supernatants were screened by indirect immunofluorescence assay (IFA), as described below. Hybridomas whose supernatants showed positive results on IFA were stabilized by two successive freeze-thaw cycles. Cells that remained positive after two cycles were subjected to two rounds of the limiting dilution method and stored in liquid nitrogen. The immunoglobulin isotypes of the mAbs were determined using the SBA Clonotyping System/HRP (Southern Biotech, Birmingham, USA), following the manufacturer's instructions.

mAb screening

Hybridomas secreting antibodies against DENV were selected by IFA on DENV-infected C6/36 cells and on control uninfected C6/36 cells (MOCK). C6/36 cells (1.0×10^5 cells/well in 96-well plates) were infected with the corresponding DENV isolate at a multiplicity of infection (MOI) of 1. Cells were fixed 72 h post-infection with methanol:acetone (1:1 v/v) for at least 30 min at -20°C. Hybridoma supernatants (100 μL) containing the first antibodies were added and incubated for 30 min at 37°C. To detect reactive antibodies, the infected cells were incubated for 1 h at 37°C with Alexa Fluor 488-conjugated anti-mouse immuno-globulins (Sigma–Aldrich). Cell nuclei were labeled with 300 nM of 4',6-diamidino-2-phenylindole (DAPI) for 5 minutes, followed by 3 washes with 1x PBS. The flavivirus-specific mAb 4G2 (hybridoma D1-4G2-4-15, ATCC HB-112) and a non-correlated mAb that recognizes hantavirus nucleoprotein (clone 572/7A) [20] were used as positive and negative controls, respectively. The immunofluorescence images were captured with a Leica AF6000 Modular System.

Table 1. Monoclonal antibody (mAb) designation and characterization.

mAb	DENV serotype for immunization	Isotype	Reactivity against				Virion protein
			DENV 1	DENV 2	DENV 3	DENV 4	
D1 463/G6/H2	DENV 1	IgG1κ	+	−	+	+	E
D1 695/12C/2H	DENV 1	IgG1κ	+	+	+	+	E
D1 606/A12/B9	DENV 1	IgG1κ	+	+	+	+	prM
D2 646/9G	DENV 2	IgG2aκ	−	+	−	−	N.D.
D2 658/9A	DENV 2	IgG2aκ	−	+	−	−	N.D.
D2 332/2D	DENV 2	IgG2aκ	−	+	−	−	E
D3 342/5G/G8	DENV 3	IgG2aκ	−	−	+	−	E
D3 388/4A/G6	DENV 3	IgG1κ	−	−	+	−	E
D3 444/4G/H3	DENV 3	IgG2bκ	−	−	+	−	E
D3 389/F4/H10	DENV 3	IgG1κ	−	−	+	−	E
D3 441/D1/H2	DENV 3	IgG2bκ	−	−	+	−	E
D3 290/4C/G9	DENV 3	IgG2aκ	−	−	+	−	E
D3 341/H9/F10	DENV 3	IgG2aκ	−	−	+	−	E
D3 344/H1	DENV 3	IgG2bκ	−	−	+	−	E*
D3 442/4E/G8	DENV 3	IgG2bκ	−	−	+	−	E
D3 242/F1/H2	DENV 3	IgG2aκ	−	+	+	−	E
D3 424/8G	DENV 3	IgG2bκ	+	+	+	+	E
D3 863/G7/H7	DENV 3	IgG2bκ	+	+	+	+	prM
D3 457/H7/H2	DENV 3	IgG2bκ	+	+	+	+	prM
D3 443/H12/H6	DENV 3	IgG2bκ	+	+	+	+	prM
D3 868/G7/H10	DENV 3	IgG2bκ	+	+	+	+	prM
D3 63/F2/G7	DENV 3	IgG2bκ	+	+	+	+	E**

N.D. not determined; − negative; + positive; E, envelope protein; prM, pre-membrane protein;
*Did not react in the western blot, but recognize recombinant DENV-3 E Δ101 protein expressed on *Drosophila* S2 cells on IFA.
**Reacted in the western blot, but did not recognize recombinant DENV-3 E Δ101 expressed on S2 cells on IFA.

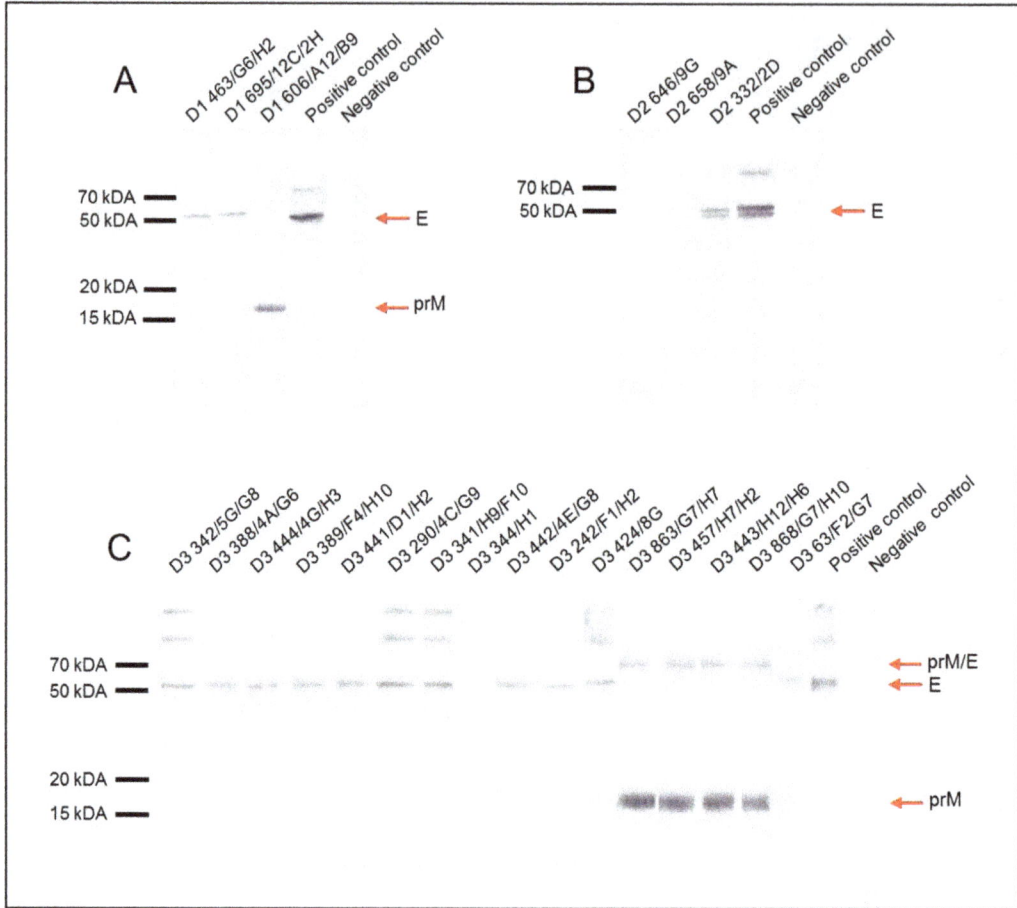

Figure 1. Western blot analysis of mAbs raised against the homologous DENV serotype. Purified gamma-irradiated DENV-1 BR/01-MR (A), DENV-2 BR/01-01 (B), and DENV-3 290-02 (C) were subjected to 13% SDS-PAGE and electroblotted onto nitrocellulose membranes. Proteins were stained with the mAbs, followed by anti-mouse IgG conjugated to alkaline phosphatase. The flavivirus-specific mAb 4G2 and a non-correlated mAb that binds to hantavirus nucleoprotein (clone 572/7A) were used as positive (+) and negative (−) controls, respectively.

Specificity of anti-dengue virus mAbs

To investigate the specificity of mAbs to DENV proteins, mAbs were used in western blot (WB) assays with the corresponding DENV serotypes. Dengue viruses were obtained from the supernatant of C6/36 cells infected with a MOI of 0.01. Each virus serotype was concentrated by polyethylene glycol precipitation using PEG 8000 at a final concentration of 7%, and purified by sedimentation through a 30%/60% sucrose (in TNE – 20 mM Tris pH 8.0, 150 mM NaCl, 2 mM EDTA) cushion. Further, purified DENV were inactivated by gamma irradiation.

Viral proteins had previously been quantified with the Micro BCA Protein Assay kit (Pierce, Rockford, USA). Three micrograms of purified gamma-irradiated DENV-1 BR/01-MR or DENV-2 BR/01-01, or 12 μg of DENV-3 290-02, were mixed with Laemmli sample buffer, boiled for 3 min and loaded into 13% SDS-PAGE gels [41]. Viral proteins were transferred to nitrocellulose membranes (GE-Healthcare, Little Chalfont, UK). Membranes were incubated first with 5% non-fat milk in TBS-T (20 mM Tris, 137 mM NaCl, pH 7.6, containing 0.05% Tween 20) and then with hybridoma supernatants. Monoclonal antibodies 4G2 and anti-hantavirus 572/7A were used as positive and negative controls, respectively. Anti-mouse IgG conjugated to alkaline phosphatase (1:7,500; Sigma-Aldrich) was used as a secondary antibody. All incubation steps were conducted for 1 h at

room temperature. The reaction was developed using a solution of NBT (nitroblue tetrazolium) and BCIP (5-bromo-4-chloro-3-indolyl-phosphate) (Promega, Madison, USA). mAbs produced against the DENV-2 isolate were also tested by WB with a recombinant domain III peptide from DENV-2 envelope protein (~12 kDa) expressed in a prokaryotic system. Furthermore, mAbs produced against DENV-3 were tested by IFA with a truncated recombinant E protein from DENV-3 (DENV-3 E Δ_{101}) expressed by transfected *Drosophila* S2 cells. S2 cells transfected with the plasmid pMt/Bip/V5-HisA containing the gene of the E protein from DENV-3 strain BR 290-02 (GenBank EF629369.1), deleted from the carboxi-terminal anchor (corresponding to the last 101 amino acids), were cultured in Schneider's medium (Gibco) with 10% FBS and 25 μg/mL of gentamicin (Gibco). Envelope protein expression was induced by 500 μM of CuSO4 for 48 h. After protein induction 1×10^5 cells/well were added to a 96-well plate. After adhesion, cells were fixed with methanol:acetone, and IFA was performed as described above.

Reactivity of mAbs against the four DENV serotypes and other flaviviruses and alphaviruses

The reactivity of the mAbs against the four serotypes of DENV was determined using the IFA. C6/36 cells were infected with the DENV-1 (BR/90), -2 (ICC 266), -3 (290-02) or -4 (TVP 360)

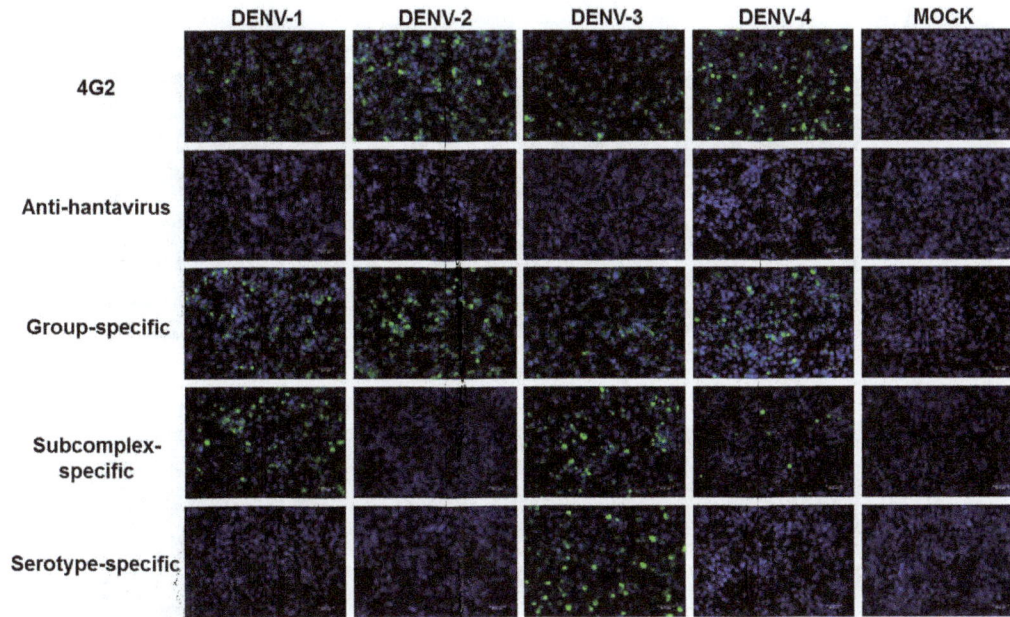

Figure 2. Representation of the reactivities of major groups of monoclonal antibodies. Indirect immunofluorescence of C6/36 cells uninfected (MOCK) or infected with DENV-1 (BR/90), DENV-2 (ICC 266), DENV-3 (290-02) and DENV-4 (TVP 360) isolates. Cells were fixed in methanol:acetone and stained with different mAbs, followed by Alexa-Fluor 488-conjugated anti-mouse immunoglobulin. Monoclonal antibody 4G2 and a non-correlated anti-hantavirus mAb (clone 572/7A) were used as positive and negative controls, respectively. Distinct groups of mAbs were raised against DENV: 1) group-specific (D3 424/8G); 2) subcomplex-specific (Anti-DENV-1, anti-DENV-3 and anti-DENV-4; clone D1 463/G6/H2); and 3) serotype-specific (anti-DENV-3 D3 290/4C/G9) mAbs. Images were produced in a Leica AF6000 Modular System. Scale bars are 30 μm.

isolates at a MOI of 1. After 72 h of infection, the cells were fixed in methanol:acetone and assayed by IFA, as previously described. The reactivity of each mAb against the Huh7.5 cells infected with the YFV 17DD strain, the SLEV 78V6507 isolate and the VEEV TC83 strain and Vero E6 cells infected with the WNV E/7229/06 isolate at MOIs of 1 (2.0×10^4 cells/well) was also assayed by IFA after 72 h, as previously described.

Conjugation of mAb to horseradish peroxidase (HRP) and application to the development of a capture ELISA

The antibodies were coupled with horseradish peroxidase (HRP) according to a modified periodate procedure [42]. Briefly, mAbs D3 424/8G, D1 606/A12/B9 and D1 695/12C/2H were purified on a protein-G column (GE-Healthcare) according to the manufacturer's instructions. HRP was structurally modified by sodium periodate and dialyzed against sodium-acetate buffer (pH 4.4) over 16 h at 4°C. The purified mAb diluted in sodium carbonate was added to the HRP solution and mixed for 2 h at room temperature, followed by the addition of a sodium borohydride solution. After 2 h, conjugated antibodies were purified by ammonium sulfate precipitation [43]. The performance of the mAbs D3 424/8G-HRP, D1 606/A12/B9-HRP and D1 695/12C/2H-HRP conjugate was evaluated by an in-house MAC-ELISA using gamma-irradiated purified DENV particles. A MAC-ELISA was performed as described by Takasaki et al. (2002) [44], with minor modifications. A total of twenty-two human serum samples from patients with dengue fever and twenty-four dengue-negative human sera kindly supplied by State Central Laboratory LACEN/PR were tested (Fiocruz Research Ethics Committee under protocol 617-11). A dengue IgM capture ELISA from PanBio (PanBio, Queensland, Australia) was used to diagnose samples for comparison with the results of the in-house assay.

Results

The fusion experiments (one for DENV-1, one for DENV-2 and another for DENV-3) generated a total of 1,100 hybridomas, which were screened by IFA to evaluate the presence of anti-DENV antibodies. One hundred forty-seven hybridomas (13.4%) were positive for antibody secretion against the corresponding DENV isolate, with different fluorescence levels. The clones were stabilized through two freeze-thaw cycles, resulting in 22 stable hybridomas. Three of these hybridomas produced antibodies against DENV-1 BR/01-MR; three produced antibodies against DENV-2 BR/01-01; and sixteen produced antibodies against DENV-3 BR 290-02. Antibody isotyping revealed ten IgG2b mAbs, seven IgG2a and five IgG1, all possessing kappa light chains (Table 1).

Western blot analysis with purified DENV particles showed that fourteen mAbs recognized the envelope protein (E) and five recognized the pre-membrane protein (prM; Figure 1; Figure S1). Additionally, mAbs D2 646/9G, D2 658/9A, and D3 344/H1 showed no reaction to the viral structural proteins on western blot assays (Figure 1). Monoclonal antibodies against DENV-2 were also tested against a recombinant peptide from domain III of the DENV-2 E protein. D2 332/2D reacted specifically to domain III of the E protein while D2 646/9G and D2 658/9A did not (Figure S1). Additionally, on IFA, mAb D3 344/H1 bound the recombinant E protein of DENV-3 expressed on *Drosophila* S2 cells, suggesting that it is directed to a conformational epitope of the E protein (Figure S2).

Interestingly, mAb D3 63/F2/G7 recognized the E protein in the western blot but not in the IFA against recombinant DENV-3 E Δ_{101} protein. From twelve mAbs that reacted against the E protein of DENV-3 by WB only D3 63/F2/G7 does not recognize E protein expressed on *Drosophila* S2 cells, suggesting that this mAb recognizes an epitope located on the carboxi-terminal of the

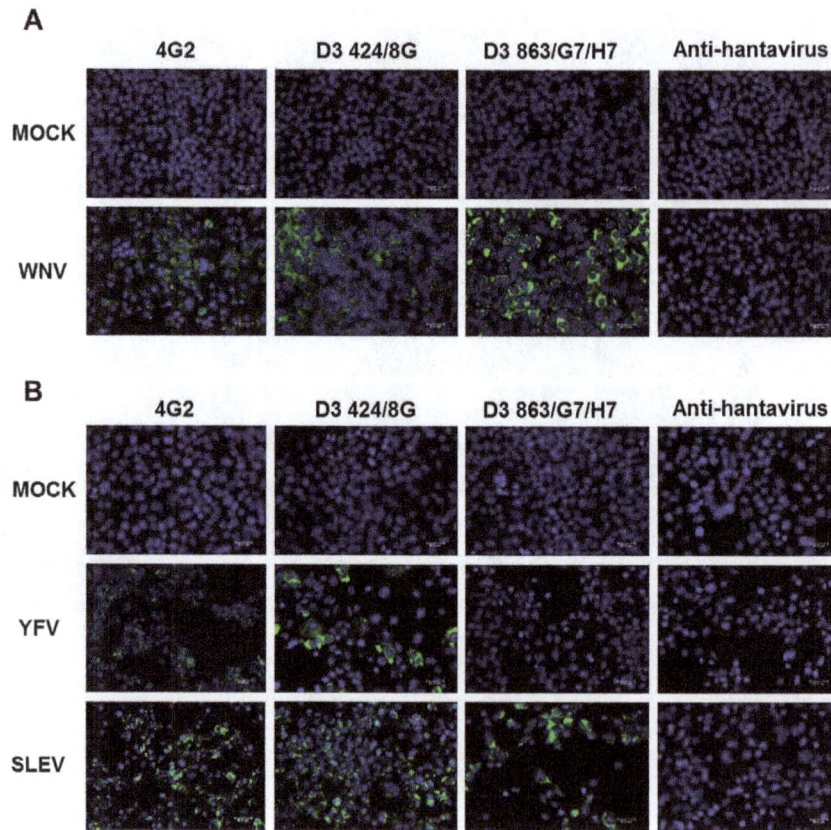

Figure 3. Cross-reactivity of mAbs D3 424/8G and D3 863/G7/H7 against WNV, SLEV and YFV. Vero E6 cells were infected with WNV (A), whereas Huh7.5 cells were infected with YFV and SLEV (B). Cells were fixed in methanol:acetone and stained with mAbs, followed by Alexa-Fluor 488-conjugated anti-mouse immunoglobulin. Monoclonal antibody 4G2 and a non-correlated anti-hantavirus mAb (572/7A) were used as positive and negative controls, respectively. Images were obtained with a Leica AF6000 Modular System. Scale bars are 30 µm.

E protein or alternatively, different epitopes conformations are available in the antigens preparations (Figure S2 and Table S1). The positive control 4G2 recognized the E protein in IFA and western blots. No reaction was observed to the anti-hantavirus mAb, which was used in both assays as a negative control (Figure 1; Figure S2).

To investigate whether the mAbs could be used for diagnostic and epidemiological purposes, the mAbs were assessed for specificity to the different DENV serotypes and to other flaviviruses. The mAbs were assayed against the DENV-1 (BR/90), -2 (ICC 266), -3 (290-02) and -4 (TVP 360) isolates. Several recognition patterns were identified: group-specific (DENV-1, -2, -3 and -4), subcomplex-specific (DENV-1, -3 and -4, and DENV-2 and -3) and serotype-specific (DENV-2 or -3). Eight mAbs recognized the four DENV serotypes. One mAb reacted with DENV serotypes 1, 3 and 4, and one reacted with serotypes 2 and 3. Three mAbs reacted specifically to serotype 2 and nine reacted to serotype 3 (Table 1 and Figure 2). All mAbs showed the same characteristic staining pattern in IFA in C6/36 infected cells, with a strong perinuclear stain, as illustrated in the reaction with mAb D3 424/8G (Figure 2).

Moreover, the reactivity of the mAbs was also tested against YFV 17DD, the SLEV 78V6507 isolate, the WNV E/7229/06 isolate and the VEEV TC38 strain. D3 424/8G recognized SLEV, WNV and YFV and did not cross-react with the alphavirus VEEV, suggesting that it is flavivirus-specific (Figure 3 and Table 2). Monoclonal antibodies directed against prM from

DENV, D3 443/H12/H6, D3 457/H7/H2, D3 863/G7/H7 and D3 868/G7/H10 recognized the four DENV serotypes, SLEV and WNV but did not react against YFV or VEEV (Table 2). The positive control 4G2 reacted with all dengue serotypes (Figure 2) and other flaviviruses (Figure 3). As expected, anti-hantavirus mAb (572/7A) did not react with any of the viruses tested (Figures 2 and 3).

Finally, mAbs D3 424/8G, D1 606/A12/B9 and D1 695/12C/2H were successfully conjugated to HRP for use in diagnostic assays. The three monoclonal antibodies were used to detect dengue virus antigen in human serum samples using an in-house MAC-ELISA (Figure 4). These results are consistent with those from the commercially available PanBio IgM capture assay kit. This method could thus be used to differentiate between negative and positive samples.

Discussion

Dengue is hyperendemic to tropical and subtropical regions of the world. In Brazil, more than seven million dengue cases have been confirmed since 1986, causing more than two thousand deaths [45]. The co-circulation of the four DENV serotypes and the wide distribution of the mosquito vector *Aedes aegypti* are most likely responsible for the increased incidence and distribution of dengue. Severe clinical manifestations have also increased in recent years, suggesting that dengue should remain a public health priority in Brazil [46]. Therefore, early and accurate diagnosis is essential to reducing morbidity and mortality related to dengue.

Table 2. Cross-reactivity of anti-dengue virus monoclonal antibodies against YFV, SLEV, WNV and VEEV.

mAb	Reactivity against			
	YFV	SLEV	WNV	VEEV
D1 463/G6/H2	–	–	–	–
D1 695/12C/2H	–	–	–	–
D1 606/A12/B9	–	–	–	–
D2 646/9G	–	–	–	–
D2 658/9A	–	–	–	–
D2 332/2D	–	–	–	–
D3 342/5G/G8	–	–	–	–
D3 388/4A/G6	–	–	–	–
D3 444/4G/H3	–	–	–	–
D3 389/F4/H10	–	–	–	–
D3 441/D1/H2	–	–	–	–
D3 290/4C/G9	–	–	–	–
D3 341/H9/F10	–	–	–	–
D3 344/H1	–	–	–	–
D3 442/4E/G8	–	–	–	–
D3 242/F1/H2	–	–	–	–
D3 424/8G	+	+	+	–
D3 863/G7/H7	–	+	+	–
D3 457/H7/H2	–	+	+	–
D3 443/H12/H6	–	+	+	–
D3 868/G7/H10	–	+	+	–
D3 63/F2/G7	–	–	–	–

–: negative;
+: positive.

Commercial kits for dengue diagnosis must be imported at great expense to the Brazilian Ministry of Health.

In this report, we describe the production and characterization of 22 mAbs against Brazilian DENV from the clinical isolates of DENV serotypes 1 (BR-01/MR), 2 (BR/01-01) or 3 (BR 290-02).

All of the mAbs showed the same characteristic staining pattern in IFA, with a strong perinuclear stain tending to spread throughout the cytoplasm in fluorescent granules. This observation is consistent with the distribution of DENV-2 proteins observed by Cardiff et al. (1973) [47], who observed an intense perinuclear

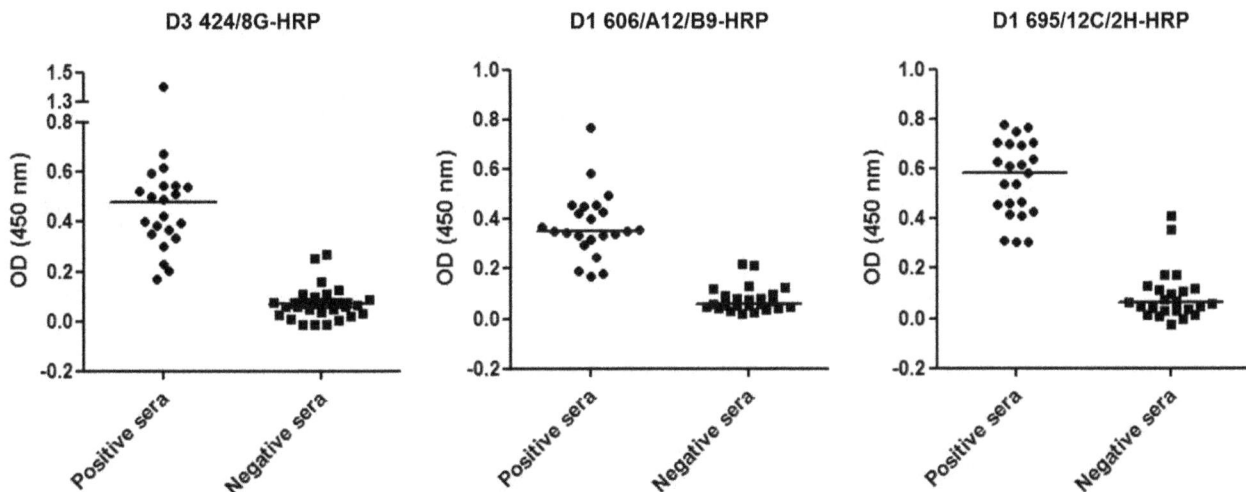

Figure 4. Application of antibodies to the development of MAC-ELISA. HRP-conjugated D3 424/8G, D1 606/A12/B9 and D1 695/12C/2H mAbs were used in an in-house MAC-ELISA assay to detect anti-dengue virus IgM in the sera of infected (N = 22) and non-infected patients (N = 24).

fluorescence radiating into the cytoplasm in a granular pattern of decreasing intensity. Henchal et al. (1982) found the same fluorescence pattern with monoclonal antibodies after infecting LLC-MK2 cells with a different flavivirus [29]. Both structural and non-structural proteins may localize in the perinuclear region before virus release, causing intense perinuclear staining in this region, whereas cytoplasmic fluorescence is associated with virion antigens [47].

Western blot and IFA analyses showed that most of the mAbs produced in this study are specific to the E or the prM proteins of DENV. The mice were immunized with the virion particle, and DENV does not replicate well in immunocompetent mice [48,49]. Usually, structural proteins are the major antigens that stimulate the immune response [50]. In humans, proteins E and prM, together with the non-structural protein 1 (NS1), are the major targets of the antibody response during DENV infection, especially in primary infection [51,52].

The envelope protein from DENV-2, recognized by both the mAbs D2 332/2D and the positive control 4G2, appeared as two bands in the WB, which may represent different glycosylation patterns of the E protein [53]. The other antibodies raised against DENV-2 (D2 646/9G and D2 658/9A) did not recognize DENV antigens in the IFA and WB assays. These mAbs may recognize a non-structural protein or a conformational epitope in structural proteins. D3 342/5G/G8, D3 290/4C/G9, D3 341/H9/F10, D3 424/G8 and the positive control, 4G2, recognized bands that may represent dimeric and trimeric forms of the DENV E protein, suggesting the presence of epitopes exposed in the three different forms of dengue E protein [54]. Also, variability on band intensities observed in WB could be due to differences in mAbs concentration since unpurified supernatants have been used in the assays.

Additionally, mAb D3 63/F2/G7 recognized DENV-3-E protein only in the WB assay and not recombinant DENV-3 E Δ_{101} protein. Since the recombinant E protein lacks the last 101 amino acids corresponding to the juxtamembrane steam region and the transmembrane anchor [55], the mAb D3 63/F2/G7 would recognize an epitope located at this domain. Also, this finding is consistent with reports describing flavivirus mAbs directed to cryptic epitopes of E protein [25,56,57]. Some epitopes are readily available on the surface of mature DENV, whereas others are partially or completely inaccessible. Denaturation of viral particles renders the cryptic epitopes accessible, allowing the antibodies to bind. Stiasny et al. (2006) isolated cross-reactive antibodies directed to a cluster of epitopes that are partially occluded in the cage-like assembly of E proteins located at the surface of infectious virions of tick-borne encephalitis virus (TBEV) [56]. Austin et al. (2012) and Chan et al. (2012), respectively, reported the isolation of a mAb able to bind to cryptic epitopes located at a CC' loop epitope on domain III (DIII) of the E protein from two different DENV-1 genotypes and the isolation of a human prM-specific antibody that bound a cryptic epitope located in the DI/DII junction on the DENV E glycoprotein [25,57].

Some flavivirus epitopes are also shared by other viruses in this family. mAbs raised against JEV E protein cross-reacted against Murray Valley encephalitis (MVE), WNV, SLE and DENV-1 and -2 [58]. Aside from the four dengue serotypes, the monoclonal antibody D3 424/8G generated in this study recognizes WNV, SLE and YFV. It thus represents a candidate for the development of flavivirus diagnostic assays. Henchal et al. (1982) developed antibodies that recognize flavivirus group-specific viruses, the four DENV serotypes, YFV, WNV, SLEV, Ntaya virus (NTA), Langat virus (LGT), Kunjin virus (Kun), Japanese encephalitis virus (JEV), Ilheus virus (ILH), Banzi virus (BAN) and Zika virus [29].

Additionally, dengue complex-specific (four DENV serotypes), subcomplex-specific (DENV-1, DENV-3) and serotype-specific mAbs were raised [29].

Serological diagnosis of flavivirus infections is difficult due to the extensive antigenic cross-reactivity among these viruses [58]. Well-characterized dengue-specific mAbs are thus powerful tools. To evaluate the applicability of mAbs to the development of immunoassays for dengue virus detection, dengue group-specific anti-E D1 695/12C/2H, anti-prM D1 606/A12/B9 and a flavivirus-specific anti-E D3 424/8G were used in an in-house IgM-capture assay. HRP-conjugated mAbs were successfully used in an anti-IgM capture immunoassay for dengue [59]. Additionally, serotype-specific mAbs (Table 1) could be valuable in an ELISA for serotyping dengue infections [60]. Furthermore, murine mAbs have also been used to detect DENV by immunohistochemistry [31], indicating another possible use for dengue mAbs conjugated to HRP. Finally, mAbs could also be labeled with other molecules such as fluorochromes or colloidal gold for routine dengue diagnosis in other formats.

In conclusion, twenty-two mAbs raised against Brazilian dengue virus isolates, including flavivirus cross-reactive, dengue-group specific, dengue subcomplex-specific and dengue serotype-specific mAbs, may be useful for the development of immunoassays such as ELISA, immunochromatographic assays, dot-blot assays and immunofluorescence assays [10,14,44]. To our knowledge, these are the first mAbs against dengue virus isolates circulating in Brazil to be developed and characterized. These mAbs thus have the potential to increase the specificity of dengue diagnosis in this region.

Supporting Information

Figure S1 Western blot analysis of DENV-2 mAbs reactivity against Domain III of E protein expressed in *E. coli*. Recombinant Domain III of E protein was subjected to 15% SDS-PAGE and electroblotted onto nitrocellulose membranes. Domain III ($\sim$12 kDa) were stained with the mAbs D2 332/2D, D2 658/9A and D2 646/9G, followed by anti-mouse IgG conjugated to alkaline phosphatase. A mouse polyclonal anti-DENV-2 serum was used as positive control.

Figure S2 Monoclonal reactivities on immunofluorescence assay (IFA) against recombinant DENV-3 E Δ_{101} protein expressed on *Drosophila* S2 cells. Indirect immunofluorescence of *Drosophila* S2 cells expressing or not (Mock) recombinant DENV-3 E Δ_{101} protein with mAbs D3 388/4A/G6, D3 344/H1 and D3 63/F2/G7. Monoclonal antibody 4G2 and a non-correlated anti-hantavirus mAb (clone 572/7A) were used as positive and negative controls, respectively. Images were produced in a Leica AF6000 Modular System. Scale bars are 75 μm.

Acknowledgments

The authors thank the Program for Technological Development in Tools for Health-PDTIS-FIOCRUZ for use of its facilities (RPT07C, Microscopy Platform at the Instituto Carlos Chagas/Fiocruz-PR, Brazil).

Author Contributions

Conceived and designed the experiments: CZ GACAM JB CNDS. Performed the experiments: CZ GACAM JB. Analyzed the data: CZ GACAM JB CNDS. Contributed reagents/materials/analysis tools: JB CNDS. Contributed to the writing of the manuscript: CZ GACAM JB CNDS.

References

1. Bhatt S, Gething PW, Brady OJ, Messina JP, Farlow AW, et al. (2013) The global distribution and burden of dengue. Nature 496(7446): 504–507.

2. Guzman A, Istúriz RE (2010) Update on the global spread of dengue. Intern J Antimicrob Agents 36: S40–S42.

3. WHO (2014) Available: http://www.who.int/topics/dengue/en/. Accessed 2014 March 30.

4. Calisher CH (1988) Antigenic classification and taxonomy of flaviviruses (family Flaviviridae) emphasizing a universal system for the taxonomy of viruses causing tick-borne encephalitis. Acta Virol 32(5): 469–478.

5. Halstead SB (1988) Pathogenesis of dengue: challenges to molecular biology. Science 239: 476–481.

6. Pierson TC, Diamond MS (2013) Flaviviruses. In: Knipe DM, Howley PM, editors. Fields Virology, 6th edition. Philadelphia, PA: Lippincott Williams & Wilkins. 747–794.

7. Wan SW, Lin CF, Wang S, Chen YH, Yeh TM, et al. (2013) Current progress in dengue vaccines. J Biomed Sci 20(37): 2–9.

8. Singh KR, Paul SD (1969) Isolation of Dengue viruses in Aedes albopictus cells cultures. Bull. World Health Organ 40(6): 982–983.

9. Lanciotti RS, Calisher CH, Gubler DJ, Chang GJ, Vorndam AV (1992) Rapid detection and typing of dengue viruses from clinical samples by using reverse transcriptase-polymerase chain reaction. J Clin Microbiol 30(3): 545–551.

10. Groen J, Koraka P, Velzing J, Copra C, Osterhaus AD (2000) Evaluation of six immunoassays for detection of dengue virus-specific immunoglobulin M and G antibodies. Clin Diagn Lab Immunol 7(6): 867–871.

11. Innis BL, Nisalak A, Nimmannitya S, Kusalerdchariya S, Chongswasdi V, et al. (1989) An enzyme-linked immunosorbent assay to characterize dengue infections where dengue and Japanese encephalitis co-circulate. Am J Trop Med Hyg 40(4): 418–427.

12. Lam SK, Devine PL (1998) Evaluation of capture ELISA and rapid immunochromatographic test for the determination of IgM and IgG antibody production during dengue infection. Clin Diagn Virol 10: 75–81.

13. Palmer CJ, King SD, Cuadrado RR, Perez E, Baum M, et al. (1999) Evaluation of the MRL Diagnostics dengue fever virus IgM ELISA and the PanBio rapid immunochromatographic test for diagnosis of dengue fever in Jamaica. J Clin Microbiol 37: 1600–1601.

14. Vaughn DW, Nisalak A, Kalayanarooj S, Solomon T, Dung NM, et al. (1998) Evaluation of a rapid immunochromatographic test for diagnosis of dengue virus infection. J Clin Microbiol 36: 234–238.

15. Wu SJ, Hanson B, Paxton H, Nisalak A, Vaughn DW, et al. (1997) Evaluation of a dipstick enzyme-linked immunosorbent assay for detection of antibodies to dengue virus. Clin Diagn Lab Immunol 4: 452–457.

16. Vazquez S, Valdes O, Pupo M, Delgado I, Alvarez M, et al. (2003) MAC-ELISA and ELISA inhibition methods for detection of antibodies after yellow fever vaccination. J Virol Methods 110: 179–184.

17. Guzman MG, Kouri G (2004) Dengue diagnosis, advances and challenges. Int J Infect Dis 8: 69–80.

18. Nybakken GE, Oliphant T, Johnson S, Burke S, Diamond MS, et al. (2005) Structural basis of West Nile virus neutralization by a therapeutic antibody. Nature 437(7059): 764–769.

19. Kobayashi Y, Hasegawa H, Yamauchi T (1985) Studies on the antigenic sctruture of Japanese ecenphalitis virus using monoclonal antibodies. Microbiol Immunol 29(11): 1069–1082.

20. Mazzarotto GACA, Raboni SM, Stella V, Carstensen S, de Noronha L, et al. (2009) Production and characterization of monoclonal antibodies against the recombinant nucleoprotein of Araucaria hantavirus. J Virol Methods 162: 96–100.

21. Chiang C-F, Lo MK, Rota PA, Spiropoulou CF, Rollin PE (2010) Use of monoclonal antibodies against Hendra and Nipah viruses in an antigen capture ELISA. Virol J 7: [115].

22. Lelli D, Moreno A, Broochi E, Sozzi E, Capucci L, et al. (2012). West Nile virus: characterization and diagnostic applications of monoclonal antibodies. Virol J 9: [81].

23. Nelson PN, Reynolds GM, Waldron EE, Ward E, Giannopoulos K, et al. (2000) Monoclonal antibodies. Mol Pathol 53(3): 111–117.

24. Sukupolvi-Petty S, Brien JD, Austin SK, Shresta B, Swayne S, et al. (2013) Functional Analysis of Antibodies against Dengue Virus Type 4 Reveals Strain-Dependent Epitope Exposure That Impacts Neutralization and Protection. J Virol 87(16): 8826–8842.

25. Austin SK, Dowd KA, Shresta B, Edeling MA, Johnson S, et al. (2012) Structural Basis of Differential Neutralization of DENV-1 Genotypes by an Antibody that Recognizes a Cryptic Epitope. PLOS Pathogens 8(10): e1002930.

26. Dittmar D, Haines HG, Castro A (1980) Monoclonal antibodies specific for dengue virus type 3. J Clin Microbiol 12(1): 74–78.

27. Romero-Vivas CM, Leake CJ, Falconar AK (1998) Determination of dengue virus serotypes in individual Aedes aegypti mosquitos in Colombia. Med Vet Entomol 12(3): 284–288.

28. Kang X, Li Y, Fan L, Lin F, Wei J, et al. (2012) Development of an ELISA-array for simultaneous detection of five encephalitis viruses. Virol J 9: [56].

29. Henchal EA, Gentry MK, McCown JM, Brandt WE (1982) Dengue virus-specific and flavivirus group determinants identified with monoclonal antibodies by indirect immunofluorescence. Am J Trop Med Hyg 31: 830–836.

30. Xu H, Biao Di, Yu-xian Pan, Li-wen Qiu, Ya-di Wang, et al. (2006) Serotype 1-Specific Monoclonal Antibody-Based Antigen Capture Immunoassay for Detection of Circulating Nonstructural Protein NS1: Implications for Early Diagnosis and Serotyping of Dengue Virus Infections. J Clin Microbiol 44(8): 2872–2878.

31. Limonta D, Capo V, Torres G, Perez A, Guzman M (2007) Apoptosis in tissues from fatal dengue shock syndrome. J Clin Virol 40: 50–54.

32. Qiu LW, Di B, Wen K, Wang XS, Liang WH, et al. (2009) Development of an Antigen Capture Immunoassay Based on Monoclonal Antibodies Specific for Dengue Virus Serotype 2 Nonstructural Protein 1 for Early and Rapid Identification of Dengue Virus Serotype 2 Infections. Clin Vaccine Immunol 16(1): 88–95.

33. Brien JD, Austin SK, Sukupolvi-Petty S, O'brien KM, Johnson S, et al. (2010) Genotype-specific neutralization and protection by antibodies against dengue virus type 3. J Virol 84(20): 10630–10643.

34. Shrestha B, Brien JD, Sukupolvi-Petty S, Austin SK, Edeling MA, et al. (2010) The Development of Therapeutic Antibodies That Neutralize Homologous and Heterologous Genotypes of Dengue Virus Type 1. PLoS Pathog 6(4): e1000823.

35. Trainor NB, Crill WD, Roberson JA, Chang GJ (2007) Mutation analysis of the fusion domain region of St. Louis encephalitis virus envelope protein. Virology 360(2): 398–406.

36. Desprès P, Frenkiel MP, Deubel (1993) Differences between cell membrane fusion activities of two dengue type-1 isolates reflect modifications of viral structure. Virology 196: 209–219.

37. Post PR, Carvalho R, Freire MS, Galler R (2001) The early use of Yellow Fever virus strain 17D for vaccine production in Brazil – a review. Mem Inst Oswaldo Cruz 96(6): 849–857.

38. Mitchell CJ, Monath TP, Sabattini MS, Cropp CB, Daffner JF, et al. (1985) Arbovirus investigations in Argentina, 1977–1980. II. Arthropod collections and virus isolations from Argentine mosquitoes. Am J Trop Med Hyg 34(5): 945–955.

39. Morales MA, Barrandeguy M, Fabbri C, Garcia JB, Vissani A, et al. (2006) West Nile Virus Isolation from Equines in Argentina, 2006. Emerg Infect Dis 12(10): 1559–1561.

40. Berge TO, Banks IS, Tiggert WD (1961) Attenuation of Venezuelan equine encephalitis virus by in vitro cultivation in guinea-pig hearts cells. Am J Epidemiol 73(2): 209–218.

41. Laemmli UK (1970) Cleavage of structural proteins during the assembly of the head of bacteriophage T4. Nature 227: 680–685.

42. Wisdom GB (2005) Conjugation of Antibodies to Horseradish Peroxidase. In: Burns R, editor. Methods in molecular biology immunochemical protocols. 3 ed, Humana Press Inc., Totowa, NJ. 127–130.

43. Perrin P (1996) Techniques for the preparation of rabies conjugates. In: Meslin, FX; Kaplan, MM; Koprowski, H (Ed.). Laboratory techniques in rabies 4. ed. Geneva: World Health Organization. 433–444.

44. Takasaki T, Nawa M, Yamada KI, Harada M, Takeda A, et al. (2002) Evaluation of dengue IgM detection tests using sera from patients with autoimmune diseases. J Virol Methods 102: 61–66.

45. Brasil. Ministério de Saúde. Secretaria de Vigilância em Saúde. Resultados preliminares da avaliação dos determinantes para ocorrência de óbitos por dengue em 2010. Available: www1.saude.ba.gov.br/entomologiabahia/dengue/apres8.ppt>. Accessed 2014 May 19.

46. Teixeira MG, Siqueira JB Jr, Ferreira GLC, Bricks L, Joint G (2013) Epidemiological Trends of Dengue Disease in Brazil (2000–2010): A Systematic Literature Search and Analysis. PLoS Negl Trop Dis 7(12): [e2520].

47. Cardiff RD, Russ SB, Brandt WE, Russell PK (1973) Cytological localization of dengue-2 antigens: an immunological study with ultrastructural correlation. Infect Immunity 7(5): 809–816.

48. Johnson AJ, Roehrig JT (1999) New mouse model for dengue virus vaccine testing. J Virol 73(1): 783–786.

49. Schul W, Liu W, Xu HY, Flamand M, Vasudevan SG (2007) A dengue fever viremia model in mice shows reduction in viral replication and suppression of the inflammatory response after treatment with antiviral drugs. J Infect Dis 195(5): 664–674.

50. Huang KJ, Li SY, Chen SC, Liu HS, Lin YS, et al. (2000) Manifestation of thrombocytopenia in dengue-2-virus-infected mice. J Gen Virol 81(Pt 9): 2177–2182.

51. Rey FA, Heinz FX, Mandl C, Kunz C, Harrison SC (1995) The envelope glycoprotein from tick borne encephalitis virus at 2 Å resolution. Nature 375: 291–298.

52. Rothman AL (2011) Immunity to dengue virus: a tale of original antigenic sin and tropical cytokine storms. Nat Rev Immunol 11(8): 532–543.

53. Mondotte JA, Lozach P-Y, Amara A, Gamarnik AV (2007) Essential Role of Dengue Virus Envelope Protein N Glycosylation at Asparagine-67 during Viral Propagation. J Virol 81(13): 7136–7148.

54. Bressanelli S, Stiasny K, Allison SL, Stura ER, Duquerroy S, et al. (2004) Structure of a flavivirus envelope glycoprotein in its low-pH-induced membrane fusion conformation. EMBO J 23: 728–738.

55. Klein DE, Choi JL, Harrison SC (2013) Structure of a dengue virus envelope protein late-stage fusion intermediate. J Virol 87(4): 2287–2293.

56. Stiasny K, Kiermayr S, Holzmann H, Heinz FX (2006) Cryptic properties of a cluster of dominant flavivirus cross-reactive antigenic sites. J Virol 80(19): 9557–9568.

57. Chan AH, Tan HC, Chow AY, Lim AP, Lok SM, et al. (2012) A human prM antibody that recognizes a novel cryptic epitope on dengue E glycoprotein. PLoS One 7(4): e33451.

58. Kuroda JK, Yasui K (1986) Antigenic Comparison of Envelope Protein E between Japanese Encephalitis Virus and Some Other Flavivirus Using Monoclonal Antibodies. J Gen Virol 67: 2663–2672.

59. Chong CF, Hgoh BL, Tan HC, Yap EH, Singh M, et al. (1994) A shortened dengue IgM capture ELISA using simultaneous incubation of antigen and peroxidase-labeled monoclonal antibody. Clin Diagn Virol 1(5–6): 335–341.

60. Kuno G, Gluber DJ, Santiago de Weil NS (1985) Antigen capture ELISA for the identification of dengue viruses. J Virol Methods 12(1–2): 93–103.

21

Phospholipase A$_2$ Isolated from the Venom of *Crotalus durissus terrificus* Inactivates *Dengue virus* and Other Enveloped Viruses by Disrupting the Viral Envelope

Vanessa Danielle Muller[1¤], **Ricardo Oliveira Soares**[3], **Nilton Nascimento dos Santos-Junior**[1], **Amanda Cristina Trabuco**[1], **Adelia Cristina Cintra**[2], **Luiz Tadeu Figueiredo**[4], **Antonio Caliri**[3], **Suely Vilela Sampaio**[2], **Victor Hugo Aquino**[1]*

1 Laboratório de Virologia, Departamento de Análises Clínicas, Toxicológicas e Bromatológicas, Faculdade de Ciências Farmacêuticas de Ribeirão Preto, Universidade de São Paulo, Ribeirão Preto, São Paulo, Brasil, 2 Laboratório de Toxinologia, Departamento de Análises Clínicas, Toxicológicas e Bromatológicas, Faculdade de Ciências Farmacêuticas de Ribeirão Preto, Universidade de São Paulo, Ribeirão Preto, São Paulo, Brasil, 3 Departamento de Física e Química, Faculdade de Ciências Farmacêuticas de Ribeirão Preto, Universidade de São Paulo, Ribeirão Preto, São Paulo, Brasil, 4 Centro de Pesquisa em Virologia, Departamento de Clínica Médica, Faculdade de Medicina de Ribeirão Preto, Universidade de São Paulo, Ribeirão Preto, São Paulo, Brasil

Abstract

The *Flaviviridae* family includes several virus pathogens associated with human diseases worldwide. Within this family, *Dengue virus* is the most serious threat to public health, especially in tropical and sub-tropical regions of the world. Currently, there are no vaccines or specific antiviral drugs against *Dengue virus* or against most of the viruses of this family. Therefore, the development of vaccines and the discovery of therapeutic compounds against the medically most important flaviviruses remain a global public health priority. We previously showed that phospholipase A$_2$ isolated from the venom of *Crotalus durissus terrificus* was able to inhibit *Dengue virus* and *Yellow fever virus* infection in Vero cells. Here, we present evidence that phospholipase A$_2$ has a direct effect on *Dengue virus* particles, inducing a partial exposure of genomic RNA, which strongly suggests inhibition via the cleavage of glycerophospholipids at the virus lipid bilayer envelope. This cleavage might induce a disruption of the lipid bilayer that causes a destabilization of the E proteins on the virus surface, resulting in inactivation. We show by computational analysis that phospholipase A$_2$ might gain access to the *Dengue virus* lipid bilayer through the pores found on each of the twenty 3-fold vertices of the E protein shell on the virus surface. In addition, phospholipase A$_2$ is able to inactivate other enveloped viruses, highlighting its potential as a natural product lead for developing broad-spectrum antiviral drugs.

Editor: Bruno Lomonte, Universidad de Costa Rica, Costa Rica

Funding: This work was supported by Fundação de Amparo à Pesquisa do Estado de São Paulo (FAPESP) grant 2005/54855-0 and 2008/50617-6. VHA, SVS and LTF hold a scholarship from the Conselho Nacional de Desenvolvimento Científico e Tecnológico (CNPq). The funders had no role in study design, data collection and analysis, decision to publish, or preparation of the manuscript.

Competing Interests: The authors have declared that no competing interests exist.

* Email: vhugo@fcfrp.usp.br

¤ Current address: Laboratório de Pesquisas em Virologia e Imunologia – LAPEVI, Instituto de Ciências Biológicas e da Saúde – ICBS, Universidade Federal de Alagoas – UFAL, Campus A.C. Simões, Av. Lourival Melo Mota s/n, 57072-900, Maceió-AL, Brasil

Introduction

The *Flaviviridae* family includes several virus pathogens associated with human diseases worldwide. Clinical conditions can vary from febrile or hemorrhagic diseases for *Dengue virus* (DENV) and *Yellow fever virus* (YFV), encephalitis for *Saint Louis encephalitis virus* (SLEV), *Japanese encephalitis virus* (JEV), *Tick-borne encephalitis virus* (TBEV), *West Nile virus* (WNV), and *Rocio virus* (ROCV) to hepatitis for *Human hepatitis C virus* (HCV) and *Human Pegivirus* (HPgV). Currently, preventative vaccines for humans are available only for YFV, TBEV, and JEV and specific antiviral treatment only for HCV [1]. Therefore, the development of vaccines and the discovery of therapeutic compounds against the medically most important flaviviruses remain a global public health priority [2].

Of the diseases caused by viruses of the *Flaviviridae* family, dengue is a major threat to public health. It is estimated that 390 million dengue infections occur per year, with 100 million manifesting some type of symptoms [3] and approximately two million requiring hospitalization [4–6]. The major goal of anti-DENV therapy is to prevent patients from developing the severe forms of the disease [7].

Members of the *Flaviviridae* family include viruses with a positive-sense, single-stranded RNA genome of approximately 11,000 nucleotides, surrounded by a nucleocapsid and covered by a lipid envelope in which viral glycoproteins are anchored. The RNA genome encodes a single polyprotein that is proteolytically cleaved into three structural proteins (C-prM/M-E) and seven non-structural proteins (NS1-NS2A-NS2B-NS3-NS4A-NS4B-NS5) [8].

Natural products offer a huge amount of compounds with a great diversity of chemical structures, the result of biosynthetic processes that have been modulated over millennia through evolution. Natural products have served as important sources of drugs for medical purposes. Tubocurarine, a toxic alkaloid with skeletal muscle relaxant properties and obtained from the bark of the South American plant *Chondrodendron tomentosum*, was the first naturally occurring toxin used in medicine [9]. Since 1970, more than 40 drugs derived from natural products have been approved for use in humans [10–12]. Among natural products, venoms are complex mixtures of many different components, such as metalloproteinases, serine proteinases, potassium channel-binding neurotoxins, proteolytic enzymes, cytotoxins, pre- and post-synaptic neurotoxins, cardiotoxins, and phospholipase A_2s, which can provide clues for designing therapeutically useful molecules [13]. Indeed, Ferreira *et al.* [14] provided a good example of the potential of snake venom components for successful drug development. These authors identified bradykinin-potentiating peptides from the Brazilian arrowhead viper (*Bothrops jararaca*) venom that were used to develop an inhibitor (captopril) of the angiotensin-converting enzyme that is widely used as an anti-hypertensive agent [15]. Two other drugs, Tirofiban and Eptifibatide, were designed based on snake venom components and are available in the market as antiplatelet agents [16,17]. In addition, snake venoms and their components have shown antiviral activity against *Measles virus* [18], *Sendai virus* [19], *Dengue virus* [20,21], and *Human immunodeficiency virus* (HIV) [22]. One of the main components of snake venom is secreted phospholipase A_2 (sPLA$_2$), which has shown systemic toxicities that include myotoxicity, cardiotoxicity, neurotoxicity, nephrotoxicity, hepatotoxicity, reprotoxicity, and systemic hemorrhage [23–28]. The sPLA$_2$ isolated from snake venoms and other sources has also shown antiviral activity against HIV [22,29,30], adenovirus [31], *Newcastle virus* [32], and *Rous virus* [33]. In addition, we have recently found a high antiviral effect of sPLA$_2$ (crotoxin, a dimeric compound composed of PLA$_2$-CB and crotapotin, isolated PLA$_2$-CB and PLA$_2$-inter-cro) from *Crotalus durissus terrificus* venom against DENV and YFV [21]. In this study, we further analyzed the antiviral effect of PLA$_2$-CB against dengue virus and three other enveloped viruses.

Materials and Methods

Cells and viruses

VERO E6 (African green monkeys kidney epithelium cell line) [34] and C6/36 (*Aedes albopictus* mosquito cell line) [35] cells were maintained in Leibovitz's medium (L-15) with 10% fetal bovine serum (FBS) at 37°C and 28°C, respectively. DENV-2 (NGC strain), *Rocio virus* (SPH 34675 strain), *Mayaro virus* (BeAn 243 strain), and *Oropouche virus* (BeAn 19991 strain) from the virus collection of the Virology Research Center of the Medical School of Ribeirao Preto, University of Sao Paulo, were used in this study. Enterovirus *Coxsackie-B5 virus* was kindly provided by Prof. Dr. Eurico Arruda Neto from the Viral Pathogenesis laboratory at the Virology Research Center, Medical School of Ribeirao Preto, University of Sao Paulo. Virus titration was performed in the Vero E6 cell line using the plaque assay, and the titer was expressed in plaque-forming units per milliliters (PFU/mL), as previously described [21].

Dengue virus RNA detection and quantification: Quantitative real-time RT-PCR (qRT-PCR)

Viral RNA detection was carried out by real-time RT-PCR using the SuperScript III Platinum SYBR Green One-Step qRT-PCR kit (Invitrogen, USA), as previously described [36]. Briefly, the 25-μL reaction mixture contained 0.5 μL of SuperScript III RT Platinum Taq Mix, 0.2 mM of each primer, 12.5 μL of 2× SYBR Green, and 5 μL of purified RNA. The amplification program was as follows: 50°C for 20 min for reverse transcription, 95°C for 5 min for reverse transcriptase inhibition and *Taq* DNA polymerase activation, followed by 45 cycles of PCR amplification with denaturation at 95°C for 15 sec, annealing at 60°C for 40 sec, and extension at 72°C for 30 sec. Finally, to verify the specificity of the PCR products, a melting curve was constructed by incubating the amplification products from 60°C to 90°C with an increase of 0.2°C/sec. The melting temperature (Tm) values of the specific amplicons were in the range of 80.57°C-81.73°C. For viral load determination, a standard curve was constructed using RNA transcribed *in vitro* from a plasmidial clone containing a fragment of 2500 base pairs (bp) corresponding to the 5' end of DENV-3 strain D3BR/RP1/2003 [37]. This plasmid was prepared as follows: the 2500-bp fragment was amplified by RT-PCR and inserted into the plasmid pXL (Invitrogen, USA), which was used to transform *Escherichia coli*. An aliquot of 250 μL of the bacteria was inoculated into 10 mL of LB+ampicillin medium, followed by incubation at 37°C for 14 h with shaking. The plasmid was purified using the QIAGEN Plasmid Mini Kit (Qiagen, Germany) following the manufacturer's recommendations. The plasmid was linearized by digestion with Bam HI, subjected to electrophoresis through a 1% agarose gel, and purified from the gel using the QIAquick Gel Extraction Kit (Qiagen, Germany) following the manufacturer's specifications. For RNA preparation, 1 μg of the linearized plasmid was transcribed using RNAMaxx High Yield Transcription Kit (Stratagene, USA) following the manufacturer's specifications. The cDNA was digested using RQ DNase (Promega, USA) at 37°C for 20 min. After this, the RNA was purified using the QIAamp Viral RNA Kit (QIAGEN, Germany), and the concentration was determined by spectrophotometry at 260 nm. Based on the concentration and size of the RNA product (2500 bp), the copy number equivalent to the genomic RNA was calculated. Serial decimal dilutions of this RNA were prepared to construct the standard curve by real-time RT-PCR for determination of the virus titer, which was expressed in copy numbers per milliliters.

Venom and toxin purification from *Crotalus durissus terrificus*

Snake venom was obtained from the serpentarium of the Medical School of Ribeirao Preto, University of Sao Paulo (authorization of the *Instituto Brasileiro do Meio Ambiente e dos Recursos Naturais Renováveis*, IBAMA: 1/35/1998/000846-1). Purification and evaluation of the enzymatic activity of PLA$_2$-CB and crotoxin were carried out as previously described [21].

Antiviral assays of PLA$_2$-CB and crotoxin against DENV-2

Virucidal assay: virus treatment before infection. To evaluate the direct effect of PLA$_2$-CB and crotoxin on viral particles, DENV-2 (2×10^3 PFU) was incubated with non-cytotoxic concentrations (8, 4, and 0.004 ng/μL) of PLA$_2$-CB and crotoxin in a final volume of 100 μL for 1 h at 37°C [21]. DENV-2 incubated with PBS was used as a control. The mixtures were diluted 100 times with L-15 serum-free medium and added to

VERO E6 cells seeded in 24-well plates (2×10^5 cells/well). After dilution, two concentrations (0.008 and 0.004 ng/µL) were above and one bellow (0.000004 ng/µL) the effective concentration that inhibits 50% (EC_{50}) of cells infection found in our previous study (EC_{50} of 0.00003 for PLA$_2$-CB and 0.001 for crotoxin) [21]. After 1 h of incubation at 37°C, the supernatant was removed, and 1 mL of L-15 medium supplemented with 2% fetal bovine serum (FBS) was added to the cells, followed by a further incubation at 37°C for 72 h. The cell culture supernatants were collected for viral inhibition evaluation by qRT-PCR, as mentioned above.

Pre-treatment assay: Treatment of cells with toxins before virus infection. This assay was carried out to evaluate whether the toxins could protect VERO E6 cells against viral infection. VERO E6 cells were seeded (2×10^5 cells/well) in a 24-wellsplate and incubated at 37°C for 24 h. The medium was then removed, and the cells were incubated with several concentrations of PLA$_2$-CB or crotoxin (0.000004, 0.04, 0.08, 0.5, 1, and 2 ng/µL). After 1 h of incubation, the supernatant was removed, and cells were washed five times with PBS at room temperature. The cells were infected with 25–100 PFU of DENV-2 in 400 µL of L-15 for 1 h. The supernatant was removed, and 1 mL of L-15m supplemented with 2% FBS was added to the cells. After 72 h of incubation at 37°C, the cell supernatants were collected for viral RNA extraction using AxyPrep Body Fluid Viral DNA/RNA Miniprep Kit (Axygen, USA) following the manufacturer's recommendations. Virus inhibition was evaluated by qRT-PCR, as mentioned above.

Evaluation of DENV-2 RNA exposure induced by PLA2-CB and crotoxin

This assay was carried out as previously proposed [38]. DENV-2 (2.0×10^3 PFU) was incubated with 8 ng/µL of PLA$_2$-CB, 8 ng/µL of crotoxin, 1 µg/µL of proteinase K (Life Technologies, USA), 1% Triton X-100 (Life Technologies, USA), or PBS in a total volume of 100 µL for 1 h and 2 h at 37°C. Then, the virus was treated with PBS or RNase A (Promega, USA) according to the manufacturer's recommendation. RNA purified from DENV-2 (2.0×10^3 PFU) was used as a control for RNA degradation induced by RNase A. After 1 h at 37°C, the viral RNA was extracted using AxyPrep Body Fluid Viral DNA/RNA Miniprep Kit (Axygen, USA), and RNA degradation was evaluated by qRT-PCR as mentioned above.

Virucidal assay of PLA2-CB and crotoxin against other enveloped and non-enveloped viruses

The enveloped viruses *Dengue virus* type 2, *Rocio virus*, *Mayaro virus*, and *Oropouche virus* and the non-enveloped *Coxsackie B5 virus* were used in this experiment. The viruses (25–100 PFU) were incubated with serial decimal dilutions of PLA$_2$-CB and crotoxin (50, 5, 0.5, 0.005, 0.0005, and 0.00005 ng/µL) for 1 h at 37°C. The treated viruses were used to infect VERO E6 cells contained in a 24-well plate for 1 h. The supernatant was removed, and the cells were overlaid with 1 mL of L-15 supplemented with 2% FBS and 1.8% carboxymethylcellulose. After 7 days at 37°C, the semisolid overlay medium was removed, and the cells were fixed and stained with naphthol blue-black in 5% acetic acid for plaque counting. The treatment of each virus was repeated three times, and the concentration that inhibited 50% of plaque formation (Effective Concentration 50%, EC_{50}) was calculated by comparison with the number of plaques observed in the PBS-treated cells.

Steric and electrostatic analysis of the interaction of PLA2-CB with the lipid bilayer of the DENV envelope

The DENV external structural model was obtained from RCSB Protein Data Bank under the PDB ID: 3J35 [39]. This model was developed by Zhang *et al.* [40] by electron microscopy analysis and reflects the structure of DENV under physiological temperature (37°C), in accordance with the experiments conducted in this work. We used this electron microscopy structure as a model to reconstruct a more refined version of the virus structure, fitting 180 high-resolution copies of DENV-2 E protein (PDB ID: 1OAN) [41]. The DENV membrane patch used to reproduce the 3-fold pore environment in the electrostatic analyses was assembled with the CHARMM-GUI program [42] and further thermalized with the GROMACS Molecular Dynamics package [43]; the lipid composition follows that described by Zhang *et al.* [44]. The resolved PLA$_2$-CB crystal structure was obtained under PDB ID: 2QOG [45]. Because this model is built as a tetramer, we extracted one monomer (including the Ca^{2+} ion) with software Visual Molecular Dynamics – VMD [46], completing the few missing atoms from residues Trp31 and Pro74 with the aid of the PyMol program [47], and finally performed an adjustment with a potential energy minimization of the side chains with the GROMACS Molecular Dynamics package [43] using the IBM BlueGene/P supercomputer hosted at Rice University. For the all-atom MD with the explicit solvent [TIP3P water model [48] constrained by the SETTLE algorithm [49]], we used the CHARMM36 force-field [50] adapted to GROMACS by Piggot and colleagues, 2012 [51], with the Particle Mesh Ewald (PME) treatment for the electrostatic interactions among the atoms, with a cut-off of non-bonded interactions of 1.0 nm. The neutral pH of the system was emulated indirectly by fixing the protonation states of ionizable side chains at their correspondent pKa values, according to Nozaki and Tanford [52]. The temperature of the system was set to 310 K, and the pressure was maintained at 1 ATM using the Nose-Hoover and Parrinello-Rahman algorithms, respectively [53–55]. The simulation protocol starts with potential energy minimizations with the steep descent method until the convergence of an energy threshold smaller than 2×10^3kJ mol^{-1} nm^{-1}. Maxwell-Boltzmann distribution assigns velocities to all atoms in the system according to the chosen initial temperature, and a position restriction was applied to the protein portion, allowing full solvation with the newly introduced water. After this step, we removed all restrains from the heavy atoms of the protein and used the P-LINCS algorithm [56] to constrain all bonded interactions, allowing us to set a time step of 2 femtoseconds. The electrostatic analyses and electrical field of the system consisting of one monomer of PLA$_2$-CB plus the extracted 3-fold pore from DENV were generated with the APBS (Adaptive Poisson-Boltzmann Solver) plugin [57] in the PyMol software [47]. The atomic individual charges of PLA$_2$-CB and the DENV 3-fold pore were attributed with aid of the pdb2pqr online server [58], and their protonation states were determined at pH 7 by PROPKA 3.1 [59]. The charges from the membrane atoms were calculated and assigned with the program *editconf* (-mead option) in the package GROMACS 4.5.5. In all cases, we set as default the solvent and protein/lipid dielectric constants to 78.0 and 2.0, respectively.

Statistics

A Mann–Whitney U test was used to compare the differences between the treated and untreated control groups. P values of < 0.05 were considered to indicate statistically significant differences. The statistical analyses were carried out using GraphPad Prism version 5.03 (GraphPad Software, La Jolla, CA).

Results

Evaluation of the direct action of PLA2-CB and crotoxin on the DENV-2 virion: Virucidal assay

To analyze whether PLA_2-CB and crotoxin have a direct effect on the virus particle, DENV-2 (2.0×10^3 PFU) was treated with 8, 4, and 0.0004 ng/µL of each toxin or PBS. One hour after treatment, the mixture was diluted 100 times (final concentration 0.08, 0.04, and 0.000004 ng/µL of toxins and 20 PFU of DENV-2) and then used to infect Vero cells. The purpose of the dilution was to reduce the concentration of toxins in contact with the cells and to use concentrations above (0.08 and 0.04 ng/µL) and below (0.000004 ng/µL) the EC_{50} found in our previous study [21]. Viral replication was evaluated in the cell culture supernatant after 72 h of infection by qRT-PCR. A significant inhibition of virus replication was observed when the virus was treated with 8 and 4 ng/µL of PLA_2-CB and crotoxin in a dose-dependent manner, suggesting a direct action of the toxins on the virus particle (Figure 1). However, despite the low concentration of toxins, some effect on Vero cells that trigger an antiviral mechanism cannot be discarded.

Pre-treatment assay: Treatment of cells with toxins before virus infection

To better analyze whether PLA_2-CB and crotoxin have some effect on Vero cells that influences DENV-2 inhibition, the cells were treated with several concentrations of PLA_2-CB and crotoxin, including those used in the virucidal assay after dilution (0.000004, 0.04, 0.08, 0.5, 1, and 2 ng/µL), before infection. One hour after treatment, the cells were washed and infected with the same amount of DENV-2 used in the virucidal assay (20 PFU). The qRT-PCR analysis of the cell culture supernatant after 72 h of infection showed that virus replication was significantly inhibited only at the higher toxin concentrations, 1 and 2 ng/µL (Figure 2). This result strongly suggests that the antiviral effect of PLA_2-CB and crotoxin observed in the virucidal assay was due to a direct action on the virus particle.

In vitro DENV-2 RNA exposure induced by PLA2-CB and crotoxin

The antiviral effect of toxins might be related to enzymatic activity by means of glycerophospholipid cleavage at the virus lipidic envelope, which could induce an exposure of the virus RNA genome. To investigate this hypothesis, DENV-2 was treated with 8 ng/µL of PLA_2-CB and crotoxin for 1 and 2 hours at 37°C and then with RNAse-A to evaluate RNA exposure. A significant viral RNA degradation was observed when DENV-2 was treated with PLA_2-CB and crotoxin, suggesting virus RNA exposure (Figure 3). However, increased RNA degradation was observed when DENV-2 was previously treated with protease (proteinase K) or detergent (Triton X-100), both of which destroy the virus envelope and induce the complete exposure of genomic RNA (Figure 4). Therefore, the lower level of genomic RNA degradation observed after PLA2-CB or crotoxin treatment suggests a partial exposure of the virus RNA by the partial disruption of the virus envelope. Incubation of DENV-2 with toxins for more than 1 hour did not increase the viral RNA degradation, suggesting that all the available glycerophospholipid on the virus envelope were already cleaved in 1 hour.

Evaluation of PLA2-CB and crotoxin antiviral activity against other enveloped viruses

The above experiments suggested that PLA_2-CB and crotoxin exert their antiviral functions via partial cleavage of the virus envelope, which has a cellular origin. Therefore, these toxins could also have an antiviral effect against other enveloped viruses. To test this hypothesis, we evaluated the antiviral activity of PLA_2-CB and crotoxin, in a virucidal assay, against other enveloped viruses, *Rocio virus* (*Flaviviridae* family), *Oropouche virus* (*Bunyaviridae* family), and *Mayaro virus* (*Togaviridae* family) and the non-enveloped virus *Coxsackie B5 virus* (*Picornaviridae* family). As expected, the toxins showed a high antiviral effect (very low EC_{50}) only against the enveloped viruses (Table 1, Figure S1–S8).

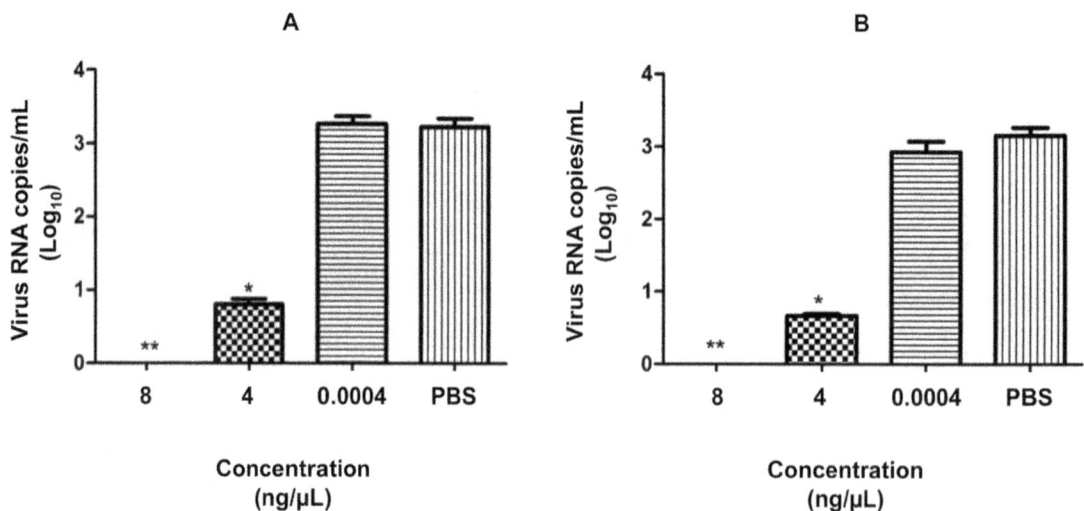

Figure 1. Virucidal assay. DENV-2 was treated with different concentrations of PLA_2-CB (a) and crotoxin (b) and then used to infect Vero cells for 72 h. The antiviral effect of the toxins was evaluated by determining the virus titer in the cell culture supernatant by qRT-PCR. The data represent mean values ± standard deviations (SD) for three independent experiments. The asterisks indicate statistically significant differences from PBS-treated viruses (*$p<0.05$, **$p<0.01$).

A

B

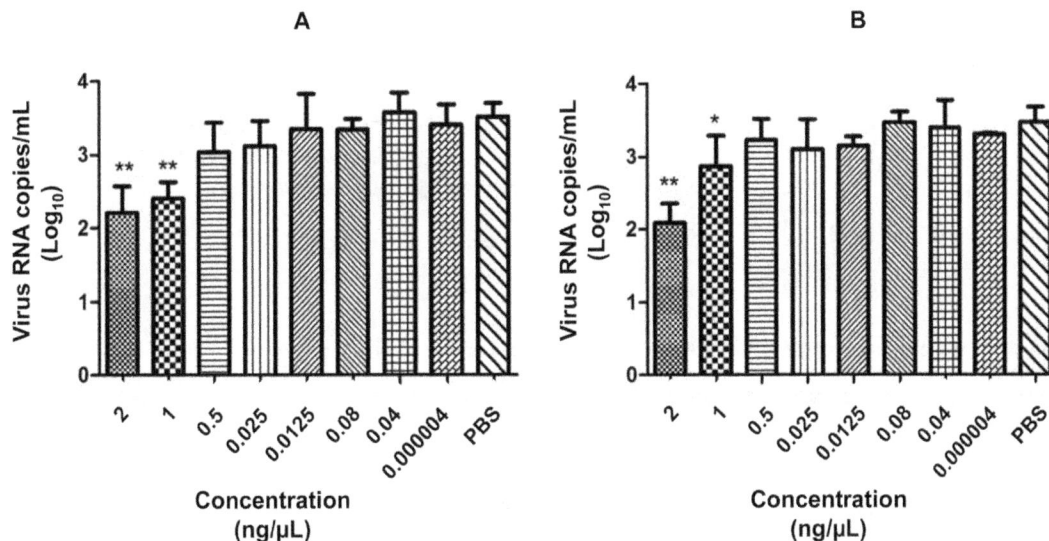

Figure 2. Pre-treatment assay. Vero cells were treated with different concentrations of PLA$_2$-CB (a) and crotoxin (b) and then infected with DENV-2 for 72 h. The antiviral effect of the toxins was evaluated by determining the virus titer in the cell culture supernatant by qRT-PCR. The data represent mean values ± standard deviations (SD) for three independent experiments. The asterisks indicate statistically significant differences from PBS-treated cells (*p<0.05, **p<0.01).

Steric and electrostatic analysis of the interaction of PLA$_2$-CB with the DENV envelope lipid bilayer

The results presented thus far consistently indicate an effective selectivity of PLA2-CB and crotoxin action in inhibiting enveloped viruses. By including structural analyses, we gained a more comprehensive knowledge of such selectivity and its process by outlining the implicated molecular mechanism of the PLA$_2$-CB/crotoxin–DENV interaction. The results concerning the non-enveloped *Coxsackie virus*, in addition to the similar success rates shared between DENV and other enveloped viruses in virucidal assays, suggest a direct catalytic action on the phospholipid bilayer. In DENV, however, this structure is not fully exposed: it lies below the protein E shell, which must be surmounted by PLA2-CB to gain access to its substrate. At physiological temperature (37°C), *Dengue virus* assumes an expanded and mostly spherical configuration, whereby E protein sub-units are arranged in such a conformation that leads to an enhanced area of lipid envelope exposure [40]. Although essentially spherical, this configuration

Figure 3. Analysis of the exposure of DENV-2 genomic RNA. DENV-2 was first treated with PLA$_2$-CB, crotoxin (8 ng/μL each) or PBS at 37°C and then with RNase-A. Virus RNA degradation was evaluated by qRT-PCR. The data represent mean values ± standard deviations (SD) for three independent experiments. The asterisks indicate statistically significant differences among groups (*p<0.05).

inherits the characteristic icosahedral symmetry from the more compact configuration at room temperature and can be described as a function of it. Three repeating sets of major gaps among the E proteins were identified in the 3-fold axis pores [60], the 5-fold axis pores, and the middle points among them (Fig. 5, a). However, cryo-electron microscopy analyses showed that the widest areas of exposure are those located on each of the twenty 3-fold axes [44]. These areas comprise the smaller radial distances from the center of the virus (~232 Å^2, as opposed to the highest value of ~264 Å^2), indicating that these regions concentrate the deepest cavities on the virus surface. Combining the properties of this pronounced cavity with its aforementioned large diameter, it becomes clear that the 3-fold pore is indeed a remarkable site of exposure of the buried DENV lipid envelope. The planar surface that surrounds the active site (i-face) from the bovine group-IB (bGIB) PLA$_2$ has an area of approximately 1500 Å^2 [61]; because snake PLA$_2$-CB shares a very similar structure with (bGIB) PLA$_2$, we assume the same i-face area for both. By structural analysis, we estimated that the 3-fold pore has an area of at least approximately 2500 Å^2, being therefore at least 60% wider than a PLA$_2$-CB monomer by superimposition at the planar orientation (Fig. 5, b). Such orientation is primarily based on taking full advantage of the interaction of the hydrophobic amino acids of PLA$_2$-CB (highlighting Trp31, Trp70, Tyr73, and Phe119) with the hydrophobic matrix just below the level of the polar phospholipid heads in the zwitterionic DENV bilayer. Electrostatic analyses of the complex PLA$_2$-CB/DENV 3-fold pore showed that the prominently positive inner surface of the 3-fold pore facing the negative charges of the membrane tends to establish a perpendicular electrical field to the plane of membrane around its periphery, whereas the centermost region displays a weaker electrical field (Fig. 5, c). We believe that because PLA$_2$-CB displays a net positive surface charge, the particular setting of these fields could slightly repel it from the pore edges. The combined repulsion of the pore edges maintains PLA$_2$-CB in the central more neutral field; at the same time, the membrane polarity could play an increasing attracting role as their distance reduces. Once PLA$_2$-CB reaches the membrane, it establishes contact with the

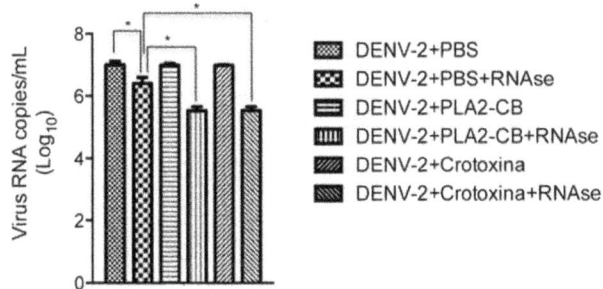

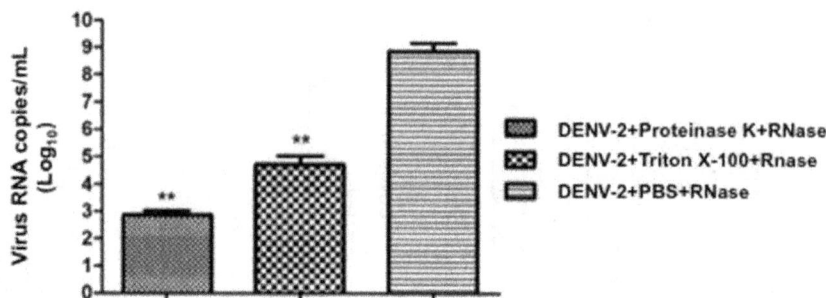

Figure 4. Analysis of the exposure of DENV-2 RNA. DENV-2 was first treated with proteinase K, Triton X-100 and PBS and then with RNase-A. Virus RNA degradation was evaluated by qRT-PCR. The data represent mean values ± standard deviations (SD) for three independent experiments. The asterisks indicate statistically significant differences from PBS-treated viruses (**p<0.01).

phospholipids, which are hydrolyzed, destabilizing the membrane and therefore the general integrity of the virus.

To further analyze if the virus external structure influence the antiviral activity of toxins, and considering that DENV acquire a "bumpy," expanded conformation when incubated at 37°C as opposed to its smooth structure at room temperature [40], DENV-2 was incubated with toxins at 28°C (temperature used to infect the mosquito C6/36 cells) and 37°C and then treated with RNase (Figure 6). A significant higher RNA degradation was observed when DENV-2 was treated with PLA$_2$-CB at 37°C, supporting the hypothesis that at this temperature the relaxed viral external structure allows an enhanced contact of PLA$_2$-CB with the glycerophospholipid on the virus envelope. However, the level of RNA degradation was the same at both temperatures for crotoxin. The last result might be related to the heterodimeric nature of this toxin (PLA$_2$-CB+crotapotin); crotapotin act as a chaperon that enhances PLA$_2$-CB activity [62].

Discussion

In a previous study, we showed that PLA$_2$s isolated from the venom of *Crotalus durissus terrificus* have a potent antiviral action against DENV-2 and YFV, especially at the early stage of the multiplication cycle [21]. Inhibition of the pathogen infectivity induced by PLA$_2$ can occur by direct action on the pathogen or as alternative processes on the host or surrounding medium [63–65]. Here, we demonstrate a dose-dependent inhibition of DENV-2

infection in Vero cells induced by crotoxin and PLA$_2$-CB in a virucidal assay, providing strong evidence of the direct action of these toxins on the virus particle. Crotoxin is a heterodimeric protein composed of the basic PLA$_2$-CB and the acidic nontoxic catalytically inactive protein crotapotin, which act as a chaperon enhancing PLA$_2$-CB activity [62]. Therefore, virus inhibition is most likely induced by the PLA$_2$-CB enzymatic activity, which relies on the hydrolysis of the sn-2 acyl ester linkage of sn-3-glycero-phospholipids, producing fatty acids and lysophospholipids as reaction products [66]. In accordance with this hypothesis, we have found previously, performing an virucidal assay, that PLA$_2$-CB lost its antiviral activity in the absence of Ca+2, which is an essential cofactor for its enzymatic activity, or by the inhibition of the enzymatic activity, suggesting that its antiviral action is due to the glycero-phospholipids cleavage on the virus envelope [67]. Glycerophospholipid hydrolysis would result in degradation of the virus envelope, leading to the exposure of the virus genomic RNA. The virus RNA degradation induced by RNase A after crotoxin and PLA$_2$-CB treatment strongly supports this hypothesis. As degradation was considerably lower when compared to that induced by detergent (Triton X-100) and protease (proteinase K) treatments, these results suggest that PLA$_2$-CB induces a partial envelope destabilization rather than full virus disassembly, in accordance with the PLA$_2$-CB enzymatic function. This hypothesis is in agreement with the results obtained when *Newcastle disease virus* (NDV), an enveloped virus of the *Paramyxoviridae* family, was treated with PLA$_2$s from different snakes [32]. NDV

Table 1. Virucidal assay.

Virus	Toxin	EC$_{50}$ (ng/μL)	95% confident limit (ng/μL)
Dengue virus type 2	PLA$_2$-CB	6.6E-5	2.56E-5-1.78E-4
	Crotoxin	0.0078	0.0042–0.015
Rocio virus	PLA$_2$-CB	0.021	0.0095–0.048
	Crotoxin	0.0046	0.0029–0.0074
Mayaro virus	PLA$_2$-CB	0.066	0.025–0.18
	Crotoxin	0.0036	0.0012–0.011
Oropouche virus	PLA$_2$-CB	0.0067	0.0023-0/019
	Crotoxin	0.0054	0.0023–0.013
Coxsackie B5 virus	PLA$_2$-CB	-	
	Crotoxin	-	

Antiviral activity of PLA$_2$-CB and crotoxin against Dengue virus type 2, Rocio virus, Mayaro virus, Oropouche virus, and Coxsackie B5 virus.

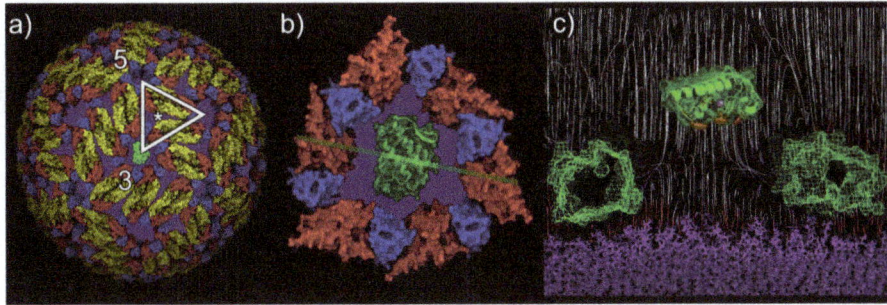

Figure 5. Structural analyses of DENV particle and PLA₂-CB. a) View of DENV at physiological temperature with one PLA₂-CB molecule shown at the putative site of interaction. The triangle shows one unit of the icosahedral symmetry, with the 5-fold and 3-fold vertices and intermediary areas indicated with an asterisk. The E protein domains I, II, and III are colored red, yellow, and blue, respectively; exposed membrane patches are colored in purple. **b)** Detailed view of the PLA₂-CB/DENV 3-fold pore complex. The green line marks the slab view on **c. c)** Electric field lines of the PLA₂-CB/DENV 3-fold pore complex; the pore domains are represented on both sides in green mesh surface, whereas PLA₂-CB is located in the middle. Hydrophobic aromatic residues in the i-face are colored in orange; the Ca^{2+} ion is colored in light purple. The membrane is colored in purple; blue and red lines indicate the proximity of positive and negative charges, respectively.

lost infectivity and cell fusing activity, which depends on envelope integrity, without significantly altering the hemagglutinin, hemolysin, or neuraminidase properties.

The fact that PLA₂-CB inactivates DENV-2 via the cleavage of envelope glycerophospholipids, which are derived from host cell membranes [8], suggests that this enzyme could also exert some effect on other enveloped viruses, as we have already observed for *Yellow fever virus* [21]. This hypothesis was confirmed: PLA₂-CB was able to inhibit other enveloped viruses such as *Rocio virus* from the same *Flaviviridae* family as DENV and YFV, *Oropouche virus* from the *Bunyaviridae* family, and *Mayaro virus* from the *Alphaviridae* family. Further support was revealed by the failure of the enzyme to inactivate the non-enveloped *Coxsackie B5 virus* from the *Picornaviridae* family.

The evidence that PLA₂-CB inhibits virus infection via glycerol-phospholipid cleavage prompted us to determine how PLA₂-CB gains access to the viral lipid-bilayer envelope if multiple copies of the E glycoprotein form a shell around it. A recent study about the extended configuration that DENV assumes at physiological temperatures revealed a series of gaps among the E proteins that provide an enhanced area of direct exposure of the virus lipid bilayer [40]. Although several channels can be identified on the E protein shell, allowing the communication between the virus lipid

membrane and the environment, we focused on the pores found on each of the twenty 3-fold vertices of the virus surface. These pores, being the widest and deepest openings of the protein envelope, could provide the primary passageway for PLA₂-CB monomers, which have been shown to be enzymatically active against glycerol-phospholipid substrates [68]. The size of the 3-fold axis pores with an area roughly twice as large as required by the enzyme's catalytic interface, provides a steric advantage to the accessibility of both PLA₂-CB and crotoxin. The crotoxin complex (PLA₂-CB and crotapotin) dissociates upon interaction with the membrane, and only the PLA₂-CB unit binds to the substrate [69]. Accordingly, the area of contact for catalysis to occur is considered to be the same for crotoxin and PLA₂-CB, which explains their similar efficiencies in virus inhibition.

Although sPLA₂s show similar activity to phospholipids composed of different fatty acids, they do have particular affinities with regard to the phospholipid headgroup [70]. In addition, PLA₂s containing tryptophan in the lipid-binding surface display the highest activity toward zwitterionic lipids [70]. PLA₂-CB (Trp31, Trp70) can reportedly act upon both phosphatidylethanolamine (PE) and phosphatidylcholine (lecithin - PC), two major components of the DENV envelope, approximately 30 and 60% molar, respectively [44]. Several studies also confirm that

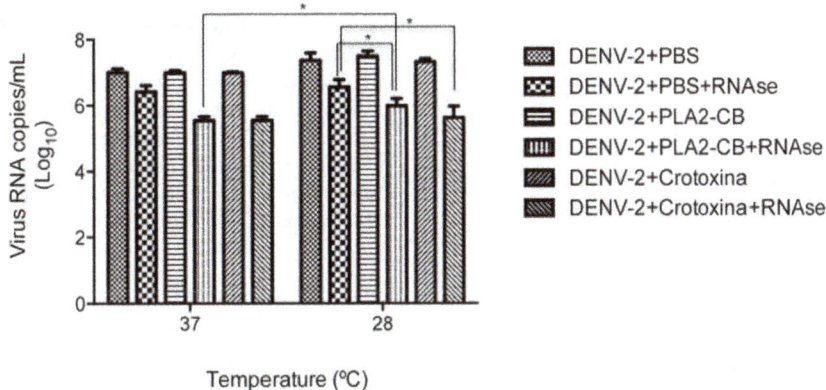

Figure 6. Analysis of the exposure of DENV-2 RNA. DENV-2 was first treated with PLA₂-CB, crotoxin (8 ng/μL each) and PBS at 37°C and 28°C and then with RNase-A. Virus RNA degradation was evaluated by qRT-PCR. The data represent mean values ± standard deviations (SD) for three independent experiments. The asterisks indicate statistically significant differences among groups (*$p < 0.05$).

PLA$_2$-CB has a high affinity for lecithin-rich vesicles [71,72], which justifies its synonym: lecithinase A or phosphatidylcholine 2-acylhydrolase [73,74]. Furthermore, target membrane curvature has been attributed as an important modulating factor for PLA$_2$ hydrolytic efficiency: the higher the curvature, the higher the enzymatic rate. Ahyayauch *et al.* [75] found increasing phosphatidylinositol-specific phospholipase C (PI-PLC) catalytic rates with decreasing curvature radii (increasing curvature) of unilamellar vesicles consisting of PI. Similarly, Berg et al. [76] showed that the fraction of total hydrolyzed substrate in the presence of pig pancreatic PLA$_2$ changes from 50% to 71% as the size of unilamellar vesicles decreased. The results appear to be similar for venom phospholipases: Kensil and Dennis [77] described higher catalytic rates for cobra *Naja naja naja* PLA$_2$ on small unilamellar PC vesicles (SUVs), with faster initial rates than those observed for large (LUVs) and multilamellar vesicles (MLVs). Interestingly, these authors detected distinctly higher catalytic rates on LUVs and MLVs at a small temperature range around the thermotropic phase transition of PC, at which a mixture of both gel and liquid crystalline phases are detected in vesicle lipid organization. Such a coexistence of two or more states triggers uneven phase boundary effects, which are loosely considered defects [78]. By observing phase boundary effects in monolayers, Grainger *et al.* [79] proposed that these prominences can be classified as defects; indeed, they provide a preferential site of action for PLA$_2$s, as opposed to more homogeneous surface areas. Such preferential sites of action for PLA2s were also detected at monolayer borders, sites where the pronounced curvature provides effects similar to those of a disordered lipid patch [80]. In fact, Ahyayauch *et al.* [75] attributed the enhancement of catalytic rates to a successful partial penetration of the enzyme into the membrane hydrophobic matrix, which is more effortlessly achieved in regions of higher curvature and/or general defects on the bilayer surface. The DENV particle structure meets several of these PLA$_2$ catalytic-enhancing conditions. Indeed, its diminutive size and spherical shape confer a relatively high curvature to its membrane (radius of curvature ~232 Å) [40], characterizing only a marginally larger vesicle than a typical SUV, which, as already stated, provides a high-affinity substrate for PLA$_2$ activity. Because of the described points of access to the bilayer on the DENV surface, PLA$_2$-CB is able to hydrolyze the outer phospholipid layer, most likely accumulating fatty acids (FAs) and lysophospholipids (LPLs) on the membrane; this, in turn, destabilizes the membrane to a point at which fundamental protein conformational changes should be impaired. Additionally, it is known that the accumulation of LPLs in a bilayer causes an enhancement on its permeability [81,82] and further activation of PLA$_2$ [83], an observable fact with critical consequences to a supporting structure, such as a viral envelope. These modifications of the membrane structure allegedly disrupt the lipid order and thus its active liquid crystalline state, which most likely unbalances fundamental parameters such as the diffusion of anchored E proteins as well as their foothold, destabilizing the virus and its infective capability. Moreover, these disturbances are likely to drive the membrane to a highly disordered state, at which regions of bilayer breakdown can give rise to RNA exposure, which we detected with RNAse treatment and real-time RT-PCR.

In summary, we provide strong evidence that crotoxin and PLA$_2$-CB have a direct effect on *Dengue virus* particles, most provably by glycerophospholipid cleavage on the virus envelope, which would lead to disruption of the lipid bilayer and destabilization of the E proteins on the virus surface, with the consequence of inactivation. Crotoxin and PLA$_2$-CB most likely gain access to the *Dengue virus* lipid bilayer through the pores found on each of the twenty 3-fold vertices in the E protein shell on the virus surface. In addition, PLA$_2$-CB was able to inactivate other enveloped viruses, highlighting its potential as a natural product lead for the development of broad-spectrum antiviral drugs.

Supporting Information

Figure S1 EC$_{50}$ of crotoxin against DENV-2 in the virucidal assay. DENV-2 (25–100 PFU) was incubated with serial decimal dilutions of crotoxin (50, 5, 0.5, 0.005, 0.0005, and 0.00005 ng/µL) for 1 h at 37°C. The treated viruses were used to infect VERO E6 cells contained in a 24-well plate. The percentage of inhibition was calculated by the reduction of the number of plaques found in the infected cells in comparison with the number of plaques in the cells infected with the untreated virus.

Figure S2 EC$_{50}$ of PLA$_2$-CB against DENV-2 in the virucidal assay. DENV-2 (25–100 PFU) was incubated with serial decimal dilutions of PLA2-CB (50, 5, 0.5, 0.005, 0.0005, and 0.00005 ng/µL) for 1 h at 37°C. The treated viruses were used to infect VERO E6 cells contained in a 24-well plate. The percentage of inhibition was calculated by the reduction of the number of plaques found in the infected cells in comparison with the number of plaques in the cells infected with the untreated virus.

Figure S3 EC$_{50}$ of crotoxin against ROCV in the virucidal assay. ROCV (25–100 PFU) was incubated with serial decimal dilutions of crotoxin (50, 5, 0.5, 0.005, 0.0005, and 0.00005 ng/µL) for 1 h at 37°C. The treated viruses were used to infect VERO E6 cells contained in a 24-well plate. The percentage of inhibition was calculated by the reduction of the number of plaques found in the infected cells in comparison with the number of plaques in the cells infected with the untreated virus.

Figure S4 EC$_{50}$ of PLA$_2$-CB against ROCV in the virucidal assay. ROCV (25–100 PFU) was incubated with serial decimal dilutions of PLA$_2$-CB (50, 5, 0.5, 0.005, 0.0005, and 0.00005 ng/µL) for 1 h at 37°C. The treated viruses were used to infect VERO E6 cells contained in a 24-well plate. The percentage of inhibition was calculated by the reduction of the number of plaques found in the infected cells in comparison with the number of plaques in the cells infected with the untreated virus.

Figure S5 EC$_{50}$ of crotoxin against MAYV in the virucidal assay. MAYV (25–100 PFU) was incubated with serial decimal dilutions of crotoxin (50, 5, 0.5, 0.005, 0.0005, and 0.00005 ng/µL) for 1 h at 37°C. The treated viruses were used to infect VERO E6 cells contained in a 24-well plate. The percentage of inhibition was calculated by the reduction of the number of plaques found in the infected cells in comparison with the number of plaques in the cells infected with the untreated virus.

Figure S6 EC$_{50}$ of PLA$_2$-CB against MAYV in the virucidal assay. MAYV (25–100 PFU) was incubated with serial decimal dilutions of PLA$_2$-CB (50, 5, 0.5, 0.005, 0.0005, and 0.00005 ng/µL) for 1 h at 37°C. The treated viruses were used to infect VERO E6 cells contained in a 24-well plate. The percentage of inhibition was calculated by the reduction of the number of plaques found in the infected cells in comparison with the number of plaques in the cells infected with the untreated virus.

Figure S7 EC$_{50}$ of crotoxin against OROV in the virucidal assay. OROV (25–100 PFU) was incubated with serial decimal dilutions of crotoxin (50, 5, 0.5, 0.005, 0.0005, and 0.00005 ng/µL) for 1 h at 37°C. The treated viruses were used to infect VERO E6 cells contained in a 24-well plate. The percentage of inhibition was calculated by the reduction of the number of plaques found in the infected cells in comparison with the number of plaques in the cells infected with the untreated virus.

Figure S8 EC$_{50}$ of PLA$_2$-CB against OROV in the virucidal assay. OROV (25–100 PFU) was incubated with serial decimal dilutions of PLA$_2$-CB (50, 5, 0.5, 0.005, 0.0005, and 0.00005 ng/µL) for 1 h at 37°C. The treated viruses were used to infect VERO E6 cells contained in a 24-well plate. The percentage of inhibition was calculated by the reduction of the number of plaques found in the infected cells in comparison with the number of plaques in the cells infected with the untreated virus.

Author Contributions

Conceived and designed the experiments: VHA VDM. Performed the experiments: VDM ROS NNdS ACT ACC. Analyzed the data: VHA AC SVS LTF. Contributed reagents/materials/analysis tools: VHA AC SVS LTF. Wrote the paper: VDM ROS NNdS ACC LTF AC SVS VHA.

References

1. Wendt A, Adhoute X, Castellani P, Oules V, Ansaldi C, et al. (2014) Chronic hepatitis C: future treatment. Clin Pharmacol 6: 1–17.
2. Ray D, Shi PY (2006) Recent advances in flavivirus antiviral drug discovery and vaccine development. Recent Pat Antiinfect Drug Discov 1: 45–55.
3. Bhatt S, Gething PW, Brady OJ, Messina JP, Farlow AW, et al. (2013) The global distribution and burden of dengue. Nature 496: 504–507.
4. Hales S, de Wet N, Maindonald J, Woodward A (2002) Potential effect of population and climate changes on global distribution of dengue fever: an empirical model. Lancet 360: 830–834.
5. Kyle JL, Harris E (2008) Global spread and persistence of dengue. Annu Rev Microbiol 62: 71–92.
6. Letson GW, Singhasivanon P, Fernandez E, Abeysinghe N, Amador JJ, et al. (2010) Dengue vaccine trial guidelines and role of large-scale, post proof-of-concept demonstration projects in bringing a dengue vaccine to use in dengue endemic areas. Hum Vaccin 6: 802–809.
7. Lim SP, Wang Q-Y, Noble CG, Chen Y-L, Dong H, et al. (2013) Ten years of dengue drug discovery: Progress and prospects. Antiviral Research 100: 500–519.
8. Lindenbach B, Thiel H, Rice C (2007) Flaviviridae: the viruses and their replication. In: Knipe D, Howley P, editors.Fields Virology. 5th ed.Philadelphia: Lippincot Williams & Wilkins. pp. 1101–1151.
9. KING H (1948) Curare alkaloids; constitution of dextro-tubocurarine chloride. J Chem Soc 174: 265.
10. Ganesan A (2008) The impact of natural products upon modern drug discovery. Curr Opin Chem Biol 12: 306–317.
11. Butler MS (2005) Natural products to drugs: natural product derived compounds in clinical trials. Nat Prod Rep 22: 162–195.
12. Butler MS (2008) Natural products to drugs: natural product-derived compounds in clinical trials. Nat Prod Rep 25: 475–516.
13. Bailey P, Wilce J (2001) Venom as a source of useful biologically active molecules. Emerg Med (Fremantle) 13: 28–36.
14. Ferreira SH, Bartelt DC, Greene LJ (1970) Isolation of bradykinin-potentiating peptides from Bothrops jararaca venom. Biochemistry 9: 2583–2593.
15. Ondetti MA, Williams NJ, Sabo EF, Pluscec J, Weaver ER, et al. (1971) Angiotensin-converting enzyme inhibitors from the venom of Bothrops jararaca. Isolation, elucidation of structure, and synthesis. Biochemistry 10: 4033–4039.
16. Scarborough RM, Rose JW, Hsu MA, Phillips DR, Fried VA, et al. (1991) Barbourin. A GPIIb-IIIa-specific integrin antagonist from the venom of Sistrurus m. barbouri. J Biol Chem 266: 9359–9362.
17. Egbertson MS, Chang CT, Duggan ME, Gould RJ, Halczenko W, et al. (1994) Non-peptide fibrinogen receptor antagonists. 2. Optimization of a tyrosine template as a mimic for Arg-Gly-Asp. J Med Chem 37: 2537–2551.
18. Petricevich VL, Mendonça RZ (2003) Inhibitory potential of Crotalus durissus terrificus venom on measles virus growth. Toxicon 42: 143–153.
19. Borkow G, Ovadia M (1999) Selective lysis of virus-infected cells by cobra snake cytotoxins: A sendai virus, human erythrocytes, and cytotoxin model. Biochem Biophys Res Commun 264: 63–68.
20. Zhang XG, Mason PW, Dubovi EJ, Xu X, Bourne N, et al. (2009) Antiviral activity of geneticin against dengue virus. Antiviral Res 83: 21–27.
21. Muller VD, Russo RR, Cintra AC, Sartim MA, Alves-Paiva ReM, et al. (2012) Crotoxin and phospholipases A$_2$ from Crotalus durissus terrificus showed antiviral activity against dengue and yellow fever viruses. Toxicon 59: 507–515.
22. Fenard D, Lambeau G, Valentin E, Lefebvre JC, Lazdunski M, et al. (1999) Secreted phospholipases A(2), a new class of HIV inhibitors that block virus entry into host cells. J Clin Invest 104: 611–618.
23. J.E. Fletcher AHSS, C.L Ownby (1997) Molecular events in the myotoxic action of phospholipases. In: Kini RM, editor. Venom phospholipase A2 enzymes: structure, function, and mechanism. Chichester; New York: John Wiley. pp. xii, 511 p.
24. Furukawa Y, Matsunaga Y, Hayashi K (1976) Purification and Characterization of a Coagulant Protein from Venom of Russells Viper. Biochimica Et Biophysica Acta 453: 48–61.
25. Huang HC, Lee CY (1984) Isolation and Pharmacological Properties of Phospholipases A2 from Vipera-Russelli (Russell Viper) Snake-Venom. Toxicon 22: 207–217.
26. Vishwanath BS, Kini RM, Gowda TV (1988) Purification and Partial Biochemical-Characterization of an Edema Inducing Phospholipase-A2 from Vipera-Russelli (Russell Viper) Snake-Venom. Toxicon 26: 713–720.
27. Thwin MM, Gopalakrishnakone P, Yuen R, Tan CH (1995) A Major Lethal Factor of the Venom of Burmese Russells Viper (Daboia-Russelli-Siamensis) - Isolation, N-Terminal Sequencing and Biological-Activities of Daboiatoxin. Toxicon 33: 63–76.
28. Mukherjee AK, Ghosal SK, Maity CR (1997) Lysosomal membrane stabilization by alpha-tocopherol against the damaging action of Vipera russelli venom phospholipase A(2). Cellular and Molecular Life Sciences 53: 152–155.
29. Fenard D, Lambeau G, Maurin T, Lefebvre JC, Doglio A (2001) A peptide derived from bee venom-secreted phospholipase A2 inhibits replication of T-cell tropic HIV-1 strains via interaction with the CXCR4 chemokine receptor. Mol Pharmacol 60: 341–347.
30. Kim JO, Chakrabarti BK, Guha-Niyogi A, Louder MK, Mascola JR, et al. (2007) Lysis of human immunodeficiency virus type 1 by a specific secreted human phospholipase A2. J Virol 81: 1444–1450.
31. Mitsuishi M, Masuda S, Kudo I, Murakami M (2006) Group V and X secretory phospholipase A2 prevents adenoviral infection in mammalian cells. Biochem J 393: 97–106.
32. Kohn A, Klibansky C (1967) Studies on the inactivation of cell-fusing property of Newcastle disease virus by phospholipase A. Virology 31: 385–388.
33. DRAYTON HA (1961) Inactivation of Rous virus by phospholipase A. Nature 192: 896.
34. Yasumura Y, Kawakita Y (1963) Studies on SV40 in tissue culture-preliminary step for cancer research in vitro. Nihon rinsho 21: 15.
35. Igarashi A (1978) Isolation of a Singh's Aedes albopictus cell clone sensitive to Dengue and Chikungunya viruses. J Gen Virol 40: 531–544.
36. Dos Santos HW, Poloni TR, Souza KP, Muller VD, Tremeschin F, et al. (2008) A simple one-step real-time RT-PCR for diagnosis of dengue virus infection. J Med Virol 80: 1426–1433.
37. Aquino VH, Anatriello E, Goncalves PF, da Silva EV, Vasconcelos PFC, et al. (2006) Molecular epidemiology of dengue type 3 virus in Brazil and Paraguay, 2002–2004. American Journal of Tropical Medicine and Hygiene 75: 710–715.
38. Kaptein SJ, De Burghgraeve T, Froeyen M, Pastorino B, Alen MM, et al. (2010) A derivate of the antibiotic doxorubicin is a selective inhibitor of dengue and yellow fever virus replication in vitro. Antimicrob Agents Chemother 54: 5269–5280.
39. Bernstein FC, Koetzle TF, Williams GJ, Meyer EF, Brice MD, et al. (1977) The Protein Data Bank. A computer-based archival file for macromolecular structures. Eur J Biochem 80: 319–324.
40. Zhang X, Sheng J, Plevka P, Kuhn RJ, Diamond MS, et al. (2013) Dengue structure differs at the temperatures of its human and mosquito hosts. Proc Natl Acad Sci U S A 110: 6795–6799.
41. Modis Y, Ogata S, Clements D, Harrison SC (2003) A ligand-binding pocket in the dengue virus envelope glycoprotein. Proc Natl Acad Sci U S A 100: 6986–6991.
42. Jo S, Kim T, Iyer VG, Im W (2008) CHARMM-GUI: a web-based graphical user interface for CHARMM. J Comput Chem 29: 1859–1865.
43. Hess B, Kutzner C, van der Spoel D, Lindahl E (2008) GROMACS 4: Algorithms for Highly Efficient, Load-Balanced, and Scalable Molecular Simulation. J Chem Theory Comput 4: 435–447.
44. Zhang Q, Hunke C, Yau YH, Seow V, Lee S, et al. (2012) The stem region of premembrane protein plays an important role in the virus surface protein rearrangement during dengue maturation. J Biol Chem 287: 40525–40534.
45. Marchi-Salvador DP, Corrêa LC, Magro AJ, Oliveira CZ, Soares AM, et al. (2008) Insights into the role of oligomeric state on the biological activities of crotoxin: crystal structure of a tetrameric phospholipase A2 formed by two isoforms of crotoxin B from Crotalus durissus terrificus venom. Proteins 72: 883–891.

46. Humphrey W, Dalke A, Schulten K (1996) VMD: visual molecular dynamics. J Mol Graph 14: 33–38, 27–38.

47. Delano W (2002) The PyMOL Molecular Graphics System. In: LLC DS, editor. San Carlos, CA, USA.

48. Jorgensen WL, Chandrasekhar J, Madura JD, Impey RW, Klein ML (1983) Comparison of simple potential functions for simulating liquid water. J Chem Phys 79: 926.

49. Miyamoto S, Kollman PA (1992) Settle: An analytical version of the SHAKE and RATTLE algorithm for rigid water models. Journal of Computational Chemistry 13: 952–962.

50. Klauda JB, Venable RM, Freites JA, O'Connor JW, Tobias DJ, et al. (2010) Update of the CHARMM all-atom additive force field for lipids: validation on six lipid types. J Phys Chem B 114: 7830–7843.

51. Piggot TJ, Piñeiro Á, Khalid S (2012) Molecular Dynamics Simulations of Phosphatidylcholine Membranes: A Comparative Force Field Study. J Chem Theory Comput 8: 4593–4609.

52. Nozaki Y, Tanford C (1967) Examination of titration behavior. In: CHW H, editor.Methods in Enzymology. 11 ed.New York: Academic Press. pp. 715–734.

53. Parrinello M, Rahman A (1980) Crystal Structure and Pair Potentials: A Molecular-Dynamics Study. Phys Rev Lett 45: 1196–1199.

54. Nosé S (1984) A unified formulation of the constant temperature molecular dynamics methods. J Chem Phys 81: 511–519.

55. Hoover WG (1985) Canonical dynamics: Equilibrium phase-space distributions. Phys Rev A 31: 1695–1697.

56. Hess B (2008) P-LINCS: A Parallel Linear Constraint Solver for Molecular Simulation. J Chem Theory Comput 4: 116–122.

57. Baker NA, Sept D, Joseph S, Holst MJ, McCammon JA (2001) Electrostatics of nanosystems: application to microtubules and the ribosome. Proc Natl Acad Sci U S A 98: 10037–10041.

58. Dolinsky TJ, Nielsen JE, McCammon JA, Baker NA (2004) PDB2PQR: an automated pipeline for the setup of Poisson-Boltzmann electrostatics calculations. Nucleic Acids Res 32: W665–667.

59. Li H, Robertson AD, Jensen JH (2005) Very fast empirical prediction and rationalization of protein pKa values. Proteins 61: 704–721.

60. Soares RO, Caliri A (2013) Stereochemical features of the envelope protein Domain III of dengue virus reveals putative antigenic site in the five-fold symmetry axis. Biochim Biophys Acta 1834: 221–230.

61. Pan YH, Epstein TM, Jain MK, Bahnson BJ (2001) Five coplanar anion binding sites on one face of phospholipase A2: relationship to interface binding. Biochemistry 40: 609–617.

62. Hendon RA, Fraenkel-Conrat H (1971) Biological roles of the two components of crotoxin. Proc Natl Acad Sci U S A 68: 1560–1563.

63. Samy RP, Gopalakrishnakone P, Stiles BG, Girish KS, Swamy SN, et al. (2012) Snake venom phospholipases A(2): a novel tool against bacterial diseases. Curr Med Chem 19: 6150–6162.

64. Ward RJ, de Azevedo WF, Arni RK (1998) At the interface: crystal structures of phospholipases A2. Toxicon 36: 1623–1633.

65. de Paula RC, Castro HC, Rodrigues CR, Melo PA, Fuly AL (2009) Structural and pharmacological features of phospholipases A2 from snake venoms. Protein Pept Lett 16: 899–907.

66. Kini RM (2003) Excitement ahead: structure, function and mechanism of snake venom phospholipase A2 enzymes. Toxicon 42: 827–840.

67. Russo RR, Müller VD, Cintra AC, Figueiredo LT, Sampaio SV, et al. (2014) Phospholipase A₂ crotoxin B isolated from the venom of *Crotalus durissus terrificus* exert antiviral effect against *Dengue virus* and *Yellow fever virus* through its catalytic activity. J Virol Antivir Res 3: 1.

68. Jain MK, Ranadive G, Yu BZ, Verheij HM (1991) Interfacial catalysis by phospholipase A2: monomeric enzyme is fully catalytically active at the bilayer interface. Biochemistry 30: 7330–7340.

69. Faure G, Harvey AL, Thomson E, Saliou B, Radvanyi F, et al. (1993) Comparison of crotoxin isoforms reveals that stability of the complex plays a major role in its pharmacological action. Eur J Biochem 214: 491–496.

70. Burke JE, Dennis EA (2009) Phospholipase A2 structure/function, mechanism, and signaling. J Lipid Res 50 Suppl: S237–242.

71. Lee CH, Bell JD, Zimmerman SS (1997) A binding study of phospholipase A2 with lecithin, lysolecithin and their tetrahedral intermediates using molecular modeling. J Pept Res 50: 25–33.

72. van Deenen L, de Haas G, Heemskerk CH (1963) Hydrolysis of synthetic mixed-acid phosphatides by phospholipase A from human pancreas. Biochim Biophys Acta 67: 295–304.

73. Tsai IH, Liu HC, Chang T (1987) Toxicity domain in presynaptically toxic phospholipase A2 of snake venom. Biochim Biophys Acta 916: 94–99.

74. Nakashima K, Nobuhisa I, Deshimaru M, Nakai M, Ogawa T, et al. (1995) Accelerated evolution in the protein-coding regions is universal in crotalinae snake venom gland phospholipase A2 isozyme genes. Proc Natl Acad Sci U S A 92: 5605–5609.

75. Ahyayauch H, Villar AV, Alonso A, Goñi FM (2005) Modulation of PI-specific phospholipase C by membrane curvature and molecular order. Biochemistry 44: 11592–11600.

76. Berg OG, Yu BZ, Rogers J, Jain MK (1991) Interfacial catalysis by phospholipase A2: determination of the interfacial kinetic rate constants. Biochemistry 30: 7283–7297.

77. Kensil CR, Dennis EA (1985) Action of cobra venom phospholipase A2 on large unilamellar vesicles: comparison with small unilamellar vesicles and multi-bilayers. Lipids 20: 80–83.

78. Yeagle PL (2011) The Structure of Biological Membranes. Boca Raton, USA: CRC Press.

79. Grainger DW, Reichert A, Ringsdorf H, Salesse C (1990) Hydrolytic action of phospholipase A2 in monolayers in the phase transition region: direct observation of enzyme domain formation using fluorescence microscopy. Biochim Biophys Acta 1023: 365–379.

80. Grandbois M, Clausen-Schaumann H, Gaub H (1998) Atomic force microscope imaging of phospholipid bilayer degradation by phospholipase A2. Biophys J 74: 2398–2404.

81. Wilschut JC, Regts J, Scherphof G (1979) Action of phospholipase A2 on phospholipid vesicles. Preservation of the membrane permeability barrier during asymmetric bilayer degradation. FEBS Lett 98: 181–186.

82. Davidsen J, Mouritsen OG, Jørgensen K (2002) Synergistic permeability enhancing effect of lysophospholipids and fatty acids on lipid membranes. Biochim Biophys Acta 1564: 256–262.

83. Jain MK, De Haas GH (1983) Activation of phospholipase A2 by freshly added lysophospholipids. Biochim Biophys Acta 736: 157–162.

Permissions

The contributors of this book come from diverse backgrounds, making this book a truly international effort. This book will bring forth new frontiers with its revolutionizing research information and detailed analysis of the nascent developments around the world.

We would like to thank all the contributing authors for lending their expertise to make the book truly unique. They have played a crucial role in the development of this book. Without their invaluable contributions this book wouldn't have been possible. They have made vital efforts to compile up to date information on the varied aspects of this subject to make this book a valuable addition to the collection of many professionals and students.

This book was conceptualized with the vision of imparting up-to-date information and advanced data in this field. To ensure the same, a matchless editorial board was set up. Every individual on the board went through rigorous rounds of assessment to prove their worth. After which they invested a large part of their time researching and compiling the most relevant data for our readers.

The editorial board has been involved in producing this book since its inception. They have spent rigorous hours researching and exploring the diverse topics which have resulted in the successful publishing of this book. They have passed on their knowledge of decades through this book. To expedite this challenging task, the publisher supported the team at every step. A small team of assistant editors was also appointed to further simplify the editing procedure and attain best results for the readers.

Apart from the editorial board, the designing team has also invested a significant amount of their time in understanding the subject and creating the most relevant covers. They scrutinized every image to scout for the most suitable representation of the subject and create an appropriate cover for the book.

The publishing team has been an ardent support to the editorial, designing and production team. Their endless efforts to recruit the best for this project, has resulted in the accomplishment of this book. They are a veteran in the field of academics and their pool of knowledge is as vast as their experience in printing. Their expertise and guidance has proved useful at every step. Their uncompromising quality standards have made this book an exceptional effort. Their encouragement from time to time has been an inspiration for everyone.

The publisher and the editorial board hope that this book will prove to be a valuable piece of knowledge for researchers, students, practitioners and scholars across the globe.

List of Contributors

Valquiria do Carmo Alves Martins
Universidade do Estado do Amazonas (UEA), Manaus, Amazonas, Brazil

Michele de Souza Bastos
Fundação de Medicina Tropical Dr. Heitor Viera Dourado (FMT-HVD), Manaus, Amazonas, Brazil
Universidade do Estado do Amazonas (UEA), Manaus, Amazonas, Brazil

Rajendranath Ramasawmy
Fundação de Medicina Tropical Dr. Heitor Viera Dourado (FMT-HVD), Manaus, Amazonas, Brazil
Universidade do Estado do Amazonas (UEA), Manaus, Amazonas, Brazil
Universidade Nilton Lins, Manaus, Amazonas, Brazil

Regina Pinto de Figueiredo
Fundação de Medicina Tropical Dr. Heitor Viera Dourado (FMT-HVD), Manaus, Amazonas, Brazil

João Bosco Lima Gimaque
Fundação de Medicina Tropical Dr. Heitor Viera Dourado (FMT-HVD), Manaus, Amazonas, Brazil

Wornei Silva Miranda Braga
Fundação de Medicina Tropical Dr. Heitor Viera Dourado (FMT-HVD), Manaus, Amazonas, Brazil
Universidade do Estado do Amazonas (UEA), Manaus, Amazonas, Brazil

Mauricio Lacerda Nogueira
Fundação de Medicina Tropical Dr. Heitor Viera Dourado (FMT-HVD), Manaus, Amazonas, Brazil
Faculdade de Medicina de São Jose do RioPreto (FAMERP), São Jose do Rio Preto, São Paulo, Brazil

Sergio Nozawa
Universidade Nilton Lins, Manaus, Amazonas, Brazil

Felipe Gomes Naveca
Instituto Leô nidas & Maria Deane (ILMD), Fundação Oswaldo Cruz (FIOCRUZ), Manaus, Amazonas, Brazil

Luiz Tadeu Moraes Figueiredo
Fundação de Medicina Tropical Dr. Heitor Viera Dourado (FMT-HVD), Manaus, Amazonas, Brazil
Centro de Pesquisas em Virologia, Faculdade de Medicina de Ribeirão Preto (FMRP-USP), Ribeirão Preto, São Paulo, Brazil

Maria Paula Gomes Mourão
Fundação de Medicina Tropical Dr. Heitor Viera Dourado (FMT-HVD), Manaus, Amazonas, Brazil
Universidade do Estado do Amazonas (UEA), Manaus, Amazonas, Brazil
Universidade Nilton Lins, Manaus, Amazonas, Brazil

Zheng Pang., Aqian Li., Jiandong Li, Jing Qu, Chengcheng He, Shuo Zhang, Chuan Li, Quanfu Zhang, Mifang Liang and Dexin Li
Key Laboratory of Medical Virology, NHFPC, National Institute for Viral Disease Control and Prevention, China CDC, Beijing, China

Faiz Ahmed Raza
Pakistan Medical Research Council, Research Centre, Punjab Medical College, Faisalabad, Pakistan

Shafiq ur Rehman
Department of Microbiology and Molecular Genetics, University of the Punjab, Quaid-e-Azam Campus, Lahore, Pakistan

Ruqyya Khalid
School of Biological Sciences, University of the Punjab, Quaid-e-Azam Campus, Lahore, Pakistan

Jameel Ahmad
Department of Pathology, Allied Hospital, Faisalabad, Pakistan

Sajjad Ashraf
Nano Bio Energy Engineering School of Integrative Engineering, Chung-Ang University, Seoul, Korea

Mazhar Iqbal
Pakistan Medical Research Council, Research Centre, Punjab Medical College, Faisalabad, Pakistan

Shahida Hasnain
Department of Microbiology and Molecular Genetics, University of The Punjab, Quaid-e-Azam Campus, Lahore, Pakistan

Suchithra Naish
School of Public Health and Social Work & Institute of Health and Biomedical Innovation, Queensland University of Technology, Kelvin Grove campus, Brisbane, Queensland, Australia

Pat Dale
Environmental Futures Centre, Australian Rivers Institute, Griffith School of Environment Griffith University, Brisbane, Queensland, Australia

John S. Mackenzie
Australian Biosecurity CRC and Faculty of Health Sciences, Curtin University, Perth, Western Australia, Australia

John McBride
School of Medicine and Dentistry, James Cook University, Cairns, Queensland, Australia

Kerrie Mengersen
Mathematical Sciences, Queensland University of Technology, Gardens Point campus, Brisbane, Queensland, Australia

Shilu Tong
School of Public Health and Social Work & Institute of Health and Biomedical Innovation, Queensland University of Technology, Kelvin Grove campus, Brisbane, Queensland, Australia

Hussin A. Rothan, Hirbod Bahrani and Rohana Yusof
Department of Molecular Medicine, Faculty of Medicine, University of Malaya, Kuala Lumpur, Malaysia

Zulqarnain Mohamed
Genetics and Molecular Biology Unit, Institute of Biological Science, Faculty of Science, University of Malaya, Kuala Lumpur, Malaysia

Noorsaadah Abd Rahman
Department of Chemistry, Faculty of Science, University of Malaya, Kuala Lumpur, Malaysia

Ru-ning Guo and Lin-hui Li
Public Health Emergency management office, Center for Disease Control and Prevention of Guangdong Province, Guangzhou, China

Chang-wen Ke
Institute of Pathogenic Microorganisms, Center for Disease Control and Prevention of Guangdong Province, Guangzhou, China

Hui-qiong Zhou
Institute of Pathogenic Microorganisms, Center for Disease Control and Prevention of Guangdong Province, Guangzhou, China

Jin-yan Lin
Center for Disease Control and Prevention of Guangdong Province, Guangzhou, China

Jian-feng He, Hao-jie Zhong, Zhi-qiang Peng, Fen Yang and Wen-jia Liang
Institute of Infectious Disease Prevention and Control, Center for Disease Control and Prevention of Guangdong Province, Guangzhou, China

Tara C. Mueller, Erna Fleischmann and Frank von Sonnenburg
Department of Tropical Medicine and Infectious Diseases, University of Munich, Munich, Germany

Sovannaroth Siv
National Center for Parasitology, Entomology, and Malaria Control, Phnom Penh, Cambodia

Nimol Khim, Saorin Kim and Didier Menard
Malaria Molecular Epidemiology Unit, Institut Pasteur in Cambodia, Phnom Penh, Cambodia

Frèdè ric Ariey
Parasitology and Mycology Department, Institut Pasteur, Paris, France

Philippe Buchy
Virology Unit, Institut Pasteur in Cambodia, Phnom Penh, Cambodia

Bertrand Guillard
Medical Laboratory, Institut Pasteur in Cambodia, Phnom Penh, Cambodia

Iveth J. Gonzá lez
Foundation for Innovative New Diagnostics (FIND), Geneva, Switzerland

Eva-Maria Christophel
WHO Regional Office for the Western Pacific (WPRO), Manila, Philippines

Rashid Abdur
WHO Country Office, Phnom Penh, Cambodia

David Bell
Intellectual Ventures Laboratory, Seattle, Washington, United States of America

Arissara Pongsiri and Alongkot Ponlawat
Department of Entomology, Armed Forces Research Institute of Medical Sciences, Bangkok, Thailand,

Butsaya Thaisomboonsuk, Richard G. Jarman
Department of Virology, Armed Forces Research Institute of Medical Sciences, Bangkok, Thailand

Thomas W. Scott
Department of Entomology and Nematology, University of California Davis, Davis, California, United States of America
Fogarty International Center, National Institutes of Health, Bethesda, Maryland, United States of America

Louis Lambrechts
Insect-Virus Interactions Group, Department of Genomes and Genetics, Institut Pasteur – Centre National de la Recherche Scientifique, Unité de Recherche Associée 3012, Paris, France

Tri Y. Setianingsih and Febrina Meutiawati, R. Tedjo Sasmono, Benediktus Yohan
Eijkman Institute for Molecular Biology, Jakarta, Indonesia

Aryati Aryati and Puspa Wardhani
Clinical Pathology Department, School of Medicine and Institute of Tropical Disease, Airlangga University, Surabaya, Indonesia

Hidayat Trimarsanto
Eijkman Institute for Molecular Biology, Jakarta, Indonesia
Agency for the Assessment and Application of Technology, Jakarta, Indonesia

Sukmal Fahri
Health Polytechnic, Jambi Provincial Health Office, Kotabaru,
Jambi, Indonesia and Graduate School in Medicine, Diponegoro University, Semarang, Indonesia

Azeem Mehmood Butt
Centre of Excellence in Molecular Biology (CEMB), University of the Punjab, Lahore, Pakistan

Izza Nasrullah
Department of Biochemistry, Faculty of Biological Sciences, Quaid-i-Azam University, Islamabad, Pakistan

Yigang Tong
State Key Laboratory of Pathogen and Biosecurity, Beijing Institute of Microbiology and Epidemiology, Beijing, Peoplés Republic of China

Panjaporn Chaichana, Tamaki Okabayashi, Orapim Puiprom and Mikiko Sasayama
Mahidol-Osaka Center for Infectious Diseases (MOCID), Faculty of Tropical Medicine, Mahidol University, Bangkok, Thailand

Tadahiro Sasaki, Akifumi Yamashita, Takeshi Kurosu and Kazuyoshi Ikuta
Department of Virology, Research Institute for Microbial Diseases, Osaka University, Osaka, Japan
JST/JICA, Science and Technology Research Partnership for Sustainable Development (SATREPS), Tokyo, Japan

Pongrama Ramasoota
Center of Excellence for Antibody Research (CEAR), Faculty of Tropical Medicine, Mahidol University, Bangkok, Thailand
JST/JICA, Science and Technology Research Partnership for Sustainable Development (SATREPS), Tokyo, Japan

Hao Zhang
Department of Infectious Diseases, Nanfang Hospital, Southern Medical University, Guangzhou, Guangdong Province, China
Key Laboratory of Prevention and Control for Emerging Infectious Diseases of Guangdong Province, School of Public Health and Tropical Medicine, Southern Medical Guangzhou, Guangdong Province, China

Yanru Zhang and Yuanping Zhou
Department of Infectious Diseases, Nanfang Hospital, Southern Medical University, Guangzhou, Guangdong Province, China

Rifat Hamoudi
Department of Pathology, Rockefeller Building, University College London, London, United Kingdom
UCL Cancer Institute, Paul O Gorman Building, University College London, London, United Kingdom

Guiyun Yan
Program in Public Health, University of California
Irvine, Irvine, California, United States of America

Xiaoguang Chen
Key Laboratory of Prevention and Control for
Emerging Infectious Diseases of Guangdong
Province, School of Public Health and Tropical
Medicine, Southern Medical Guangzhou,
Guangdong Province, China

**Vivaldo G. da Costa, Ariany C. Marques-Silvam
and Marcos L. Moreli**
Virology Laboratory, Federal University of Goiás,
Jataí, Brazil

**Jing Liu-Helmersson, Hans Stenlund and Joacim
Rocklö v**
Department of Public Health and Clinical Medicine,
Epidemiology and Global Health, Umea° University,
Umea°, Sweden

Annelies Wilder-Smith
Department of Public Health and Clinical Medicine,
Epidemiology and Global Health, Umea° University,
Umea°, Sweden
Lee Kong Chian School of Medicine, Nanyang
Technological University, Singapore, Singapore

Md Abu Choudhury and John Aaskov
Institute of Health and Biomedical Innovation,
Queensland University of Technology, Brisbane,
Queensland, Australia

William B. Lott
Institute of Health and Biomedical Innovation,
Queensland University of Technology, Brisbane,
Queensland, Australia
School of Chemistry, Physics, and Mechanical
Engineering, Science and Engineering Faculty,
Queensland University of Technology, Brisbane,
Queensland, Australia

Karina Alves Toledo
Department of Biological Sciences, Universidade
Estadual Paulista – UNESP (FCL-Assis), Assis,
Brazil

**Marise Lopes Fermino, Camillo del Cistia
Andrade, Thalita Bachelli Riul, Marcelo Dias-
Baruffi, Renata Tomé Alves, Victor Hugo Aquino,
Vanessa Danielle Menjon Muller and Raquel
Rinaldi Russo**
Departmento de Análises Clínicas, Toxicoló
gicas e Bromatoló gicas, Faculdade de Ciências
Farmaceˆuticas de Ribeirão Preto, Universidade de
São Paulo, Ribeirão Preto, Brazil

Sean R. Stowell and Richard D. Cummings
Emory University School of Medicine, Atlanta,
Georgia, United States of America

Caroline Petitdemange
Sorbonne Universites, UPMC, Univ Paris 06, CR7,
CIMI-Paris, Paris, France
INSERM, U1135, CIMI-Paris, Paris, France Centre
International de Recherches Medicales de
Franceville, Unite des maladies Emergentes,
Franceville, Gabon

Nadia Wauquier
Sorbonne Universites, UPMC, Univ Paris 06, CR7,
CIMI-Paris, Paris, France,
Metabiota Inc., San Francisco, California, United
States of America

Jean-Michel Jacquet
AP-HP Hopital Pitiè-Salpêtrière, Departement
d'Immunologie, Paris, France

Ioannis Theodorou
Sorbonne Universites, UPMC, Univ Paris 06, CR7,
CIMI-Paris, Paris, France
INSERM, U1135, CIMI-Paris, Paris, France
AP-HP Hopital Pitie-Salpe triere, Departement
d'Immunologie, Paris, France

Eric Leroy
Centre International de Recherches Medicales de
Franceville, Unite des maladies Emergentes,
Franceville, Gabon
IRD, Maladies Infectieuses et Vecteurs: Ecologie,
Genetique, Evolution et Contro le, Montpellier,
France

Vincent Vieillard
Sorbonne Universites, UPMC, Univ Paris 06, CR7,
CIMI-Paris, Paris, France
INSERM, U1135, CIMI-Paris, Paris, France
CNRS, ERL8255, CIMI-Paris, Paris, France

Camila Zanluca
Laborato rio de Virologia Molecular, Instituto
Carlos Chagas (ICC/Fiocruz/PR), Curitiba, Parana,
Brasil
Programa de Po s-Graduacao em Biologia Celular e
Molecular Universidade Federal do Parana
(UFPR), Curitiba, Parana, Brasil

**Giovanny Augusto Camacho Antevere Mazzarotto,
Juliano Bordignon and Claudia Nunes Duarte dos
Santos**
Laborato rio de Virologia Molecular, Instituto
Carlos Chagas (ICC/Fiocruz/PR), Curitiba, Parana,
Brasil

**Vanessa Danielle Muller, Nilton Nascimento dos
Santos-Junior, Victor Hugo Aquino and Amanda
Cristina Trabuco**
Laborató rio de Virologia, Departamento de
Análises Clínicas, Toxicoló gicas e Bromatoló gicas,
Faculdade de Ciências Farmacêuticas de Ribeirão
Preto, Universidade de São Paulo, Ribeirao Preto,
Sao Paulo, Brasil

Adelia Cristina Cintra and Suely Vilela Sampaio
Laborató rio de Toxinologia, Departamento de Aná
lises Clínicas, Toxicoló gicas e Bromatoló gicas,
Faculdade de Ciências
Farmace^uticas de Ribeirão Preto, Universidade de
São Paulo, Ribeirão Preto, São Paulo, Brasil

Luiz Tadeu Figueiredo
Centro de Pesquisa em Virologia, Departamento de
Clínica Mé dica, Faculdade de Medicina de Ribeirão
Preto, Universidade de São Paulo, Ribeirão Preto,
São Paulo, Brasil

Antonio Caliri and Ricardo Oliveira Soares
Departamento de Física e Química, Faculdade
de Ciências Farmacêuticas de Ribeirão Preto,
Universidade de São Paulo, Ribeirão Preto, São
Paulo, Brasil

Index

www.ingramcontent.com/pod-product-compliance
Lightning Source LLC
Chambersburg PA
CBHW061248190326
41458CB00011B/3608

Dengue: Diagnosis, Treatment and Control